Tumor Ablation

Tumor Ablation

Principles and Practice

Eric vanSonnenberg, MD

William N. McMullen

Luigi Solbiati, MD

Editors

Tito Livraghi, MD
Peter R. Müeller, MD
Stuart G. Silverman, MD

Associate Editors

With 200 Illustrations in 457 Parts

Springer

Eric vanSonnenberg, MD
formerly:
Chief of Radiology
Dana-Farber Cancer Institute
Harvard Medical School
Interventional Radiologist
Brigham and Women's Hospital
Children's Hospital
Boston, MA 02115
USA

William N. McMullen
Interventional Oncology Consultant
Boston, MA 02115
USA

Luigi Solbiati, MD
Chairman
Department of Radiology
Ospedale Civile Busto Arsizio
21052 Busto Arsizio
Italy

ISBN 978-1-4419-3046-0 e-ISBN 978-0-387-28674-7

Library of Congress Cataloging-in-Publication Data
Tumor ablation: principles and practice / [edited by] Eric vanSonnenberg, William McMullen, Luigi Solbiati.
p. ; cm.
Includes bibliographical references and index.

1. Cancer—Thermotherapy. 2. Catheter ablation. I. vanSonnenberg, Eric. II. McMullen, William. III. Solbiati, L. (Luigi)
[DNLM: 1. Neoplasms—therapy. 2. Catheter Ablation—methods. QZ 266 T9232 2004]
RC271.T5T865 2004
616.99′40632—dc22

Printed on acid-free paper.

9 8 7 6 5 4 3 2 1

springeronline.com

Foreword I

There is an enormous sense of excitement in the communities of cancer research and cancer care as we move into the middle third of the first decade of the 21st century. For the first time, there is a true sense of confidence that the tools provided by the human genome project will enable cancer researchers to crack the code of genomic abnormalities that allow tumor cells to live within the body and provide highly specific, virtually non-toxic therapies for the eradication, or at least firm control of human cancers. There is also good reason to hope that these same lines of inquiry will yield better tests for screening, early detection, and prevention of progression beyond curability.

While these developments provide a legitimate basis for much optimism, many patients will continue to develop cancers and suffer from their debilitating effects, even as research moves ahead. For these individuals, it is imperative that the cancer field make the best possible use of the tools available to provide present day cancer patients with the best chances for cure, effective palliation, or, at the very least, relief from symptoms caused by acute intercurrent complications of cancer. A modality that has emerged as a very useful approach to at least some of these goals is tumor ablation by the use of physical or physiochemical approaches. Tumor ablation by means of other than traditional surgical approaches, as noted in the excellent Introduction to this text, is a methodology attempted with modest success for a number of years. Modern approaches take advantage of the vastly superior armamentarium of imaging strategies now available. These permit pinpoint localization of tumors causing distressing symptoms, such as pain, obstruction, compression, etc. Advances in materials science, and methods for delivery of ablating agents such as intense cold, ultrasound, etc., combined with improved localization now make it possible to be much more aggressive and effective in attempting to achieve local ablation of primary or metastatic tumors that cause morbidity.

This book represents an outstanding effort on the part of the editors and authors to gather in one place a review of the advances in tumor ablation methods as well as a clear, practical, and readable description of specific applications in different organ systems. The sections on imaging of tumors for the purposes of localizing targets for the ablation methodologies that are covered in the next section, provide physicians involved in cancer research, regardless of orientation, with an indispensable resource for understanding the rationale, capabilities, limitations, benefits, and toxicities of these approaches. Readers of this volume will no doubt find a strong basis for an increased, but much more appropriate, use of this method for the benefit of their patients with cancers that are either advanced or located in spots difficult to reach by surgery, radiation therapy, or chemotherapeutic drugs. In this regard, the final section offers perspectives from cancer care experts who approach the care of these patients from a variety of perspectives: the medical oncologist's, the surgical oncologist's, the radiation therapist's, etc. are especially valuable. It provides a good balance between those who are immersed in developing and advancing this modality and the "end users," who must balance the use of these methods with a variety of other complex options. The final section of this text is also valuable, because it provides a basis for approaching the difficult issue of how to integrate a novel modality of therapy into the totality of cancer care to the benefit of the individual patients.

In my view, this book provides a comprehensive yet incisive overview of a field that has reached a highly appropriate stage for this kind of resource. Tumor ablation, at least in its present form, is still a relatively young field that can be adequately captured in a volume of this size. On the other hand, it has grown sufficiently large in its methods and applications that a summary is needed both within and outside the field. Dr. vanSonnenberg is to be complimented for taking on this difficult challenge and meeting it so effectively.

Edward J. Benz, Jr, MD
President of Dana-Farber
Cancer Institute
Professor of Medical Oncology
& Hematology
Harvard Medical School

Foreword II

Drs. vanSonnenberg, McMullen, and Solbiati have produced a truly timely and comprehensive textbook on a topic that is coming of age. While the last few decades have seen the development and establishment of safe surgery for malignant tumors, forward thinking surgeons, radiologists, and interventional radiologists have now begun to consider and realize the potential to treat solid tumors with ablative techniques. Although not a new concept, the use of extreme temperatures to kill tumors but preserve normal cells has exploded in recent years. As with any new treatment modality, more questions are often raised than answers. This textbook provides the basis from which one can draw information on virtually any topic related to ablative procedures for tumors, and should be an essential resource for anyone who treats solid tumors potentially amenable to ablation.

This textbook is not only timely, but it is comprehensive. It addresses all aspects of ablation through contributions from the leading experts in the field. The spectrum of topics addressed by the editors is appropriate and is exemplary for its implicit understanding that this is a multidisciplinary field that requires the teamwork of specialists in many fields for the ultimate success of ablative techniques. From basic science, to the logistics of practice, to imaging, to specific tumors, and to psychosocial issues, this book has tremendous breadth of coverage, giving it extraordinary value to students and practitioners. As we embark on more and more innovative approaches to the treatment of solid tumors, textbooks such as this are an essential reference for anyone interested in practicing or researching ablative techniques.

Leslie H. Blumgart, MD
Michael I. D'Angelica, MD
Department of Surgery
Memorial Sloan-Kettering Hospital
Cornell Medical School

Foreword III

Radiofrequency ablation (thermal tissue coagulation) has evolved rapidly in the decade since I was first enticed to use two simple bipolar needle electrodes in the laboratory in an attempt to produce coagulative necrosis of liver tissue. Important preclinical and clinical work from the authors included in this book paved the way for the clinical trials utilizing radiofrequency ablation as a treatment for unresectable primary and secondary hepatic malignancies. As I predicted to many of the engineers in the industry involved with radiofrequency ablation equipment, "build it and they will come"; investigators have subsequently employed local thermal destruction of tumors in many additional body sites and organs. Several chapters in this book describe the current status of radiofrequency ablation of tumors in organs other than the liver.

Technologic advances have produced an ever-growing array of multiple needle and hook electrode arrays. Ongoing research in industry and academic centers is designed to produce larger zones of thermal necrosis in a safe and reproducible fashion. The geometry of zones of thermal necrosis produced by radiofrequency is a complex issue, and numerous mathematical models have been developed in an attempt to understand the overlap of zones of thermal necrosis necessary to treat larger hepatic malignancies. Unfortunately, many of these models fail to account for the effect of large blood vessels near the treated tumors or the differences in the blood flow between tumor and normal tissue. Like many novel treatments that involve technical skill and the manipulation of instruments, there is a learning curve when utilizing radiofrequency ablation to treat malignancies in any body site. Another important aspect of radiofrequency ablation that is reviewed in this book is the role and limitations of imaging modalities to monitor and predict the completeness of tumor destruction during radiofrequency ablation, and the role and limitations of diagnostic imaging modalities to diagnose local recurrence (incomplete tumor destruction) following radiofrequency ablation.

The challenges in the next decade regarding radiofrequency ablation include establishing long-term disease-free and overall survival rates following radiofrequency ablation of primary and metastatic hepatic malignancies, developing criteria to better define those patients who are candidates for treatment with a percutaneous approach versus those who are better treated with a laparoscopic or open surgical radiofrequency ablation procedure, defining the role and the relative risks and benefits in treating non hepatic malignancies in other organs and body sites, and developing and completing clinical trials involving advances in radiofrequency ablation equipment and combined modalities to improve the reliability and reduce local recurrence rates after treatment. The role, benefits, risks, and complications of radiofrequency ablation to treat malignant tumors must be identified and defined. Radiofrequency as a part of multimodality therapies, including surgical resection of large liver tumors combined with radiofrequency ablation of additional small lesions, and the use of neoadjuvant and adjuvant treatments with radiofrequency ablation of hepatic malignancies are being explored. Exciting results should be forthcoming in the next several years. The field is truly "heating up," as other forms of thermal ablation treatments have been introduced into the market place; the role of these modalities also will be studied in the coming decade. The rapid progress in radiofrequency ablation of hepatic and other tumors indicates that a significant patient population is in need of a safe and reliable treatment to produce complete destruction of measurable tumors.

Steven A. Curley, MD
Department of Surgery
M. D. Anderson Hospital
University of Texas

Preface

So much good is happening on so many fronts in the battle against cancer—from powerful new drugs to complex anti-angiogenesis strategies to creative research unlocking the mysteries of molecular biology to thermal and mechanical methods of tumor destruction. The specialty of radiology is contributing in integral and multifaceted ways in this anticancer crusade. Remarkable advances in the precision and speed of CT, MRI diffusion and spectroscopy, metabolic assessment by PET, and *avant garde* fusion imaging with PET/CT, as well as percutaneous methods to kill tumors, all have a powerful impact in the fight against cancer.

The time is both ripe and right for a book on *Tumor Ablation.* There is a rapidly growing acceptance, if not excitement, that this method adds a new dimension to the therapeutic oncologic armamentarium. While some forms of percutaneous ablation have been in existence for more than ten years, a certain maturity has been achieved, such that referrals from oncologists, surgeons, and radiation therapists are now common—not to mention patient self-referral. While research in the ablation field expands and innovations are constantly made, there has been a leveling off of the exponential growth and changes in the ablation field. Hence, larger series are now being accumulated, the procedures are proliferating in many hospitals, and there is multidisciplinary acceptance of ablation as a viable alternative for select patients with cancer. The book focuses on tumor ablation, largely but not exclusively percutaneous, with guidance and monitoring by a variety of imaging modalities.

Section I covers the background and foundations of tumor ablation. The building of a practice, anesthesia, and the various instruments for ablation are described in Section II. Section III discusses imaging for ablation. Section IV deals with the various methods of ablation. Section V reviews the clinical experience by leaders in the field about a variety of tumors in different organ systems. Section VI offers perspectives by nonradiology oncologic physicians, along with future directions in the field. *Tumor Ablation* contains forewords by oncologists and surgeons from three prestigious cancer centers with frank insights into the role of tumor ablation in oncology. A chapter that depicts the cancer journey by patients and their families provides unique perspectives.

Our goal was to assemble the pioneers and world's experts in the field of tumor ablation to contribute to the book; we succeeded, but more importantly, they succeeded in conveying their marvelous creativity and contributions. Extensive experience is provided by numerous authors from Europe and Asia, where much of the seminal work originated. The many North American experts highlight their pushing of the envelope, reflected in many of the major advances in the field of tumor ablation. Contributors include radiologists, surgeons, oncologists, anesthesiologists, nonphysician scientists, and internists, thereby reflecting the multidisciplinary nature of tumor ablation.

Finally, our appreciation to those who facilitated this endeavor. First to our publisher, Rob "Louie" Albano, for his wise counsel, and to his associate, Michelle Schmitt-DeBonis. Our thanks to our local assistants for their help, Kristen Rancourt and Sue Ellen Lynch. Our appreciation to all our contributing authors for sharing their expertise, experience, and enlightenment. Finally to our patients and families—it has been, and is, a privilege to have offered and delivered hope and benefit to their care.

Eric vanSonnenberg, MD
William N. McMullen
Luigi Solbiati, MD

Contents

Contributors

Fateh Ahmed, MBBS
Surgical Research Fellow, Department of Surgery, Leicester Royal Infirmary, University Hospitals, Leicester, UK

Muneeb Ahmed, MD
Research Assistant in Radiology, Harvard Medical School, Beth Israel Deaconess Medical Center, Boston, MA, USA

Thomas D. Atwell, MD
Senior Associate Consultant, Department of Radiology, Mayo Clinic College of Medicine, Rochester, MN, USA

Ramsey D. Badawi, PhD
Assistant Professor, Department of Radiology, University of California Davis, University of California Davis Medical Center, Sacramento, CA, USA

Daniel T. Boll, MD
Research Associate, Department of Radiology, Case Western Reserve University and University Hospitals of Cleveland, Cleveland, OH, USA

Stephen D. Brown, MD
Instructor in Radiology, Harvard Medical School, Staff Radiologist, Children's Hospital, Boston, MA, USA

Matthew R. Callstrom, MD, PhD
Assistant Professor of Radiology, Department of Radiology, Mayo Clinic College of Medicine, Rochester, MN, USA

Vito Cantisani, MD
Department of Radiology, Brigham and Women's Hospital, Boston, MA, USA

J. William Charboneau, MD
Professor of Radiology, Department of Radiology, Mayo Clinic College of Medicine, Rochester, MN, USA

Lawrence Cheung
Medical Student, Harvard Medical School, Boston, MA, USA

Luca Cova, MD
Department of Radiology, Ospedale Civile Busto Arsizio, Busto Arsizio, Italy

Laura Crocetti, MD
Research Fellow, Department of Oncology, Transplants, and Advanced Technologies in Medicine, University of Pisa, Pisa, Italy

Thierry de Baère, MD
Staff Radiologist, Institut Gustave Roussy, Villejuif, France

Gerald D. Dodd III, MD, FACR
Professor of Radiology, University of Texas, San Antonio, Chairman of Radiology, University of Texas Health Science Center, San Antonio, TX, USA

Damian E. Dupuy, MD
Professor of Diagnostic Imaging, Brown Medical School, Director of Ultrasound and Office of Minimally Invasive Therapy, Rhode Island Hospital, Providence, RI, USA

Craig Earle, MD, PhD
Assistant Professor of Medicine, Harvard Medical School, Department of Medical Oncology, Dana-Farber Cancer Institute, Boston, MA, USA

Beth S. Edeiken, MD
Professor of Radiology, Department of Radiology, M. D. Anderson Cancer Center, Houston, TX, USA

Katrin Eichler, MD
Institute for Diagnostic and Interventional Radiology, Department of Radiology, University Hospital, Frankfurt, Germany

Judah Folkman, MD
Professor of Surgery, Harvard Medical School, Children's Hospital, Boston, MA, USA

Bruno D. Fornage, MD
Professor of Radiology, University of Texas, Houston, Department of Radiology, M. D. Anderson Cancer Center, Houston, TX, USA

John A. Fox, MD
Staff Anesthesiologist, Department of Anesthesiology, Perioperative and Pain Medicine, Brigham and Women's Hospital, Boston, MA, USA

Debra A. Gervais, MD
Assistant Professor of Radiology, Harvard Medical School, Department of Radiology, Massachusetts General Hospital, Boston, MA, USA

Allison Gillams, MD
Senior Lecturer, University College of London Medical School, Honorary Consultant, Imaging, Middlesex Hospital, London, UK

Matthew P. Goetz, MD
Assistant Professor of Oncology, Mayo Clinic College of Medicine, Rochester, MN, USA

S. Nahum Goldberg, MD
Associate Professor of Radiology, Harvard Medical School, Director, Abdominal Intervention and Tumor Ablation, Director, Minimally Invasive Tumor Therapy Laboratory, Department of Radiology and Abdominal Imaging, Beth Israel Deaconess Medical Center, Boston, MA, USA

Alan M. Harvey, MD, MBA
Director of Quality Assurance/Quality Improvement, Department of Anesthesiology, Perioperative and Pain Medicine, Brigham and Women's Hospital, Boston, MA, USA

John V. Heymach, MD, PhD
Assistant Professor of Medicine, Harvard Medical School, Children's Hospital, Boston, MA, USA

Kullervo Hynynen, PhD
Professor of Radiology, Harvard Medical School, Director of Therapeutic Research, Department of Radiology, Brigham and Women's Hospital, Boston, MA, USA

David A. Iannitti, MD
Assistant Professor of Surgery, Brown University, Department of Surgery, Rhode Island Hospital, Providence, RI, USA

Tiziana Ierace, MD
Department of Radiology, Ospedale Civile Busto Arsizio, Busto Arsizio, Italy

David A. Israel, MD, PhD
Instructor in Radiology, Harvard Medical School, Staff Radiologist, Dana-Farber Cancer Institute, Boston, MA, USA

Sapna K. Jain, MD
Resident in Radiology, University of California, San Francisco, Department of Radiology, University Hospital, San Francisco, CA, USA

Pasi A. Jänne, MD
Assistant Professor of Medicine, Harvard Medical School, Department of Medical Oncology, Dana-Farber Cancer Center, Boston, MA, USA

Bruce E. Johnson, MD
Professor of Medicine, Harvard Medical School, Director of Thoracic Oncology, Department of Medical Oncology, Dana-Farber Cancer Center, Boston, MA, USA

Ferenc A. Jolesz, MD
B. Leonard Holman Professor of Radiology, Harvard Medical School, Vice Chairman for Research, Director, Division of MRI and Image Guided Therapy Program, Department of Radiology, Brigham and Women's Hospital, Boston, MA, USA

Anthony Kam, MD
Staff Clinician, Diagnostic Radiology Department, Clinical Center, National Institutes of Health, Bethesda, MD, USA

Robert A. Kane, MD, FACR
Professor of Radiology, Harvard Medical School, Associate Chief of Administration, Director of Ultrasound, Department of Radiology, Beth Israel Deaconess Medical Center, Boston, MA, USA

Lily Y. Kernagis, MD
Instructor in Radiology, University of Pennsylvania, Department of Radiology, University Hospital, Philadelphia, PA, USA

Matthew Kulke, MD
Assistant Professor of Medical Oncology, Dana-Farber Cancer Institute, Harvard Medical School, Boston, MA, USA

Stanislav Lechpammer, MD, PhD
Department of Orthopedic Surgery, Brigham and Women's Hospital, Boston, MA, USA

Fred T. Lee, Jr., MD
Professor of Radiology, University of Wisconsin, Chief, Division of Abdominal Imaging, Department of Radiology, University Hospital, Madison, WI, USA

William R. Lees, MD
Professor of Medical Imaging, University College of London Medical School, Department of Medical Imaging, Middlesex Hospital, London, UK

Riccardo Lencioni, MD
Associate Professor of Radiology, University of Pisa, Department of Oncology, Transplants, and Advanced Technologies in Medicine, University of Pisa, Pisa, Italy

Jonathan S. Lewin, MD
Martin W. Donner Professor and Chairman, The Johns Hopkins School of Medicine, Radiologist-in-Chief, The Russell H. Morgan Department

of Radiology and Radiological Science, The Johns Hopkins Hospital, Baltimore, MD, USA

Tito Livraghi, MD
Chairman Consultant, Department of Interventional Radiology, Ospedale Civile Vimercate, Vimercate-Milano, Italy

David M. Lloyd, MBBS, FRCS (Lond.), MD
Honorary Lecturer in Medicine, Consultant Hepatobiliary and Laparoscopic Surgeon, Department of Surgery, Leicester Royal Infirmary, Leicester, UK

Nathan MacDonold, MD
Department of Radiology, Brigham and Women's Hospital, Boston, MA, USA

Martin Mack, MD, PhD
Deputy Medical Director, Institute for Diagnostic and Interventional Radiology, Department of Radiology, University Hospital, Frankfurt, Germany

John P. McGahan, MD
Professor of Radiology, University of California, Davis, Director of Ultrasound, University of California, Davis Medical Center, Sacramento, CA, USA

Maria Franca Meloni, MD
Radiologist, Department of Interventional Radiology, Ospedale Civile Vimercate, Vimercate-Milano, Italy

Elmar M. Merkle, MD
Associate Professor, Duke University School of Medicine, Director of Body MRI, Department of Radiology, Duke University Hospital and Medical Center, Durham, NC, USA

Paul R. Morrison, MS
Medical Physicist, Harvard Medical School, Department of Radiology, Brigham and Women's Hospital, Boston, MA, USA

Koenraad J. Mortele, MD
Assistant Professor of Radiology, Harvard Medical School, Staff Radiologist, Department of Radiology, Brigham and Women's Hospital, Boston, MA, USA

Peter R. Müeller, MD
Professor of Radiology, Harvard Medical School, Director of Abdominal Imaging and Interventional Radiology, Department of Radiology, Massachusetts General Hospital, Boston, MA, USA

David M. Nagorney, MD
Consultant, Division of Gastroenterologic and General Surgery, Mayo Clinic; Professor of Surgery, Mayo Clinic College of Medicine, Rochester, MN, USA

Ziv Neeman, MD
Staff Clinician, Diagnostic Radiology Department, Clinical Center, National Institutes of Health, Bethesda, MD, USA

Sherif G. Nour, MD
Assistant Professor, Case Western Reserve University, Director of Interventional MRI, Research, Department of Radiology, Case Western Reserve University and University Hospitals of Cleveland, Cleveland, OH, USA

Masao Omata, MD
Department of Gastroenterology, University of Tokyo, Tokyo

Gary Onik, MD
Director of Surgical Imaging, Center for Surgical Advancement, Celebration Health/Florida Hospital, Celebration, FL, USA

Hugue Ouellette, MD
Department of Radiology, Massachusetts General Hospital, Boston, MA, USA

Florencia G. Que, MD
Consultant, Division of Gastroenterologic and General Surgery, Mayo Clinic; Assistant Professor of Surgery, Mayo Clinic College of Medicine, Rochester, MN, USA

John C. Rewcastle, PhD
Adjuvant Assistant Professor, University of Calgary, Department of Radiology, Chief Scientific Officer, Sanarus Medical, Pleasanton, CA, USA

Daniel I. Rosenthal, MD
Professor of Radiology, Harvard Medical School, Vice Chairman, Department of Radiology, Massachusetts General Hospital, Boston, MA, USA

Joseph Rubin, MD
Professor of Oncology, Mayo Clinic College of Medicine, Rochester, MA, USA

Toshihito Seki, MD
Professor of Medicine, Kansai Medical University, Division of Hepatology, Third Department of Internal Medicine, Kansai Medical University, Osaka, Japan

Sridhar Shankar, MD
Assistant Professor of Radiology, University of Massachusetts, Worcester, Department of Radiology, University of Massachusetts Medical Center, Worcester, MA, USA

William E. Shiels II, DO
Associate Professor of Radiology, Ohio State University College of Medicine, Chairman of Radiology, Columbus Children's Hospital, Columbus, OH, USA

Shuichiro Shiina, MD
Associate Professor of Medicine, University of Tokyo, Department of Gastroenterology, University Hospital, Tokyo, Japan

Stuart G. Silverman, MD
Associate Professor of Radiology, Harvard Medical School, Director, Abdominal Imaging and Intervention, Director, CT Scan, Director, Cross-sectional Interventional Service, Brigham and Women's Hospital, Boston, MA, USA

Luigi Solbiati, MD
Chairman, Department of Radiology, Ospedale Civile Busto Arsizio, Busto Arsizio, Italy

Michael C. Soulen, MD
Professor of Radiology and Surgery, University of Pennsylvania, Department of Radiology, University Hospital, Philadelphia, PA, USA

Elizabeth A. Stewart, MD
Associate Professor of Obstetrics, Gynecology, and Reproductive Biology, Harvard Medical School, Clinical Director, The Center for Uterine Fibroids, Brigham and Women's Hospital, Boston, MA, USA

Ralf Straub, MD
Institute for Diagnostic and Interventional Radiology, Department of Radiology, University Hospital, Frankfurt, Germany

Andrew D. Strickland, MD, MRCS
Specialist Registar in Surgery, Department of Surgery, Leicester Royal Infirmary, Leicester, UK

Clare Tempany, MD
Professor of Radiology, Harvard Medical School, Director of Clinical MRI and Clinical Focused Ultrasound, Department of Radiology, Brigham and Women's Hospital, Boston, MA, USA

Takuma Teratani, MD
Department of Gastroenterology, University of Tokyo, Tokyo

Massimo Tonolini, MD
Department of Radiology, Ospedale Civile Busto Arsizio, Busto Arsizio, Italy

Kemal Tuncali, MD
Instructor in Radiology, Harvard Medical School, Department of Radiology, Brigham and Women's Hospital, Boston, MA, USA

Annick D. Van den Abbeele, MD
Acting Clinical Director of Radiology, Director of Nuclear Medicine, Dana-Farber Cancer Institute, Director, Nuclear Medicine Oncologic Program, Brigham and Women's Hospital, Boston, MA, USA

Vanessa A. van Raalte, MD
Victoria Radiology Consulting Group, Victoria, BC, Canada

Eric vanSonnenberg, MD
formerly: Chief of Radiology, Dana-Farber Cancer Institute, Harvard Medical School, Interventional Radiologist, Brigham and Women's Hospital, Children's Hospital, Boston, MA, USA

Thomas J. Vogl, MD, PhD
Professor, Johann Wolfgang Goethe University, Chairman of Radiology, Institute for Diagnostic and Interventional Radiology, Department of Radiology, University Hospital, Frankfurt, Germany

Sharon M. Weber, MD
Associate Professor of Surgery, University of Wisconsin, Department of Surgery, University Hospital, Madison, WI, USA

Bradford J. Wood, MD
Senior Clinical Investigator and Director, Interventional Radiology Research, Adjunct Investigator, Diagnostic Radiology Department, Clinical Center, National Institutes of Health, Bethesda, MD, USA

Robert L. Worthington-Kirsch, MD, FSCVIR, FASA
Clinical Professor of Radiology, Philadelphia College of Osteopathic Medicine, President, Image Guided Surgery Associates, PC, Director, Section of Interventional Radiology, Tenet Roxborough Memorial Hospital, Philadelphia, PA, USA

Stefan Zangos, MD
Institute for Diagnostic and Interventional Radiology, Department of Radiology, University Hospital, Frankfurt, Germany

Section I
Introduction to Ablation

1
History of Ablation

John P. McGahan and Vanessa A. van Raalte

Numerous techniques have been developed for tissue ablation. Techniques to kill tumor cells include heating, freezing, radiation, chemotherapy, occluding the tumor blood supply, injection of caustic agents directly into the tumor, as well as various combinations of these. While most of these were introduced in the late 20th century, at least one dates back to the 19th century. This chapter reviews the general historical perspectives of these different methods, with particular emphasis on radiofrequency ablation.

Radiofrequency Ablation

While percutaneous methods of radiofrequency ablation (RFA) are relatively new, the basic technique for RFA was described over a century ago by D'Arsonval (1), who, in 1891, first demonstrated that when RF waves passed through tissue, they caused an increase in tissue temperature. In the early 1900s, RF was used in relatively few medical applications (2,3). In 1910 Beer (2) described a new method for the treatment of bladder neoplasms using cauterization through a cystoscope. In 1911 Clark (3) described the use of oscillatory dessication in the treatment of malignant tumors that were accessible for minor surgical procedures.

However, RF for medical applications was not widely popularized until after the introduction of the Bovie knife in 1928 by Cushing and Bovie (4) (Liebel Florsheim, Cincinnati, Ohio). This instrument could be used either for cauterization or for cutting tissue by varying the RF current. A pulsed or damped current would cauterize tissue, whereas a more continuous current could be used to cut through tissue. The amount of tissue cauterized was limited to only a few millimeters because charred tissue adhered to the tip of the knife. This first-generation Bovie knife was a monopolar electrode similar to that used for contemporary percutaneous RF techniques. Consequently, the grounding pads that were used were placed on the patient in a fashion similar to that employed with most modern percutaneous RF techniques. The current passing through the Bovie knife into the body is ultimately dispersed over the wide area provided by the grounding pads.

The fact that RF works by causing ionic agitation of the tissues surrounding the needle was first demonstrated by Organ (5). The shaft of the needle does not produce heat. Rather, the heat is produced in the tissues, and that leads to coagulation and cellular necrosis. Fairly rapid application of current leads to a small region of coagulation as well as local tissue charring. Charring acts to inhibit further ionic agitation, thus limiting the amount of surrounding coagulation necrosis. In 1990, two independent investigators used a modification of prior RF techniques to create coagulation necrosis that could be applied via the percutaneous route. McGahan et al (6) described their research in the English literature, and in the same year Rossi et al (7) described a similar technique in the Italian literature. These investigators replaced the Bovie knife with specially designed needles insulated to the distal tip. This

A

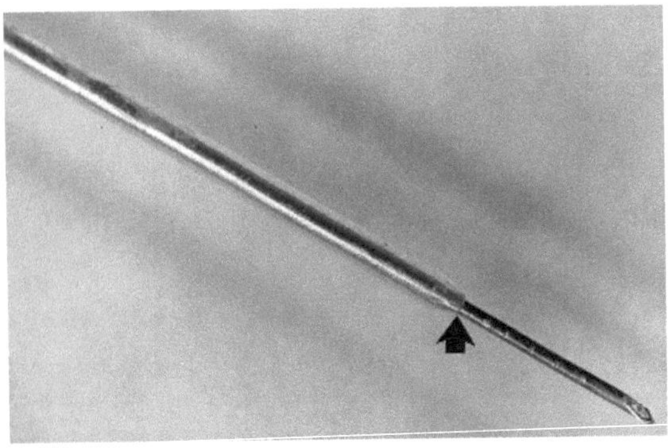

B

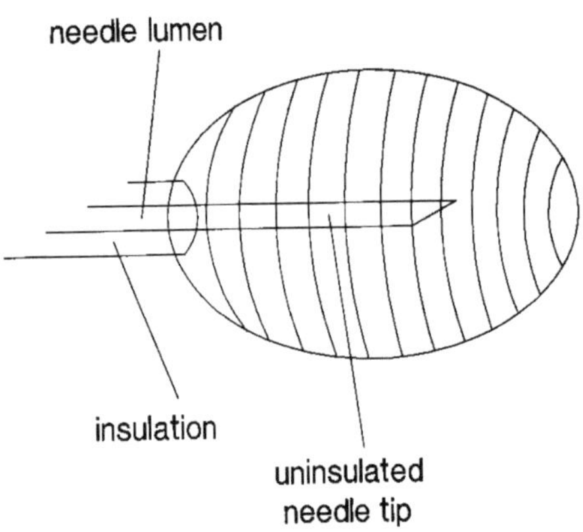

FIGURE 1.1. (A) Original needle design. Photograph of original needle design shows standard stock needle that is insulated (arrow) up to distal tip. Needle tip is not insulated. (B) Original needle design. Drawing shows theoretic lesion that would be produced if noninsulated needle tip were used during monopolar radiofrequency electrocautery. (Reprinted with permission from The American Journal of Roentgenology.)

design directed the flow of current into the target tissue. Thus, an insulated needle could be percutaneously placed deep into a target organ such as the liver to produce an area of focal necrosis (Fig. 1.1). The length of the central axis of the lesion could be increased by exposing the tissue to a larger area of uninsulated needle. A limitation of this original needle design was that the diameter of the lesion to be ablated needed to be 1.5 cm or less. Grounding pads were placed in a similar manner to that used for the Bovie knife.

In 1992 McGahan et al (8) showed that ultrasound could be used both to monitor the RF needle placement and to assess the echogenic response in the tissue surrounding the RF needle during ablation. They documented increased echogencity surrounding the exposed needle tip following the application of current (Fig. 1.2). This echogenic response was ellipsoid in appearance and roughly corresponded to the volume of coagulation necrosis seen on pathologic examination. There was a central zone of char around the needle tip and an accompanying larger zone of coagulation necrosis. There was also a zone of hemorrhage at the interface between the coagulated tissue and normal liver (Fig. 1.3).

In 1993 this technique was used for RFA of liver tumors in humans (9). It was soon investigated by others and shortly thereafter became commercially available. RF generators and needles were developed that could be used for percutaneous, laparoscopic, or open ablation. A problem with initial needle design is that the volume of tissue necrosis was limited to approximately 2 cm^3 when using an uninsulated needle length of approximately 2 cm. Multiple applications with this type of needle could ablate a 2-cm-diameter tumor, with a volume slightly greater than 4 cm^3 (Fig. 1.4). The lesion was elongate, with the long axis of the necrosis parallel to the shaft of the needle. However, most lesions that are treatable by RF are oval rather than elongate in shape, and smaller lesions are the exception rather than the rule. To ablate a lesion of approximately 4 cm in diameter with a tumor volume greater than 36 cm^3, one would need at least 18 separate optimal placements of the originally designed needle to eradicate the tumor completely. Even more treatments would be needed if a volume of normal tissue had to be destroyed to ensure tumor-free margins and prevent recurrence.

There have been a number of commercially available technical advances intended to solve the problem of the limited volume of tissue necrosis associated with percutaneous RF needles. Early RF generators for percutaneous applications produced a maximum of 50 W of power, whereas modern generators can produce between 150 and 200 W. Recent improvements in software designs and methods of power deposition ensure maximal energy

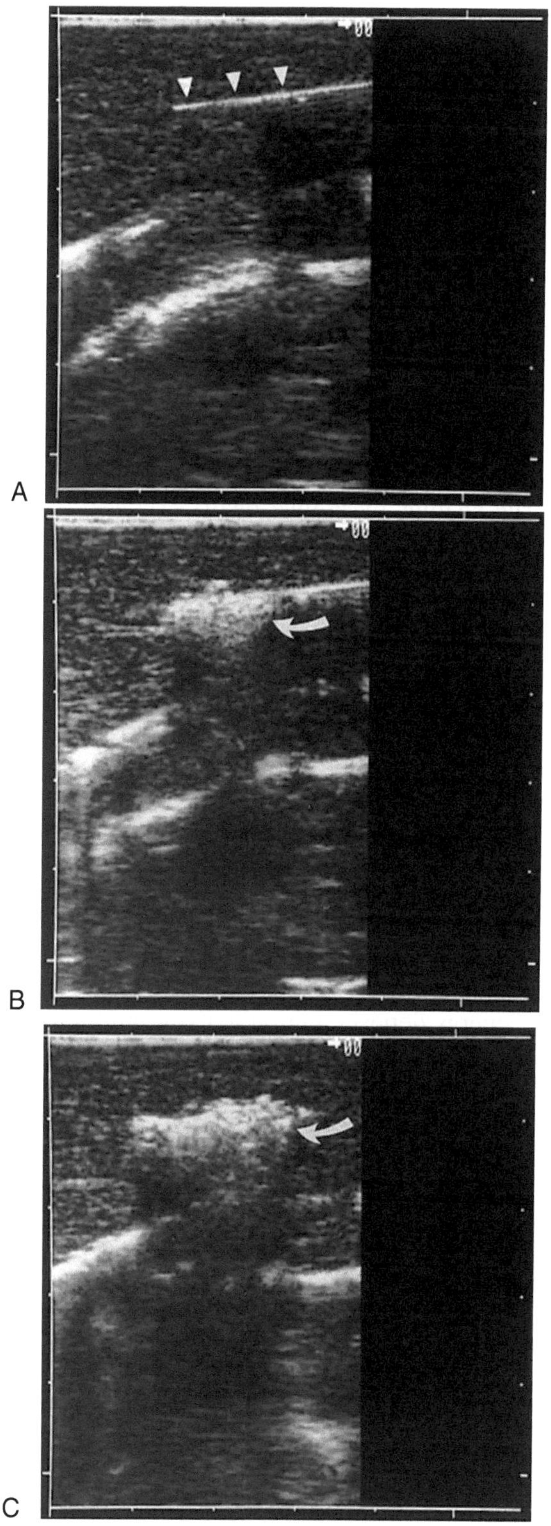

FIGURE 1.2. In vitro radiofrequency coagulation of bovine liver. (A) Needle being placed under ultrasound guidance showing uninsulated needle tip (arrowhead 5). (B,C) With increasing power deposition, there is increased echogenicity of liver surrounding the needle tip (curved arrow).

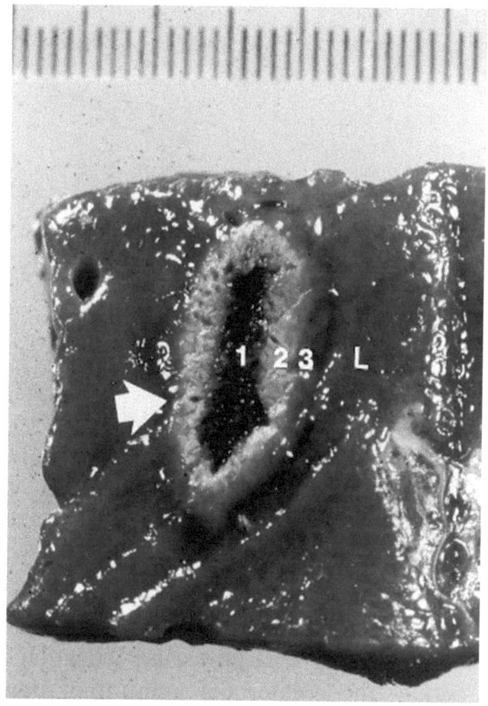

FIGURE 1.3. In vivo histologic correlation for radiofrequency coagulation of swine liver. Photograph of in vivo liver reveals central area of charred tissue (1) surrounded by coagulative necrosis (2) and hyperemic rim (arrow, 3). L, healthy liver. (Reprinted with permission from J.P. McGahan, J.M. Brock, H. Tesluk et al. "Hepatic ablation with use of radiofrequency electocautery in the animal model." JVIR 19923: 291–297.)

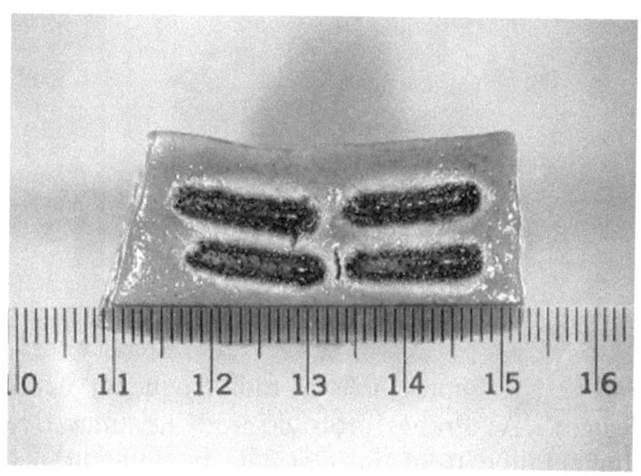

FIGURE 1.4. Overlapping coagulation. One method of increasing coagulation is to produce multiple regions of necrosis by repositioning the needle.

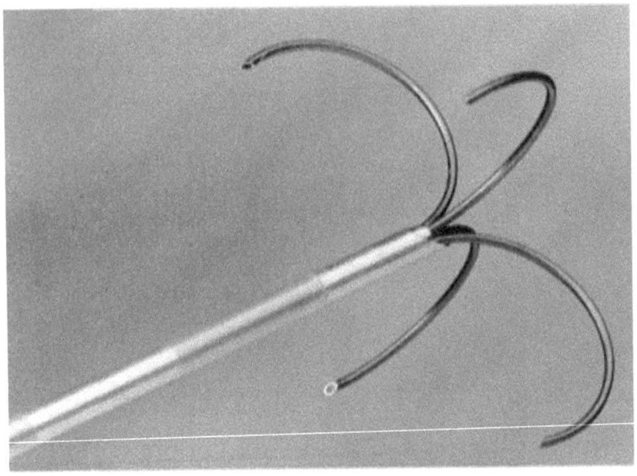

FIGURE 1.5. Some of the original self-expanding needles had only a few prongs that deployed. This could lead to an uneven distribution of coagulation necrosis.

transmission to the target organ before discontinuance of current flow and coagulation. Generally, the greater the amount of power disposition to the target area, the greater the volume of tissue destroyed. Additionally, several different types of needles have been designed to increase the volume of tissue necrosis. In 1997 LeVeen (10) described an approach for a monopolar needle or electrode that had separate prongs deployable from the needle tip. Each of these prongs is uninsulated and functions as an RF antenna for dispersion of current (Fig. 1.5). By increasing the energy output of the generators, the regions of coagulation surrounding each prong coalesce, resulting in increased volumes of necrosis. Other needle designs enable the operator to deploy an even greater number of prongs from the needle tip, producing a larger uniform volume of necrosis (Fig. 1.6).

In 1996 and 1997 Goldberg et al (11) and Lorentzen et al (12) described an innovative approach in which the needle tip was cooled by chilled saline pumped through the shaft of the needle. While it may seem counterintuitive to cool the needle tip in an attempt to create a larger region of coagulation necrosis from tissue heating, these investigators showed that cooling of the needle tip prevented tissue charring that occurred with the original needle designs by McGahan and Rossi. A cooled needle allows for a decrease in the temperature of the tissue surrounding the needle tip, thereby producing tissue coagulation without significant charring. The reduction in charring results in further ionic agitation with increased volume of tissue necrosis. A variation of this technology utilizes three or more cooled tip needles ("clustered") to increase the volume of tissue necrosis (13) (Fig. 1.7).

Further research has shown that several factors can alter the amount of tissue necrosis. Coagulation necrosis is a function of the total RF energy deposited into the tissue, multiplied

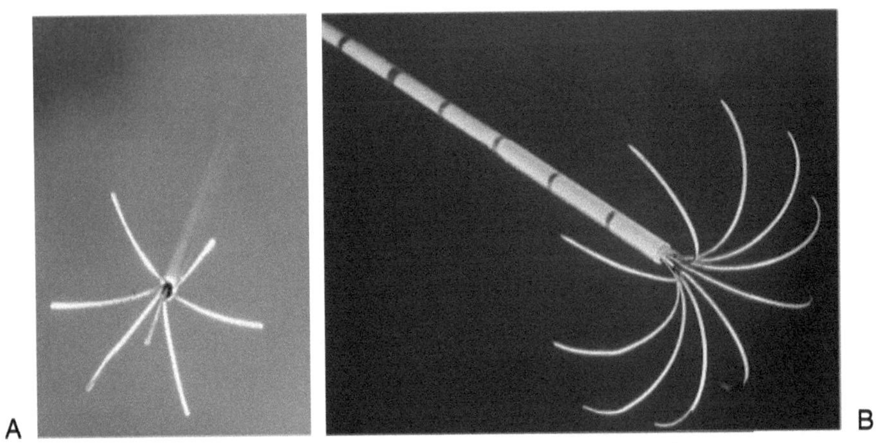

FIGURE 1.6. Photographs of radiofrequency needle designs. (A) Prongs protrude in "Christmas tree" configuration from tip of needle manufactured by RITA Medical Systems, Mountain View, CA. (B) Ten prongs protrude in umbrella configuration from tip of needle manufactured by Radiotherapeutics. (Boston Scientific, Natick, MA.)

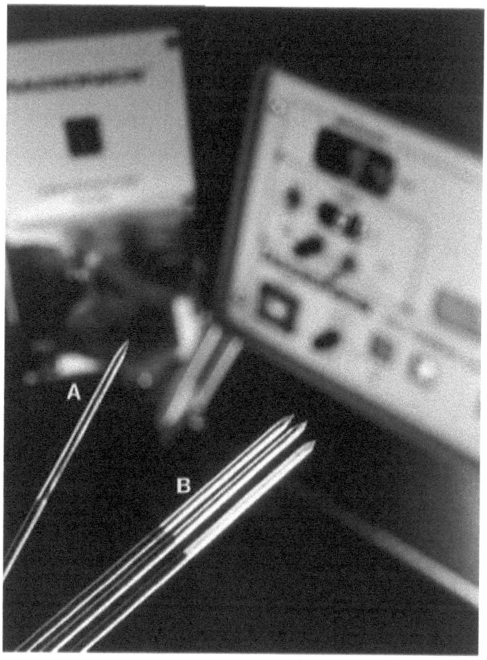

FIGURE 1.7. Photographs of radiofrequency needle designs. Single (A) and clustered (B), cooled-tip needles manufactured by Valleylab. (Photos printed with permission from Valleylab.)

by local tissue interactions, minus the local and systemic heat lost (14–16). Modern RF generators with higher wattages can increase the power deposition with a resulting increase in tissue necrosis. Local tissue characteristics and tissue interaction with RF current are important parameters in creating regions in necrosis. For instance, rapid application of current creates charring that reduces the water content of the tissue and ionic agitation, thereby limiting the amount of tissue necrosis.

In 1997 Livraghi et al (17) performed RF application on animal liver both ex vivo and in vivo. Their studies were conducted both with and without intraparenchymal saline injection. Radiofrequency application with continuous saline infusion also was evaluated. Livraghi et al found the largest volume of coagulation necrosis resulted from RF performed with continuous saline perfusion, while the smallest volumes were associated with RF performed without saline. Based on these data, they performed continuous saline-enhanced RF in 14 patients with liver metastases and one patient with primary cholangiocarcinoma. They documented complete necrosis in 13 of 25 liver lesions with diameters up to 3.9 cm. They concluded that this continuous saline infusion technique had promise in RF treatment of larger tumors. Curley and Hamilton (18) increased coagulation diameters from 1.4 to 2.6 cm by infusion of 10 mL/min of *normal* saline into ex vivo liver for 4 minutes during RF application. Miao et al (19) achieved coagulation diameters up to 5.5 cm by infusion of 1 mL/min of *hypertonic* saline into ex vivo liver for 12 minutes. As a direct consequence of this research and that performed by other investigators, saline-perfused RF has become a promising treatment option in management of liver tumors (20) (Fig. 1.8).

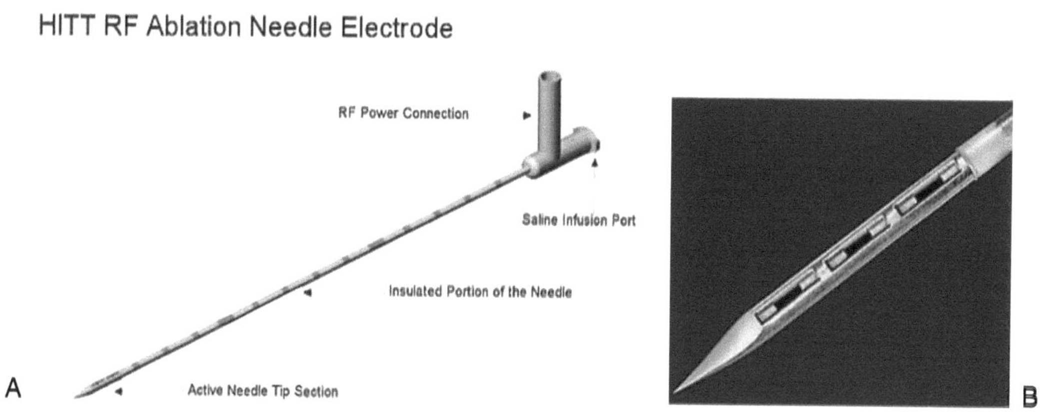

FIGURE 1.8. (A) Diagram of needle design HITT RF ablation needle in which saline is infused through infusion port at proximal end. (B) Distal end of needle with channels for dispersion of saline during RF application (BerCHTOLD Medical Electronic, Tuttlingen, Germany).

Optimal ablation results are achieved when local temperature is maintained between 60° and 100°C, with nearly instantaneous tissue coagulation necrosis (14–16). Lower temperatures require longer exposure time to achieve the desired result. For example, at 46°C, at least 1 hour is required to ensure cell damage. Conversely, a rapid increase in local tissue temperature above 100°C causes tissue charring that limits effective coagulation necrosis. Some manufacturers have devices in the needle tips that measure local tissue temperature during RF application.

Decreased Blood Flow and RF

To compensate for the "heat sink" effect of large vessels within tumors, several investigators have described methods intended to decrease blood flow to the organ of interest, before or during RF application. This approach was first presented by Buscarini et al (21), who, in 1999, described the use of RF combined with transcatheter arterial embolization for treatment of large hepatocellular carcinomas (HCC). Rossi et al (22) used balloon occlusion of the hepatic artery during RFA to treat larger HCCs. In 81% of HCCs averaging 4.7 cm in size treated by Rossi et al, there was no local recurrence at 1 year after this combined therapy.

Another method of decreasing the blood supply to hepatic tumors is use of the Pringle maneuver, which is performed during open surgical application of RF. After the RF needle is positioned within the tumor, the surgeon temporarily occludes the portal vein and the hepatic artery, thereby temporarily interrupting the blood supply to the liver, which significantly reduces the "heat sink" effect. Goldberg et al (23) used this technique in a limited series reported in 1998. They were able to achieve an increase in the volume of the tumor necrosis in patients when employing the Pringle maneuver compared to patients being treated with similar RF parameters but without the Pringle maneuver. The tumor necrosis diameter without the Pringle maneuver was 2.5 cm compared with 4.1 cm when using this maneuver.

Clinical results using the Pringle maneuver are reported to be excellent. In 1999 Curley et al (24) reported the results of RF in 123 patients. The Pringle maneuver was used in the majority of the 92 patients who were treated with RF intraoperatively. Tumor recurrence was detected in only three of the 169 lesions that were treated at a median follow-up of 15 months (24).

Chemotherapy and RF

There has been considerable interest in combining RF with chemotherapy. In 1999 Kainuma et al (25) combined intraarterial infusion of chemotherapy with RF electrocautery to treat hepatic metastases from colon cancer. Other investigators have shown there is an enhanced effect when chemotherapeutic agents are heated to hyperthermic temperatures between 42° and 45°C prior to infusion into the target tissue (26). In an initial report by Goldberg et al (27), increased coagulation necrosis was documented when RFA was combined with intratumoral injection of doxyrubicin. The volume of necrosis with the injection of doxyrubicin alone was 2 to 3 mm in an R3230 mammary adenocarcinoma model, whereas RFA alone produced 6.7 mm of necrosis. When RF was combined with injection of doxorubicin, a necrosis diameter of 11.4 mm was achieved (27), a marked improvement in monotherapy.

Summary

Over the past 10 years there has been a rapid advancement in the utilization of RF electrocautery for percutaneous, laparoscopic, and open surgical applications in the treatment of a number of different tumors. It was only in the early 1990s that McGahan et al and Rossi et al independently described the pioneering application of the percutaneous use of RF energy in the animal liver model. Over the past 10 years, manufacturers have designed more powerful generators, developed special programs for heat deposition, and achieved improved needle designs that enable the creation of larger volumes of tissue necrosis. Most recently, a number of investigators have explored other methods for increasing the amount of RF-induced tissue necrosis including catheter arterial occlusion during performance of RF, as well as intraoperative performance of the Pringle maneuver. Others have used chemotherapy in combination with RF to increase the volume of tumor ablated. Some investigators have demonstrated that injection of saline into the tumor during RF application can increase tumor necrosis. There is little doubt that RF alone or in combination with other technologies will find further utilization and wider application in percutaneous treatment of tumors and other diseases throughout the body.

Percutaneous Ethanol Injection

Percutaneous tissue ablation using ethanol is not new. One of the first descriptions of its use was in the treatment of renal cysts by Bean (28) in 1981. He treated 34 benign renal cysts in 29 patients using direct injection of 95% ethanol. The technique used by Bean more than 20 years ago has not changed significantly to the present. After confirming with contrast fluoroscopy that there was no leakage from a benign cyst, 4.6-French polyethylene catheters were placed into the cyst. Approximately 3% to 44% of the cyst volumes were replaced with 95% ethanol that was maintained in the cyst for 10 to 20 minutes. In this series, there was only one recurrence at 3 months. During the past two decades, other agents have been used to sclerose renal cysts. In 1985 Bean and Rodan (29) described a similar technique for treatment of hepatic cysts.

In 1985 Solbiati et al (30) injected absolute alcohol into enlarged parathyroids in patients with secondary hyperparathyroidism. This technique was useful in reducing the size of the parathyroid glands in those patients in whom surgery was contraindicated. The following year, Livraghi et al (31) described the use of ultrasound-guided needle placement into 14 hepatic lesions. These included nine patients with HCC, four with hepatic metastasis from gastric carcinoma, and one peritoneal metastasis from transitional cell carcinoma. All patients were treated with percutaneous injection of 95% ethanol into tumors that were less than 4 cm in diameter. From three to nine sessions were performed for each lesion, according to size. This work established the feasibility and value of percutaneous intratumoral alcohol injection to treat selected small hepatic neoplasms.

In 1988, Livraghi et al (32) published findings involving a series of 23 patients with HCC with tumor diameters less than 4.5 cm; 32 lesions were treated by ethanol injections performed under percutaneous ultrasound guidance. A total of 271 treatment sessions achieved a 1-year survival rate in 12 patients of 92%. All the lesions were smaller at 6 to 27 months' follow-up. In the early 1990s, other authors began using intratumoral ethanol for ablation of liver tumors. These efforts established the efficacy of percutaneous ethanol injection (PEI) in the treatment of hepatocellular carcinoma (33,34). In 1991, Livraghi et al (35) demonstrated that while PEI could be used to treat focal metastatic disease, its benefits are limited by the natural course of the disease.

In 1995 Livraghi et al (36) demonstrated PEI to be safe, effective, low cost, and easily reproducible in the treatment of patients with HCC. They performed this technique in 746 patients with HCC. The survival rates of patients were generally good, but dependent on the severity of accompanying cirrhosis. Patients with Child's A cirrhosis had a much better survival than their counterparts with Child's B or C cirrhosis. Livraghi et al believed that the survival after PEI was comparable to that of surgery, in part due to the increased mortality from surgery and liver damage associated with resection.

Other Injectables

Other injected liquids have been used to treat tumors. In 1986 Livraghi et al (37) performed what they called percutaneous intratumoral chemotherapy (PIC) under ultrasound guidance in 12 selected patients with tumors that had been unresponsive to conventional treatment. They injected a single agent or a combination of either 5-fluorouracil, methotrexate, or cyclophosphamide depending on the histology of the tumor. There were 119 sessions of PIC in which the authors achieved either partial or total pain control and stable disease response in 60% of the patients. During that same year, Livraghi et al (38) described the treatment of inoperable HCCs smaller than 3 cm with percutaneous interstitial chemotherapy using 5-fluorouracil injected under ultrasound guidance. They documented some fibrosis in the region of treatment at 3 months, and they suggested that this type of therapy could be useful as an alternative treatment for HCC.

In the early 1990s Honda and his coauthors advocated use of percutaneous hot saline injection therapy (PSITN) as an alternative to percutaneous ethanol treatment for hepatic tumors. One hundred twenty-three patients with HCC were treated with PSITN. A therapeutic effect occurred in all patients. Even so, hot saline therapy did not become widely utilized.

Another percutaneous therapy advocated in the 1990s was injection of acetic acid under sonographic guidance (41–43). For example, in 1994 Ohnishi et al (41) performed ultrasound-guided percutaneous acetic acid injection (PAI) in the treatment of hepatocellular carcinoma. PAI with 50% acetic acid was performed in 25 patients with solitary HCCs 3 cm or less in diameter. There was a total of 82 sessions with no significant complications and no evidence of viable HCC on follow-up biopsy. The survival rate among their 23 patients was 100% at 1 year and 92% at 2 years. In the future, research into these and other injectable agents for the treatment of focal neoplasms seems likely.

Lasers

A neodymium: yttrium-aluminum-garnet (Nd: YAG) laser system with ceramic rods was initially developed and tested in animals, then later used in clinical practice to treat head and neck tumors. This method was initially used to produce an "incision," rather than for tumor destruction. It was thought to be a precise method of surgical dissection, with reduced bleeding and minimal damage to adjacent tissue (44). In 1986 in the Japanese literature, Fujishima et al (45) published an experiment using the Nd:YAG laser as a possible treatment of deep-seated brain tumors. Hashimoto (46) published an experiment on the clinical application of the effects of lasers for hyperthermia of liver neoplasms. In 1998 Tajiri et al (47) induced local interstitial hyperthermia using the Nd:YAG laser to treat gastrointestinal and pancreatic carcinomas that had been transplanted into mice. These authors demonstrated there were areas of ischemic infarction and marked necrosis of the pancreatic tumor in the region of laser treatment.

In 1990 Hahl et al (48) treated seven patients with malignant tumors using the Nd:YAG laser during open laparotomy. They used sapphire probes with the power settings between 6 and 8 W. Even though only limited necrosis was produced by these lasers, they believed that selective destruction of malignant tumors was possible using laser-induced hyperthermia. In 1991 Van Hillegersberg et al (49) studied the use of laser coagulation in rat liver metastases and again demonstrated selective necrosis using this technique. In 1992 Dowlatshahi et al (50) reported in situ focal hyperthermia that was generated by an Nd:YAG laser. The laser was introduced through a 19-gauge needle inserted percutaneously into the liver under ultrasound guidance. This process was monitored under ultrasound and confirmed by computed tomography. Tumor growth was halted at 3 months, indicating partial response in humans.

In 1993 Nolsoe et al (51) used laser hyperthermia in 11 patients with 16 colorectal liver metastases. Real-time ultrasound was utilized to monitor this technique. They demonstrated in this larger patient group that laser hyperthermia was feasible, effective, and safe. Following that publication, others have obtained wider experience using these techniques in clinical practice in the treatment of primary and secondary liver tumors. Some investigators have used interstitial laser hyperthermia to treat neck tumors, in various neurosurgical applications, and in limited animal experimentation with mammary tumors (52–54).

Microwave Hyperthermia

Compared to other techniques, percutaneous microwave coagulation of tumors arrived somewhat late on the scene. In 1994 Seki et al (55) described a single case of percutaneous transhepatic microwave coagulation therapy for a patient with HCC with bile duct involvement. That same year, they described how percutaneous microwave coagulation therapy (PMCT) was used in the local treatment of unresectable HCC (56). This was performed in 18 patients with small diameter (less than 2cm) HCCs. A microwave electrode 1.6mm in thickness was inserted percutaneously under ultrasound guidance into the tumor region. The microwave was generated using 60W for 120 seconds. As with other thermal techniques, an echogenic response around the tumor was detected on ultrasound. Complete necrosis of the tumor area was documented in one patient who underwent hepatectomy after PMCT. In a short follow-up period lasting from 11 to 33 months, the patients had no local recurrence following treatment of these tumors.

In 1995 Murakami et al (57) used PMCT therapy in nine HCCs less than 3cm in diameter, and it was found to be a useful alternative to other forms of interstitial therapy for treatment of small HCCs. Hamazoe et al (58) also reported the use of microwave tissue coagulation (MTC) during laparotomy in eight patients with nonresectable HCCs. They found that intraoperative MTC appeared to be an effective method for inducing tumor necrosis that could be used in combination with local surgical resection for multiple HCCs when radical liver resection was not feasible.

In 1996 others reported using microwave hyperthermia guided by ultrasound in the percutaneous treatment of HCCs. These included limited results in 12 patients reported by Dong et al (59), two patients with long-term survival reported by Sato et al (60), and eight patients treated by Yamanaka et al (61). The patients in the Yamanaka series were treated both under laparoscopic and open methods. More recent and larger series describe the utility of microwave hyperthermia in the treatment of focal masses. Currently there are limitations on the volume of tissue necrosis that can be achieved utilizing microwave. Improvements in needle design and technology should address this problem.

Cryotherapy

Some of the initial work in cryotherapy was undertaken in the late 1970s, and most of it was experimental (62–66). In 1987 Ravikumar and his associates (67) reported their surgical experience with hepatic cryosurgery for metastatic colon cancer to the liver. Their development of 8 to 12mL liquid nitrogen–cooled probes, suitable for surgical placement within the liver, established the advent of interstitial hepatic cryosurgery. Real-time ultrasound was used to verify the extent of treatment and to measure the size of the increasing iceball that was created by freezing. Freezing and thawing for three cycles was an effective means of ensuring tumor necrosis. The average size of these lesions was in the range of 3cm. Further experimentation by Onik et al (68) in 1995 confirmed in the animal model the efficacy of sonography for monitoring hepatic cryotherapy.

By the late 1980s and early 1990s, investigators such as Charnley et al (69) and Onik et al (68) demonstrated the usefulness of this technique. However, the disadvantages of cryotherapy included that the technique required open surgery and that fairly large probes had to be placed into the lesions. Consequently, the surgical risks must be factored into analysis of morbidity and mortality for this patient group. In addition to the usual pleural effusions and the morbidity associated with the open technique, there were certain unique complications or imaging findings that occurred specifically with cryosurgery. These include posttreatment "cracking" of the hepatic parenchyma, air or hemorrhage in the lesion, and subcapsular hemorrhage. Smaller percutaneous cryotherapy probes have been developed that eliminate the risk associated with open surgical exploration (68). The techniques and various applications of modern cryotherapy will be explained in further detail in the accompanying chapter on that topic.

High-Intensity Focused Ultrasound

Documenting the first published research on the cavitation effects of ultrasound has been difficult. High-intensity focused ultrasound was described in 1989 as a method to treat discrete liver tumors. This was investigated in both in vivo and excised liver samples by ter Harr and associates (72). They performed both qualitative and quantitative studies to demonstrate the feasibility of this technique, with particular attention devoted to the lesion shape, position, and volume in relation to the duration of the ultrasound exposure.

Further research in this area was carried out in the early 1990s by Chapelon et al (73), Prat et al (74), and Yang et al (75). At least two of these investigators reviewed the use of high-intensity focused ultrasound (HIFU) in the treatment of hepatic lesions. One study (75) examined the use of HIFU to treat hepatomas implanted into the livers of rats. A total of 112 rats with liver tumors were divided into two groups—those that had HIFU and those that did not. A significant inhibition of tumor growth of 65% was seen in the HIFU-treated group on the third day posttreatment, with 93% growth inhibition on the 28th day following treatment. There was evidence of both tumor necrosis and fibrosis. This is one of the first studies on the use of HIFU for treatment of liver tumors.

In 1992 and in 1993 Yang et al (76,77) produced further work demonstrating that HIFU could destroy targeted deep-seated tissue within the liver without causing damage to nontargeted tissue. These experiments demonstrated the potential usefulness of this therapy for ablation of liver cancer without the need for laparotomy.

Similar experimentation was performed by Sibille et al (78) in 1993. They demonstrated that in the in-vivo rabbit liver a relationship exists among HIFU intensity levels, exposure times, and the posttreatment lesion appearance. This work demonstrated the need to adapt intensity to the depth of the target tissue.

This technique for the ablation of liver tumors is not without its challenges. For example, the movement of the liver associated with respiration will require gating of HIFU for transcutaneous applications to ensure that the target lesion remains within the zone of maximum intensity of the ultrasound beam to minimize collateral damage to nonneoplastic tissue.

Where organ movement is not a problem, HIFU has been more successful. For example, when used in the prostate or when used intraoperatively, the ultrasound can be directly applied to the organ of interest and kept in one position for the duration of HIFU application. There has been research involving HIFU applications in the genitourinary system including ablation of renal and prostatic lesions (79–81). Gelet et al (80) demonstrated the utility of HIFU to induce coagulation necrosis in the canine prostate. They determined the different levels of HIFU required to achieve varying amounts of tissue ablation within the prostate. There was homogeneous coagulation necrosis within the lesions that later progressed to inflammatory fibrosis and finally to sclerosis with cavity formation. This study in animals demonstrated the potential for creating irreversible prostate lesions using HIFU without damaging the rectal wall. In the same year, Gelet et al (81) successfully used a similar technique in nine patients with prostate hypertrophy. Finally, as was mentioned previously, some of the problems resulting from organ motion can be eliminated when HIFU is used intraoperatively.

Summary

Modern medicine is constantly evolving less invasive methods for the treatment of disease. While some of this research with tissue ablation was documented over 100 years ago, the majority of investigative efforts have taken place within the past 20 years. In the future there will undoubtedly be additional research into these techniques and the development of new methods of tissue ablation.

References

1. D'Arsonval MA. Action physiologique des courants alternatifs. C R Soc Biol 1891; 43:283–286.
2. Beer E. Removal of neoplasms of the urinary bladder: a new method employing high frequency (oudin) currents through a cauterizing cystoscope. JAMA 1910;54:1768–1769.
3. Clark WL. Oscillatory desiccation in the treatment of accessible malignant growths and minor surgical conditions. J Adv Ther 1911;29:169–183.
4. Cushing H, Bovie WT. Electro-surgery as an aid to the removal of intracranial tumors. Surg Gynecol Obstet 1928;47:751–784.
5. Organ LW. Electrophysiologic principles of radiofrequency lesion making. Appl Neurophysiol 1976–1977;39:69–76.
6. McGahan JP, Browing PD, Brock JM, Tesluk H. Hepatic ablation using radiofrequency electrocautery. Invest Radiol 1990;25:267–270.
7. Rossi S, Fornari F, Pathies C, Buscarini L. Thermal lesions induced by 480 KHz localized current field in guinea pig and pig liver. Tumori 1990;76:54–57.
8. McGahan JP, Brock JM, Tesluk H, et al. Hepatic ablation with use of radiofrequency electrocautery in the animal model. J Vasc Intervent Radiol 1992;3:291–297.
9. McGahan JP, Scheider P, Brock JM, Teslik H. Treatment of liver tumors by percutaneous radiofrequency electrocautery. Semin Intervent Radiol 1993;10(2):143–149.
10. LeVeen RF. Laser hyperthermia and radiofrequency ablation of hepatic lesions. Semin Intervent Radiol 1997;14:313–324.
11. Goldberg SN, Gazelle GS, Solbiati L, Rittman WJ, Mueller PR. Radiofrequency tissue ablation: increased lesion diameter with a perfusion electrode. Acad Radiol 1996;3:636–644.
12. Lorentzen T, Christensen NE, Nolsoe CP, Torp-Pedersen ST. Radiofrequency tissue ablation with a cooled needle in vitro: ultrasonography, dose response, and lesion temperature. Acad Radiol 1997;4:292–297.
13. Goldberg SN, Solbiati L, Hahn PF, et al. Large volume tissue ablation with radiofrequency by using a clustered, internally cooled electrode technique: laboratory and clinical experience in liver metastases. Radiology 1998;209:371–379.
14. Goldberg SN, Dupuy DE. Image-guided radiofrequency tumor ablation: challenges and opportunities—part I. J Vasc Intervent Radiol 2001;12:1021–1032.
15. McGahan JP, Dodd GD III. Radiofrequency ablation of the liver: current status. AJR 2001; 176:3–16.
16. Zevas NT, Kuwayama A. Pathological characteristics of experimental thermal lesions: comparison of induction heating and radiofrequency electrocoagulation. J Neurosurg 1972;37:418–422.
17. Livraghi T, Goldberg SN, Lazzaroni S, et al. Saline-enhanced radiofrequency tissue ablation in the treatment of liver metastases. Radiology 1997;202:205–210.
18. Curley MG, Hamilton PS. Creation of large thermal lesions in liver using saline-enhanced RF ablation. Proceedings of the 19th International Conference IEEE/EMBS, Chicago, October 30–November 2, 1997.
19. Miao Y, Ni Y, Mulier S, et al. Ex vivo experiment on radiofrequency liver ablation with saline infusion through a screw-tip cannulated electrode. J Surg Res 1997;71:19–24.
20. Hansler J, et al. Percutaneous ultrasound guide radiofrequency tissue ablation (RFTA) with perfused needle applicators—treatment of hepatocellular carcinoma and liver metastases—first results. Proceedings of EMBEC 1999;pt II:1576–1577.
21. Buscarini L, Buscarini E, Stasi M, Quaretti P, Zangrandi A. Percutaneous radiofrequency thermal ablation combined with transcatheter arterial embolization in the treatment of large hepatocellular carcinoma. Ultraschall Med 1999; 20:47–53.
22. Rossi S, Garbagnati F, Lencioni R. Unresectable hepatocellular carcinoma: percutaneous radiofrequency thermal ablation after occlusion of tumor blood supply. Radiology 2000;217:119–126.
23. Goldberg SN, Hahn PF, Tanabe KK, et al. Percutaneous radiofrequency tissue ablation: Does perfusion-mediated tissue cooling limit coagulation necrosis? J Vasc Intervent Radiol 1998;9: 101–111.
24. Curley SA, Izzo F, Delrio P, et al. Radiofrequency ablation of unresectable primary and metastatic hepatic malignancies: results in 123 patients. Ann Surg 1999;230:1–8.
25. Kainuma O, Asano T, Aoyama H, et al. Combined therapy with radiofrequency thermal ablation and intra-arterial infusion chemotherapy for hepatic metastases from colorectal cancer. Hepatogastroenterology 1999;46(26):1071–1077.
26. Seegenschmiedt MH, Brady LW, Sauer R. Interstitial thermo-radiotherapy: a review on techni-

cal and clinical aspects. Am J Clin Oncol 1990; 13:352–363.
27. Goldberg SN, Saldinger PF, Gazelle GS, et al. Percutaneous tumor ablation: increased coagulation necrosis with combined radiofrequency and percutaneous doxorubicin injection. Radiology 2001.
28. Bean WJ. Renal cysts: treatment with alcohol. Radiology 1981;138(2):329–331.
29. Bean WJ, Rodan BA. Hepatic cysts: treatment with alcohol. AJR 1985;144(2):237–241.
30. Solbiati L, Giangrande A, De Pra L, Bellotti E, Cantu P, Ravetto C. Percutaneous ethanol injection of parathyroid tumors under US guidance: treatment for secondary hyperparathyroidism. Radiology 1985;155(3):607–610.
31. Livraghi T, Festi D, Monti F, Salmi A, Vettori C. US-guided percutaneous alcohol injection of small hepatic and abdominal tumors. Radiology 1986;161(2):309–312.
32. Livraghi T, Salmi A, Bolondi L, Marin G, Arienti V, Monti F. Small hepatocellular carcinoma: percutaneous alcohol injection—results in 23 patients. Radiology 1998;168(2):313–317.
33. Ebara M, Otho M, Sugiura N, Okuda K, Kondo F, Kondo Y. Percutaneous ethanol injection for the treatment of small hepatocellular carcinoma: study of 95 patients. J Gastroenterol Hepatol 1990;5:616–626.
34. Shiina S, Tagawa K, Unuma T, et al. Percutaneous ethanol injection therapy for hepatocellular carcinoma: a histopathologic study. Cancer 1991;68: 1524–1530.
35. Livraghi T, Vettori C, Lazzaroni S. Liver metastases: results of percutaneous ethanol injections in 14 patients. Radiology 1991;179(3):709–712.
36. Livraghi T, Giorgio A, Marin G, et al. Hepatocellular carcinoma and cirrhosis in 746 patients: long-term results of percutaneous ethanol injection. Radiology 1995;197(1):101–108.
37. Livraghi T, Bajetta E, Matricardi L, Villa E, Lovati R, Vettori C. Fine needle percutaneous intratumoral chemotherapy under ultrasound guidance: a feasibility study. Tumori 1986;72(1): 81–87.
38. Livraghi T, Ravetto C, Solbiati L, Suter F. Percutaneous interstitial chemotherapy of a small hepatocellular carcinoma under ultrasound guidance. Tumori 1986;72(5):525–527.
39. Honda N, Guo Q, Uchida H, et al. Percutaneous hot water injection therapy (PhoT) for hepatic tumors: a clinical study. Nippon Igaku Hoshasen Gakkai Zasshi 1993;53(7):781–789.
40. Honda N, Guo Q, Uchida H, Ohishi H, Hiasa Y. Percutaneous hot saline injection therapy for hepatic tumors: an alternative to percutaneous ethanol injection therapy. Radiology 1994; 190(1):53–57.
41. Ohnishi K, Ohyama N, Ito S, Fujiwara K. Small hepatocellular carcinoma: treatment with US-guided intratumoral injection of acetic acid. Radiology 1994;193(3):747–752.
42. Ohnishi K, Yoshioka H, Ito S, Fujiwara K. Treatment of nodular hepatocellular carcinoma larger than 3 cm with ultrasound-guided percutaneous acetic acid injection. Hepatology 1996;24(6): 1379–1385.
43. Ohnishi K, Nomura F, Ito S, Fujiwara K. Prognosis of small hepatocellular carcinoma (less than 3 cm) after percutaneous acetic acid injection: study of 91 cases. Hepatology 1996;23(5): 994–1002.
44. Ohyama M, Katsuda K, Nobori T, et al. Treatment of head and neck tumors by contact Nd-YAG laser surgery. Auris Nasus Larynx 1985;12(suppl 2):S138–142.
45. Fujishima I, et al. Experimental study of deep brain radiation with the Nd-YAG laser. A possible new treatment for deep-seated brain tumor. Neurol Med Chir (Tokyo) 1986;26(8):621–627.
46. Hashimoto D. Clinical application of the thermal effect of lasers. 2. Application of the laser thermal effect to the therapy of liver neoplasms. Nippon Rinsho 1987;45(4):888–896.
47. Tajiri H, Oguro Y, Egawa S, Sugimura T. Local hyperthermia using a low powered Nd:YAG laser for pancreatic and gastric carcinoma. Hokkaido Igaku Zasshi 1998;63(6):889–896.
48. Hahl J, Haapiainen R, Ovaska J, Puolakkainen P, Schroder T. Laser-induced hypothermia in the treatment of liver tumors. Lasers Surg Med 1990; 10(4):319–321.
49. Van Hillegersberg R, Kort WJ, ten Kate FJ, Terpstra OT. Water-jet-cooled Nd:YAG laser coagulation: selective destruction of rat liver metastases. Lasers Surg Med 1991;11(5):445–454.
50. Dowlatshahi K, Bhattacharya AK, Silver B, Matalon T, Williams JW. Percutaneous interstitial laser therapy of a patient with recurrent hepatoma in a transplanted liver. Surgery 1992;112(3):603–606.
51. Nolsoe CP, Torp-Pedersen S, Burcharth F, et al. Interstitial hyperthermia of colorectal liver metastases with a US-guided Nd-YAG laser with a diffuser tip: a pilot clinical study. Radiology 1993;187(2):333–337.

52. Panjehpour M, Overholt BF, Frazier DL, Klebanow ER. ND:YAG laser-induced hyperthermia treatment of spontaneously occurring veterinary head and neck tumors. Lasers Surg Med 1991;11(4):351–355.
53. Dowlatshahi K, Babich D, Bangert JD, Kluiber R. Histologic evaluation of rat mammary tumor necrosis by interstitial Nd:YAG laser hyperthermia. Lasers Surg Med 1992;12(2): 159–164.
54. Sakai T, Fujishima I, Sugiyama K, Ryu H, Uemura K. Interstitial laserthermia in neurosurgery. J Clin Laser Med Surg 1992;10(1):37–40.
55. Seki T, Kubota Y, Wakabayashi M, et al. Percutaneous transhepatic microwave coagulation therapy for hepatocellular carcinoma proliferating in the bile duct. Dig Dis Sci 1994;39(3): 663–666.
56. Seki T, Wakabayashi M, Nakagawa T, et al. Ultrasonically guided percutaneous microwave coagulation therapy for small hepatocellular carcinoma. Cancer 1994;74(3):817–825.
57. Murakami R, Yoshimatsu S, Yamashita Y, Matsukawa T, Takahashi M, Sagara K. Treatment of hepatocellular carcinoma: value of percutaneous microwave coagulation. AJR 1995;164(5): 1159–1164.
58. Hamazoe R, Hirooka Y, Ohtani S, Katoh T, Kaibara N. Intraoperative microwave tissue coagulation as treatment for patients with nonresectable hepatocellular carcinoma. Cancer 1995;75(3):794–800.
59. Dong B, Liang P, Yu X. US-guided microwave in the treatment of liver cancer: experimental study and preliminary clinical application. Zhonghua Yi Xue Za Zhi 1996;76(2):87–91.
60. Sata M, Watanabe Y, Ueda S, et al. Two long-term survivors after microwave coagulation therapy for hepatocellular carcinoma: a case report. Hepatogastroenterology 1996;43(10):1035–1039.
61. Yamanaka N, Tanaka T, Oriyama T, Furukawa K, Tanaka W, Okamoto E. Microwave coagulonecrotic therapy for hepatocellular carcinoma. World J Surg 1996;20(8):1076–1081.
62. Cahan WG. Cryosurgery of massive recurrent cancer. Panminerva Med 1975;17(11–12):359–361.
63. Dutta P, Montes M, Gage AA. Large volume freezing in experimental hepatic cryosurgery. Avoidance of bleeding in hepatic freezing by an improvement in the technique. Cryobiology 1979;16(1):50–55.
64. Grana L, Airan M, Gordon M, Johnson R. Cryogenic technique for resection of carcinoma of the colon. Int Surg 1978;63(5):53–56.
65. Walzel C. Current status of cryogenic surgery. [Article in German] Chirurg 1978;49(4):202–208.
66. Zhou XD. Cryosurgery for liver cancer: experimental and clinical study (author's trans). [Article in Chinese] Zhonghua Wai Ke Za Zhi 1979;17(6):480–483.
67. Ravikumar TS, Kane R, Cady B, et al. Hepatic cryosurgery with intraoperative ultrasound monitoring for metastatic colon carcinoma. Arch Surg 1987;122:403.
68. Onik G, Gilbert J, Hoddick W, et al. Sonographic monitoring of hepatic cryosurgery in an experimental animal model. AJR 1985;144(5):1043–1047.
69. Charnley RM, Dorn J, Morris DL. Cryotherapy for liver metastases: a new approach. Br J Surg 1989;76(10):1040–1041.
70. Onik G, Rubinsky B, Zemel R, et al. Ultrasound-guided hepatic cryosurgery in the treatment of metastatic colon carcinoma. Preliminary results. Cancer 1991;67(4):901–907.
71. Onik GM, Atkinson D, Zemel R, et al. Cryosurgery of liver cancer. Semin Oncol 1993; 9:309.
72. ter Harr G, Sinnett D, Rivens I. High intensity focused ultrasound—a surgical technique for the treatment of discrete liver tumours. Phys Med Biol 1989;34(11):1743–1750.
73. Chapelon JY, Margonari J, Bouvier R, Cathignol D, Gorry F, Gelet A. [Tissue ablation by focused ultrasound] [Article in French]. Prog Urol 1991;1(2):231–243.
74. Prat F, Ponchon T, Berger F, Chapelon JY, Gagnon P, Cathignol D. Hepatic lesions in the rabbit induced by acoustic cavitation. Gastroenterology 1991;100(5 pt 1):1345–1350.
75. Yang R, Reilly CR, Rescorla FJ, et al. High-intensity focused ultrasound in the treatment of experimental liver cancer. Arch Surg 1991; 126(8):1002–1009; discussion 1009–1010.
76. Yang R, Sanghvi NT, Rescorla FJ, et al. Extracorporeal liver ablation using sonography-guided high-intensity focused ultrasound. Invest Radiol 1992;27(10):796–803.
77. Yang R, Kopecky KK, Rescorla FJ, Galliani CA, Wu EX, Grosfeld JL. Sonographic and computed tomography characteristics of liver ablation lesions induced by high-intensity focused ultrasound. Invest Radiol 1993;28(9):796–801.

78. Sibille A, Prat F, Chapelon JY, et al. Extracorporeal ablation of liver tissue by high-intensity focused ultrasound. Oncology 1992;50(5):375–379.
79. Chapelon JY, Margonari J, Theillere Y, et al. Effects of high-energy focused ultrasound on kidney tissue in the rat and the dog. Eur Urol 1992;22(2):147–152.
80. Gelet A, Chapelon JY, Margonari J, et al. Prostatic tissue destruction by high-intensity focused ultrasound: experimentation on canine prostate. J Endourol 1993;7(3):249–253.
81. Gelet A, Chapelon JY, Margonari J, et al. High-intensity focused ultrasound experimentation on human benign prostatic hypertrophy. Eur Urol 1993;23(suppl 1):44–47.

2
Epidemiology: How to Appraise the Ablation Literature Critically

Craig Earle

Example of an Abstract

PURPOSE: To evaluate the effectiveness of ablation for hepatic tumors. METHODS: The medical records of patients with either primary or secondary hepatic tumors who underwent ablative procedures from February 1991 to May 2001 at a single institution were retrospectively reviewed. One hundred nine patients with 140 tumors ranging in size from 0.5 to 12 cm in diameter were treated. The diagnoses were colorectal cancer (n = *69), hepatoma* (n = *15), ovarian cancer* (n = *8), cholangiocarcinoma* (n = *4), carcinoid* (n = *7), one each of leiomyosarcoma, testicular cancer, and endometrial cancer, and other tumors* (n = *3). Ablation was used to treat 90 tumors: 47 percutaneously, 23 laparoscopically, and 20 intraoperatively. Additional tumors were identified by intraoperative ultrasound in 37% of the patients taken to surgery despite extensive preoperative imaging. In 45%, radiofrequency ablation (RFA) was combined with resection or cryoablation or both. Alcohol ablation was performed on those patients who were found to have residual tumor after the initial ablative procedure. Ten patients underwent a second procedure and three had a third for progressive or recurrent disease. Neoadjuvant chemotherapy was used in 19 cases, intrahepatic treatment in 10, and postoperative chemotherapy was given to 33 patients. Follow-up ranged between 12 and 28 months. RESULTS: If we exclude the six cases in which it was clearly impossible to destroy the liver tumors and the one death due to postprocedure myocardial infarction, median progression-free survival was 13 months. Tumor response was seen in 87% of cases. Median time to death or last follow-up was 18 months: 16 months for nonsurvivors, and 20 months for survivors. Complications occurred in 27% of patients and included one skin burn, one postoperative hemorrhage from hepatic parenchyma cracking, and two hepatic abscesses. Only 4.7% locally recurred, although 37% have died of their cancer, and another 28% developed metastatic disease at other sites. CONCLUSION: Ablation may be effective in allowing patients to undergo liver surgery and achieve better survival.*

Clinical epidemiology spans the breadth of health and disease, from evaluating causation and risk, to strategies for disease prevention, to establishing diagnosis and prognosis, and to evaluating interventions. As the focus of this book is on techniques of tumor ablation, the focus here is on the evaluation of this form of intervention, in particular looking at pitfalls the reader may encounter when trying to read the ablation literature. The composite abstract above was extracted from abstracts of published papers describing clinical studies of tumor ablation. Although no single study was this uninterpretable, it illustrates the challenges a reader faces when trying to make sense of ablation studies. In the end, clinicians must be able to take the results reported in a study and evaluate whether the intervention in question is likely to benefit the patient they have before them.

When assessing a medical article, the reader must first judge whether the results are valid, and then try to fit them into the greater context of the field. A review conducted in June 2002 of clinical trials in adults reported in English in the past 10 years of the MEDLINE database using the intersection of key words "tumor ablation", "radiofrequency ablation", or "cryoablation" with "neoplasms", yielded 95 citations, of which 49 were relevant original studies. All but one was an uncontrolled case series. These ranged in size from four to 308 patients. There were large variations in reported outcomes, much of which likely is due to differing characteristics of the patients, different ablative techniques, other interventions the patients received, or the way the outcomes were assessed, analyzed, or reported. As a result, it is clear that understanding the ablation literature requires the ability to evaluate such noncomparative studies and to recognize their strengths and limitations.

Appraising Noncomparative Studies

One of the main strengths of randomized controlled trials is that randomization provides the appropriate control group for comparison of outcomes, as patients in the intervention and control arms should be similar in all ways except for the random allocation to the different treatment groups. If randomization is carried out correctly in a study of sufficient sample size, both known and unknown prognostic features should be balanced between the intervention and control groups. Nonrandomized studies with a control group attempt to do the same thing, although there is always a risk that the control group is different from the intervention group in some way that could influence the results. For example, more robust patients are generally more likely to have been selected to undergo aggressive therapy. Even in studies without an explicit control group, however, such as the bulk of the ablation literature, implicit comparison of outcomes is usually being made with the reader's sense of what the outcomes of such patients would have been without the intervention being studied. This, in a sense, is a form of historic controls. If the outcomes of the study exceed these expectations, the treatment can be judged to be promising; however, the reader must be careful to question at least three important components of the study: (1) Who were the patients? (2) What was the intervention? (3) What are the outcomes, and how are they assessed?

Who Were the Patients?

Selection Bias

The first concern about encouraging results in a nonrandomized trial is usually that the patients have been "cherry picked," meaning that selection bias has influenced the results. Because no study can observe every patient in the world with a given clinical problem, the patients in trials are a *sample* of the entire universe of patients. It is critical to determine how representative this sample is of the population of interest. For example, patients with better performance status are known to tolerate interventions better, are more likely to have favorable outcomes like response to treatment, and tend to have longer survival than those who are more ill. Patients with a lesser disease burden usually do better in these respects, while those who have been heavily pretreated do worse. Patients drawn entirely from academic referral centers tend to be younger and more proactive and health conscious than those in the community. A study consisting only of patients with characteristics making them likely to have good outcomes anyway, can almost guarantee promising results. Taken to extremes, exclusion of patients who are less likely to respond to treatment can theoretically eventually lead to 100% response rate. Authors should provide enough information for readers to know the entry criteria and patient characteristics to assess whether the sample is representative of their patients.

Assembly of the Inception Cohort

An important safeguard against selection bias is a clear description of how the inception cohort was assembled. This involves communicating an understanding of the number of eligible and ineligible patients seen within the study period so that the reader can estimate the degree of selection used to obtain the study population (1). The reader must be able to follow the flow of patients including referral patterns, seeing that consecutive patients (not selected patients) were approached for the study, noting how many of those refused and how many were later excluded, and the reasons for their exclusion. Ultimately, one should be able to account for all patients who did or did not participate, and know the denominator used for analyses at all times.

Entry Criteria

Another safeguard against selection bias is to have rigorously defined entry criteria that ensure that the patient group is relatively homogeneous. For example, although it seems obvious, histologic confirmation of disease should be required for entry into an ablation study. However, several relatively large series have not required this, leading at least one reviewer to wonder, "How many of the survivors . . . may have had cryotherapy for lesions that were not in fact metastases?" (2). This must be kept in mind when comparing outcomes to those for surgical resection, as a resected tumor will always be pathologically confirmed, while the same is not necessarily true of an ablated lesion.

The way a study sample is constructed depends in part on whether the primary goal of the study is to demonstrate internal validity and efficacy (Can something work under ideal conditions?) versus external validity and effectiveness (Does it work? Are the results generalizable to the real world?). Selection of patients in clinical trials always involves trade-offs between these concepts. Ideally, to prove that an intervention works in a specific situation, investigators would select patients who were very similar in all clinical and demographic characteristics. If the intervention is demonstrated to work and the trial is done well, it is efficacious in that particular clinical situation with those patients (internal validity). However, it may be unclear whether the results could be extrapolated to other scenarios. To demonstrate real-world effectiveness, the study would be designed to take consecutive patients with perhaps less strict entry criteria to include the breadth of patients to whom the intervention is likely to be applied, and carry out the intervention outside of highly specialized settings. While it may be more difficult to obtain a positive result in such a study, the generalizability of these results makes them much more compelling.

Excluded Patients

The fewer the patients who refuse to be included or are excluded from analysis, the better. There are many examples from the medical literature showing that patients who agree to participate in clinical trials and who are compliant with therapy tend to have better outcomes than those who do not. For example, if patients who suffer complications from a procedure or for whom the procedure is considered technically incomplete are excluded from the analysis for being "inevaluable", the results are likely to be biased. The easiest way to improve the results of a trial are to exclude the patients who didn't tolerate or respond to treatment! Once again, patients with the best underlying performance status and biology tend to be more likely to tolerate medical interventions successfully. Thus, a study with very few patients excluded is likely to provide more valid results.

What Was the Intervention?

Ablative technologies are relatively new and are still undergoing development. As a result, trials may not be comparable because of the different techniques, instruments and manufacturers, and operator abilities. Furthermore, this continuous evolution means that the results of trials are often obsolete by the time they are published. Also, unless ablation is followed by surgical resection, it is usually not possible to assess the adequacy of the ablation, unlike the ability to pathologically assess surgical margins. A related consideration is whether the technique is likely to be adequately performed when brought out of a highly specialized setting into general use. Problems with translating a procedure into practice can greatly reduce the *effectiveness* of an *efficacious* intervention.

Study protocols also differ widely in whether multiple lesions are ablated, the maximum size of lesion to be attempted, and whether there is co-intervention. For example, several studies examined above allowed patients following ablation to subsequently receive chemotherapy. As a result, it is impossible to discern whether observed stable disease is primarily due to innate biology, ablation, or subsequent systemic therapy. This heterogeneity in intervention makes much of the ablation literature difficult to interpret.

What Are the Outcomes, and How Were They Assessed?

The only outcomes that really matter to patients are the quantity and quality of life (*primary end points*). Anything else is a *surrogate or intermediate* end point that may correlate to a greater or lesser extent with primary end points (Table 2.1).

Response

Response to therapy, particularly the control of single lesions, has been shown many times to be a poor surrogate for either survival or quality of life. If response is used as an outcome, it must be clearly defined a priori in terms of the stringency of criteria (e.g., evaluated on high-quality scans at prespecified intervals), the threshold for measurements that were used (e.g., 50% decrease in the sum of the bidimensional areas of all tumors required to be deemed a response), and whether the response had to be "durable", that is, maintained for a prespecified period of time (e.g., on two computed tomography [CT] scans at least 2 months apart). This is important because minor responses of short duration can occur entirely on the basis of measurement error in diagnostic imaging alone (3,4). In ablation studies, response is a difficult end point because the ablation procedure often results in radiographic abnormalities that make it difficult to measure the tumor. Measuring decreased uptake of a lesion on positron emission tomography (PET) scan has not been adequately validated.

Time to Progression

Time to progression often is evaluated in ablation studies. However, it has little meaning unless it is of long duration. As Baar and Tannock (1) point out, any tumor with exponential growth and a volume doubling time of 2 months (an average value for human solid tumors) will require at least 1 month to increase its cross-sectional area by 25%. CT scans also may lack the sensitivity to determine when an ablated liver metastasis has started to grow again until its size increases substantially. Last, the time to progression depends very much on how often it is assessed. A study that does

TABLE 2.1. Considerations when evaluating the ablation literature.

1. Who were the patients? Is there evidence of selection bias?
   a. How was the inception cohort assembled? What were the referral patterns? Were consecutive patients considered for study? Is the sample size large enough?
   b. Were there clearly defined entry criteria: disease type, histologic confirmation of lesions, restrictions on tumor size and number? Are the patients representative of the population usually considered for this procedure?
   c. Can you follow all patients approached and excluded to reach the final denominator?
2. What was the intervention?
   a. Was the protocol specifically defined and uniformly followed?
   b. How was the adequacy of ablation evaluated?
   c. What co-interventions were permitted?
3. What were the outcomes, and how were they measured? Was there objective, preferably blinded assessment of prespecified intermediate outcomes?
   a. Was there a definition of how response to treatment would be defined, and how often it would be assessed?
   b. Was there adequate follow-up time to evaluate survival?
   c. Were toxicity and complications reported in detail?

scans every 2 months is likely to have shorter times to progression than one that evaluates patients only every 3 months. Such studies cannot easily be compared. For these reasons, the way outcomes are measured should be as objective as possible, specified a priori, and, when possible, evaluated blindly. For example, radiologists could be asked to evaluate lesions out of chronologic order to get objective measures of size. In this way, any optimism about the effectiveness of treatment that could systematically affect the results of the study can be minimized.

Survival

Evaluation of survival can be divided into two general situations: those in which treatment is potentially curative, and those in which it is palliative only. In a situation in which the disease is considered uniformly and predictably fatal without treatment, such as that of a solitary liver metastasis from colon cancer, demonstration of disease-free survival 5 years after an intervention is a strong indication of efficacy. However, there is a small proportion of patients with indolent disease who may survive at least 5 years without intervention. While such a situation is more likely in prostate cancer than lung cancer, it has been described in both (5,6). Therefore, although the results may be provocative, any possibility of selection bias still must be evaluated. It is important to know not only that a number of such patients exists, but what proportion of the population of interest they represent. In this case, *overall survival*, including death from any cause, must be reported.

Cause-specific survival, which evaluates only whether patients died of recurrent or progressive cancer, can be misleading, as judgment is required in assigning the cause of death, potentially leading to misclassification of the outcome. Furthermore, even though the literature suggests that ablation generally is safer than surgical procedures (2), any patients who die from complications of the procedure should be included in survival analyses. Last, it is crucial that adequate follow-up time be allowed to evaluate survival after potentially curative ablations to ensure that patients have had an adequate time to manifest recurrent disease.

Survival in the palliative setting is even more difficult to assess. Here it is very likely that patients will undergo some form of co-intervention because of the severity of their disease. It is also very difficult to compare patients if they are in different places in their disease course (e.g., newly diagnosed versus heavily pretreated), making eligibility criteria an important consideration. Moreover, if patients with more than one type of cancer were included, they may have very different prognoses. Comorbid diseases and competing risks also become important in this situation. Such potentially confounding factors must be taken into account in the analysis through stratification (comparing like patients only with like) or statistical adjustment. Analyses or survival by response ("patients who responded to treatment lived longer") are usually not considered valid because the patients who respond are usually those with better prognostic features as well.

Quality of Life

There has been little research into the quality-of-life effects of tumor ablation. In potentially curative settings, if ablation can be shown to be as effective as surgery, it would likely avert much of the trauma and morbidity associated with many operative procedures. Most patients with incurable metastatic disease have relatively small tumors that are not causing specific symptoms such as pain. As a result, it is difficult to show that a procedure that usually causes at least some discomfort actually improves overall quality of life. Advanced cancer, however, is associated with several constitutional symptoms such as anorexia, weight loss, fatigue, and anemia. These effects, mediated through cytokines such as tumor necrosis factor (TNF), correlate with overall body tumor burden. If ablation could decrease tumor burden, it is possible that it could ameliorate some of these more subtle cancer-related symptoms and improve psychological well-being, thereby improving quality of life. However, there have been no studies looking at these outcomes. Whether delay or prevention of later progressive symptoms provides overall benefit would need to be evaluated in a randomized trial.

The toxicity of treatment should be described explicitly in reports of tumor ablation results. Any serious event, even if it could have been due to the underlying disease or an unrelated cause, should be reported in detail. Over time, and with randomized studies, it will become apparent whether these are truly attributable to the procedure or not. Subjective statements, such as "the treatment was generally well tolerated", are not useful and may have very different meanings for different readers.

Statistical Considerations

Regarding the analysis of results, sample size is the most important factor for determining the precision of results. For example, a positive outcome for six patients in a study of 10 patients is interesting, but much less certain than a good result for 60 patients out of 100. Statistically, this manifests by being able to draw more narrow confidence limits around an estimate of response rate derived from the larger study. Chance, or random variation, is less likely to cause the point estimate to be different from the true underlying response rate for the entire population of patients in a larger study.

Conclusion

Techniques for tumor ablation are promising and becoming more refined with time. However, the current literature is dominated by small case series that are difficult to interpret and compare with each other. Evaluation of different ablative procedures through comparison of nonrandomized studies requires, in addition to assessment of the quality of the study, synthesis of whether the patients undergoing the procedures were representative, whether the intervention was applied correctly, and whether the important outcomes were measured in a valid way. For the reader, all of this is also dependent on the quality of the reporting of the trial.

The role of ablation in almost all clinical situations needs more study in large prospective trials with rigorous entry criteria, uniform treatment protocols, and precise outcome measurements over adequate follow-up time. Attempts to synthesize existing data are useful, but are prone to publication bias: series with poor results are less likely to be published, and if published, are usually in less prominent journals. If warranted, based on such studies, randomized trials will be needed in most applications before ablation can rightly take its place among the other standard treatments for cancer. As promising as these techniques are, we must ensure that they do not become entrenched in medical practice before they are studied rigorously, as this can make randomization in trials very difficult. The history of medicine tells us that we have been wrong before about interventions that seem as if they should work. Therefore, it is imperative that the benefits be proven before subjecting large numbers of patients to the risks and expense of ablation. At that time, added considerations such as cost-effectiveness and health policy will need to be addressed as well.

References

1. Baar J, Tannock IF. Analyzing the same data in two ways: a demonstration model to illustrate the reporting and misreporting of clinical trials. J Clin Oncol 1989;7:969–978.
2. Tandan VR, Harmantas A, Gallinger S. Long-term survival after hepatic cryosurgery versus surgical resection for metastatic colorectal carcinoma: a critical review of the literature. Canadian Journal of Surgery 1997;40:175–181.
3. Moertel CG, Hanley JA. The effect of measuring error on the results of therapeutic trials in advanced cancer. Cancer 1976;38:388–394.
4. Warr D, McKinney S, Tannock IF. Influence of measurement error on assessment of response to anticancer chemotherapy: Proposal for new criteria of tumor response. J Clin Oncol 1984;2:1040–1046.
5. Marcus PM, Bergstralh EJ, Fagerstrom RM, et al. Lung cancer mortality in the Mayo Lung Project: impact of extended follow-up. J Natl Cancer Inst 2000;92:1308–1316.
6. Holmberg L, Bill-Axelson A, Helgesen F, et al. A randomized trial comparing radical prostatectomy with watchful waiting in early prostate cancer. N Eng J Med 2002;347:781–789.

3
Image-Guided Tumor Ablation: Basic Science

Muneeb Ahmed and S. Nahum Goldberg

Minimally invasive strategies in image-guided tumor ablation are gaining increasing attention as viable therapeutic options for focal primary and secondary hepatic malignancies (1–3). Although liver transplantation continues to be the standard for cure of hepatocellular carcinoma (HCC), there remains a clear need for treatment alternatives in the large population of HCC patients unable to qualify for liver transplantation surgery (4). For hepatic metastases, while conventional surgical resection has demonstrated acceptable rates of success (5) in carefully selected patient populations, several classes of minimally invasive, image-guided therapeutic strategies are being vigorously explored as practical alternatives (2,3). Possible advantages of minimally invasive therapies compared to surgical resection include the anticipated reduction in morbidity and mortality, lower cost, the ability to perform procedures on outpatients, and the potential application in a wider spectrum of patients, including nonsurgical candidates. The role of these strategies in the HCC patient population is further amplified by the presence of severe underlying hepatic dysfunction and coagulopathy in many patients, which complicates or obviates potential surgery; the absence of adequate alternative therapeutic options; and the favorable initial equivalent treatment response of HCC compared to surgical resection (2,6). Furthermore, the availability of various techniques allows treatment tailored to patient-specific disease, which is anticipated to further increase long-term success rates. These techniques will also need to be modified for the increasing use of ablation to treat tumors in such locations as the kidney (7,8), lung (9,10), bone (11), and breast (12).

Current percutaneous tumor ablation techniques can be divided into two broad categories, chemical and thermal, based on differences in mechanisms of inflicting tissue injury. Chemical ablation strategies involve the percutaneous intratumoral administration (or instillation) of ablative substances, such as ethanol and acetic acid. Thermal ablation strategies utilize alterations in tissue temperature to induce cellular disruption and tissue coagulation necrosis. Potential strategies within this latter group include ablation via thermal energy (radiofrequency, microwave, laser, ultrasound) and freezing via cryotherapy. Given that a wide range of technologies is being applied, this chapter provides a conceptual framework for the principles and theories that underlie focal tumor ablation therapies. Furthermore, the basic principles and tissue–therapy interactions of widely accepted modalities are reviewed. Finally, current and future directions of research also will be discussed.

Overview: Theory of Image-Guided Tumor Ablation

Principles of Minimally Invasive Focal Tumor Ablation

The ultimate strategy of image-guided tumor ablation therapies encompasses two specific objectives: First and foremost, all tumor ablation therapies, through applications of energy or chemical substances, attempt to completely eradicate all viable malignant cells within a designated area. Based on earlier studies examining tumor progression for patients undergoing surgical resection, and the demonstration of the presence of viable malignant cells beyond visible tumor boundaries, tumor ablation therapies also attempt to include a 1.0 cm "ablative" margin of seemingly normal tissue that is presumed to also contain viable malignant cells (1). Second, while complete tumor eradication is of primary importance, specificity and accuracy of therapy also are required. One of the significant advantages of these therapies over conventional standard surgical resection is the potential minimal amount of normal tissue loss that occurs. For example, in primary liver tumors, in which functional hepatic reserve is a primary predictive factor in long-term patient survival outcomes, image-guided tumor ablation therapies have documented success in minimizing iatrogenic damage to cirrhotic parenchyma surrounding focal malignancies. Therefore, one of the objectives of tumor ablation therapies is maintaining a balance between adequate tumor destruction and minimal damage to normal tissue and surrounding structures.

Chemical Ablation

Intratumoral administration of chemically ablative substances, such as ethanol and acetic acid, has documented efficacy as a method for percutaneous focal tumor destruction. Ethanol instillation has had widely reported success in the treatment of focal hepatocellular carcinoma. More recently, several investigators also have documented similar or greater efficacy with intratumoral instillation of acetic acid.

Ethanol

Ethanol ablation, classically known as percutaneous ethanol instillation (PEI), is used principally to treat HCC in patients with cirrhosis (13,14). Ethanol ablation has been utilized for the longest period of all image-guided ablative therapies, with the largest number of studies reporting long-term follow-up. Injected alcohol achieves its effect on tumor cells by two primary mechanisms: (a) as it diffuses into neoplastic cells, alcohol results in immediate dehydration of the cytoplasm, protein denaturation, and consequent coagulation necrosis; and (b) alcohol entering the local circulation leads to necrosis of the vascular endothelium and subsequent platelet aggregation, that results in vascular thrombosis and ultimately ischemic tissue necrosis (15,16).

The treatment of primary HCC with ethanol injection has been considerably more successful than the treatment of liver metastases because of tumor characteristics, including softer tumor composition and a delineated capsule surrounded by cirrhotic liver that results in limited diffusion and increased concentration within the target (17). Hepatic tumors can be treated with ethanol ablation using either multiple treatment sessions (1), or a single session in which a large volume of alcohol is injected, usually via many separate needle punctures (18). However, this latter approach has been largely abandoned in favor of thermal therapies, as it is performed only under general anesthesia, and has higher reported complication rates. Furthermore, studies have demonstrated that the efficacy of percutaneous chemical ablation with ethanol is variable and significantly influenced by tumor type. In cases of secondary hepatic malignancies, the heterogeneous and dense fibrous nature of the tumor tissue limits the diffusion of ethanol within the tumor (19). Efficacy rates of ethanol instillation for hepatic metastases are poor, and therefore ethanol is not recommended for the treatment of such malignancies.

Acetic Acid

Intratumoral instillation of acetic acid recently has received increased attention as another chemical substance with documented efficacy in percutaneous chemical tumor ablation. Given several limitations of ethanol instillation, including poor and uneven distribution, and limited success in a wider range of tumor types, several studies have investigated the use of acetic acid as a viable alternative to ethanol for cases undergoing chemical ablation (20,21). The mechanisms of tissue injury, including direct cellular damage through the induction of intracellular dehydration and vascular endothelial injury and resultant thrombosis, are similar for both acetic acid and ethanol (22). However, in preliminary animal studies, Ohnishi et al (22) have demonstrated significantly greater coagulation necrosis diameters for acetic acid solutions with concentrations above 20%, compared to 100% ethanol. This suggests that the diffusion ability of acetic acid solutions may exceed those of ethanol, likely based on the effects of acetic acid on dissolving fibrous interstitial tissue; this factor may potentially result in improved tumor ablation efficacy compared to ethanol (23). However, further research is required to fully characterize and understand the interactions of acetic acid with tumor tissue.

Thermal Ablation Therapies

Thermal ablation strategies attempt to destroy tumor tissue in a minimally invasive manner by increasing or decreasing temperatures sufficiently to induce irreversible cellular injury. These strategies can be broadly divided into two groups, based on whether they utilize tissue freezing or heating: cryoablation or hyperthermic ablation therapies.

Cryoablation

Cryoablation, used successfully in the focal treatment of several types of tumors, achieves focal tissue destruction by alternating between sessions of freezing followed by tissue thawing (24–28). These reductions in tissue temperatures are achieved through specially constructed probes that are placed within the target tissue. Liquid forms of inert gases are then cycled through the hollow probes, resulting in tissue cooling. In the past, liquid nitrogen was placed directly on tissue, but with the exception of dermatologic applications, this agent no longer is used. In the neck, chest, abdomen/pelvis, and extremities, cryoablation is performed using a closed cryoprobe that is placed on or inside a tumor. The two main types of systems use either gas or liquid nitrogen, or argon gas. Temperatures are measured either at the tip of the cryoprobe or in the handle. Although in the past, cryoablation needed to be performed in the setting of an open procedure, technologic developments have led to smaller probes that can be placed percutaneously under magnetic resonance imaging (MRI) or computed tomography (CT) guidance (29).

Several mechanisms have been identified through which cryoablation induces tissue injury (30). First, cryoablation induces direct cellular injury through tissue cooling. At low cooling rates, freezing primarily propagates extracellularly, which draws water from the cell and results in osmotic dehydration (31). The intracellular high solute concentration that develops leads to damage to enzymatic systems and proteins, and injury to the cellular membrane (32,33). At faster cooling rates, water is trapped within the cell, intracellular ice formation occurs, and organelle and membrane injury results (31,34). A second hypothesized mechanism of cryoablative tissue destruction is that of vascular injury, manifested as mechanical injury to the vessel wall, direct cellular injury to various cells lining the vessel, and post-thaw injury from reperfusion (30). Mechanical injury to the vessel wall from intravascular ice formation results in increased vessel leakiness, reduced plasma oncotic pressure, and perivascular edema (35). Endothelial injury further results in exposure of underlying connective tissue and subsequent thrombus formation (36). Damage to endothelial cells occurs in a fashion similar to the direct cellular injury described above. Reperfusion injury results from the release of vasoactive factors after the tissue thaws, which leads to vasodilation and increased blood flow into treated areas. Subsequent high oxygen delivery (37) and neutrophil migration (38) into the damaged area result in increased free radical formation, and ultimately, through peroxidation of membrane lipids, further endothelial damage.

The degree to which each of the above mechanisms of cellular and tissue injury determine overall tissue destruction is governed by characteristics of the administration algorithm, that include freezing and thawing rate, the nadir (i.e., coldest) temperature reached, and the duration that the temperature is maintained (30). At low and high tissue cooling rates, osmotic dehydration and intracellular ice formation, respectively, induce direct cellular injury, while cooling rates in between these extremes do not inflict as much tissue injury (31). Maintaining freezing temperatures for longer durations also may increase the amount of damage by facilitating recrystalization, whereby smaller ice crystals coalesce to create larger and more damaging crystals to reduce overall surface area and minimize free energy (39). Similarly, thawing rate maximizes the time spent at lower temperatures. The effect of nadir freezing temperature also determines the ability of cryoablative therapies to effectively destroy tumor tissue. Studies on the effects of freezing temperatures have demonstrated that minimum lethal temperature is both variable and cell-type specific (30).

While the algorithmic parameters detailed above influence overall tissue destruction, clinical outcomes are highly variable (30). Rates of tissue cooling and thawing vary and are nonlinear throughout treated tissue. Furthermore, tissue inhomogeneities, including differences in vascularity, make it difficult to achieve similar cooling characteristics throughout the tissue. Several biologic and physical characteristics of the cell and surrounding microenvironment also influence the degree of injury that occurs. These include oxygen tension and metabolites in the tissue, cell cycle stage, state of membrane proteins before and after freezing, and the presence of minerals and proteins inside the bloodstream.

High-Temperature Ablation

Tumor cells also can be destroyed effectively by cytotoxic heat from different sources. As long as adequate heat can be generated throughout the tumor volume, it is possible to accomplish the objective of eradicating the tumor. Multiple energy sources have been used to provide the heat necessary to induce coagulation necrosis. Focal high temperature (>50°C) hyperthermic ablation therapies use microwave, radiofrequency (RF), laser, or ultrasound energies to generate isolated increases in tissue temperature. This focal heating primarily is achieved through the placement of applicators in the center of the target, around which heating occurs. This approach is similar for all thermal ablation strategies, regardless of the type of energy source used. Currently, the greatest number of both clinical and experimental studies have been performed using RF-based ablative devices. Therefore, our review of basic principles of focal high-temperature ablative therapies primarily uses RF systems as a representative model to describe the basic principles of focal thermal ablation, followed by brief discussions of the principles of heat generation for other energy sources.

Radiofrequency

Induction of Coagulation Necrosis

Thermal strategies for ablation attempt to destroy tumor tissue in a minimally invasive manner, while limiting injury to nearby structures (1,2,40,41). Treatment also includes a 5- to 10-mm ablative margin of normal tissue, based on the uncertainty concerning the exact tumor margin and the possibility of potential microscopic disease in the rim of tissue immediately surrounding visible tumor (1,40). Cosman et al (42) have shown that the resistive heating produced by RF ablation techniques leads to heat-based cellular death via thermal coagulation necrosis. Therefore, generated temperatures, and their pattern of distribution within treated tissues, determine the amount of tumor destruction.

Prior work has shown that cellular homeostatic mechanisms can accommodate slight increases in temperature (to 40°C). Although increased susceptibility to damage by other mechanisms (radiation, chemotherapy) is seen at hyperthermic temperatures between 42° and 45°C, cell function and tumor growth continue even after prolonged exposure (43,44). Irreversible cellular injury occurs when cells are heated to 46°C for 60 minutes, and occurs more rapidly as temperature rises (45). The basis for immediate cellular damage centers on protein coagulation of cytosolic and mitochondrial enzymes, and nucleic acid–histone protein complexes (46–48). Damage triggers cellular death over the course of several days. *Coagulation necrosis* is the term used to describe this thermal damage, even though ultimate manifestations of cell death may not fulfill strict histopathologic criteria of coagulative necrosis. This has significant implications with regard to clinical practice, as percutaneous biopsy with histopathologic interpretation may not be a reliable measure of adequate ablation. Optimal desired temperatures for ablation range from 50° to 100°C. Extremely high temperatures (>105°C) result in tissue vaporization, which in turn impedes the flow of current and restricts total energy deposition (49).

Principles of the Bioheat Equation

Success of thermal ablative strategies, whether the source is RF, microwave, laser, or high-intensity focused ultrasound, is contingent on adequate heat delivery. The ability to heat large volumes of tissue in different environments is dependent on several factors that include both RF delivery and local physiologic tissue characteristics. Pennes (50) first described the relationship between this set of parameters as the bioheat equation:

$$\rho_t c_t \partial \mathbf{T}(\mathbf{r},\mathbf{t})/\partial \mathbf{t} = \nabla(\mathbf{k}_t \nabla \mathbf{T}) - \mathbf{c}_b\, \rho_b\, \mathbf{m}\, \rho_t (\mathbf{T} - \mathbf{T}_b) + \mathbf{Q}_p(\mathbf{r},\mathbf{t}) + \mathbf{Q}_m(\mathbf{r},\mathbf{t})$$

where:

ρ_t, ρ_b = density of tissue, blood (kg/m^3)
c_t, c_b = specific heat of tissue, blood (W s/kg C)
k_t = thermal conductivity of tissue
m = perfusion (blood flow rate/unit mass tissue) (m^3/kg s)
Q_p = power absorbed/unit volume of tissue
Q_m = metabolic heating/unit volume of tissues

This complex equation was further simplified to a first approximation by Goldberg et al (2) to describe the basic relationship guiding thermal ablation induced coagulation necrosis as, *"coagulation necrosis = energy deposited × local tissue interactions – heat loss"*. Based on this, several strategies have been pursued to increase the amount of coagulation necrosis by improving tissue–energy interactions during thermal ablation. Discussed below, these strategies have centered on altering one of the three parameters of the simplified bioheat equation, either by increasing RF energy deposition, or by modulating tissue interactions or blood flow.

RF Techniques to Improve Potential Outcome

Complete and adequate destruction by RF ablation requires that an entire tumor be subjected to cytotoxic temperatures. The studies described in the previous section demonstrated that early use of RF as a strategy for percutaneous thermal ablation was inadequate for tumors larger than 1.8 cm (49). Of the strategies to improve results of RF ablation, enhancement of the electrode design has played an essential role in achieving acceptable tissue tumor coagulation.

Modification of Probe Design

Multiprobe Arrays

Although lengthening the RF probe tip increased the volume of coagulation necrosis, the cylindrical lesion shape does not correspond well with the spherical geometry of most tumors. In an attempt to address this inadequacy, several groups tried to insert multiple RF electrodes into tissue to increase heating in a more uniform manner (51,52). However, for complete ablation, this requires multiple overlapping treatments in a contiguous fashion to treat tumors adequately. Hence, the time and effort required for this strategy make it impractical for clinical use.

Subsequent work centered on using several conventional monopolar RF electrodes utilized simultaneously in an array, to determine the effect of probe spacing, configuration, and RF application method (53). Spacing no greater than 1.5 cm between individual probes produced uniform and reproducible tissue coagulation, with simultaneous application of RF energy that produced more necrosis than sequential application. Coagulation shape was further dependent on spacing and the number of probes, and most often corresponded to the array shape. This improvement in RF application technique results in a significant increase in the volume of inducible tissue necrosis, augmenting coagulation volume by up to 800% over RF application with a single conventional probe with similar tip exposure.

Working to overcome the technical challenges of multiprobe application, multi-tined expandable RF electrodes have been developed. These systems, produced by two commercial vendors, involve the deployment of a varying number of multiple thin, curved tines in the shape of an umbrella or more complex geometries from a central cannula (54,55). This surmounts earlier difficulties by allowing placement of multiple probes to create large, reproducible volumes of necrosis. LeVeen (56), using a 12-hook array, was able to produce lesions measuring up to 3.5 cm in diameter in in vivo porcine liver by administering increasing amounts of RF energy from a 50 W RF generator for 10 minutes. More recently, high-power systems (up to 250 W) have been developed with complex, multi-tine electrode geometries. With these, preliminary reports claim coagulation up to 3.5 cm in diameter (57,58). Furthermore, with the injection of adjuvant NaCl solution into tissue surrounding the RF electrode, increases in achievable coagulation up to 5 to 7 cm in diameter now have been reported.

Bipolar Arrays

Several groups have worked with bipolar arrays, compared to the conventional monopolar system to increase the volume of coagulation created by RF application. In these systems, applied RF current runs from an active electrode to a second grounding electrode in place of a grounding pad. Heat is generated around both electrodes, creating elliptical lesions. McGahan et al (59) used this method in exvivo liver to induce necrosis of up to 4.0 cm in the long axis diameter, but could only achieve 1.4 cm of necrosis in the short diameter. Although this system results in an overall increase in coagulation volume, the shape of necrosis is unsuitable for actual tumors, making the gains in coagulation less clinically significant.

Desinger et al (60) described another bipolar array that contains both the active and return electrodes on the same 2 mm-diameter probe. This arrangement of probes eliminates the need for surface grounding pads and the risk of grounding pad burns (see below). Although there has been limited clinical experience with this device, studies report coagulation of up to 3 cm in ex vivo liver. Last, Lee's group (61,62) reports using two multi-tined electrodes as active and return, to increase coagulation during bipolar RF ablation, and a switching technique between electrodes to increase ablation efficiency.

Internally Cooled Electrodes

One of the limitations to greater RF energy deposition has been overheating that surrounds the active electrode and leads to tissue charring, rising impedance, and RF circuit interruption. To address this, internally cooled electrodes have been developed that are capable of greater coagulation compared to conventional monopolar RF electrodes. These electrodes contain two hollow lumina that permit continuous internal cooling of the tip with a chilled perfusate, and the removal of warmed effluent to a collection unit outside of the body. This reduces heating directly around the electrode, tissue charring, and rising impedance, allowing greater RF energy deposition. Goldberg et al (63) studied this modification using an 18-gauge electrode. With internal electrode tip cooling (of 15 ± 2°C using 0°C saline perfusate), RF energy deposited into tissue and resultant coagulation necrosis were significantly greater ($p < .001$) than that achieved without electrode cooling. With this degree of cooling, greater RF current could be applied without observing tissue charring. Maximum diameters of coagulation measured 2.5, 3.0, 4.5, and 4.4 cm for the 1-, 2-, 3-, and 4 cm electrode tips, respectively. With tip temperatures of 25° to 35°C (less cooling), tissue charring occurred with reduced RF application, and resulting necrosis decreased from 4.5 to 3.0 cm in diameter. Similar results have been reported by Lorentzen (64), who applied RF to ex vivo calf liver using a 14-gauge internally cooled electrode and 20°C perfusate.

Subsequent in vivo studies were performed in normal porcine liver and muscle tissue. Within muscle tissue, lesion diameter increased from 1.8 to 5.4 cm for 12 minutes of RF. Nevertheless, in normal liver only 2.3 cm of coagulation was observed, regardless of current applied or treatment duration (to 30 minutes). Thus, in vivo necrosis was significantly less than that observed for ex vivo liver using identical RF parameters ($p < .01$). In clinical studies, Solbiati et al (65) demonstrated 2.8 ± 0.4 cm of coagulation for liver metastases.

Cluster RF

Based on success in inducing greater volumes of necrosis by using both multiprobe arrays and cooling, initial experiments were performed to study the use of internally cooled electrodes in an array (66). Three 2 cm tip exposure internally cooled electrodes were placed at varying distances in ex vivo liver for simultaneous RF application (1100 mA for 10 minutes). At spacing distances of 0.5 to 1.0 cm apart, a uniform circular cross-sectional area of coagulation necrosis measuring 4.1 cm in diameter was achieved. In contrast, electrode spacing of 1.5 to 2.5 cm resulted in cloverleafed lesions with areas of viable tissue within the treatment zone.

Using an optimized 0.5 cm spacing distance between probes, Goldberg et al (66) proceeded to study variations in electrode tip length and duration of application on coagulation volume. Tip lengths of 1.5 to 3.0 cm were used in ex vivo liver and in vivo porcine liver and muscle systems for varied RF application (1400–2150 mA) and duration (5–60 minutes). In ex vivo liver, simultaneous RF application to internally cooled electrode clusters for 15, 30, and 45 minutes produced 4.7, 6.2, and 7.0 cm of coagulation, respectively. In contrast, RF application for 45 minutes to a single internally cooled electrode resulted in only 2.7 cm of coagulation ($p < .01$).

Radiofrequency applied for 12 minutes to electrode clusters produced 3.1 cm of coagulation in in vivo liver, and 7.3 cm in in vivo muscle. This was significantly greater than the 1.8- and 4.3 cm sized lesions in in vivo liver and muscle, respectively, that was seen with the use of single internally cooled electrodes with similar technique ($p < .01$). When RF current (2000 mA) was applied for 30 minutes in in vivo muscle, 9.5 cm of coagulation was observed, including extension into the retroperitoneum and overlying tissues.

In the initial clinical use of this clustered electrode device, 10 patients with large solitary intrahepatic colorectal metastases (4.2–7.0 cm) were treated with a single RF application (12–15 minutes, 1600–1950 mA) (66). Contrast-enhanced CT postablation showed induced coagulation necrosis that measured 5.3 ± 0.6 cm, with a minimum short axis diameter of 4.2 cm. The overall shape of coagulation was not spherical in several cases, and generally conformed to the tumor shape. In two cases, large blood vessels limited the size of induced coagulation.

The use of the internally cooled cluster electrode array offers the potential of large-volume coagulation for clinical tumor ablation compared to conventional monopolar RF electrodes or single internally cooled electrodes. Spacing distances of less than 1 cm between individual electrodes produces more spherical zones of necrosis with no intervening viable tissue, compared to greater spacing distances. While these results appear counterintuitive, postulating that these electrodes function as a single large electrode can explain this phenomenon of greater coagulation necrosis with relatively closely spaced electrodes.

Pulsed RF Application

Pulsing of energy is another strategy that has been used with RF and other energy sources such as laser to increase the mean intensity of energy deposition. When pulsing is used, periods of high-energy deposition are rapidly alternated with periods of low-energy deposition. If a proper balance between high- and low-energy deposition is achieved, preferential tissue cooling occurs adjacent to the electrode during periods of minimal energy deposition without significantly decreasing heating deeper in the tissue. Thus, even greater energy can be applied during periods of high-energy deposition, thereby enabling deeper heat penetration and greater tissue coagulation (66). Synergy between a combination of both internal cooling and pulsing has resulted in greater coagulation necrosis and tumor destruction than either method alone (66).

Clearly, optimization is required for each system. Currently, at least one manufacturer has incorporated a pulsing algorithm into its generator design (67). An optimal algorithm with a variable peak current for a specified minimum duration was designed. Maximum coagulation, which measured 4.5 cm in diameter, was achieved using initial currents greater than 1500 mA, a minimum RF duration of 10 seconds of maximum deliverable current, with a 15-second reduction in current to 100 mA following impedance rises. This latter algorithm produced 3.7 ± 0.6 cm of necrosis in in vivo liver, compared to 2.9 cm without pulsing ($p < .05$). Remote thermometry further demonstrated more rapid temperature increases and higher tissue temperatures when pulsed-RF techniques were used. Ramping of RF deposition based on impedance also is used with some multi-tined expandable electrodes. Thus, an optimized algorithm for pulsed-RF deposition can increase coagulation over other pulsed and conventional RF ablation strategies.

Perfused Electrodes

Perfusion electrodes also have been developed that have small apertures at the active tip to allow fluids (i.e., normal or hypertonic saline) to be infused or injected into the tissue before, during, or after the ablation procedure. Curley and Hamilton (68) infused up to 10 mL/min of normal saline in ex vivo liver for 4 minutes during RF application and achieved coagulation that measured 2.6 cm in diameter. Similarly, Livraghi et al (69) have reported coagulation of up to 4.1 cm in diameter using continuous infusion of normal saline at 1 mL/min in experimental animal models and human liver tumors. Miao et al (70,71) used a novel "cooled-wet" technique to significantly increase RF-induced coagulation in both ex vivo and in vivo tissue using a continuous saline infusion combined with an expandable electrode system. Kettenbach et al (72) have reported clinical use of these devices in 26 patients. In these studies, the mechanisms responsible for the increase in coagulation were not well characterized. This strategy seemed to confirm an initial hypothesis that high local ion concentration from NaCl injection could increase the extent of coagulation necrosis by effectively increasing the area of the active surface electrode. Other possible explanations for the increase in coagulation include reduced effects of tissue vaporization (i.e., allowing for the probe to contact tissue despite the formation of electrically insulating gases), or improved thermal conduction caused by diffusion of boiling solution into the tissues.

Overcoming Physiologic Limitations

While modifications in electrode design and application protocols have yielded increases in coagulation volume compared to conventional monopolar RF systems, further gains through RF equipment modifications have not produced equivalent increases in clinical settings. This is largely due to multiple and often tissue-specific limitations that prevent heating of the entire tumor volume (41,49). Most important is the heterogeneity of heat deposition throughout a given lesion to be treated. Recent attention has centered on altering underlying tumor physiology as a means to advance RF thermal ablation. Based on the simplified bioheat equation described earlier, these efforts can be divided into two broad categories. One examines altering local tissue interactions to permit greater RF energy input by changing tissue conductivity or increasing local heat conduction, while the other explores reducing heat loss by modulating blood flow within treatment zones. As will be shown, certain modifications can have several simultaneous effects. For example, saline and iron compounds have been useful for improving energy deposition (73), while continuous injection of saline during ablation has facilitated the spread of heat from the RF electrode into deeper tissues (70). Modulation of blood flow during RF application can improve ablation by limiting perfusion-mediated tissue cooling (74).

Local Tissue Interactions

The effect of local tissue characteristics is defined by thermal and electrical conductivity of surrounding tissue. Altering both of these, either separately or simultaneously, can alter the pattern of thermal distribution with treated tissue.

Improved Tissue Heat Conduction

As discussed for perfusion electrodes, improved heat conduction within the tissues by injection of saline and other compounds has been proposed (68,70,71). The heated liquid spreads thermal energy farther and faster than heat conduction in normal "solid" tissue. An additional potential benefit of simultaneous saline injection is increased tissue ionicity that enables greater current flow. Similarly, amplification of current shifts with iron compounds, injected or deposited in the tissues prior to ablation, has been used for RF and microwave. Increased ferric ions, in the form of high doses of supraparamagnetic iron oxide MRI contrast agent, can raise the temperature of polyacrylamide phantoms during RF ablation (75).

Altered Tissue Thermal and Electrical Conductivity

For a given RF current, the power deposition at each point in space is strongly dependent on the local electrical conductivity. Several investigators have demonstrated the ability to increase coagulation volume by altering electrical conductivity in tissues through saline injection prior to or during RF ablation. In both experimental animal models and human liver tumors, Livraghi et al (60) achieved 4.1 cm of coagulation when continuous infusion of normal saline at 1 ml/min was administered during RF application. Additionally, Curley et al (68) and Miao et al (70,71) reported significant increases in coagulation with normal saline infusion during RF ablation in ex vivo and invivo tissue.

Saline can have multiple effects, and in relevant studies the mechanisms responsible for the increase in coagulation were not well characterized.

More recent study has centered on exploring the effects of volume and concentration of NaCl on the RF coagulation volume. In normal porcine liver and agar tissue phantom models, Goldberg et al (73) have demonstrated that both NaCl concentration and volume influenced RF coagulation. These experiments demonstrated that increased NaCl concentration increases electrical conductivity (which is inversely proportional to the measured impedance) and enables greater energy deposition in tissues without inducing deleterious high temperatures at the electrode surface. However, this effect is nonlinear with markedly increased tissue conductivity that decreased tissue heating. Under many circumstances (i.e., in the range of normal tissue conductivities) the increased conductivity can be beneficial for RF ablation in that it enables increased energy deposition that increases tissue heating. However, given less intrinsic electrical resistance, increased tissue conductivity also increases the energy required to heat a given volume of tissue. When this amount of energy cannot be delivered (i.e., it is beyond the maximum generator output), the slope is negative and less tissue heating (and coagulation) will result. Thus, to achieve clinical benefit (i.e., an increase in RF-induced coagulation), optimal parameters for NaCl injection need to be determined both for each type of RF apparatus used and for the different tumor types and tissues to be treated.

In an attempt to optimize the effects of altered conductivity using injectable therapies, Goldberg et al (73) initially investigated the effect of injecting different volumes of high-concentration NaCl on the extent of RF-induced coagulation. Using an iterative, nonlinear simplex optimization strategy, parameters for NaCl injection were studied in in vivo porcine liver over varying concentrations (0.9–38%) and injection volume (0–25 mL) using internally cooled electrodes following pulsed-RF algorithms for 12 minutes. Significant increases in generator output, tissue heating, and coagulation volume were seen when NaCl was injected ($p < .001$), with maximum heating and coagulation occurring with 6mL of 36% NaCl solution. Regression analysis demonstrated that both volume and concentration of NaCl injected significantly influenced tissue heating and coagulation.

In a subsequent study, Lobo et al (76) explored the relationship between NaCl volume and concentration in a reproducible, static agar tissue phantom model. Using a protein gel with varying NaCl concentration (0–35%) in different-sized wells (0–38cc) surrounding the electrode to simulate tissue injection, various parameters of RF application (power, current, impedance, temperature) were recorded. Using mathematical modeling, they derived two equations, one describing the multivariate relationship to a peak point that represented maximum generator output. The other describes the relationship when temperature decreases as generator output is exceeded. Both equations predict the effect of volume and concentration of NaCl with an $R^2 = .96$. Based on this, the investigators reexamined the earlier reported trials in normal porcine liver to correlate results with these equations. Though the constants changed, the equations were able to account for 86% of the variance seen in those data. This mathematic characterization is a significant step toward reliably predicting the effects of NaCl when combined with RF ablation.

Reducing Blood Flow

Biophysical aspects of tumor–heat interaction must be taken into account when performing thermal ablation therapies. Based on the simplified form of the bioheat equation, the third component defining thermal induced coagulation necrosis is heat loss. Radiofrequency ablation outcomes in in vivo models have been less successful and more variable compared to reported reproducible ex vivo results for identical RF protocols. Radiofrequency-induced necrosis in vivo is often shaped by the presence of hepatic vasculature in the vicinity of the ablation. This reduced RF coagulation necrosis in in vivo settings is most likely a result of both visible and perfusion-mediated tissue cooling (capillary vascular flow) that functions as a heat sink. By drawing heat from the treatment zone, this effect reduces the volume of tissue that receives the required minimal thermal dose for coagulation. Several studies that explored altering tissue perfusion to increase the ablative zone through either mechanical occlusion or pharmacologic agents strongly support the contention that perfusion-mediated tissue cooling is responsible for this reduction in observed coagulation.

Mechanical Occlusion

Using internally cooled electrodes, Goldberg et al applied RF to normal in vivo porcine liver without and with balloon occlusion of the portal vein, celiac artery, or hepatic artery, and to ex vivo calf liver (77). Increased coagulation was observed with RF ablation combined with portal venous occlusion, compared to RF without occlusion ($P < .01$). The differences seen in coagulation correlated to an approximate reduction in hepatic blood flow.

Several clinical studies provide additional data supporting the role of mechanical blood flow reduction to improve RF ablation efficacy. Goldberg et al performed mechanical blood flow occlusion in three patients with hepatic colorectal metastases undergoing intraoperative RF ablation (77). Two similar sized hepatic colorectal metastases (2.2–4.2cm) were treated with identical RF parameters in each patient. In each case, one lesion was treated with normal blood flow, while the second was treated during portal flow occlusion (Pringle maneuver) by clamping the hepatic artery and portal vein to eliminate all intrahepatic blood flow. In each case, coagulation was increased with inflow occlusion (4.0cm vs 2.5cm, $P < .05$). Hepatic inflow occlusion was performed in additional patients undergoing intrahepatic RF ablation for hepatic colorectal metastases. In these cases, remote thermometry demonstrated increases in temperature at 10mm (62°C–72°C) and 20mm (39°C–50°C) distances from the RF probe within 5 minutes of portal vein occlusion during constant RF application. This increase at the 20 mm distance holds particular significance as the threshold for induction of coagulation necrosis (50°C) was achieved with blood flow reduction.

In a second study, Patterson et al have confirmed the strong predictive nature of hepatic blood flow on the extent of RF induced coagulation in normal in vivo porcine liver using a hooked electrode system (78). The coagulated focus created by RF during a Pringle maneuver was significantly larger in all three dimensions than coagulation with unaltered blood flow. Minimum and maximum diameters were significantly increased from 1.2 cm to 3.0 cm and 3.1 cm to 4.5 cm, respectively, when the Pringle maneuver was performed ($P = .002$). Coagulation volume was increased from 6.5 cm^3 to 35.0 cm^3 with hepatic inflow occlusion. Additionally, the number of blood vessels within a 1 cm radius of the electrode strongly predicted minimum lesion size and lesion volume. In a subsequent study in an in vivo porcine model, Lu et al examined the effect of hepatic vessel diameter on RF ablation outcome (79). Using CT and histopathologic analyses, the authors documented more complete thermal heating and a reduced heat-sink effect when hepatic vessels within the heating zone were <3 mm in diameter. In contrast, vessels >3 mm in diameter had higher patency rates, less endothelial injury, and greater viability of surrounding hepatocytes after RF ablation.

Pharmacologic Modulation of Blood Flow

Goldberg et al modulated hepatic blood flow using intraarterial vasopressin and high dose halothane in conjunction with RF ablation in in vivo porcine liver (74). Laser Doppler techniques identified a 33% increase and 66% decrease in hepatic blood flow after administration of vasopresson and halothane, respectively. Correlation of blood flow to coagulation diameter produced was excellent as $R^2 = .78$.

Clearly, several strategies to reduce blood flow during ablation therapy have been proposed. Total portal inflow occlusion (Pringle maneuver) has been used at open laparotomy. Angiographic balloon occlusion can be used, but may not prove adequate for intrahepatic ablation given the dual hepatic blood supply with redirection of compensated flow. Embolotherapy prior to ablation with particulates that occlude sinusoids such as Gelfoam and Lipiodol may overcome this limitation, as has been reported by Rossi et al (80). Pharmacologic modulation of blood flow and antiangiogenesis therapy are theoretically possible, but should currently be considered experimental. Another proposal is to combine RF with arsenic trioxide to increase ablation efficacy via decreased blood flow.

Microwave

Microwaves are a second thermal energy source that has been used for percutaneous image-guided tumor ablation, and thus far largely used in the Far East. In contrast to RF, in which the inserted electrode functions as the active source, in microwave ablation the inserted probes (usually 14 gauge) function as antennae for externally applied energy at 1000 to 2450 mHz (81). The microwave energy applied to the tissues results in rotation of polar molecules that is opposed by frictional forces. As a result, there is conversion of rotational energy into heat (82). One potential advantage of microwave over RF and laser is that investigational ex vivo studies have shown greater tissue penetration and larger zones of coagulation-necrosis with microwave technology. This finding is most pronounced with cooling of the microwave antenna in a fashion similar to cooled-tip RF (83). In clinical practice, however, arrays of microwave antennas or multiple insertions of a single microwave probe have been necessary to treat lesions greater than 2 cm in diameter (84–87). However, research likely will adapt advances in RF technology to microwave systems, such as cooling, pulsing, and higher power (83,88,89).

Laser

Laser ablation or laser photocoagulation is another method to induce thermally mediated coagulation necrosis that has been employed for percutaneous tumor ablation. For this procedure, flexible thin optic fibers are inserted into the target through percutaneously placed needles using imaging guidance. The laser provides sufficient energy to allow for significant heat deposition surrounding the fiber tip, inducing protein denaturation and cellular death (90). As with RF systems, thermal profiles have been demonstrated to correlate well with the extent of coagulation necrosis that is observed histopathologically (91,92), as well as with ultrasound (92,93) and T1-weighted MRI (94,95).

Most devices use a standard laser source (neodymium: yttrium-aluminum-garnet [Nd: YAG], erbium, holmium, etc.) that produces precise wavelengths. Additional device modifications on a conventional laser applicator device have been developed to increase the size of the heated volume. These developments include: (a) different types of laser fibers (flexible/glass dome); (b) modifications to the tip (i.e., flexible diffusor tip or scattering dome); (c) length of applicator and diameter of the optic fiber; and (d) the number of laser applicators used (i.e., single versus multiple applicators) (96). Similar to RF technologies, additional device modifications such as pulsing algorithms and internal cooling of the applicator have been reported (97).

Ultrasound

High-intensity focused ultrasound (HIFU) is a transcutaneous technique that has been studied as a potential method for minimally invasive treatment of localized benign and malignant tumors (98,99). This technique uses a parabolic transducer to focus the ultrasound energy at a distance that creates a focused beam of energy with very high peak intensity. This focusing of energy has been likened to using a magnifying glass to focus sunlight (100). The focused energy is transmitted transcutaneously into the target tissue without requiring percutaneous insertion of an electrode or transducer. The ultrasound energy is absorbed by tissue and is converted to heat. Ablation occurs by coagulation necrosis.

Using a 4-MHz transducer and a power intensity of 550 W/cm^2 for 5 seconds, temperature in excess of 80°C can be produced in rat liver (101). Areas of coagulation necrosis have been shown at histopathology to have a spatially sharp demarcation between regions of normal and necrotic tissue. By using a suitable acoustic frequency, regions of tissue destruction can be induced at depths of up to at least 10 cm with exposure times on the order of 1 second (102). One main potential benefit of HIFU is that the focused ablative energy can destroy a selected target without causing damage to the intervening tissues. Although hampered by small focal zones in the past, this technique is gaining further enthusiasm as larger zones of coagulation are produced by using array transducers and other advancing technologies. Furthermore, since insertion of a percutaneous probe is not required, HIFU can be considered the least invasive of the minimally invasive therapies.

Combination Therapies

The ultimate goal of tumor therapy is complete eradication of all malignant cells within a focal tumor. Given the high likelihood of incomplete treatment by heat-based modalities alone, the case for combining thermal ablation with other therapies such as chemotherapy or chemoembolization cannot be overstated. The belief that tumors can reliably destroyed using only one technique is likely overly optimistic, given the variety of tumor types and organ sites. Combination therapy is a key focus of current ablation research. A multidisciplinary approach that includes surgery, radiation, and chemotherapy is used for the treatment of most solid cancers.

Thermal Ablation with Adjuvant Chemotherapy

Strategies that decrease tumor tolerance to heat are not well studied. Theoretically, previous insult to the tumor cells by cellular hypoxia (caused by vascular occlusion or antiangiogenesis factor therapy), or prior tumor cell damage from chemotherapy or radiation could be used to increase tumor sensitivity to heat (9,10). Alternatively, tumor cells that undergo heat-induced reversible cell injury may demonstrate increased susceptibility to secondary chemotherapy. Synergy between chemotherapy and hyperthermic temperatures (42–45°C) has been established (44,103).

In one study, Goldberg et al (104) treated 1.2- to 1.5 cm R3230 rat mammary adenocarcinoma with RF and/or intratumoral injection of doxorubicin chemotherapy. Tumors were treated with combinations of RF alone (monopolar, 70°C for 5 minutes), direct intratumoral doxorubicin injection (250 µL; 0.5 mg in total) alone, intratumoral doxorubicin followed by RF, and no treatment. RF alone, RF with distilled water, and intratumoral doxorubicin alone produced 6.7 mm, 6.9 mm, and 2 mm of coagulation, respectively. Significantly increased coagulation occurred with combined RF and intratumoral doxorubicin (11.4 mm; $p < .001$). Additional experiments conducted to examine the effect and timing of doxorubicin adminstration demonstrated greatest effect when the drug was given 30 minutes after RF application. In particular, the increased necrosis seen when the doxorubicin was injected after RF points to a potential two-hit effect, with initial reversible cell injury inflicted by sublethal doses of heat in the more peripheral ablation zone, followed by irreversible injury by doxorubicin on already susceptible cells.

Subsequently, investigators explored intravenous doxorubicin use as a means to achieve greater delivery to the zone surrounding RF-induced coagulation. Recent study has focused on the use of a commercially available, sterically stabilized liposomal preparation of doxorubicin (Doxil, Alza Pharmaceuticals). Liposomes function as delivery vehicles for a variety of chemotherapeutic agents through increased circulating time and greater tumor specificity, with the added advantage of reduced drug toxicity. Goldberg et al (105) combined RF ablation with intravenous Doxil (0.5 mL, 1.0 mg in total) in a rat mammary adenocarcinoma model. A significant increase in coagulation (13.1 mm) was seen with this particular approach compared to either RF alone (6.7 mm) or RF plus direct intratumoral free doxorubicin injection (11.4 mm) ($p < .01$). In more recent follow-up studies in the same animal tumor model, Monsky et al (106) documented a fivefold increase in intratumoral doxorubicin concentration for tumors receiving RF ablation, while D'Ippolito et al (107) demonstrated reduced tumor growth in animals receiving combination RF/Doxil treatment over either RF ablation or Doxil alone.

Recently, Goldberg et al (108) conducted a pilot clinical study combining RF ablation with adjuvant Doxil therapy in 10 patients with liver malignancies. Patients with at least one liver lesion (mean size 4.0 ± 1.8 cm) were randomized into two groups for treatment with RF alone ($n = 5$) versus RF with pretreatment single-dose intravenous Doxil (24 hours pre-RF, 20 mg/kg). Several tumor types were treated, including primary hepatocellular carcinoma ($n = 4$), colorectal metastases ($n = 3$), neuroendocrine tumors ($n = 2$), and breast cancer metastases ($n = 1$). Patients receiving Doxil therapy with RF ablation demonstrated a 25% increase in coagulation volume 2 to 4 weeks postablation. Two Doxil/RF ablation–treated tumors with incomplete initial treatment denoted by contrast enhancement at the periphery of the ablation zone on baseline post-RF scans were converted to complete ablation within 4 weeks of treatment. Similar incompletely ablated tumors treated with RF alone did not show a similar conversion. Additionally, in the tumors treated incompletely with combination Doxil and RF ablation, large blood vessels traversing the ablation zone were present on baseline scans, but were absent on follow-up imaging. These preliminary results highlight the potential of combining RF ablation with adjuvant liposomal chemotherapeutic agents for greater and more complete treatment.

Several separate mechanisms likely underlie this considerable synergy between RF and Doxil. Postulated reasons for this adjuvant effect can be divided into two distinct categories. The first involves increased delivery of Doxil into tumor tissue peripheral to the central RF coagulation zone. Monsky et al (106) explored intratumoral distribution using radiolabeled liposomal doxorubicin preparations identical to Doxil. They were able to visualize the distribution of liposomes within the tumor post-RF ablation, which concentrated in a thick rim of tumor surrounding the central RF zone. Quantitation of doxorubicin content of RF-treated tumors compared to untreated tumors revealed a fivefold increase in Doxil uptake ($p < .01$). Potential explanations for this increased delivery include nonspecific RF-induced inflammation in surrounding tissue leading to hyperthermic vasodilation and increased vascular permeability and increased cellular uptake and retention of doxorubicin due to disruption of cellular defense mechanisms. Kruskal et al (109) used dynamic intravital video microscopy to study microvascular and cellular alterations in normal livers of live nude mice treated with RF ablation. At temperatures well below those required for irreversible thermal damage, several distinct changes conducive to increased liposome delivery were identified beyond the central coagulation necrosis, including alterations in permeability, reversible microvascular stasis, and increased endothelial leakiness.

A second likely means of synergy between RF ablation and Doxil concerns the tumoricidal effect of both the liposome and doxorubicin components of Doxil. Interestingly, tumors treated with RF in combination with empty liposome preparations (identical formulation to Doxil without doxorubicin) also demonstrated significantly greater necrosis than RF alone (10.9mm, $p < .01$) (105). Prior studies investigating synergy between lipid preparations and low-level hyperthermia have identified free radical generation as a cause of cellular injury (110). Further research may focus on optimizing liposome structure to foster this effect for greater RF coagulation gain.

Conclusion

Several different percutaneous and minimally invasive therapies, both chemical and thermal, have been well described to treat focal malignancies. Investigators have begun to characterize many of the basic principles underlying the tumor ablative features of these treatments. We have provided an overview of the basic principles of each of the widely used strategies and described the recent technologic modifications that have been developed to further improve clinical success of these therapies. Future directions of research are now looking to combination therapies, such as combining liposomal chemotherapy with thermal ablation, as the next step to further improve the clinical effectiveness of such therapies.

References

1. Dodd GD III, Soulen MC, Kane RA, et al. Minimally invasive treatment of malignant hepatic tumors: at the threshold of a major breakthrough. Radiographics 2000;20:9–27.
2. Goldberg SN, Gazelle GS, Mueller PR. Thermal ablation therapy for focal malignancy: a unified approach to underlying principles, techniques, and diagnostic imaging guidance. Am J Radiol 2000;174:323–331.
3. Goldberg SN, Dupuy DE. Image-guided radiofrequency tumor ablation: challenges and opportunities—Part I. J Vasc Intervent Radiol 2001;12:1021–1032.
4. Colella G, Bottelli R, De Carlis L, et al. Hepatocellular carcinoma: comparison between liver transplantation, resective surgery, ethanol injection, and chemoembolization. Transpl Int 1998;11(suppl 1):S193–196.
5. Liver Cancer Study Group of Japan. Survey and follow-up study of primary liver cancer in Japan: report 14. Kyoto: Shinko-Insatsu, 2000.
6. Ahmed M, Goldberg SN. Thermal ablation therapy for hepatocellular carcinoma. J Vasc Intervent Radiol 2002;13(9 suppl):S231–244.
7. Pautler SE, Pavlovich CP, Mikityansky I, et al. Retroperitoneoscopic-guided radiofrequency ablation of renal tumors. Can J Urol 2001;8: 1330–1333.
8. Pavlovich CP, Walther MM, Choyke PL, et al. Percutaneous radio frequency ablation of small renal tumors: initial results. J Urol 2002;167: 10–15.
9. Dupuy DE, Zagoria RJ, Akerley W, Mayo-Smith WW, Kavanaugh PV, Safran H. Percutaneous RF ablation of malignancies in the lung. AJR 2000;174:57–60.

10. Zagoria RJ, Chen MY, Kavanagh PV, Torti FM. Radio frequency ablation of lung metastases from renal cell carcinoma. J Urol 2001;166: 1827–1828.
11. Woertler K, Vestring T, Boettner F, Winkelmann W, Heindel W, Lindner N. Osteoid osteoma: CT-guided percutaneous radiofrequency ablation and follow-up in 47 patients. J Vasc Intervent Radiol 2001;12:717–722.
12. Jeffery SS, Birdwell RL, Ikeda DM. Radiofrequency ablation of breast cancer: first report of an emerging technology. Arch Surg 1999;134: 1064–1068.
13. Livraghi T, Giorgio A, Marin A. Hepatocellular carcinoma and cirrhosis in 746 patients: long-term results of percutaneous ethanol injection. Radiology 1995;197:101–108.
14. Shiina S, Tagawa K, Niwa Y. Percutaneous ethanol injection therapy for hepatocellular carcinoma: results in 146 patients. AJR 1993; 160:1023–1025.
15. Kawano M. An experimental study of percutaneous absolute ethanol injection therapy for small hepatocellular carcinoma: effects of absolute ethanol on healthy canine liver. Gastroenterol Jpn 1989;24:663–669.
16. Shiina S, Tagawa K, Unuma T. Percutaneous ethanol injection therapy for hepatocellular carcinoma: a histopathologic study. Cancer 1991;68:1524–1530.
17. Giovannini M, Seltx UF. Ultrasound guided percutaneous alcohol injection of small liver metastases. Cancer 1994;73:294–297.
18. Livraghi T, Vettori C, Torzilli G, Lazzaroni S, Pellicano S, Ravasi S. Percutaneous ethanol injection of hepatic tumors: single-session therapy under general anesthesia. AJR 1993; 160:1065–1069.
19. Livraghi T. Percutaneous ethanol injection in the treatment of hepatocellular carcinoma in cirrhosis. Hepatogastroenterology 2001;48: 20–24.
20. Liang HL, Yang CF, Pan HB, et al. Small hepatocellular carcinoma: safety and efficacy of single high-dose percutaneous acetic acid injection for treatment. Radiology 2000;214: 769–774.
21. Ohnishi K, Yoshioka H, Ito S, Fujiwara K. Treatment of nodular hepatocellular carcinoma larger than 3 cm with ultrasound-guided percutaneous acetic acid injection. Hepatology 1996;24:1379–1385.
22. Ohnishi K, Ohyama N, Ito S, Fujiwara K. Small hepatocellular carcinoma: treatment with US-guided intratumoral injection of acetic acid. Radiology 1994;193:747–752.
23. Ohnishi K, Yoshioka H, Ito S, Fujiwara K. Prospective randomized controlled trial comparing percutaneous acetic acid injection and percutaneous ethanol injection for small hepatocellular carcinoma. Hepatology 1998;27: 67–72.
24. Cooper IS. Cryogenic surgery: a new method of destruction or extirpation of benign or malignant tissue. N Engl J Med 1963;268:743–749.
25. Onik G, Kane RA, Steele G. Monitoring hepatic cryosurgery with sonography. AJR 1986;147:665–669.
26. Lee FT, Mahvi DM, Chosy SG, et al. Hepatic cryosurgery with intraoperative US guidance. Radiology 1997;202:624–632.
27. Cozzi PJ, Stewart GJ, Morris DL. Thrombocytopenia after hepatic cryosurgery for colorectal metastases: correlates with hepatic injury. World J Surg 1994;18:774–777.
28. Rubinsky B, Lee CY, Bastacky J, Onik G. The process of freezing and the mechanism of damage during hepatic cryosurgery. Cryobiology 1990;27:85–97.
29. Silverman SG, Tuncali K, Adams DF, et al. MR image-guided percutaneous cryotherapy of liver tumors: initial experience. Radiology 2000; 217:657–664.
30. Hoffmann NE, Bischof JC. The cryobiology of cryosurgical injury. Urology 2002;60:40–49.
31. Mazur P. Freezing of living cells: mechanisms and implications. Am J Physiol 1984;247:125–142.
32. Lovelock JE. The hemolysis of human red blood cells by freezing and thawing. Biochem Biophys Acta 1953;10:414–426.
33. Steponkus PL. Role of plasma membrane in freezing injury and cold acclimation. Annu Rev Plant Physiol 1984;35:543–584.
34. Toner M. Nucleation of ice crystals inside biological cells. In: Steponkus PL, ed. Advances in Low-Temperature Biology. 1993:1–52.
35. Pollock GA, Pegg DE, Hardie IR. An isolated perfused rat mesentery model for direct observation of the vasculature during cryopreservation. Cryobiology 1986;23:500–511.
36. Hoffmann NE, Bischof JC. Cryosurgery of normal and tumor tissue in the dorsal skin flap chamber. II. J Biomech Eng 2001;123:310–316.
37. Barker JH, Bartlett R, Funk W. The effect of superoxide dismutase on ths skin microcirculation after ischemia and reperfusion. Prog Appl Microcirc 1987;12:276–281.

38. Zook N, Hussmann J, Brown R. Microcirculatory studies of frostbite injury. Ann Plast Surg 1998;40:246–253.
39. Asahina E, Shimada K, Hisada Y. A stable state of frozen protoplasm with invisible intracellular ice crystals obtained by rapid cooling. Exp Cell Res 1970;59:349–358.
40. Gazelle GS, Goldberg SN, Solbiati L, Livraghi T. Tumor ablation with radiofrequency energy. Radiology 2000;217:6333–6346.
41. McGahan JP, Dodd GD III. Radiofrequency ablation of the liver: current status. AJR 2001; 176:3–16.
42. Cosman E, Nashold B, Ovelman-Levitt J. Theoretical aspects of radiofrequency lesions in the dorsal root entry zone. Neurosurgery 1984;15: 945–950.
43. Seegenschmiedt M, Brady L, Sauer R. Interstitial thermoradiotherapy: review on technical and clinical aspects. Am J Clin Oncol 1990;13: 352–363.
44. Trembley B, Ryan T, Strohbehn J. Interstitial hyperthermia: physics, biology, and clinical aspects. In: Hyperthermia and Oncology, vol 3. Utrecht: VSP, 1992:11–98.
45. Larson T, Bostwick D, Corcia A. Temperature-correlated histopathologic changes following microwave thermoablation of obstructive tissues in patients with benign prostatic hyperplasia. Urology 1996;47:463–469.
46. Zervas N, Kuwayama A. Pathologic analysis of experimental thermal lesions: comparison of induction heating and radiofrequency electrocoagulation. J Neurosurg 1972;37:418–422.
47. Thomsen S. Pathologic analysis of photothermal and photomechanical effects of laser tissue interactions. Photochem Photobiol 1991;53: 825–835.
48. Goldberg SN, Gazelle GS, Compton CC, Mueller PR, Tanabe KK. Treatment of intrahepatic malignancy with radiofrequency ablation: radiologic-pathologic correlation. Cancer 2000;88:2452–2463.
49. Goldberg SN, Gazelle GS, Halpern EF, Rittman WJ, Mueller PR, Rosenthal DI. Radiofrequency tissue ablation: importance of local temperature along the electrode tip exposure in determining lesion shape and size. Acad Radiol 1996;3:212–218.
50. Pennes H. Analysis of tissue and arterial blood temperatures in the resting human forearm. J Appl Physiol 1948;1:93–122.
51. Rossi S, DiStasi M, Buscarini E. Percutaneous RF interstitial thermal ablation in the treatment of hepatic cancer. AJR 1996;167: 759–768.
52. Solbiati L, Ierace T, Goldberg SN. Percutaneous US-guided RF tissue ablation of liver metastases: long-term follow-up. Radiology 1997;202: 195–203.
53. Goldberg SN, Gazelle GS, Dawson SL, Rittman WJ, Mueller PR, Rosenthal DI. Tissue ablation with radiofrequency using multiprobe arrays. Acad Radiol 1995;2:670–674.
54. Rossi S, Buscarini E, Garbagnati F. Percutaneous treatment of small hepatic tumors by an expandable RF needle electrode. AJR 1998; 170:1015–1022.
55. Siperstein AE, Rogers SJ, Hansen PD, Gitomirsky A. Laparoscopic thermal ablation of hepatic neuroendocrine tumor metastases. Surgery 1997;122:1147–1155.
56. Leveen RF. Laser hyperthermia and radiofrequency ablation of hepatic lesions. Semin Intervent Radiol 1997;12:313–324.
57. Berber E, Foroutani A, Garland AM, et al. Use of CT Hounsfield unit density to identify ablated tumor after laparoscopic radiofrequency ablation of hepatic tumors. Surg Endosc 2000;14:799–804.
58. de Baere T, Denys A, Johns Wood B, et al. Radiofrequency liver ablation: experimental comparative study of water-cooled versus expandable systems. AJR 2001;176:187–192.
59. McGahan JP, Gu WZ, Brock JM, Tesluk H, Jones CD. Hepatic ablation using bipolar radiofrequency electrocautery. Acad Radiol 1996;3:418–422.
60. Desinger K, Stein T, Muller G, Mack M, Vogl T. Interstitial bipolar RF-thermotherapy (REITT) therapy by planning by computer simulation and MRI-monitoring—a new concept for minimally invasive procedures. Proc SPIE 1999;3249:147–160.
61. Haemmerich DG, Lee FTJ, Chachati L, Wright AS, Mahvi DM, Webster JG. A device that allows for multiple simultaneous radiofrequency (RF) ablations in separated areas of the liver with impedance-controlled cool-ip probes: an ex vivo feasibility study [abstract]. Radiology 2002;225(p):242.
62. Haemmerich DG, Lee FTJ, Mahvi DM, Wright AS, Webster JG. Multiple probe radiofrequency: rapid switching versus simultaneous power application in a computer model. Radiology 2002;225(p):639.
63. Goldberg SN, Gazelle GS, Solbiati L, Rittman WJ, Mueller PR. Radiofrequency tissue abla-

tion: increased lesion diameter with a perfusion electrode. Acad Radiol 1996;3:636–644.
64. Lorentzen T. A cooled needle electrode for radiofrequency tissue ablation: thermodynamic aspects of improved performance compared with conventional needle design. Acad Radiol 1996;3:556–563.
65. Solbiati L, Ierace T, Tonolini M, Osti V, Cova L. Radiofrequency thermal ablation of hepatic metastases. Eur J Ultrasound 2001;13:149–158.
66. Goldberg SN, Solbiati L, Hahn PF, et al. Large-volume tissue ablation with radiofrequency by using a clustered, internally-cooled electrode technique: laboratory and clinical experience in liver metastases. Radiology 1998;209:371–379.
67. Goldberg SN, Stein M, Gazelle GS, Sheiman RG, Kruskal JB, Clouse ME. Percutaneous radiofrequency tissue ablation: optimization of pulsed-RF technique to increase coagulation necrosis. J Vasc Intervent Radiol 1999;10:907–916.
68. Curley MG, Hamilton PS. Creation of large thermal lesions in liver using saline-enhanced RF ablation. Proc 19th International Conference IEEE/EMBS 1997:2516–2519.
69. Livraghi T, Goldberg SN, Monti F, et al. Saline-enhanced radiofrequency tissue ablation in the treatment of liver metastases. Radiology 1997; 202:205–210.
70. Miao Y, Ni Y, Yu J, Marchal G. A comparative study on validation of a novel cooled-wet electrode for radiofrequency liver ablation. Invest Radiol 2000;35:438–444.
71. Miao Y, Ni Y, Yu J, Zhang H, Baert A, Marchal G. An ex vivo study on radiofrequency tissue ablation: increased lesion size by using an "expandable-wet" electrode. Eur Radiol 2001; 11:1841–1847.
72. Kettenbach J, Kostler W, Rucklinger E, et al. Percutaneous saline-enhanced radiofrequency ablation of unresectable liver tumors: initial experience in 26 patients. AJR 2003;180:1537–1545.
73. Goldberg SN, Ahmed M, Gazelle GS, et al. Radiofrequency thermal ablation with adjuvant saline injection: effect of electrical conductivity on tissue heating and coagulation. Radiology 2001;219:157–165.
74. Goldberg SN, Hahn PF, Halpern EF, Fogle R, Gazelle GS. Radiofrequency tissue ablation: effect of pharmacologic modulation of blood flow on coagulation diameter. Radiology 1998; 209:761–769.
75. Merkle E, Goldberg SN, Boll DT, et al. Effect of supramagnetic MR contrast agents on radiofrequency induced temperature distribution: in vitro measurements in polyacrylamide phantoms and in vivo results in a rabbit liver model. Radiology 1999;212:459–466.
76. Lobo SM, Afzal SK, Kruskal JB, Lenkinski RE, Gazelle GS, Goldberg SN. Radiofrequency thermal ablation using an adjuvant NaCl gel: effect of electrical conductivity on tissue coagulation [abstract]. Radiology 2001;201(suppl): 398.
77. Goldberg SN, Hahn PF, Tanabe KK, et al. Percutaneous radiofrequency tissue ablation: does perfusion-mediated tissue cooling limit coagulation necrosis? J Vasc Intervent Radiol 1998;9:101–111.
78. Patterson EJ, Scudamore CH, Owen DA, Nagy AG, Buczkowski AK. Radiofrequency ablation of porcine liver in vivo: effects of blood flow and treatment time on lesion size. Ann Surg 1998;227:559–565.
79. Lu DS, Raman SS, Vodopich DJ, Wang M, Sayre J, Lassman C. Effect of vessel size on creation of hepatic radiofrequency lesions in pigs: assessment of the "heat sink" effect. AJR 2002; 178:47–51.
80. Rossi S, Garbagnati F, Lencioni R, et al. Percutaneous radiofrequency thermal ablation of nonresectable hepatocellular carcinoma after occlusion of tumor blood supply. Radiology 2000;217:119–126.
81. King RWP, Shen LC, Wu TT. Embedded insulated antenna for communication and heating. Electromagnetics 1981;1:51–72.
82. Foster KR, Schepps JL. Dielectric properties of tumor and normal tissues at radio through microwave frequencies. J Microwave Power 1981;16:107–119.
83. Moriyama E, Matsumi N, Shiraishi T, et al. Hyperthermia for brain tumors: improved delivery with a new cooling system. Neurosurgery 1988;23:189–195.
84. Saitsu H, Mada Y, Taniwaki S, et al. Investigation of microwave coagulo-necrotic therapy for 21 patients with small hepatocellular carcinoma less than 5 cm in diameter. Nippon Geka Gakkai Zasshi 1993;94:356–365.
85. Saitsu H, Nakayama T. Microwave coagulo-necrotic therapy for hepatocellular carcinoma. Nippon Rinsho 1993;51:1102–1107.
86. Watanabe Y, Sato M, Abe Y, et al. Laparoscopic microwave coagulo-necrotic therapy for hepatocellular carcinoma: a feasible study of an

alternative option for poor-risk patients. J Laparoendosc Surg 1995;5:169–175.
87. Sato M, Watanabe Y, Ueda S, et al. Microwave coagulation therapy for hepatocellular carcinoma. Gastroenterology 1996;110:1507–1514.
88. Shibata T, Iimuro Y, Yamamoto Y, et al. Small hepatocellular carcinoma: comparison of radiofrequency ablation and percutaneous microwave coagulation therapy. Radiology 2002;223: 331–337.
89. Dong B, Liang P, Yu X, et al. Percutaneous sonographically guided microwave coagulation therapy for hepatocellular carcinoma: results in 234 patients. AJR 2003;180:1547–1555.
90. Brown S. Laser-tissue interactions. Krausner N 1991;Lasers in Gastroenterology:37–50.
91. Dachman AH, McGehee JA, Beam TE, Burris JA, Powell DA. US-guided percutaneous laser ablation of liver tissue in a chronic pig model. Radiology 1990;176:129–133.
92. Jiao LR, Hansen PD, Havlik R, Mitry RR, Pignatelli M, Habib N. Clinical short-term results of radiofrequency ablation in primary and secondary liver tumors. Am J Surg 1999; 177:303–306.
93. Nolsoe CP, Torp-Pedersen S, Burcharth F, et al. Interstitial hyperthermia of colorectal liver metastases with an US-guided Nd-YAG laser with a diffuser tip: a pilot clinical study. Radiology 1993;187:333–337.
94. Diederich CJ, Nau WH, Deardorff DL. Prostate thermal therapy with interstitial and transurethral ultrasound applicators: a feasibility study. In: Ryan TP, ed. Surgical Applications of Energy, Proceedings of SPIE Vol. 3249. 1998:2–13.
95. Vogl TJ, Muller PK, Hammerstingl R, et al. Malignant liver tumors treated with MR imaging-guided laser-induced thermotherapy: technique and prospective results. Radiology 1995;196:257–265.
96. Vogl T, Eichler K, Straub R, et al. Laser-induced thermotherapy of malignant liver tumors: general principles, equipment, procedure—side effects, complications and results. Eur J Ultrasound 2001;13:117–127.
97. Vogl TJ, Mack MG, Roggan A, et al. Internally cooled power laser for MR-guided interstitial laser-induced thermotherapy of liver lesions: initial clinical results. Radiology 1998;209: 381–385.
98. Yang R, Sanghvi NT, Rescorla FJ, Kopecky KK, Grosfeld JL. Liver cancer ablation with extracorporeal high-intensity focused ultrasound. Eur Urol 1993;23(suppl 1):17–22.
99. Jolesz FA, Hynynen K. Magnetic resonance image-guided focused ultrasound surgery. Cancer 2002;8(suppl 1):S100–112.
100. Sanghvi NT, Hawes RH. High-intensity focused ultrasound. Gastrointest Endosc Clin North Am 1994;4:383–395.
101. Reilly CR, Yang R, Reilly WM. Tissue heating measurements during high intensity focused ultrasound cancer therapy. J Ultrasound Med 1991;10:S26.
102. Hill CR, ter Haar GR. Review article: high intensity focused ultrasound—potential for cancer treatment. Br J Radiol 1995;68:1296–1303.
103. Christophi C, Muralidharan V. Treatment of hepatocellular carcinoma by percutaneous laser hyperthermia. J Gastroenterol Hepatol 2001;16:548–552.
104. Goldberg SN, Saldinger PF, Gazelle GS, et al. Percutaneous tumor ablation: increased coagulation necrosis with combined radiofrequency and percutaneous doxorubicin injection. Radiology 2001;220:420–427.
105. Goldberg SN, Girnan GD, Lukyanov AN, et al. Percutaneous tumor ablation: increased necrosis with combined radio-frequency ablation and intravenous liposomal doxorubicin in a rat breast tumor model. Radiology 2002;222:797–804.
106. Monsky WL, Kruskal JB, Lukyanov AN, et al. Radio-frequency ablation increases intratumoral liposomal doxorubicin accumulation in a rat breast tumor model. Radiology 2002;224: 823–829.
107. D'Ippolito G, Ahmed M, Girnan GD, et al. Percutaneous tumor ablation: increased endpoint survival with combined radiofrequency ablation and liposomal doxorubicin in a rat breast tumor model. Radiology; in press.
108. Goldberg SN, Kamel IR, Kruskal JB, et al. Radiofrequency ablation of hepatic tumors: increased tumor destruction with adjuvant liposomal doxorubicin therapy. AJR 2002;179: 93–101.
109. Kruskal JB, Oliver B, Huertas JC, Goldberg SN. Dynamic intrahepatic flow and cellular alterations during radiofrequency ablation of liver tumors in mice. J Vasc Intervent Radiol 2001; 12:1193–1201.
110. Kong G, Dewhirst MW. Hyperthermia and liposomes. Int J Hyperthermia 1999;15:345–370.

4 Tumor Angiogenesis: General Principles and Therapeutic Approaches

John V. Heymach and Judah Folkman

Tumor growth is dependent on angiogenesis, the process by which new capillary blood vessels are recruited and sustained. In recent years, key steps in the angiogenic process have been identified, and various angiogenesis inhibitors have been developed. These agents are now in clinical testing for cancer and a number of other diseases. In the majority of cases, angiogenesis inhibitors are being tested alone and in combination with chemotherapy for advanced or metastatic cancers. Recent evidence suggests, however, that they potentially may be beneficial in earlier stage disease (i.e., chemoprevention) or in combination with other modalities such as radiation therapy. Furthermore, tumor ablation techniques such as hyperthermia and chemoembolization work, at least in part, through effects on the tumor vasculature. Understanding mechanisms of tumor angiogenesis, therefore, may shed light on ways to inhibit tumor growth and increase the effectiveness of existing treatment modalities.

Historical Background

It was observed more than a century ago that tumors have a rich vascular supply, and are often more vascularized than normal tissues (1,2). This was initially attributed to a simple dilation of existing host blood vessels (3), stimulated by factors secreted by the tumor. Three studies in the 1930s and 1940s suggested that tumor hyperemia could be related to new blood vessel growth stimulated by the tumor. Using a transparent rabbit ear chamber, Ide and colleagues (4) showed in 1939 that wound-associated vessels regressed during the healing process, whereas a tumor implant caused progressive growth of new vessels. Algire and coworkers (5) showed in the mid-1940s that new vessels in the neighborhood of a tumor implant arose from existing vessels in the host, and not from the tumor itself. These studies were largely overlooked, and it was generally assumed that tumors could expand by simply living on preexisting vessels. Tumor-induced changes such as those seen in the rabbit ear chamber were assumed to be a nonspecific inflammatory reaction to the tumor (6).

In the 1960s, it was shown that tumor growth in an isolated organ perfusion system was severely restricted in the absence of tumor neovascularization (7,8). Based on these observations, in 1971 it was proposed that tumor growth is angiogenesis dependent, and that inhibiting angiogenesis might therefore be a therapeutic strategy for fighting cancer (9). Furthermore, it was proposed that tumors secreted diffusible factors that activated the normally quiescent host endothelial cells, stimulating their proliferation and migration. This hypothesis was supported by the observations that in the absence of neovascularization, tumors failed to grow beyond several millimeters and remained in a dormant state (10,11).

Experimental confirmation and acceptance of this hypothesis were slow, as they required a number of scientific developments, including: (a) the development of in vitro methods for culturing endothelial cells, (b) the discovery of angiogenesis inhibitors, and (c) identification of tumor-derived proteins that stimulated angiogenesis (12–17), particularly basic fibroblast growth factor (bFGF) and vascular endothelial growth factor (VEGF) (16–20). Because of these early efforts, the nascent field of angiogenesis research began and has subsequently undergone explosive growth through the 1980s and 1990s. The field encompasses a broad range of basic science and clinical disciplines, with active areas of investigation including oncology, cardiology, dermatology, gynecology, ophthalmology, and developmental biology. To illustrate this growth, in 1980 there were fewer than 40 publications with angiogenesis in the title or abstract, whereas in 2002 there were approximately 3800. More importantly, there are currently more than 100 clinical trials of angiogenesis inhibitors for cancer patients in the United States alone.

Key Steps in the Angiogenic Process

In the adult, angiogenesis normally occurs during wound healing and in the female reproductive system. With these exceptions, endothelium is typically quiescent with turnover times measured in the hundreds of days. Bone marrow cells, in contrast, maintain an average turnover time of less than 1 week. Pathologic neovascularization occurs in a number of diseases, including diabetic retinopathy, rheumatoid arthritis (21), and cancer.

Tumor angiogenesis is a complex, multistep process regulated by the local balance of endogenous pro- and antiangiogenic factors (22–25). The molecular mechanisms underlying these processes are now understood in some detail, and each step is being investigated as a potential therapeutic target (Fig. 4.1). The

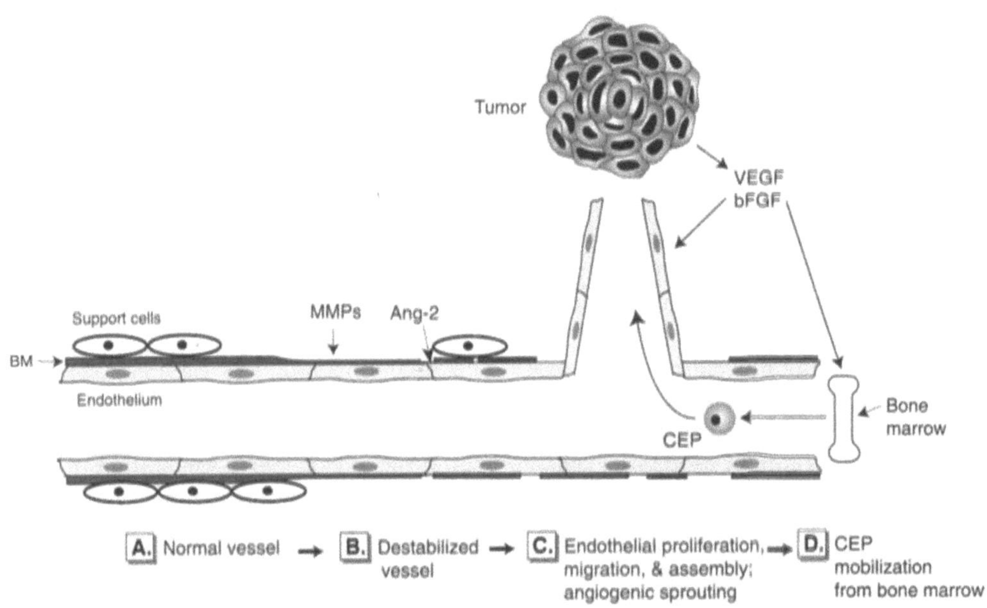

FIGURE 4.1. Steps in tumor angiogenesis. A: Normal vessel with intact basement membrane, surrounded by support cells (i.e., pericyctes, smooth muscle cells). B: The tumor stimulates breakdown of the basement membrane by matrix metalloproteinases (MMPs) and other proteases. Interactions between support cells and endothelium are disrupted by angiopoietin-2 (Ang-2). C: In response to tumor-derived factors such as basic fibroblast growth factor (bFGF) and vasculature endothelial growth factor (VEGF), endothelial cells proliferate, migrate, and assemble into capillary tubes that form tumor vasculature. D: Bone marrow–derived circulating endothelial precursors (CEPs) are mobilized in response to VEGF and other factors, and may provide a second source of endothelial cells for tumor vasculature. (Reprinted with permission from J.V. Heymach. "Angiogenesis and antiangiogenic approaches to sarcomas." Current Opinion in Oncology 2001;13:261–269.)

TABLE 4.1. Endogenous stimulators and inhibitors of angiogenesis.

Stimulators	Inhibitors
Vascular endothelial growth factor-A, B, C	Thrombospondin-1, 2
Basic fibroblast growth factor	Endostatin
Acidic fibroblast growth factor	Angiostatin
Transforming growth factor-α	Tumstatin
Transforming growth factor-β	Canstatin
Platelet-derived growth factor	Antiangiogenic antithrombin III
Interleukin-8	Interferon-α, β, γ
Hepatocyte growth factor	Platelet factor-4
EG-VEGF	
Angiopoietin-1	
Matrix metalloproteinases (MMPs)	
Proangiogenic oncogenes: *K-ras*, *H-ras*, *Src*, *p53*, *EGFR*, *Her-2*, *c-myb*, etc.	

EG-VEGF, endocrine gland–derived vascular endothelial growth factor; EGFR, epidermal growth factor receptor.

initial step involves degradation of the underlying extracellular matrix and basement membrane by matrix metalloproteinases (MMPs), particularly MMP-2 and MMP-9, and other proteinases (26,27). The host vessel is further destabilized by angiopoietin-2 (Ang-2), a natural antagonist for the endothelial-specific Tie-2 receptor (28,29). Tie-2 plays a critical role in promoting and maintaining the interaction between endothelial and supporting cells (30). Freed from the constraints of their surrounding basement membrane and support cells, endothelial cells then proliferate, migrate, and assemble into tubes. A number of molecules contribute to these processes (Table 4.1), although VEGF and bFGF are thought to play a preeminent role. VEGF also acts as a survival factor for endothelial cells (Ecs) (31), regulates vascular permeability (32), and promotes the recruitment of circulating endothelial precursors (see below). Migration and assembly are dependent on adhesion molecules such as integrin αvβ3, vascular endothelial cadherin, vascular cell adhesion molecule-1 (VCAM-1), and members of the selectin family. Finally, stabilization and maturation of the new vessels require recruitment of pericytes and smooth muscle cells and production of a new basement membrane, processes involving Ang-1, platelet-derived growth factor (PDGF), transforming growth factor-β (TGF-β), and other factors (23,25,29,30).

Contribution of Circulating Endothelial Cells to Tumor Vascularization

In the above model, endothelial cells in tumor vasculature arise through the proliferation of ECs in local vessels. In the 1990s, however, studies by Isner and colleagues (33–35) revealed another potential supply of cells to participate in tumor neovascularization: bone marrow–derived circulating endothelial precursors (CEPs). Using animal models in which bone marrow cells were labeled with lacZ as a marker, CEPs were found to contribute to neovascularization occurring during wound healing, limb ischemia, and tumor growth (35). These cells were mobilized by VEGF (35). The contribution of CEPs to tumor neovascularization and growth was further established by a study in which mice rendered incapable of undergoing normal angiogenesis through targeted disruption of one allele of Id1 and two alleles of Id3 (36). In these mice, three different types of implanted tumors failed to induce angiogenesis, their growth was severely restricted, and they did not metastasize. However, when these mice were injected with bone marrow from wild-type mice, circulating endothelial precursors from the donor marrow were recruited to the tumor vascular bed and restored the ability of these tumors to undergo angiogenesis and grow at essentially the same rate as in wild-type mice (37). This established that bone marrow–derived cells were capable of differentiating into endothelial cells, becoming tumor vasculature, and restoring tumor growth. Subsequent animal studies suggest that tumor types vary in their ability to recruit and incorporate circulating endothelial precursors (38).

In humans, the contribution of bone marrow–derived endothelial cells to tumor vasculature in humans remains to be determined. Circulating endothelial cells can be detected in the blood using cell surface markers (39), and they are known to be elevated in cancer patients (40,41) and to change in response to antiangiogenic therapy (41), raising the possibility that they may be useful as a surrogate marker for trials of angiogenesis inhibitors (42). They are also elevated in patients with limb ischemia or inoperable coronary artery disease who undergo gene therapy with a VEGF expression vector (43,44). Furthermore, human bone marrow stem cells were able to differentiate and contribute substantially to tumor vasculature in a mouse model (45). Taken together, these studies suggest that bone marrow–derived endothelial cells are likely to make at least some contribution to tumor vasculature in humans, although the relative contribution is likely to depend on the specific tumor type and local balance of angiogenic factors.

Role of Angiogenesis in Tumor Progression and Metastatic Spread

The development of cancer is a multistage process, and angiogenesis may play an important role at one or more points in the development of cancer (Fig. 4.2). During the premalignant (avascular) phase, when angiogenic activity is absent or insufficient, tumors remain small (1–2 mm^3). These premalignant lesions, which may be categorized as hyperplasia, metaplasia, dysplasia, or carcinoma in situ, often have genetic changes and proliferation rates comparable to larger, rapidly growing tumors. This suggests that the difference between the two tumors is that in the premalignant lesion, the generation of new tumor cells is balanced by tumor apoptosis (46). A relatively small percentage of these lesions undergo an "angiogenic switch," reflecting a change in the net balance between angiogenic stimulators and inhibitors (22). This appears to be a critical step for sustained tumor growth

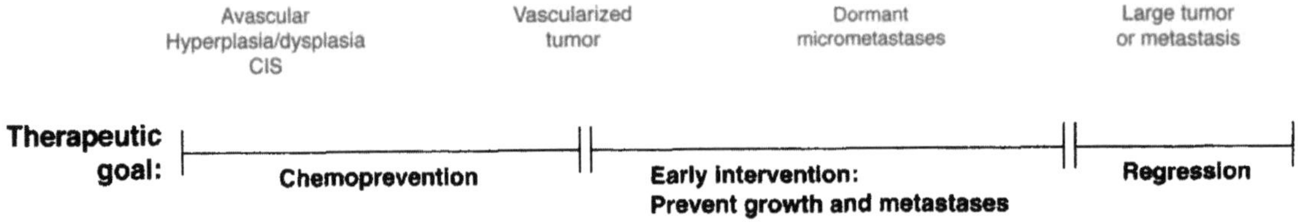

FIGURE 4.2. The role of angiogenesis in the progression of cancer. Premalignant lesions must acquire a vascular supply to progress to macroscopic lesions. Vascularization also increases the likelihood of metastatic spread. CIS, carcinoma in situ.

and metastatic spread (Fig. 4.2). The angiogenic stimulus arising from preneoplastic lesions can be observed clinically: biopsies from patients with preneoplastic bronchial, colonic, or cervical lesions ranging from hyperplasia and metaplasia to carcinoma in situ often are associated with increased microvessel density in the surrounding mucosa (47–49). The specific factors controlling this switch have not been fully elucidated and probably vary depending on the tumor type, but elevated levels of proangiogenic factors including VEGF, epidermal growth factor receptor (EGFR), and cyclooxygenase-2 (Cox-2) have been observed (50) in preneoplastic lesions.

The majority of cancer deaths are caused by metastases, not by the primary tumor. Evidence from preclinical and clinical studies suggests that the metastatic spread of cancer is also angiogenesis dependent (1). For a tumor to enter the circulation and successfully metastasize, it must first overcome several obstacles: it must invade through the basement membrane, which is often fragmented and leaky in tumors; survive in the circulation; arrest in the target organ; and induce angiogenesis to resume growth (51–55). In animal models, tumor cells are rarely detectable in the circulation before a primary tumor is vascularized, but can be detected (at levels as high as 10^6 cells per gram of tumor) after vascularization (56,57). Angiogenic factors such as VEGF and bFGF increase endothelial motility and induce production of proteinases that degrade the basement membrane, further facilitating the entry of tumor cells into the circulation (56). Fortunately, the vast majority of tumor cells that gain entry into the circulation do not develop into macroscopic tumors. Such metastases may lack angiogenic activity for a number of reasons, and therefore remain as a microscopic tumor of 100 to 200 μm indefinitely (21,58).

Angiogenesis inhibitors, therefore, may offer benefit when used for chemoprevention as well as in treatment of early stage, occult metastatic, or advanced disease (59). This hypothesis has been supported by a transgenic murine model of pancreatic islet carcinogenesis. In this model, lesions in mice harboring an oncogene expressed in the β-islet cells of the pancreas reproducibly undergo a transition from normal islets to hyperplasia (60). A small percentage of these hyperplastic lesions become angiogenic, leading to the development of tumors. Interestingly, different antiangiogenic agents (TNP-470, endostatin, angiostatin, or the matrix metalloproteinase inhibitor BB-94) had distinct activity profiles in terms of their ability to prevent tumor formation (chemoprevention), slow the growth of small tumors (early intervention), and regress established tumors (61). This highlights the importance of investigating the most appropriate applications for specific angiogenesis inhibitors.

Potential Advantages of Antiangiogenic Therapy

The approach of targeting the endothelium instead of, or in addition to, the tumor cell has a number of advantages over traditional approaches focused on tumor cells alone. Tumor endothelium appears to be distinct from normal endothelium at a molecular level, but endothelium from different tumor types appear to share tumor endothelium-specific markers (TEMs) (62) and other important characteristics, such as high proliferation rates. This raises the possibility that agents directed against tumor endothelium will be active for a broad range of tumor types, a hope that has been supported by animal studies (63–65). It is important to note, however, that recent studies have highlighted the heterogeneity of different endothelial beds in terms of markers and responsiveness to proangiogenic factors (66,67). It is likely that tumor endothelium from different tumor types will vary in their responsiveness to both angiogenic stimulators and inhibitors.

Resistance to conventional chemotherapy occurs, in large part, because genetic instability and high mutation rates inevitably lead to the selection of resistant clones. Angiogenesis inhibitors, by contrast, target activated endothelial cells that are diploid and presumably genetically stable. This led to the prediction that resistance will develop more slowly, or not at all, to angiogenesis inhibitors. Consistent with this hypothesis, resistance was not observed in three different murine tumor models even after six cycles of therapy with endostatin (68). It is clear, however, that different tumor types do not respond identically to antiangiogenic therapy and that genetic changes in the tumor can alter this responsiveness. For example, p53 mutations are known to cause increased tumor angiogenesis through several mechanisms, including VEGF upregulation and a reduction in the thrombospondin-1 (TSP-1). p53 mutations also render tumor cells relatively resistant to hypoxia-induced apoptosis. Not surprisingly, tumors derived from a p53-null human colorectal cell line responded less well to antiangiogenic therapy than their p53 wild-type counterparts, although their growth was still inhibited (69).

Antiangiogenic therapy differs from traditional cytotoxic therapies in at least two other important ways. First, because tumors have high interstitial pressures, tumor blood flow is often compromised, resulting in markedly diminished penetration of cytotoxic drugs into tumor tissues (70). In contrast, antiangiogenic agents target endothelium that is in direct contact with circulation and do not, therefore, need to penetrate tissues to exert their effects. Second, the side-effect profiles of antiangiogenic agents have typically been quite favorable, and non-overlapping with chemotherapy. Two exceptions to this have been rare life-threatening side effects such as hemoptysis (71) and blood clots (72) that occurred primarily when VEGF pathway antagonists were given in combination with chemotherapy. These side effects are discussed below.

Types of Angiogenesis Inhibitors

Research into the molecular mechanisms underlying tumor angiogenesis has catalyzed a rapid growth in the number of angiogenesis inhibitors developed over the past decade. An exhaustive review of the large number of agents entering clinical trials is beyond the scope of this chapter. Instead, we will briefly review several representative examples and discuss a conceptual framework for considering these drugs.

Direct vs. Indirect Inhibitors

It is useful to separate antiangiogenic agents into two broad categories: direct and indirect inhibitors (Fig. 4.3) (73). Direct inhibitors, such as TNP-470, angiostatin, vitaxin, and others, act directly on vascular endothelial cells to prevent them from proliferating, migrating, or surviving in response to a spectrum of proangiogenic factors such as VEGF, bFGF, and PDGF (Table 4.2). Direct angiogenesis inhibitors should in theory be less prone to resistance because they target genetically stable cells. Indirect inhibitors, on the other hand, block the expression or activity of factors produced by tumor. For example, ZD1839 (Iressa) and Herceptin are agents developed to inhibit the EGFR and

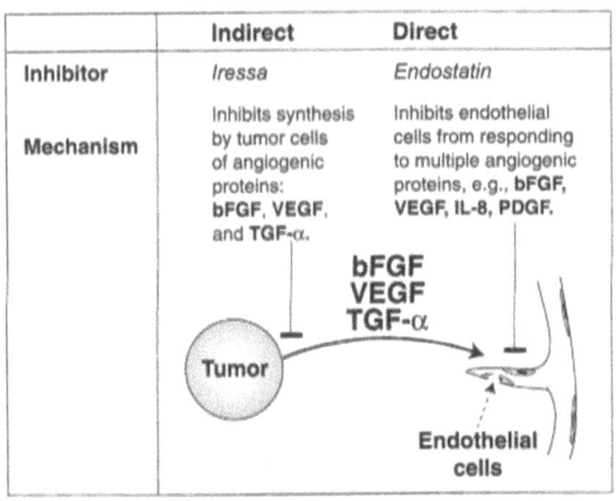

FIGURE 4.3. Direct vs. indirect angiogenesis inhibitors. Direct angiogenesis inhibitors, such as endostatin, target tumor endothelial cells and prevent them from responding to various tumor-derived factors that stimulate angiogenesis. Indirect inhibitors such as Iressa (ZD1839) target proteins that are produced by tumor cells, such as VEGF, bFGF, and TGF-α, or inhibit their receptors on endothelium. bFGF, basic fibroblast growth factor; VEGF, vascular endothelial growth factor; TGF-α, transforming growth factor-α; IL-8, interleukin-8; PDGF, platelet-derived growth factor. (Reproduced with permission from Nature Reviews Cancer, Vol. 2, No. 10, pp. 727–739, copyright 2002, Macmillan Magazines Ltd.)

TABLE 4.2. Examples of direct and indirect angiogenesis inhibitors in clinical trials.

Agent	Proposed mechanism	Clinical trials
Direct		
Angiostatin	Binds to ATP synthase and annexin II to inhibit EC proliferation and migration	Phase I
Combretastatin, ZD6126	Microtubule inhibitor (VTA)	Phase I
Vitaxin, cilengitide	Inhibit $\alpha v\beta 3$ integrin	Phase I
Endostatin	Binds to several EC targets including $\alpha 5$ and αv integrin, MMP2, eNOS; prevents loss of adhesion to BM induced by VEGF and bFGF	Phase II
NM-3	Inhibits EC proliferation, sprouting, and tube formation	Phase I
Thalidomide	Inhibits bFGF-angiogenesis; may also inhibit production of VEGF, bFGF, TNF-α	Phase II
Indirect		
ZD1839	Inhibits EGFR leading to decreased production of VEGF, bFGF, TGF-α	Phase III
Herceptin	Inhibits *Her-2*, decreasing VEGF, TGF-α, Ang-1, etc	Phase III
Celecoxib, rofecoxib	Inhibit COX-2	Phase III

VTA, vascular targeting agent; mAb, monoclonal antibody; EC, endothelial cell; BM, basement membrane; VEGF, vascular endothelial growth factor; bFGF, basic fibroblast growth factor; TNF, tumor necrosis factor; EGFR, epidermal growth factor receptor; TGF, transforming growth factor; Ang, angiopoietin; Cox, cyclooxygenase.

Her-2 pathways on tumor cells. Recent studies have established that blockade of these oncogenic pathways also decreases the expression of proangiogenic factors such as VEGF, and increases the effects of endogenous angiogenesis inhibitors such as thrombospondin-1 (74). It is worth noting that these categories are not mutually exclusive; a number of drugs, such as interferon-α, have both direct effects on endothelium and indirect effects on the production of cytokines.

Endogenous Angiogenesis Inhibitors

In the early 1980s it was demonstrated that interferon-α/β, a cytokine initially identified as an antiviral agent, inhibited endothelial proliferation (75). Other endogenous proteins such as platelet factor-4 (76,77) later were identified to have antiangiogenic activity as well. Interestingly, angiogenesis inhibitors also were produced by tumors themselves. This led to the proposal that the angiogenic phenotype of a tumor was determined by the net balance of angiogenesis inhibitors and stimulators (22,78). While the production of angiogenesis inhibitors by tumors may seem counterintuitive, it suggests a molecular basis for the longstanding clinical observation that removal of a primary tumor often results in an acceleration in the growth of metastases. This led to an intensive search for additional tumor-derived antiangiogenic agents.

Angiostatin was initially purified from the urine of mice bearing Lewis lung carcinoma, a tumor that when implanted subcutaneously suppressed the growth of lung metastases via inhibition of angiogenesis (79). It was found to be a 38-kd internal fragment of plasminogen. Tumors do not appear to directly produce angiostatin, but rather they release proteases that cleave circulating plasminogen. In addition to potent antiangiogenic activity in a variety of tumor models, angiostatin potentiates the effects of radiation (80).

A similar strategy has been used to identify a number of other inhibitors, including endostatin (81), tumstatin (82), canstatin (83), and antiangiogenic antithrombin-III (84), which are reviewed in detail elsewhere (1). In phase I testing, endostatin was found to be safe, and evidence of antitumor and antiangiogenic activity was observed (85,86). Angiostatin and endostatin are currently in phase II testing.

VEGF Pathway Antagonists

VEGF is expressed in the vast majority of human tumors, and levels of VEGF protein have been correlated with poor prognosis in a variety of malignancies including lung, breast, colon, and prostate cancer (87–90). VEGF expression is regulated physiologically by hypoxia, and in tumors a number of oncogenes have been found to regulate VEGF production including *H-Ras, K-Ras, v-src, p53, Her-2*, and *bcl-2* (91,92). It performs a number of roles in the angiogenic process (Fig. 4.1), such as inducing endothelial migration and proliferation and promoting ECs survival. In addition to these important roles, VEGF also mobilizes bone marrow–derived circulating ECs precursors, induces the expression of matrix metalloproteinases, and increases vascular permeability—it was, in fact, initially identified by Dvorak's group (20) in the 1980s as a vascular permeability factor. Because of its widespread expression in tumors and its central role in angiogenesis, VEGF has been the subject of intense investigation, and a number of inhibitors of the VEGF pathway are being tested in clinical trials (Table 4.3).

The activity of VEGF appears to be primarily mediated by the tyrosine kinase receptor VEGFR-2, although other receptors such as VEGFR-1, VEGFR-3, and neuropilin-1 likely play a role as well. Approaches to inhibiting these pathways include antibodies to the ligand (bevacizumab), antibodies to the receptor that blocks ligand binding (IMC-1C11), and small molecule receptor tyrosine kinase inhibitors (RTKIs). The newest generation of RTKIs, such as PTK787, ZD6474, and SU11248, are oral drugs, an important advantage for therapies that may need to be taken for sustained periods of time (Table 4.3).

In early clinical testing, some VEGF pathway inhibitors have shown promising activity both as a single agent and in combination with chemotherapy. For example, in a randomized phase II trial in patients with renal cell cancer, bevacizumab significantly prolonged the time for tumor progression compared to placebo, and objective tumor shrinkage was observed in 8% of patients (93). In another randomized phase II trial, patients with colon cancer were treated with a standard chemotherapy 5-fluorouracil/leucovorin (5-FU/LV) regimen with or without the addition of the VEGF monoclonal antibody bevacizumab (BV) (94). Patients receiving the combination containing low-dose BV had a higher objective response rate (40% vs. 17% for control arm), longer time to progression (5.2 vs. 9 months), and prolonged survival (13.8 vs. 21.5 months) than the control arm (94). Phase III trials of bevacizumab are ongoing.

Two serious toxicities observed with VEGF pathway inhibitors have been thrombosis (94,95), and hemoptysis (71), which occurred in the setting of rapid tumor necrosis. Both toxicities are likely related to endothelial damage that occurred when angiogenesis inhibitors were given in combination with chemotherapy. This highlights the need for further investigations

TABLE 4.3. Inhibitors of the VEGF pathway in clinical trials.

Agent	Main target(s)	Type	Company	Clinical trials
Bevacizumab	VEGF	mAb	Genentech	Phase III
SU5416	VEGFR-2	RTKI	Sugen	Phase III (discontinued)
SU6668	VEGFR-2, PDGF	RTKI (oral)	Sugen	Phase II (discontinued)
SU11248	VEGFR-2, PDGF	RTKI (oral)	Sugen	Phase II
PTK787	VEGFR-2, PDGF	RTKI (oral)	Novartis	Phase II
ZD6474	VEGFR-2, PDGF	RTKI (oral)	Astra Zeneca	Phase II
IMC-1C11	VEGFR-2	mAb	Imclone	Phase I
VEGF trap	VEGF	Soluble VEGFR-2	Regeneron	Phase I
Angiozyme	VEGFR-1	ribozyme	Ribozyme Pharmaceuticals	Phase II

VEGF, vascular endothelial growth factor; VEGFR, VEGF receptor; PDGF, platelet-derived growth factor; RTKI, receptor tyrosine kinase inhibitor; mAb, monoclonal antibody.

into the optimal means for combining these inhibitors with other treatment modalities.

Role of Angiogenesis in Other Therapeutic Modalities: "Incidental" Antiangiogenesis

Most therapeutic approaches to fighting cancer were developed with the goal of attacking the cancer cell. Evidence suggests that many of these treatment modalities actually exert their effects, at least in part, though inhibition and damage to tumor endothelial cells and vasculature (96–99). Examples of this are chemotherapy and radiofrequency ablation, discussed below; today a number of "antiangiogenic" or "metronomic" chemotherapy regimens are undergoing clinical testing. Another example is radiation therapy. Endothelial damage and apoptosis induced by ionizing radiation appear to play a crucial role in both the antitumor and toxic effects (100). Consistent with this hypothesis, antiangiogenic agents such as angiostatin (80) and an antibody to VEGF act synergistically with radiotherapy (101). Combinations of antiangiogenic agents and radiotherapy are now undergoing clinical testing as well.

Antiangiogenic Effects of Chemotherapy

Chemotherapeutic agents traditionally have been selected based on their antitumor activity. However, there is now substantial evidence that endothelial cells also may be an important target for these drugs. Some cytotoxic agents have been shown to exert antiangiogenic effects via their ability to induce endothelial apoptosis or interfere with the key steps in the angiogenic cascade that include endothelial proliferation, migration, or capillary tube formation (96). The chemotherapeutic agents that interfere with microtubule formation such as paclitaxel (102–104), docetaxel (105,106), and vinca alkaloids (92,107) appear to be particularly potent antiangiogenic agents in vitro and in vivo, often exerting toxicity against endothelial cells at concentrations one to two orders of magnitude lower than those required for antitumor effects (106,108,109).

The antiangiogenic effects of cytotoxics appear to be highly dependent on the dosing schedule. We developed a cyclophosphamide dosing schedule (170mg/kg every 6 days) that inhibited the growth of highly cyclophosphamide-resistant Lewis lung carcinoma through the induction of endothelial apoptosis (99). The combination of the angiogenesis inhibitor TNP-470 with cyclophosphamide administered by this schedule caused tumors to regress completely for longer than 600 days (Fig. 4.2). Other investigators have subsequently confirmed that frequent administration of low doses of chemotherapeutics (i.e., vinblastine, cisplatin, or Adriamycin given every 3 days) (92,108) can damage tumor endothelium with limited host toxicity in murine models. Based on these observations such regimens are often referred to as antiangiogenic or metronomic dosing. This effect is heightened by combination with VEGF antagonists such as the monoclonal VEGFR antibody DC101 (92,108). The rationale is that such frequent dosing damages or inhibits rapidly dividing tumor endothelium with greater efficacy than conventional regimens, without allowing time for recovery.

VEGF is an important survival factor for endothelial cells damaged by chemotherapy (110). Consistent with this observation, a recombinant human monoclonal antibody against VEGF (rhuMab VEGF) augments chemotherapy-induced endothelial cell death (106). Conventional regimens, by contrast, are typically based on the maximum tolerated dose (MTD) with an interval for recovery from toxicity and bone marrow suppression; this interval appears to allow time for recovery of tumor endothelial function as well (99). Because endothelial cells, like other normal tissues such as gut epithelium, are more genetically stable, they are less likely to acquire drug resistance through genetic mutation. Therefore, they are likely to remain sensitive to chemotherapy regardless of whether the tumor is resistant.

Antivascular Effects of Radiofrequency Ablation and Hyperthermia

Radiofrequency ablation provides a means to induce local hyperthermia. There is a direct effect of heat on tumor cells, but in preclinical models tumors may be cured despite the fact that a significant percentage of tumor cells remain viable at the end of therapy (111–114). The effects of hyperthermia, therefore, extend beyond direct damage to tumor cells. Investigations into the changes in tumor microvasculature after hyperthermia have shown a brief initial increase in blood flow followed by a prolonged decrease and in some cases a cessation of perfusion that leads to tissue hypoxia and necrosis (98,113,115). These changes are accompanied by intravascular thrombosis, microvessel rupture, endothelial apoptosis, and an inhibition of angiogenesis (114,116). Proliferating endothelial cells in tumor vasculature, appear to be more sensitive than endothelium from normal tissues (98,117,118). This has led to the identification of tumor microvasculature as an important target for hyperthermia (97,98, 119).

Tissue hypoxia induced by these antivascular effects appears to induce the expression of proangiogenic factors such as VEGF and bFGF (120). These factors are likely responsible for a compensatory wave of angiogenesis sometimes observed after hyperthermia. With this in mind, it is not surprising that angiogenesis inhibitors such as TNP-470 augment the antitumor efficacy of hyperthermia (121–123). One would expect that newer agents such as the VEGF pathway antagonists (discussed above) could also potentiate the effects of hyperthermia, a hypothesis that merits further investigation as these agents move forward in clinical testing.

Summary

Tumor growth is angiogenesis dependent, and currently various antiangiogenic agents are being tested in clinical trials for cancer and other diseases. Furthermore, it is now appreciated that many therapies initially developed with intention of attacking cancer cells—such as chemotherapy, radiotherapy, and radiofrequency ablation—actually exert their effects, at least in part, through effects on angiogenesis and tumor vasculature. Understanding the mechanisms by which different treatment modalities exert their antitumor and antivascular effects, therefore, is important for designing appropriate preclinical models, choosing other agents to be combined with these modalities, and optimizing schedules of administration. In the near future, approaches aimed at targeting both tumor cells and tumor vasculature may lead to more effective—and less toxic—treatments for cancer.

References

1. Folkman J, Kalluri R. Tumor angiogenesis. In: Kufe DW, Pollock RE, Weichselbaum RR, Bast RC Jr, Holland JF, Frei III E, eds. Cancer Medicine. 6th ed. Hamilton, Ontario: B.C. Decker, 2003.
2. Warren BA. The vascular morphology of tumors. In: Peterson HI, ed. Tumor Blood Circulation: Angiogenesis, Vascular Morphology, and Blood Flow of Experimental Human Tumors. Florida: CRC Press, 1979:1–47.
3. Coman DR, Sheldon WF. The significance of hyperemia around tumor implants. Am J Pathol 1946;22:821–831.
4. Ide AG, Baker NH, Warren SL. Vascularization of the Brown-Pearce rabbit ephithelioma transplant as seen in the transparent ear chamber. AJR 1939;42:891–899.
5. Algire GH, Chalkely HW, Legallais FY, Park H. Vascular reactions of normal and malignant tumors in vivo: I. Vascular reactions of mice to wounds and to normal and neoplastic transplants. J Natl Cancer Inst 1945;6:73–85.
6. Folkman J. Toward an understanding of angiogenesis: search and discovery. Perspect Biol Med 1985;29:10–36.
7. Folkman J, Cole P, Zimmerman S. Tumor behavior in isolated perfused organs: in vitro growth and metastases of biopsy material in rabbit thyroid and canine intestinal segment. Ann Surg 1966;164:491–502.
8. Folkman J, Long DM, Becker FF. Growth and metastasis of tumor in organ culture. Cancer 1963;16:453–467.

9. Folkman J. Tumor angiogenesis: therapeutic implications. N Engl J Med 1971;285:1182–1186.
10. Gimbrone MA, Leapman SB, Cotran RS, Folkman J. Tumor dormancy in vivo by prevention of neovascularization. J Exp Med 1972; 136:261–276.
11. Holmgren L, O'Reilly MS, Folkman J. Dormancy of micrometastases: balanced proliferation and apoptosis in the presence of angiogenesis suppression. Nat Med 1995;1: 149–153.
12. Gimbrone MA Jr, Cotran RS, Folkman J. Endothelial regeneration: studies with human endothelial cells in culture. Ser Haematol 1973; 6:453–455.
13. Jaffe EA, Nachman RL, Becker CG, Minick CR. Culture of human endothelial cells derived from umbilical veins. Identification by morphologic and immunologic criteria. J Clin Invest 1973;52:2745–2756.
14. Folkman J, Haudenschild CC, Zetter BR. Long-term culture of capillary endothelial cells. Proc Natl Acad Sci USA 1979;76:5217–5221.
15. Taylor S, Folkman J. Protamine is an inhibitor of angiogenesis. Nature 1982;297:307–312.
16. Shing Y, Folkman J, Sullivan R, Butterfield C, Murray J, Klagsbrun M. Heparin affinity: purification of a tumor-derived capillary endothelial cell growth factor. Science 1984;223:1296–1299.
17. Klagsbrun M, Sasse J, Sullivan R, Smith JA. Human tumor cells synthesize an endothelial cell growth factor that is structurally related to basic fibroblast growth factor. Proc Natl Acad Sci USA 1986;83:2448–2452.
18. Leung DW, Cachianes G, Kuang WJ, Goeddel DV, Ferrara N. Vascular endothelial growth factor is a secreted angiogenic mitogen. Science 1989;246:1306–1309.
19. Ferrara N, Henzel WJ. Pituitary follicular cells secrete a novel heparin-binding growth factor specific for vascular endothelial cells. Biochem Biophys Res Commun 1989;161:851–858.
20. Senger DR, Galli SJ, Dvorak AM, Perruzzi CA, Harvey VS, Dvorak HF. Tumor cells secrete a vascular permeability factor that promotes accumulation of ascites fluid. Science 1983;219: 983–985.
21. Folkman J. Angiogenesis in cancer, vascular, rheumatoid and other disease. Nat Med 1995; 1:27–31.
22. Hanahan D, Folkman J. Patterns and emerging mechanisms of the angiogenic switch during tumorigenesis. Cell 1996;86:353–364.
23. Carmeliet P, Jain RK. Angiogenesis in cancer and other diseases. Nature 2000;407:249–257.
24. Liekens S, De Clercq E, Neyts J. Angiogenesis: regulators and clinical applications. Biochem Pharmacol 2001;61:253–270.
25. Heymach JV. Angiogenesis and antiangiogenic approaches to sarcomas. Curr Opin Oncol 2001; 13:261–269.
26. Bergers G, Brekken R, McMahon G, et al. Matrix metalloproteinase-9 triggers the angiogenic switch during carcinogenesis. Nat Cell Biol 2000;2:737–744.
27. Moses MA, Wiederschain D, Loughlin KR, Zurakowski D, Lamb CC, Freeman MR. Increased incidence of matrix metalloproteinases in urine of cancer patients. Cancer Res 1998;58:1395–1399.
28. Maisonpierre PC, Suri C, Jones PF, et al. Angiopoietin-2, a natural antagonist for Tie2 that disrupts in vivo angiogenesis. Science 1997;277:55–60.
29. Yancopoulos GD, Davis S, Gale NW, Rudge JS, Wiegand SJ, Holash J. Vascular-specific growth factors and blood vessel formation. Nature 2000;407:242–248.
30. Suri C, Jones PF, Patan S, et al. Requisite role of angiopoietin-1, a ligand for the TIE2 receptor, during embryonic angiogenesis. Cell 1996; 87:1171–1180.
31. Gerber HP, Hillan KJ, Ryan AM, et al. VEGF is required for growth and survival in neonatal mice. Development 1999;126:1149–1159.
32. Senger DR, Perruzzi CA, Feder J, Dvorak HF. A highly conserved vascular permeability factor secreted by a variety of human and rodent tumor cell lines. Cancer Res 1986;46: 5629–5632.
33. Asahara T, Masuda H, Takahashi T, et al. Bone marrow origin of endothelial progenitor cells responsible for postnatal vasculogenesis in physiological and pathological neovascularization. Circ Res 1999;85:221–228.
34. Asahara T, Murohara T, Sullivan A, et al. Isolation of putative progenitor endothelial cells for angiogenesis. Science 1997;275:964–967.
35. Asahara T, Takahashi T, Masuda H, et al. VEGF contributes to postnatal neovascularization by mobilizing bone marrow-derived endothelial progenitor cells. EMBO J 1999;18: 3964–3972.
36. Lyden D, Young AZ, Zagzag D, et al. Id1 and Id3 are required for neurogenesis, angiogenesis and vascularization of tumour xenografts. Nature 1999;401:670–677.

37. Lyden D, Hattori K, Dias S, et al. Impaired recruitment of bone-marrow-derived endothelial and hematopoietic precursor cells blocks tumor angiogenesis and growth. Nat Med 2001; 7:1194–1201.
38. Rafii S, Meeus S, Dias S, et al. Contribution of marrow-derived progenitors to vascular and cardiac regeneration. Semin Cell Dev Biol 2002;13:61–67.
39. Peichev M, Naiyer AJ, Pereira D, et al. Expression of VEGFR-2 and AC133 by circulating human CD34(+) cells identifies a population of functional endothelial precursors. Blood 2000;95:952–958.
40. Mancuso P, Burlini A, Pruneri G, Goldhirsch A, Martinelli G, Bertolini F. Resting and activated endothelial cells are increased in the peripheral blood of cancer patients. Blood 2001;97:3658–3661.
41. Bertolini F, Mingrone W, Alietti A, et al. Thalidomide in multiple myeloma, myelodysplastic syndromes and histiocytosis. Analysis of clinical results and of surrogate angiogenesis markers. Ann Oncol 2001;12:987–990.
42. Monestiroli S, Mancuso P, Burlini A, et al. Kinetics and viability of circulating endothelial cells as surrogate angiogenesis marker in an animal model of human lymphoma. Cancer Res 2001;61:4341–4344.
43. Kalka C, Tehrani H, Laudenberg B, et al. VEGF gene transfer mobilizes endothelial progenitor cells in patients with inoperable coronary disease. Ann Thorac Surg 2000;70:829–834.
44. Kalka C, Masuda H, Takahashi T, et al. Vascular endothelial growth factor(165) gene transfer augments circulating endothelial progenitor cells in human subjects. Circ Res 2000;86: 1198–1202.
45. Reyes M, Dudek A, Jahagirdar B, Koodie L, Marker PH, Verfaillie CM. Origin of endothelial progenitors in human postnatal bone marrow. J Clin Invest 2002;109:337–346.
46. Udagawa T, Fernandez A, Achilles EG, Folkman J, D'Amato RJ. Persistence of microscopic human cancers in mice: alterations in the angiogenic balance accompanies loss of tumor dormancy. FASEB J 2002;16:1361–1370.
47. Fontanini G, Calcinai A, Boldrini L, et al. Modulation of neoangiogenesis in bronchial preneoplastic lesions. Oncol Rep 1999;6:813–817.
48. Smith-McCune KK, Weidner N. Demonstration and characterization of the angiogenic properties of cervical dysplasia. Cancer Res 1994;54: 800–804.
49. Keith RL, Miller YE, Gemmill RM, et al. Angiogenic squamous dysplasia in bronchi of individuals at high risk for lung cancer. Clin Cancer Res 2000;6:1616–1625.
50. Wolff H, Saukkonen K, Anttila S, Karjalainen A, Vainio H, Ristimaki A. Expression of cyclooxygenase-2 in human lung carcinoma. Cancer Res 1998;58:4997–5001.
51. Fidler IJ, Gersten DM, Hart IR. The biology of cancer invasion and metastasis. Adv Cancer Res 1978;28:149–250.
52. Nicolson GL. Organ specificity of tumor metastasis: role of preferential adhesion, invasion and growth of malignant cells at specific secondary sites. Cancer Metastasis Rev 1988;7:143–188.
53. Zebrowski BK, Yano S, Liu W, et al. Vascular endothelial growth factor levels and induction of permeability in malignant pleural effusions. Clin Cancer Res 1999;5:3364–3368.
54. Zetter BR. Angiogenesis and tumor metastasis. Annu Rev Med 1998;49:407–424.
55. Dvorak HF, Nagy JA, Dvorak JT, Dvorak AM. Identification and characterization of the blood vessels of solid tumors that are leaky to circulating macromolecules. Am J Pathol 1988;133: 95–109.
56. Liotta LA, Tryggvason K, Garbisa S, Hart I, Foltz CM, Shafie S. Metastatic potential correlates with enzymatic degradation of basement membrane collagen. Nature 1980; 284:67–68.
57. Chang YS, di Tomaso E, McDonald DM, Jones R, Jain RK, Munn LL. Mosaic blood vessels in tumors: frequency of cancer cells in contact with flowing blood. Proc Natl Acad Sci USA 2000;97:14608–14613.
58. Chambers AF. The metastatic process: basic research and clinical implications. Oncol Res 1999;11:161–168.
59. Herbst RS, Hidalgo M, Pierson AS, Holden SN, Bergen M, Eckhardt SG. Angiogenesis inhibitors in clinical development for lung cancer. Semin Oncol 2002;29:66–77.
60. Folkman J, Watson K, Ingber D, Hanahan D. Induction of angiogenesis during the transition from hyperplasia to neoplasia. Nature 1989;339: 58–61.
61. Bergers G, Javaherian K, Lo KM, Folkman J, Hanahan D. Effects of angiogenesis inhibitors on multistage carcinogenesis in mice. Science 1999:284:808–812.
62. St Croix B, Rago C, Velculescu V, et al. Genes expressed in human tumor endothelium. Science 2000;289:1197–1202.

63. Wedge SR, Ogilvie DJ, Dukes M, et al. ZD6474 inhibits vascular endothelial growth factor signaling, angiogenesis, and tumor growth following oral administration. Cancer Res 2002; 62:4645–4655.
64. Fong TA, Shawver LK, Sun L, et al. SU5416 is a potent and selective inhibitor of the vascular endothelial growth factor receptor (Flk-1/KDR) that inhibits tyrosine kinase catalysis, tumor vascularization, and growth of multiple tumor types. Cancer Res 1999;59:99–106.
65. Wood JM, Bold G, Buchdunger E, et al. PTK787/ZK 222584, a novel and potent inhibitor of vascular endothelial growth factor receptor tyrosine kinases, impairs vascular endothelial growth factor-induced responses and tumor growth after oral administration. Cancer Res 2000;60:2178–2189.
66. Lin R, LeCouter J, Kowalski J, Ferrara N. Characterization of endocrine gland-derived vascular endothelial growth factor signaling in adrenal cortex capillary endothelial cells. J Biol Chem 2002;277:8724–8729.
67. Arap W, Kolonin MG, Trepel M, et al. Steps toward mapping the human vasculature by phage display. Nat Med 2002;8:121–127.
68. Boehm T, Folkman J, Browder T, O'Reilly MS. Antiangiogenic therapy of experimental cancer does not induce acquired drug resistance. Nature 1997;390:404–407.
69. Yu JL, Rak JW, Coomber BL, Hicklin DJ, Kerbel RS. Effect of p53 status on tumor response to antiangiogenic therapy. Science 2002;295:1526–1528.
70. Jain RK. Normalizing tumor vasculature with anti-angiogenic therapy: a new paradigm for combination therapy. Nat Med 2001;7:987–989.
71. DeVore RF, Fehrenbacher L, Herbst RS, et al. A randomized phase II trial comparing Rhumab VEGF (recombinant humanized monoclonal antibody to vascular endothelial cell growth factor) plus carboplatin/paclitaxel (CP) to CP alone in patients with stage IIIB/IV NSCLC. Proc Am Soc Clin Oncol 2000;19:1896.
72. Kuenen BC, Rosen L, Smit EF, et al. Dose-finding and pharmacokinetic study of cisplatin, gemcitabine, and SU5416 in patients with solid tumors. J Clin Oncol 2002;20:1657–1667.
73. Kerbel R, Folkman J. Clinical translation of angiogenesis inhibitors. Nature Rev 2002;2: 727–739.
74. Ciardiello F, Caputo R, Bianco R, et al. Inhibition of growth factor production and angiogenesis in human cancer cells by ZD1839 (Iressa), a selective epidermal growth factor receptor tyrosine kinase inhibitor. Clin Cancer Res 2001; 7:1459–1465.
75. Brouty-Boye D, Zetter BR. Inhibition of cell motility by interferon. Science 1980;208:516–518.
76. Maione TE, Gray GS, Petro J, et al. Inhibition of angiogenesis by recombinant human platelet factor-4 and related peptides. Science 1990;247: 77–79.
77. Rastinejad F, Polverini PJ, Bouck NP. Regulation of the activity of a new inhibitor of angiogenesis by a cancer suppressor gene. Cell 1989; 56:345–355.
78. Bouck N. Tumor angiogenesis: the role of oncogenes and tumor suppressor genes. Cancer Cells 1990;2:179–185.
79. O'Reilly MS, Holmgren L, Shing Y, et al. Angiostatin: a novel angiogenesis inhibitor that mediates the suppression of metastases by a Lewis lung carcinoma. Cell 1994;79:315–328.
80. Mauceri HJ, Hanna NN, Beckett MA, et al. Combined effects of angiostatin and ionizing radiation in antitumour therapy. Nature 1998; 394:287–291.
81. O'Reilly MS, Boehm T, Shing Y, et al. Endostatin: an endogenous inhibitor of angiogenesis and tumor growth. Cell 1997;88:277–285.
82. Maeshima Y, Colorado PC, Torre A, et al. Distinct antitumor properties of a type IV collagen domain derived from basement membrane. J Biol Chem 2000;275:21340–21348.
83. Kamphaus GD, Colorado PC, Panka DJ, et al. Canstatin, a novel matrix-derived inhibitor of angiogenesis and tumor growth. J Biol Chem 2000;275:1209–1215.
84. O'Reilly MS, Pirie-Shepherd S, Lane WS, Folkman J. Antiangiogenic activity of the cleaved conformation of the serpin antithrombin. Science 1999;285:1926–1928.
85. Herbst RS, Tran HT, Mullani NA, et al. Phase I clinical trial of recombinant human endostatin (rHE) in patients (Pts) with solid tumors: pharmacokinetic (PK), safety and efficacy analysis using surrogate endpoints of tissue and radiologic response. Proc Am Soc Clin Oncol 2001; 20:9.
86. Eder JP Jr, Supko JG, Clark JW, et al. Phase I clinical trial of recombinant human endostatin administered as a short intravenous infusion repeated daily. J Clin Oncol 2002;20:3772–3784.
87. Fontanini G, Vignati S, Boldrini L, et al. Vascular endothelial growth factor is associated with neovascularization and influences progression

of non-small cell lung carcinoma. Clin Cancer Res 1997;3:861–865.
88. Yuan A, Yu CJ, Chen WJ, et al. Correlation of total VEGF mRNA and protein expression with histologic type, tumor angiogenesis, patient survival and timing of relapse in non-small-cell lung cancer. Int J Cancer 2000;89: 475–483.
89. George DJ, Halabi S, Shepard TF, et al. Prognostic significance of plasma vascular endothelial growth factor levels in patients with hormone-refractory prostate cancer treated on Cancer and Leukemia Group B 9480. Clin Cancer Res 2001;7:1932–1936.
90. Gasparini G. Prognostic value of vascular endothelial growth factor in breast cancer. Oncologist 2000;5(suppl 1):37–44.
91. Rak J, Mitsuhashi Y, Bayko L, et al. Mutant ras oncogenes upregulate VEGF/VPF expression: implications for induction and inhibition of tumor angiogenesis. Cancer Res 1995;55:4575–4580.
92. Kerbel RS, Viloria-Petit A, Klement G, Rak J. 'Accidental' anti-angiogenic drugs. anti-oncogene directed signal transduction inhibitors and conventional chemotherapeutic agents as examples. Eur J Cancer 2000;36:1248–1257.
93. Yang JC, Haworth L, Steinberg SM, Rosenberg SA, Novotny W. A randomized double-blind placebo-controlled trial of bevacizumab (anti-VEGF antibody) demonstrating a prolongation in time to progression in patients with metastatic renal cancer. NEJM 2003;349(5): 427–434.
94. Kabbinavar F, Hurwitz HI, Fehrenbacher L, et al. Phase II, randomized trial comparing bevacizumab plus fluorouracil (FU)/leucovorin (LV) with FU/LV alone in patients with metastatic colorectal cancer. J Clin Oncol 2003; 21:60–65.
95. Kuenen BC, Levi M, Meijers JC, et al. Analysis of coagulation cascade and endothelial cell activation during inhibition of vascular endothelial growth factor/vascular endothelial growth factor receptor pathway in cancer patients. Arterioscler Thromb Vasc Biol 2002;22:1500–1505.
96. Miller KD, Sweeney CJ, Sledge GW Jr. Redefining the target: chemotherapeutics as antiangiogenics. J Clin Oncol 2001;19:1195–1206.
97. Denekamp J. Inadequate vasculature in solid tumours: consequences for cancer research strategies. BJR Suppl 1992;24:111–117.
98. Reinhold HS, Endrich B. Tumour microcirculation as a target for hyperthermia. Int J Hyperthermia 1986;2:111–137.
99. Browder T, Butterfield CE, Kraling BM, et al. Antiangiogenic scheduling of chemotherapy improves efficacy against experimental drug-resistant cancer. Cancer Res 2000;60:1878–1886.
100. Paris F, Fuks Z, Kang A, et al. Endothelial apoptosis as the primary lesion initiating intestinal radiation damage in mice. Science 2001;293:293–297.
101. Gorski DH, Beckett MA, Jaskowiak NT, et al. Blockage of the vascular endothelial growth factor stress response increases the antitumor effects of ionizing radiation. Cancer Res 1999; 59:3374–3378.
102. Belotti D, Vergani V, Drudis T, et al. The microtubule-affecting drug paclitaxel has antiangiogenic activity. Clin Cancer Res 1996; 2:1843–1849.
103. Klauber N, Parangi S, Flynn E, Hamel E, D'Amato RJ. Inhibition of angiogenesis and breast cancer in mice by the microtubule inhibitors 2-methoxyestradiol and taxol. Cancer Res 1997;57:81–86.
104. Lau DH, Xue L, Young LJ, Burke PA, Cheung AT. Paclitaxel (Taxol): an inhibitor of angiogenesis in a highly vascularized transgenic breast cancer. Cancer Biother Radiopharm 1999;14:31–36.
105. Vacca A, Ribatti D, Iurlaro M, et al. Docetaxel versus Paclitaxel for antiangiogenesis. J Hematother Stem Cell Res 2002;11:103–118.
106. Sweeney CJ, Miller KD, Sissons SE, et al. The antiangiogenic property of docetaxel is synergistic with a recombinant humanized monoclonal antibody against vascular endothelial growth factor or 2-methoxyestradiol but antagonized by endothelial growth factors. Cancer Res 2001;61:3369–3372.
107. Vacca A, Iurlaro M, Ribatti D, et al. Antiangiogenesis is produced by nontoxic doses of vinblastine. Blood 1999;94:4143–4155.
108. Klement G, Huang P, Mayer B, et al. Differences in therapeutic indexes of combination metronomic chemotherapy and an anti-VEGFR-2 antibody in multidrug-resistant human breast cancer xenografts. Clin Cancer Res 2002;8:221–232.
109. Wang J, Lou P, Lesniewski R, Henkin J. Paclitaxel at ultra low concentrations inhibits angiogenesis without affecting cellular microtubule assembly. Anticancer Drugs 2003;14:13–19.

110. Tran J, Master Z, Yu JL, Rak J, Dumont DJ, Kerbel RS. A role for surviving in chemoresistance of endothelial cells mediated by VEGF. Proc Natl Acad Sci USA 2002;99:4349–4354.
111. Song CW, Kang MS, Rhee JG, Levitt SH. Effect of hyperthermia on vascular function in normal and neoplastic tissues. Ann NY Acad Sci 1980; 335:35–47.
112. Song CW, Kang MS, Rhee JG, Levitt SH. Vascular damage and delayed cell death in tumours after hyperthermia. Br J Cancer 1980;41:309–312.
113. Fajardo LF, Egbert B, Marmor J, Hahn GM. Effects of hyperthermia in a malignant tumor. Cancer 1980;45:613–623.
114. Fajardo LF, Prionas SD, Kowalski J, Kwan HH. Hyperthermia inhibits angiogenesis. Radiat Res 1988;114:297–306.
115. Eikesdal HP, Bjorkhaug ST, Dahl O. Hyperthermia exhibits anti-vascular activity in the s.c. BT4An rat glioma: lack of interaction with the angiogenesis inhibitor batimastat. Int J Hyperthermia 2002;18:141–152.
116. Nishimura Y, Hiraoka M, Jo S, et al. Microangiographic and histologic analysis of the effects of hyperthermia on murine tumor vasculature. Int J Radiat Oncol Biol Phys 1988;15:411–420.
117. Badylak SF, Babbs CF, Skojac TM, Voorhees WD, Richardson RC. Hyperthermia-induced vascular injury in normal and neoplastic tissue. Cancer 1985;56:991–1000.
118. Song CW. Effect of hyperthermia on vascular functions of normal tissues and experimental tumors; brief communication. J Natl Cancer Inst 1978;60:711–713.
119. Fajardo LF, Prionas SD. Endothelial cells and hyperthermia. Int J Hyperthermia 1994;10: 347–353.
120. Kanamori S, Nishimura Y, Okuno Y, Horii N, Saga T, Hiraoka M. Induction of vascular endothelial growth factor (VEGF) by hyperthermia and/or an angiogenesis inhibitor. Int J Hyperthermia 1999;15:267–278.
121. Ikeda S, Akagi K, Shiraishi T, Tanaka Y. Enhancement of the effect of an angiogenesis inhibitor on murine tumors by hyperthermia. Oncol Rep 1998;5:181–184.
122. Nishimura Y, Murata R, Hiraoka M. Combined effects of an angiogenesis inhibitor (TNP-470) and hyperthermia. Br J Cancer 1996;73:270–274.
123. Yano T, Tanase M, Watanabe A, et al. Enhancement effect of an anti-angiogenic agent, TNP-470, on hyperthermia-induced growth suppression of human esophageal and gastric cancers transplantable to nude mice. Anticancer Res 1995;15:1355–1358.

Section II
Operations for Tumor Ablation

5 Image-Guided Tumor Ablation: How to Build a Practice

Gary Onik

Integrating the occasional tumor ablation procedure into a thriving radiology practice is not a particularly difficult job. Patient preoperative workup, billing, and patient follow-up need not change from the usual handling of other interventional radiology or cross-sectional imaging patients. If the intent, however, is to build a large, thriving tumor ablation service, many issues need to be addressed if the venture is to be successful, without placing undue time and financial burden on a radiology practice. My practice is image-guided tumor ablation exclusively, and therefore this chapter focuses on problems and pitfalls associated with building a successful tumor ablation practice.

Many concepts in this chapter are a work in progress, since many difficult issues have yet to be satisfactorily resolved. There are two major subject areas to be addressed when growing such an ablation practice: acquiring the patients, and receiving adequate reimbursement to make the effort worthwhile. It is truly problematic to lose money on the treatment of each patient, while trying to make up for the shortfall in income with the increased volume as the ablation practice grows. We will first discuss the ins and outs of building the ablation practice, and then address the more difficult aspect of adequate reimbursement.

Getting Started

The most basic step in starting an ablation practice is to become an expert in the overall management of the cancer you will be treating. When I first started treating prostate cancer, I had an enormous amount of information to digest about the treatment of the disease. Since the most useful prostate imaging modality, transrectal ultrasound, is generally carried out by urologists, I, as with most radiologists, had little experience with this organ or modality. Except for reading the occasional prostate magnetic resonance imaging (MRI) or perusing a bone scan to rule out prostate metastasis, radiologists have few instances in which knowledge of the clinical and pathologic aspects of prostate cancer is relevant.

It was not until I started actively managing these patients myself that I found it necessary to become conversant with the patient selection for the various prostate cancer treatments, the significance of both staging and pathologic grading of prostate cancer, the benchmark success rates, and the possible outcomes and complications of alternative procedures. Without that knowledge it was impossible to give adequate information to patients as to how this new ablation treatment fit into treatment options. In addition, since there was now competition from other physicians practicing more traditional prostate cancer therapies, I had to defend the right to treat these patients in one forum or another (the institutional review board [IRB] or the committee overseeing privileges). Only by having a firm grasp of prostate cancer was I able to expose the weaknesses in the arguments of those trying to defend their turf. Secondarily, my ability to converse in the "language" of prostate cancer markedly increased my credibility with referring primary physicians and sophisticated patients, who are extremely well informed through the Internet.

Along with the need to become broadly clinically proficient, a commitment to establish an "ablation clinic" almost certainly will have to be made. In this clinic, patients will be seen for their preprocedure evaluation, given informed consent forms, and perhaps even undergoing a problem-directed physical exam prior to scheduling the procedure. Doing a procedure on the same day as seeing the patient for the first time should be avoided, since it does not allow development of an adequate physician–patient relationship. This relationship is critical to help defend malpractice suits when an inevitable ablation complication occurs.

A decision also has to be made at the outset as to whether to practice alone or establish a team approach with the other specialties at your institution. Such an approach would be akin to the Miami Vascular Institute concept so successfully instituted by Dr. Barry Katzen.

Establishing, for instance, a liver cancer institute in which the medical and surgical oncologists are represented has certain advantages, and has the potential to provide more coordinated and therefore superior patient care. Such an approach can simplify political issues, widen the scope of the patients to be treated (doing intraoperative ablations with surgical oncologists), and provide collegial backup for the complications that may occur. Take for instance the treatment of patients with liver metastasis from colon carcinoma. In our experience, an overwhelming number of patients in this situation will not be amenable to a percutaneous ablation therapy in the radiology department. Limiting factors to treating patients with a percutaneous approach include too many lesions, lesions that are too large, and a lesion adjacent to a structure that is at risk for thermal injury, such as bowel. Many of these patients, however, can be treated in an intraoperative environment that allows larger ablations or even resection combined with ablation. A good case can be made that since intraoperative (maybe even laparoscopic) ultrasound is still the most sensitive means to find lesions in these patients, the best overall outcome can be obtained by treating these unsuspected lesions as early as possible before they appear on nonoperative cross-sectional imaging.

Another factor is that at least one recent study has shown a survival advantage in treating hepatic resection patients with adjuvant long-term intraarterial infusional chemotherapy delivered by implantable pump combined with systemic chemotherapy (1). We found it a compelling argument that the same advantage would be realized in ablation patients as well. Since almost all of our patients are going to have at least a minilaparotomy for the pump placement, it makes sense to do an intraoperative ultrasound and ablation at the same time. In practicality, in our team approach, after the laparotomy is performed, the radiologist is called in to carry out the intraoperative ultrasound. Decisions are made jointly between surgeons and radiologists as to which lesions will be resected and which will be ablated. The pump is placed, any lesions to be resected are carried out first, since radiofrequency ablation (RFA) or cryosurgery can increase clotting times and decrease platelet counts, and then the radiologist is called back to do the ablation. In other words, if a real commitment is going to made to a liver ablation program, it is almost inevitable that radiologists will have to do some work intraoperatively and interact on a coordinated basis with both medical and surgical oncologists.

Another decision that needs to be dealt with when starting a program is the choice of ablation equipment. Since each ablation method has its own advantages and disadvantages, having both RFA and cryosurgery available can be advantageous. There is much hype and misinformation in the marketplace as to lesion size, shape, etc. created by the various RF systems. At the very least, a side-by-side comparison of the three systems that are currently available should be carried out. Whenever I am evaluating new ablation technology, I use a large rump roast as my experimental model. The relative size and shape, as well as time needed to make the lesion, will all become clear as the lesions are created with the various systems.

The final consideration when starting the program is data collection. Clinical data are the currency by which the program will grow and gain legitimacy. As soon as the program is started, therefore, a database should be initiated in which the patient's clinical, procedural, and postprocedure data are entered prospectively. With such a database, valuable information will be sure to be collected on every patient, with the result that patients are far less likely to be lost to follow-up, and trends that affect patient care such as local recurrence rates will be tracked without fail. Such a database also allows new patients to know when the test results can be expected. If the results are available sooner than those reported by more traditional treatment, your practice will be in a good position in competing for patients. Also, without this prospective data collection, it is much less likely that your data will be published, since nothing cools the ardor for writing like the thought of poring though a huge stack of charts to extract data.

Growing the Practice

The traditional model of growing a specialty practice by patient referral from local practicing physicians is undergoing a revolution, as patients gain more access to information through the Internet, patient support groups, and the media. More and more patients are supplementing the information their physician gives them with information from these sources, and are taking more responsibility for the ultimate treatment decisions. The greater acceptance of alternative medicine also has made patients more receptive to newer treatments if they are properly informed. A physician wishing to build a tumor ablation practice beyond the occasional liver ablation will eventually have to address the issue of direct patient marketing.

Sources of Local Patients

As already stated, a team approach that provides comprehensive cancer care is a foundation for building the practice and for attracting referrals for ablation, particularly when clinicians learn that ablation therapy does not preclude traditional therapy, but rather often augments it.

Initially, when starting the program other noninterventional members of the radiology department should be informed of the cases that would be amenable for treatment. The "ablationist" can then contact the referring physician to explain that a new treatment modality is available. This is the single most effective means of initially gaining access to the local patient population.

The Internet

If the most important mantra for the real estate industry is "location, location, location", then the equivalent for building an ablation practice is "the Internet, the Internet, the Internet". The Internet is revolutionizing the delivery of medical care. For the first time, patients have ready access to health information without the physician being the filter. It is therefore much more likely that a patient will learn of an emerging treatment. Coupled with a growing skepticism of the medical profession and a growing acceptance of alternative medical treatments, it follows that patients can research their own illness through the Internet and choose newer treatments despite a negative bias of their treating physician. The impact that this can have on an ablation practice can be enormous. About 75% of patients that I treat have learned of tumor ablation through the Internet, and have heard about my practice on the Internet. But on the downside, clinicians become more motivated to improve the delivery of patient care because they realize that a disgruntled patient can reach the whole world by posting on patient-oriented Web sites and disease-specific patient chat rooms negative comments about your lack of expertise, poor bedside manner, and bad breath.

Don't skimp on the development of an engaging and informative Web site; this is a job for a professional. Usually, your institution can be counted on to contribute significantly to this endeavor if its name is prominently displayed and incorporated into the site. Once the Web site is up and running, it is important to hire a professional to maintain it and to continually improve its visibility among the various search engines. How search engines rank their various results is critical. The Web site consultant should be included in the process of choosing the site name and Internet address, as these are important for a successful ranking. An ongoing fee will have to be paid to this consultant to maintain the Web site, explore links to advantageous sites, continually monitor the Web site activity, and make adjustments to maintain your ranking.

We get a monthly report of Internet traffic at our site and on our ranking, based on various key words for the different search engines. One can fall from a number one or two ranking in a key area on a major search engine to number ten within less than a week. On a practical level, we all save time and money by referring interested patients for more information to the Web site first, rather than sending out expensive brochures. On a cost versus benefit basis, a good Web site has great value.

The Media

As someone who has the dubious distinction of having had two articles written about his work in the tabloid press, I feel like an expert on the positive and negative aspect of media exposure. Just to set the record straight, the standard of journalism associated with medical reporting in the tabloid paper was among the highest I have encountered, with all facts being checked and the final article being read back to me before publication to verify its accuracy. This is a standard I have found lacking in other more prestigious outlets.

At the very least, the local media should be contacted (with the help of the hospital public relations department), announcing the start of the ablation program and the implications for medical care in the community. Often, the company that sells the ablation equipment will have a media program that helps gain local exposure. I was chagrined recently to find competitors across town being hailed by the local newspaper as "pioneers in this new cancer treatment", after they treated just one case. If you desire national media exposure, the only reliable avenue is through publication of an article in a media-recognized journal (*JAMA*, *New England Journal of Medicine*, or a subspecialty journal) or presentation of an abstract at a major meeting such as the Radiological Society of North America (RSNA). Some of the best media exposure has occurred through the excellent work of the RSNA public relations staff, which organizes press releases and press conferences based on abstracts presented at the meeting.

Media exposure can be a double-edged sword, however, particularly if the topic is considered controversial and has opponents in the particular subspecialty of the traditional treatment. Any major national program will seek out and present the negative view of your treatment from a well-known "expert" in the field. This expert usually has a vested interest in seeing that your new ablation procedure is considered about as credible as reading the bumps on a patient's head to diagnosis prostate cancer, and will undoubtedly cast a negative light on this new major treatment advance. The worst media experience I had was engineered by a prominent orthopedic surgeon who was vehemently opposed to a new procedure I had invented that was capturing a lot of attention at the time (percutaneous discectomy). Unfortunately, he had a friend who was a producer at a major television network whom he was able to convince that percutaneous discectomy was an untested procedure that was being foisted on an unsuspecting public for purely financial gain. This was despite its approval from the National Blue Cross/Blue Shield Technology Assessment Committee, and the rigorous review it had undergone. No amount of contrary information we provided was going to change the slant of that story. On the whole, though, national media exposure can have a dramatic positive impact on an ablation practice, and should be pursued if at all feasible.

There is another strategy for large-scale nationwide exposure. Most local news stations don't have the time, expertise, or money to develop medical news content. Therefore, they are amenable to using any credible content that is provided to them in a form that can be tailored to their needs. Television production companies will produce a news segment in its appropriate form to be sent to local news affiliates across the country. The local affiliates then take the footage provided and add their own commentary. This is an expensive option, but it usually produces significant results.

Payment

Dealing with Current Procedural Terminology (CPT) codes are beyond the scope of this chapter, but proper planning can have a major impact on the financial viability of an ablation program. The reimbursement provided by standard insurance contracts for ablation procedures is poor. If balance billing is precluded by the radiology group's contract, then certain ablation procedures may become financially unfeasible. If an attempt to grow an ablation program is being planned, an effort should be made to carve tumor ablation out of the contract, to at least allow balance billing. Ironically, the financial environment is often much better when cash payment is possible, before the approval of a procedure with a CPT code. For instance, the approval of prostate cryosurgery by Medicare has set reimbursement so low as to make performance of the procedure barely viable financially, if at all. Many patients would gladly pay cash to be treated, but federal law prohibits this approach.

Conclusion

Image-guided tumor ablation is going to have a major impact on the practice of oncology in the future. As with any new image-guided treatment, radiologists will have to rapidly enter the field to prevent it from being usurped by other specialties. As already stated, a cooperative approach with the other oncology subspecialties can offer advantages, but radiologists should be aware that ultimately an independent flow of patients directly to the practice is the only assurance of a viable long-term program.

Reference

1. Kemeny N, Huang Y, Cohen AM, et al. Hepatic arterial infusion of chemotherapy after resection of hepatic metastases from colorectal cancer. N Engl J Med 1999;341(27):2039–2047.

6 Anesthesia for Ablation

John A. Fox and Alan M. Harvey

This chapter provides a short primer on anesthesiology for clinicians who are involved in the care of tumor ablation patients, but who have not been trained in one of the surgical subspecialties. Anesthesiologists, in the role of pain treatment specialists, have long been asked to care for patients with metastatic tumors; the role of anesthesiologists in tumor ablation therapy represents a continuation of a recent trend that has seen anesthesiologists perform their conventional services (i.e., to make the patient insensible to pain) in areas outside of the operating room. Anesthesiologists have expanded their roles in the past several years in angiography, endoscopy, and magnetic resonance imaging (MRI)-guided surgical suites, in which they interact with physician and nonphysician personnel who are as unfamiliar with what the anesthesiologist needs to deliver patient care as the anesthesiologist is with the needs of the team members in these non–operating-room settings. Many other chapters in this book discuss the goals of the tumor ablation team. This chapter discusses the goals of the anesthesiologist. Thus, this chapter will be as instructive for interventional radiologists as the remaining chapters were for us, the anesthesiologists.

Advantages of Anesthesiology Involvement

The role of the anesthesiologist in tumor ablation therapy is to facilitate patient safety and patient satisfaction.

First, patients with more extensive tumors can be selected for treatment. During tumor ablation using computed tomography (CT) or MRI guidance, the interventional radiologist is involved in a myriad of tasks to localize the lesion, accurately place the device delivering the treatment, and then monitor the treatment results. Each of these tasks requires numerous careful steps often coupled with multiple scans; the attention of the interventionalist is, of necessity, on these steps and scans. In patients with significant cardiopulmonary disease, it may be inappropriate to assign the task of vital sign monitoring to nonphysician personnel. Additionally, should any complication occur, all anesthesiologists, who, by the nature of their subspecialty, are already experts in the "airway" section of Advanced Cardiac Life Support, would already be present, on site, to treat airway events and to assist in the treatment of cardiac events.

Second, anesthesiology has made a point of emphasizing patient safety in its practice. Accordingly, it has advocated the use of physiologic monitors and practice standards, and it encourages discussing ways of improving patient outcomes. These attributes can serve as a guide for the interventional radiologist when initiating and evaluating the safety and results of a tumor ablation program.

Third, the presence of an anesthesiologist in the care of the tumor ablation patient ensures that the patient will have minimal pain during the procedure. In most hospitals, anesthesiologists are the only clinicians who can supersede the sedative and narcotic dosage outlined in conscious sedation protocols and have the familiarity with the pharmacology of these medications to adjust the dosage according to the patient's prior medical condition. Specifically, tumor patients will often be on other medications that could increase their resistance to standard doses of pain medications. In patients who have large tumors that would require multiple treatments, this could lead to increased patient satisfaction by minimizing the anxiety of the patient about repeated visits and treatments.

Fourth, tumor ablation therapy outside of the operating room is, in most institutions, a new program involving new equipment and new treatment plans. Inherent in new programs are unforeseen equipment and patient issues that may entail prolonged periods of time in which the patient must lie still in the CT or MRI tube. Active participation by an anesthesiologist would allow the treatment plan to be carried out in a safe, painless, and expeditious way.

Disadvantages of Anesthesiology Involvement

Involving an anesthesiologist in the care of the tumor ablation patient increases the logistics of care before, during, and after the procedure, and thereby adds costs to the program. But the increase in patient safety and patient satisfaction, along with the ability to care for patients with more complex conditions, should offset this cost to the hospital with increased patient volume and safer practices.

Once an anesthesiologist is consulted, specific guidelines toward the care of the patient must be met. These guidelines, codified by the American Society of Anesthesiology, describe components for (a) a preoperative visit, (b) physiologic monitoring during the anesthesia, (c) a proper postanesthesia care unit for recovery, and (d) a postoperative visit (1). Failure to meet these guidelines would be unsafe for the patient and would subject the anesthesiology practitioner to the risk of malpractice claims. If proper planning has not incorporated these requirements for anesthesia care, the treatment plan may be canceled for the day or be significantly delayed. If the care is to be in the CT or MRI suite, this could lead to long waits by other patients needing the scanners, the waste of valuable technician time, and other costly inefficiencies.

Additionally an anesthesiology department needs to allocate an individual to administer the anesthesia during the ablation procedure. Of necessity this requires that the individual not be available for the care of other patients in the practice, and, depending on the clinical load of the hospital, may require recruitment and hiring of additional anesthesiology practitioners.

Anesthesia Standards

Preoperative Visit

The preoperative visit serves several purposes and is the standard of care in the preoperative preparation of the patient (2). On either the day of the procedure or, ideally, several days before the anticipated procedure, the anesthesia options are explained to the patient and consent for the anesthesia is signed. A history is taken and a physical examination is performed, both focusing on the anesthesia priorities. The findings are documented, as is the need for the patient to fast for 6 to 8 hours before the anesthesia (3). Overall, the preanesthesia interview addresses the following disease areas, which can be included by the ablation team in its routine interview. This would ensure that patients who are potentially an anesthesia risk would be identified for further consultation by the anesthesia team.

Cardiovascular Disease

Cardiovascular disease is a risk factor for complications in patients who are undergoing anesthesia; therefore, any questions that would elicit a cardiovascular problem would be appropriate in the initial history. Although this may include atherosclerotic stroke, hypertension, or claudication, the patients at highest risk for cardiovascular complications are those who are either in congestive heart failure at the time of procedure or who had a myocardial infarction within the past 6 months. Accordingly, questions about these conditions need to be asked, and if the anesthesiologist indicates that the patient is at high risk for a cardiac event, then one should consider whether the benefits of the procedure are warranted. Other comorbid conditions that are markers for cardiovascular disease, such as diabetes and hypercholesterolemia, also should be noted (4).

Pulmonary Disease

A history of shortness of breath, smoking, bronchospastic pulmonary disease (asthma) or documented chronic obstructive pulmonary disease will lead the clinician or anesthesiologist to document if the patient can withstand positioning for the tumor ablation. This history would also guide the anesthesiologist in deciding whether other pulmonary function tests and other preoperative preparations of the patient are indicated. Patients with an acute upper respiratory infection may be well served by having their procedure postponed until this acute event resolves. It is essential to identify any reversible component of bronchospastic disease so that proper treatment may be initiated preoperatively and continued intra- and postoperatively.

Anesthesia History

Many patients give a history of problems during their prior anesthesias. These may include a history of severe nausea and vomiting postanesthesia in which the treatment would include use of antiemetics (ondansetron, ephedrine, metoclopramide) in the perioperative period or of using of anesthesia agents that are purported to produce less nausea. Some patients give a history of other severe reactions to anesthesia, such as cardiac or respiratory arrest. In this case, obtaining the old anesthesia record documenting this problem would help in avoiding this situation, whatever the cause.

Finally, there is a rare genetic disorder, triggered by many anesthesia drugs, called malignant hyperthermia. This condition, caused by a disorder of calcium metabolism in the skeletal muscle, causes a hypercontractile state of the muscle that results in high fever, increased carbon dioxide production, and potential life-threatening arrhythmias. With prompt treatment with the calcium blocker dantrolene, which should be available wherever anesthesia is being administered, malignant hyperthermia can be stopped. Every institution in which anesthesia is given should have a protocol and a kit readily available for the quick treatment of this rare but potentially life-threatening disorder.

History and Physical Examination of the Airway

The anesthesiologist is best qualified to determine by physical examination if a patient has an abnormal airway that would lead to problems with ventilation once anesthesia is administered. All anesthesiologists view a history of prior airway problems as significant. Specifically, this includes a history of difficult intubation, a history of mandibular or neck surgery in which range of motion of the neck could potentially be decreased, or a history of sleep apnea. In the case of sleep apnea, it may be difficult to ventilate the patient by mask or to secure the airway by an endotracheal tube once airway reflexes are lost. Here, special precautions to secure the airway in an awake patient may be needed.

In terms of physical examination, anesthesiologists look at the length of the mandible (patients with smaller mandibles are more difficult to intubate), the distance between the mandible and the hyoid bone (smaller distances are more difficult to intubate), and a grading of the view of the hypopharynx when the patient opens the mouth. If there is a large tongue and no view of the soft palate and the epiglottis, this patient is at higher risk for a difficult intubation than are patients with an unencumbered view of the hypopharynx.

The American Society of Anesthesiology has specific recommendations for the potentially difficult airway (5).

Monitoring During the Procedure

The American Society of Anesthesiology codified intraoperative monitoring for all anesthesias about 20 years ago, with a revision in 1998 (6). Monitoring includes a continuous display of electrocardiogram (ECG), checking blood pressure at least every 5 minutes while the anesthesia is in progress, and a measure of respiratory function. As of 2003, this includes a method of capnography and pulse oximetery for every patient. Finally, an individual trained in the administration of anesthesia medications should be continuously present throughout the anesthesia. When asking an anesthesia team member to be included in the care of the tumor ablation patient, these monitors will need to be included in the anesthetizing site.

Postanesthesia Care Unit

The postanesthesia care unit, where patients recover from their anesthesia, has been shown to decrease anesthesia morbidity and mortality. In this area, personnel who have advanced airway training are available should respiratory difficulties arise. Additionally, this area provides a place where additional tests such as postprocedure chest x-rays, ECG, or blood work can be performed. Discharge from this area should be after examination by the anesthesiologist or by the patient meeting protocol criteria for discharge.

Postoperative Visit

The postoperative visit provides a mechanism whereby the patient can give feedback to the anesthesiologist on the conduct of the procedure and anesthesia. During the visit, potential problems routinely discussed are the event of recall during the procedure, nerve injuries due to positioning, or other reasons for patient dissatisfaction with the procedure. Pain relief during the procedure and immediately postoperation are frequently reviewed for continuous quality improvement.

Pain of the Procedure and the Selection of Anesthesia Techniques

The administration of anesthesia involves assessing the patient's preexisting pain and anxiety from the medical condition, the pain of the procedure itself, and the amount of postoperative pain expected. The level of anesthesia is balanced with the stimulus of the procedure.

In analyzing the stimulus for liver tumor ablation, there is a body wall component of somatic pain, extending from T5 to T9 skin dermatomes, where the needles are passed through the skin, which can be well anesthetized by a long-acting local anesthetic in all patients for patient comfort. Even if the patient is under general anesthesia, the routine use of a skin local anesthetic is encouraged, as this reduces the somatic stimuli of the procedure, allows lower levels of anesthetic agents, and may allow quicker wake-up. Local anesthetic supplementation may result in less postoperative pain, thus increasing patient satisfaction and facilitating discharge.

The visceral pain pathways transmit stimuli from the liver and upper abdominal organs during tumor ablation procedures. Visceral pain is described as a diffuse, dull, aching, cramping-type pain (7). The celiac plexus innervates most of the abdominal viscera, including the stomach, liver, biliary tract, pancreas, spleen, kidneys, adrenals, omentum, and small and large bowel. According to most standard anatomic textbooks, there are three splanchnic nerves—great, lesser, and least (8). The great splanchnic nerve arises from the roots of T5 or T6 to T9 or T10, runs paravertebrally into the thorax, through the crus of the diaphragm to enter the abdominal cavity, and ends in the celiac ganglion on that side. The lesser splanchnic nerve arises from the T10 to T11 segments and passes lateral to, or with the great nerve to the celiac ganglion. It sends postganglionic fibers to the celiac and renal plexuses. The least splanchnic nerve arises from T11 and T12 and passes through the diaphragm to the celiac ganglion. The plexus varies anatomically in relation to the vertebral column from the bottom of T12 to the middle of L2. It is important to emphasize that a celiac plexus block does not provide total anesthesia of all upper abdominal visceral sensation or reflexes. A celiac plexus block may be combined with sedation or light general anesthesia, and with local anesthesia/intercostal nerve blocks for the skin for tumor ablation procedures on the upper abdominal organs.

After needles are inserted, the ablation procedure itself produces painful sensations. Tumors are ablated by radiofrequency, absolute alcohol, and cryotherapy.

Radiofrequency is the heating and destruction of tissues in which a high-frequency alternating current raises the temperature of the tissues beyond 60°C, resulting in a region of necrosis surrounding the electrode. This ultrasonic energy is an intense stimuli that requires greater anesthesia levels during the radiofrequency procedure. The injection of absolute alcohol can induce tumor necrosis and shrinkage by a mechanism of action that involves cytoplasmic dehydration with subsequent coagulation necrosis and a fiberous reaction. Absolute alcohol causes a neurologic and tissue-destructive effect, with significant pain during its administration, thus requiring higher anesthesia levels. Cryotherapy, which involves the formation of an ice ball and ice crystals with necrosis of tissue, stimulates the pain fibers to a lesser extent than the other modalities mentioned. During the time of administration of radiofrequency and absolute alcohol, one may see a rise in pulse rate and blood pressure, indicating a sympathetic response to the stimuli. Deepening of the anesthesia level or control of the hypertension and tachycardia by beta blockade is needed at this point in the anesthesia course.

Many centers have been able to accomplish ablation of liver tumors under local anesthesia for the skin and body wall and intravenous conscious sedation that extends to intravenous general anesthesia for the visceral pain component of the procedure. The requirements of the procedure, however, suggest that the patient should not be moving during the time of needle placement to reduce the risk of pneumothorax or tearing of the liver capsule during needle placement, and to provide clearer imaging. General anesthesia, with securing and control of the airway and respiratory movements, may offer benefits for these liver tumor ablation cases.

Anesthesia for renal tumor ablation is similar to that for liver tumors due to the similar innervation of the kidneys and upper abdominal viscera. It can be accomplished under both general anesthesia and local/intravenous analgesia, progressing to intravenous general anesthesia depending on patient requirements.

Spinal cord metastases and tumors tend to be treated under local anesthesia and lighter sedation, to allow for patient feedback and functional assessment of lesion size during radiofrequency procedures.

Types of Anesthesia

Anesthesia care for tumor ablation can be divided into four types: conscious sedation, monitored anesthesia care, regional anesthesia, and general anesthesia. No hard rules for the type of anesthesia are presented here. Each patient is different, and the best anesthesia plan is one that is tailored to the procedure and the patient's medical condition.

Conscious Sedation

Conscious sedation involves the administration of sedative and pain medication by a practitioner who is not performing the procedure. This practitioner could be a physician or a registered nurse, and the purpose of conscious sedation is to provide the patient with anxiolysis as well as pain medication. All conscious sedation modalities rely on the use of local anesthesias by the interventional radiologist prior to proceeding. Each institution has established training standards for privileges in conscious sedation, which are most likely supervised and written by members of the anesthesiology department. Medications most commonly used for conscious sedation are the shorter-acting benzodiazepines (midazolam) and narcotics (fentanyl) because of their relatively quick onset and quick offset, along with their ability to be reversed by the appropriate medication (flumazenil and naloxone). Most institutions set upper limits on the dosage of conscious sedation medications that can be given by nonanesthesia staff before a consultation by the anesthesiology team is required. Additionally, if the patients have a history of airway complications, a complex medical history, or a history of severe anxiety, most conscious sedation staff will consult their anesthesiology backup prior to proceeding.

Monitored Anesthesia Care

Monitored anesthesia care (MAC) involves a deeper level of sedation. In this type of care, more potent hypnotic medications are used alone or in combination, which could compromise the patient's airway or depress the patient's respiratory drive. Staff who are trained in anesthesia care should be present whenever a MAC is given, and precautions to secure the patient's airway should be taken prior to embarking on this type of anesthesia. Many medications can be used in a MAC from increased doses of narcotics (fentanyl) and benzodiazepenes (midazolam) to the common barbiturate thiopental, or to the newer, shorter acting propofol.

A common philosophical approach is to think in terms of a building block technique in which a base of anxiolysis and sedation is achieved with benzodiazepines (midazolam), a small amount of narcotic (fentanyl) is given for the anticipated discomfort of the positioning and analgesia for the stimulus of the procedure with propofol administration, either as small boluses or drug pump infusion technique as the fine-tuning to decrease patient awareness. By using this building-block technique of short acting drugs with specific selection of doses based on the component of anxiolysis, analgesia, and patient's request for decreased awareness, one is able to more easily maintain the patient's spontaneous respiration without respiratory depression or obstruction.

Regional Anesthesia

Regional anesthesia can be used for liver tumor ablation procedures once one understands the neural pathway of stimulation. Epidural anesthesia can be accomplished with a catheter to control and extend the spread of a local anesthesia agent so that T4-L1 is covered. This would block both the somatic body wall and visceral pain pathways. Spinal anesthesia with hyperbaric local anesthesia to obtain a T4–T5 level also is a possibility. Another regional anesthesia technique is a combination of celiac plexus block for the visceral component of the pain with intercostal nerve block for the body wall and somatic components.

General Anesthesia

General anesthesia, during which the patient is made completely unconscious, requires specialized equipment to administer. The practice of general anesthesia is divided into induction, maintenance, and emergence. Induction agents include intravenous drugs like barbiturates (thiopental or propofol) or etiomidate. Intravenous induction agents are usually more tolerated by the patient. There are conditions in which an inhalational medication may be indicated to induce general anesthesia. These inhalational agents, which are halogenated hydrocarbons, can be either longer acting or shorter acting, but all are given into the lungs and taken up into the brain to produce and maintain unconsciousness. Most of these agents are monitored by the use of end-tidal expiration levels. At the end of the procedure, the patient awakens by cessation of continuous administration of these medications. Given that most patients who undergo tumor ablation therapy will need to have multiple CT or MRI scans, patients who undergo general anesthesias most likely have their airway secured with an endotracheal tube, which provides higher security against aspiration or airway loss while the patient is in the scanner.

When indicated, an anesthesiologist may elect to place a device called a laryngeal mask airway. This tool, which resides in the hypopharynx, can be connected to the anesthesia machine and, during either spontaneous or controlled ventilation, inhalational anesthesia may be given. Laryngeal mask airways do not provide total airway protection, but are easily tolerated by patients. For both endotracheal and laryngeal mask airway anesthetics, end-tidal CO_2 is monitored while the procedure is performed.

Procedure Room Design and Anesthesia Equipment Selection and Checkout

In designing facilities for tumor ablation, it is important to plan for the administration of anesthesia in a way that meets the American Society of Anesthesiologists' guidelines for non–operating-room anesthetizing locations (9,10). The location for the anesthesia machine should have oxygen and suction outlets as well as air outlets for ventilator use. A backup supply of oxygen should include the equivalent of at least a full E cylinder. The key monitors in the administration of anesthesia are an ECG, noninvasive blood pressure (BP) cuff, pulse oximeter, and end-tidal CO_2 capnometry. Sufficient electrical outlets need to be available for these monitors, and there should be a reserve of outlets for other equipment, including clearly labeled outlets connected to an emergency power supply.

As a systems philosophy, the anesthesia workstation should be the same configuration as other anesthetizing locations in the main operating room for ease and comfort of use from a human factor perspective. All anesthesia locations in the operating rooms are set up with the anesthesia machine placed to the right of the patient's head prior to induction of the anesthesia (Fig. 6.1). In the planning of the tumor ablation facilities, consultation with the anesthetizing team will result in the best working conditions for all involved in patient care. At times, the anesthesiologist may be called upon to initiate a program within the constraints of existing resources. In these situations, where an existing CT scanner room is modified as an ablation room (Fig. 6.2), the only place for the anesthesia equipment to be placed might be to the left of the patient. If

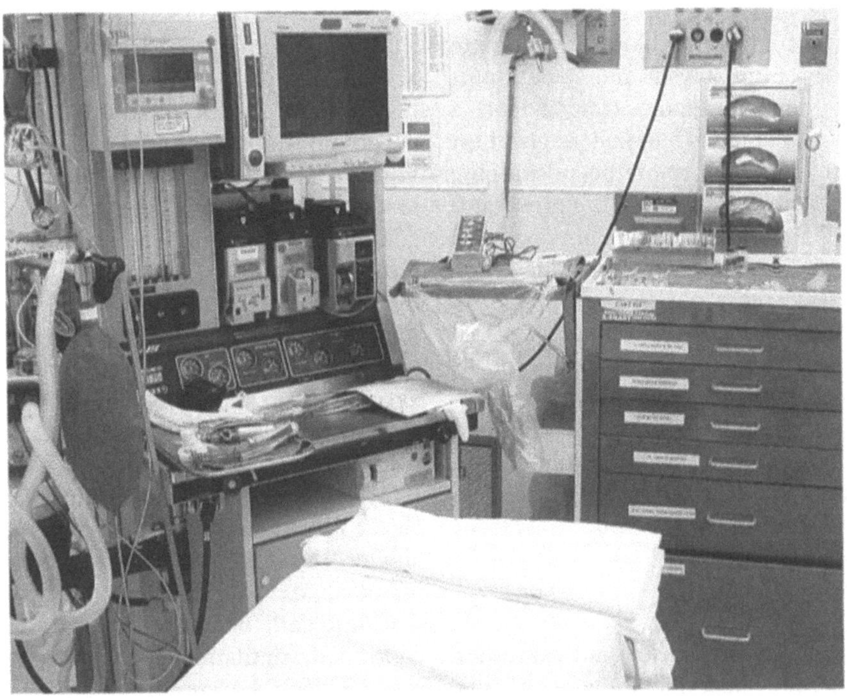

FIGURE 6.1. An anesthesia workstation in a standard operating suite, illustrating the usual positioning of an operating room table in relation to the anesthesiologist's workstation. The operating room table is at the bottom. The anesthesia machine, with its physiologic monitoring screens and attached airway circuit and ambu bag, resides to the right of the patient's head. If general anesthesia is induced, a mask fit is maintained by the anesthesiologist's left hand while ventilation is carried on through the ambu with the right hand.

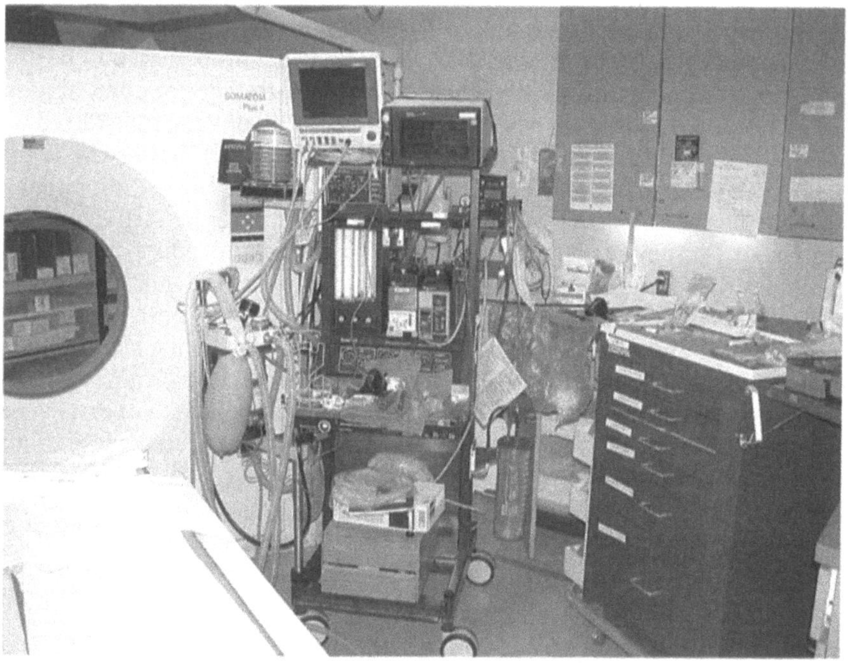

FIGURE 6.2. An anesthesia workstation in a computed tomography (CT) scan suite, illustrating a standard CT scan suite that has been converted into a room for CT-guided ablation procedures. Because of space constraints in this conversion, the anesthesia machine is at the left of the patient's head. This is the reverse from the usual work position of the anesthesiologist and should be communicated to the anesthetizing team. Some anesthesiologists may prefer to design an induction room in which general anesthesia is performed and the patient is then moved into the CT scanner, or they may wish to arrange assistance while induction is performed in this "reversed" room. With proper communication, patients may be anesthetized safely.

this is necessary, the interventional team must consult the anesthesia team and inform them of this situation, as assistance during the induction of general anesthesia might be required. Finally, the ideal anesthesia workstation has an anesthesia cart with drawers for supplies in the same configuration as any other anesthetizing location (Fig. 6.3). An MRI-compatible anes-

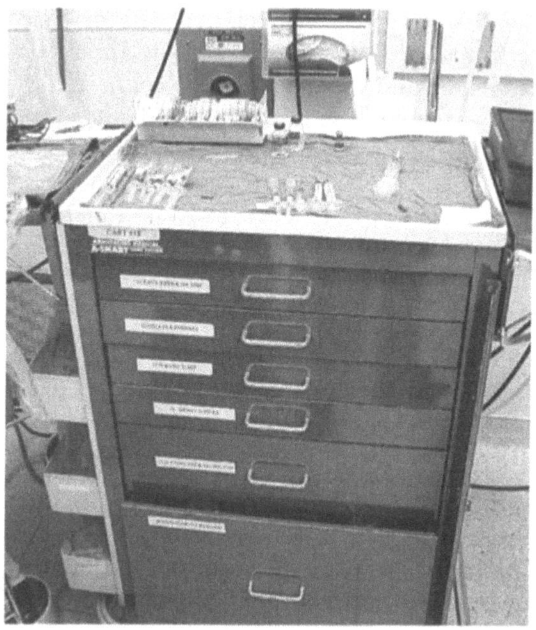

FIGURE 6.3. An anesthesia equipment cart. In addition to the anesthesia machine, specialized equipment is required that is stored on the cart, as illustrated here. The top center of the cart usually holds anesthetic and resuscitative medications that are drawn into syringes for ready administration. The other drawers hold airway supplies, intravenous and central vein placement supplies, and other items deemed necessary for the conduct of the anesthesia. Additionally, gloves and a needle disposal box should be readily available.

thesia machine, MRI-compatible anesthesia cart, and equipment should be available for tumor ablation procedures in the MRI environment. A large trash disposal for medical wastes as well as a wide-mouth, deep, hard-wall sharps disposal receptacle should be within arm's reach for needle safety.

Unique equipment for long-distance administration of anesthesia includes long breathing circuit tubing, intravenous tubing extensions, end-tidal CO_2 sampling tubing extensions, as well as sufficient lengths of pulse oximetry, noninvasive blood pressure, and ECG cables.

As most anesthestizing locations for tumor ablation do not have a permanently installed anesthesia machine, it is even more critical that the machine and equipment have an appropriate checkout before each use for key index connection to the medical gas supply (11). The Food and Drug Administration (FDA) published a simplified anesthesia machine checkout and inspection procedure in 1993 (12). A copy of the checkout procedure should be available at the point of use, attached to and visible on the machine. Complete equipment checkout and a rigid suction catheter with adequate pressure should be present before proceeding with patient care. A good guiding philosophy to prioritize actions for these remote-site procedures is patient safety is number one, patient comfort is number two, and on-time performance is number three. An anesthetic gas scavenging system should be connected to wall suction to meet Occupational Safety and Health Administration (OSHA) workplace standards for waste anesthetic gases (13). Ideally, the waste-scavenging suction should be a separate outlet and not Y-connected, since the latter decreases the force of suction power available to clear the patient's airway during critical airway events. Anesthesia equipment should meet current standards. Preventive and routine maintenance of the anesthesia equipment and monitors with appropriate record keeping should be the same standard as for all anesthesia equipment in the institution.

Specific equipment needs include easy access to the head of the patient for induction and intubation, with adjustable table height. If this is not possible on the radiologic table, then induction and intubation must be accomplished on another stretcher or adjustable surface with the patient then being transferred to the radiologic surface after the airway is in place and secured. The patient and monitors need to be visualized during the frequent breath holding and scanning procedures when all personnel leave the room. The ventilator and respiratory alarms should have both a visual and auditory component so all members of the procedure and anesthesia teams know when ventilations have been suspended, either for needle placement or radiologic scanning. Adequate illumination of the patient, anesthesia machine, and monitoring equipment must be available, with a backup of a battery-powered form of illumination. Distractors in the environment that divert the attention of the anesthesiologist away from the patient's care must be identified. Tasks not requiring performance by the anesthesiologist should be accomplished by other personnel so that the anesthesiologist can focus on the patient and his or her care. Extraneous noise and tasks need to be reduced to a minimum. For example, door openings and closings for the scanning period should be minimized, and table positioning and patient positioning tasks need to be unloaded from the anesthesiologist so that he or she can devote full attention to the patient, the monitors, and airway and anesthesia management.

In establishing the same system of care for remote-site administration of anesthesia, two-way communication to request assistance with phone access and phone numbers for anesthesia technicians and biomedical support should be available at the point of care. As anesthesiology is a time-based service and to coordinate procedure events on a timeline, a wall clock that is visualized by all members of the procedure team is important to coordinate timed events. Specialized anesthesia carts for difficult airway management should be immediately available with additional trained personnel to assist the anesthesiologists for all off-site anesthetizing locations. An emergency cart with defibrillator, emergency drugs, and other equipment adequate to provide cardiopulmonary resuscitation should be available. Code policies and procedures with special consideration for a surgical airway code for the hospital should be uniform for all off-site locations. Evacuation procedures should be planned for moving the patient out of the scanner with ambu bag ventilation, oxygen or air ventilation, and portable physiologic monitoring with pulse oximetry. Medications to decrease patient awareness, such as midazolam and propofol, can be administered during these unplanned evacuation procedures.

Quality Assurance and Continuous Quality Improvement

The goals for any quality assurance activity are the improvement in health care and patient safety for the patients we serve. For anesthesia for tumor ablation, a quality assurance program should look at the structure, process, function, and outcomes of patient care (14). Data should be captured on all adverse events and near-miss events so that an interdisciplinary team of interventional radiologists, anesthesiologists, nurses, and administrators can analyze and improve the tumor ablation system of care. After any adverse event, patient data are retrieved, and the members of the tumor ablation team are interviewed and debriefed to obtain the various perspectives of the case and event. A timeline is created so that all observations and multiple dimensions of contributing factors can be placed in this two-dimensional structure. A physiologic theory of the event or injury is created, along with a systems theory that analyzes the contribution of the environment of care and human factors to the event. Anytime equipment malfunction is suspected in adverse patient events in remote locations, an impartial investigation protocol should be followed for analysis of the event (15). The literature is reviewed to fully define the event and see if this event has been described before. The team then makes its recommendations for improved care in a nonpunitive educational approach, with the systems of care improved so that the event does not recur. The patient and family are fully informed of medical events, as is currently recommended by patient safety advocates and required by the Joint Commission on Accreditation of Healthcare Organizations (JCAHO) patient reporting standards.

Complications

The most common complication of these procedures is pneumothorax. Any inadvertent needle insertion into the visceral pleura, during either liver or renal tumor ablation techniques, can initiate a slow leakage of air from the pulmonary parenchyma. If the patient is sedated, the occurrence may be heralded by the onset of chest pain, coughing, shortness of breath, or pulse oximetry desaturation. With pneumothorax, physical examination may show either hyperresonance or loss of breath sounds on the side of the procedure. Agitated, coughing patients or those with chronic obstructive pulmonary disease (COPD) or emphysema are at increased risk for pneumothorax. Under general anesthesia, suspending positive pressure ventilation so the lungs are deflated at the time of needle and radiofrequency probe or cryoprobe placement may decrease the risk of this event. If a pneumothorax is suspected, positive pressure ventilation and nitrous oxide may worsen the pneumothorax and cause the development of a tension pneumothorax. If the needle passage is close to the diaphragm or signs and symptoms of pneumothorax occur, as the patient is already in the scanning radiologic device, imaging to rule out a pneumothorax is warranted. With lung tumor ablation, pneumothorax is anticipated.

A second potential complication is positioning injuries to nerves (16,17). Care should be taken whenever the angulation of the arms and shoulders is greater than 90 degrees axially, as this puts stretch forces on the brachial plexus. Anesthetized patients are susceptible to brachial plexus injury as they are unable to respond to pain, numbness, paresthesia, or weakness. Muscle relaxants used during these procedures may reduce the protective effect of normal muscle tone against nerve stretch injuries. Strategies to prevent brachial plexus injuries include positioning the arms across the chest with adequate padding to slightly raise them from skin contact of the chest wall, positioning the arms above the head only during the actual imaging stage, and frequently changing the arm position, especially in prolonged procedures.

Reimbursement for Providing Anesthesia Services

Adequate reimbursement for anesthesia services needs to be considered in order to obtain the resources of an anesthesiologist in the care of these patients. One needs to understand anesthesia billing for tumor ablation services so that the patient, procedure, and time of the case can be documented and income can be generated. Anesthesia is a time-based service as the anesthesiologist has no control over the length of the procedure. Typically, the procedure has a "base" unit value, which includes the value of all usual anesthesia services except the time actually spent in delivering anesthesia care. The base units include the usual preoperative and postoperative visits, the preoperative introduction, review of chart, IV start, administration of fluids incident to the anesthesia care, and interpretation of monitoring (ECG, BP, oximetry, capnography, gas monitoring, and temperature). The "start time" and time units begin when the anesthesiologist is in constant personal attendance, and time is measured in 15-minute intervals. One time unit is 15 minutes or a portion thereof. The "end time" is when the patient is signed out to the postanesthesia care unit (PACU), with intensive care unit (ICU) nursing care or its equivalent.

Facility and interventional radiologists will typically use two codes for submission, a surgical or procedure component code and the guidance code. Only two tumor ablation codes are specific at this time for liver tumor ablation, that being for Current Procedural Terminology (CPT) code 47382, ablation, one or more tumor(s), percutaneous, radiofrequency; and CPT 47381, ablation, one or more tumor(s), cryosurgical. All other sites for tumor ablation (abdomen CPT 20999, retroperitoneal CPT 20999, lung CPT 32999, bone CPT 20999, soft tissue CPT 20999, and spinal cord CPT 99) have to use a nonspecific "99" code with a specific detailed report sent with the submitted encounter form and bill (18). The guidance codes that also are submitted include a CT guidance code (CPT 76360), MRI guidance (CPT 76393), and ultrasound guidance (CPT 76942).

The associated common CPT codes for anesthesia for liver tumor ablation is 00790, with a seven-base-units-plus-time billing. The American Society of Anesthesiologists (ASA) also has a relative value guide (RVG), which is also used for billing (19). The ASA RVG code for anesthesia for intraperitoneal upper abdominal procedures is 00790, also of seven-base-unit-plus-time valuation. Anesthesia for tumor ablation for renal lesions is ASA code 00862; anesthesia for tumor ablation for a lung lesion is ASA code 00520; and for anesthesia for tumor ablation for spinal cord lesions 99; the cervical ASA code is 00600, the thoracic ASA code is 00620, and the lumbar ASA code is 00630.

In the submission of anesthesia billing, it is important to accurately define the anesthesia services provided. General anesthesia is defined as a loss of consciousness and protective reflexes; MAC is an intermediate plane of anesthesia; and conscious sedation is a lighter plane of anesthesia, in which patients can respond to verbal commands and can protect their own airway. Conscious sedation provided by nonanesthesiologists, such as an independent trained person to assist the physician in monitoring the patient's level of consciousness and physiologic status, can be billed under CPT codes 99141 (intravenous, intramuscular, or inhalational) and CPT 99142 (oral, rectal, or intranasal).

Medicare and some private payers need to have justification for MAC billing with regard to medical status, ASA classification, underlying medical disease, anxiety, or inability to accomplish the procedure under conscious sedation analgesia before the payer will reimburse for MAC services. Constant monitoring of the billing and receipts for anesthetic procedures for tumor ablation are needed to assure clinic income to support the anesthesia needs of the patient undergoing these procedures and to maintain the services of an anesthesiologist to assist in anesthesia for tumor ablation.

References

1. Standards of the American Society of Anesthesiologists: basic standards for preanesthetic care (1987), standards for post anesthesia care (1994). ASA Executive Office, 520 N. Northwest Highway, Park Ridge, IL 60068-2573.
2. Practice advisory for preanesthetic evaluation. Anesthesiology 2002;96:485–496.
3. Warner MA, et al. Practice guidelines for preoperative fasting. Park Ridge, IL: American Society of Anesthesiologists. Anesthesiology 1999;90: 896–905.
4. Roizen MA, Foss JF, Fischer SP. Peroperative evaluation. In: Miller RA, ed. Anesthesia. 5th ed. New York: Churchill Livingstone, 2000:824–883.
5. Practice guidelines for management of the difficult airway. Park Ridge, IL: American Society of Anesthesiologists. Anesthesiology 2003. www.asahq.org
6. Standards for basic anesthesia monitoring. 1998. ASA Executive Office, 520 N. Northwest Highway, Park Ridge, IL 60068-2573.
7. Bonica JJ. In: Loeser JD, ed. Management of Pain. Philadelphia: Lippincott Williams & Wilkins, 2001;679:1293–1296.
8. Cousins MJ, Bridenbaugh PO. Neural Blockade in Clinical Anesthesia and Management of Pain. 3rd ed. Philadelphia: Lippincott-Raven, 1998: 463–470.
9. Guidelines for nonoperating room anesthetizing locations. 1994. ASA Executive Office, 520 N. Northwest Highway, Park Ridge, IL 60068–2573.
10. Dorsch JA, Dorsch SE. Operating room design and equipment selection. In: Understanding Anesthesia Equipment. 4th ed. Baltimore: Williams & Wilkins, 1999:1015–1036.
11. Dorsch JA, Dorsch SE. Equipment checking and maintenance. In: Understanding Anesthesia Equipment. 4th ed. Baltimore: Williams & Wilkins, 1999:937–965.
12. Morrison JL. FDA anesthesia apparatus checkout recommendations, 1993. American Society of Anesthesiologists Newletter 1994;58(6): 25–26.
13. U.S. Department of Health, Education, and Welfare. Criteria for a recommended standard; occupational exposure to waste anesthesia gases and vapors. (DHEW [NIOSH] publication No.77-140). Washington, DC: US Government Printing Office, 1977.
14. Dodson BA. In: Miller RA, ed. Quality Assurance/Quality Improvement in Anesthesia. 5th ed. New York: Churchill Livingstone, 2000: 2597–2612.
15. Dorsch JA, Dorsch SE. Chapter 26. In: Understanding Anesthesia Equipment. 4th ed. Baltimore: Williams & Wilkins, 1999:960–961.
16. Warner MA, et al. Practice advisory for the prevention of perioperative peripheral neuropathies. Park Ridge, IL: American Society of Anesthesiologists. Anesthesiology 2000;92:1168–1182.
17. Shankar S, vanSonnenberg E, Silverman SG, Tuncali K, Flanagan HL, Whang EE. Brachial plexus injury from CT-guided RF ablation under general anesthesia. (CVIR in press)
18. CPT 2003. American Medical Association, 515 N. State Street, Chicago IL 60610.
19. ASA Relative Value Guide, 2003. ASA Executive Office, 520 N. Northwest Highway, Park Ridge, IL 60068-2573.

7
Devices, Equipment, and Operation of Ablation Systems

Paul R. Morrison and Eric vanSonnenberg

This chapter reviews the operation of each of several medical systems that is used to deliver local thermal therapy. Each system provides its own mechanism for the transfer of energy within tissue that results in cytotoxic effects. This targeted destruction of cells is referred to as *tissue ablation*. This chapter concentrates on the medical system itself, and not the principles behind the various mechanisms of tissue ablation. It is concerned with the physician as a user, or *operator*, of the ablation system during a procedure. Accordingly, emphasis is placed on the following: the thermal *applicator*, the *main control panel*, user-defined *parameters and settings*, and *feedback* to the operator.

The *applicator* is the "working end" of the system. Examples include an electrode wired to a radiofrequency (RF) generator, a light-diffusing tip on an optical fiber connected to a infrared laser, a microwave antenna, a cryogenic probe, and a high-intensity ultrasound transducer. The "thinking end" of the system includes a control panel, by which the user can communicate with the device to conduct the ablation. The control panel is used by the operator to set and adjust treatment parameters that include the energy delivered, the rate of energy deposition, the duration of an exposure, or the temperatures within tissue. Observation of these and other parameters on the control panel during ablation serves as data feedback to the user on the progress of the procedure. This feedback may be an electronic display of the temperature of the applicator, the electrical resistance of the tissue, or simply the elapsed time. Importantly, such data affect the course of the procedure, as they are indicative of whether or not a therapeutic end point has been reached; for example, a planned protocol might be altered should the temperature reading be too low, the resistance too high, or the time too short.

Radiofrequency Ablation Systems

Radiofrequency ablation (RFA) is performed with the patient and an RF generator serving as the primary components of an electrical circuit. The generator is the source of current in the circuit and the human body serves as a resistor, all connected by wire leads. It is the resistance in the tissue to the RF current that generates heat and creates a thermal ablation effect. The electrical resistance of the body's tissue is referred to as the *impedance*, and is measured in ohms (Ω). Impedance, rather than *resistance*, is a term more appropriate when dealing with alternating current.

In monopolar-type RFA systems, the ablation is confined to a targeted volume of tissue by inserting an RF electrode that is connected to the generator directly into the tissue. The electrically noninsulated tip of the electrode is relatively small, and thus the current density surrounding this tip is high; this creates a localized thermal effect due to ionic agitation. A *return* connection to the RF generator is required to complete the circuit. This return is established by placing dispersive electrodes in contact with the skin, usually on the patient's thighs. These *grounding pads* offer a large surface area, keeping the current density low to eliminate heating at the sites of contact.

For tumor ablation, generally, there are two types of monopolar RFA electrodes: *needle* and *array*. As noted above, both provide segments of a noninsulated conductor that can be placed into tissue and through which the RF current flows. The needle-type electrode is a thin cylindrical conductor, usually beveled at the tip, making it sharp so as to penetrate into tissue. It is electrically insulated along its shaft up to the exposed tip; the latter is usually 1 cm or a few centimeters long, which is referred to as the "active length". This tip provides an extended source of heat (compared to a single point source just at the very tip), the length of which can be selected to best match the dimensions of the target. The array-type electrode also serves as an extended source; from a needle-like cannula a number of individual noninsulated wire electrodes splay out radially into tissue away from the long axis of the cannula. The diameter of the radial extension also can be chosen to best match the target volume.

The RFA systems produced by several manufacturers are presented in the following sections. Manufacturers are presented not in alphabetical order, but rather in chronologic order based on when the technology first became available in the marketplace.

Radionics

The Radionics RFA electrode (Cool-Tip, Radionics, Burlington, MA) is shown in Figure 7.1. The single 17-gauge electrode is a needle-type design. The overall length of the electrode is selected (10, 15, 20, or 25 cm) to provide the appropriate depth of penetration into the body. Separate consideration is given to the selection of the active length of the electrode (1, 2, or 3 cm). As noted above, this choice of the length of the exposed tip establishes the physical dimension of the RF source, allowing the user to best match the ablation to the target. The Radionics cluster electrode, also shown in Figure 7.1, consists of three single electrodes fixed in one handle, each with a 2.5-cm exposed tip. The cluster design adds to the extended source of RF energy and is intended to yield a volume of ablation (on the order of 4 cm in diameter), larger than that for a single elec-

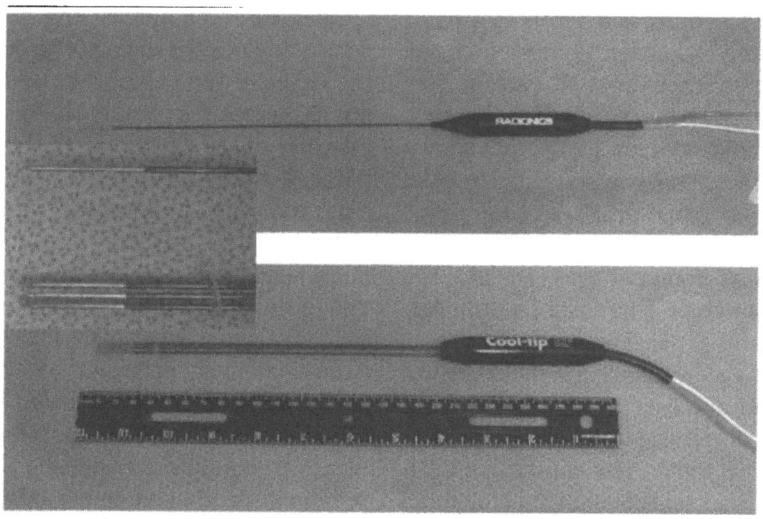

FIGURE 7.1. Valleylab needle-type RF electrodes. A "single" electrode (top) with a 3-cm noninsulated active length is internally cooled during ablation by a closed-loop flow of water. Cooling reduces tissue char that might impede RF current flow into tissue. The "cluster" electrode (bottom) combines three single electrodes with 2.5-cm active lengths to induce larger volume lesions. Needle-like tips provide penetration into tissue (inset). (Photos printed with permission from Valleylab.)

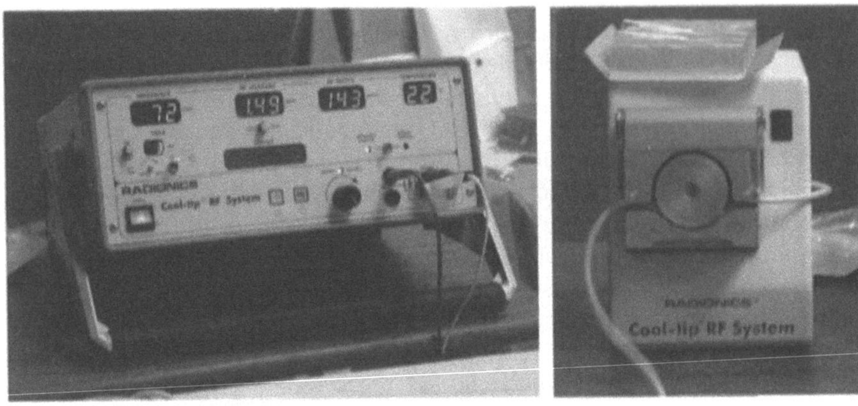

A B

Figure 7.2. Valleylab RF generator and coolant pump. Running in "impedance control" mode, power is adjusted automatically by the system to maintain the level of baseline tissue impedance measured in ohms. The main control panel (A) displays impedance, elapsed time, current, power, and temperature. Wires lead from panel to electrode and grounding pads. A rotary pump (B) sends water to the electrode. Water-cooled tips read cool water temperatures, 22°C in the figure. The ablation end point is based on time, that is, duration of exposure. (Photos printed with permission from Valleylab.)

trode. The device operates at a frequency of 480 kHz (1).

A salient feature of the Radionics Cool-Tip system is that, as the name suggests, the electrode is cooled by a continuous flow of cold water (~20°C). This flow is done in a closed loop; no water is deposited into tissue as the water flows internally to, and returns from, the tip. The cool tip temperatures are intended to prevent excessive heating and carbonization of tissue immediately adjacent to the electrode that can pose high impedance to current flow and prevent optimal penetration of the energy. The generator and coolant pump are shown in Figure 7.2. The main control panel on the generator includes visual displays of the tissue impedance (Ω), the current (amps), the power (watts, W), probe temperature (I), and the elapsed time (minutes). There is a potentiometer (knob) to control the power output.

The device has a switch on the main control panel that allows the user to select a mode of operation. The device typically is operated in *impedance control mode*. The coolant pump is switched on, a timer on the main control panel is started, and the power knob is rotated to its maximum. The ablation at that location is completed when the timer reaches a set time (12 minutes). There are no adjustments made by the operator to any parameters during ablation in this mode. The power and current are automatically lowered to reverse any large increase in impedance. With this device, the latter is understood to indicate gas formation in tissue that is counterproductive to the conduction of RF into tissue.

Consider these sample readings from the main control panel in Figure 7.2 at 3 minutes of RFA: 72 Ω, 1.49 A, 143 W, 22°C. Note that the temperature reading is low due to the cool water flowing through the probe. Thus, while the tissue around the probe is heated, there is no temperature feedback that provides a measure of the elevated temperatures. The end point for the procedure is, as noted above, a duration (i.e., 12 minutes). The tumor tissue is indeed heated, as there is considerable energy being deposited. The heating is observed at the end of the procedure just prior to the end of the exposure when the coolant flow is turned off to expose tissues immediately adjacent to the electrode to an uncooled probe. With the pump off, the static water in the electrode quickly comes to equilibrium with the tissue, and temperatures on the order of 100°C typically are seen.

Alternatively, the device can be operated in a *manual mode* to control the output via manipulation of the power knob. No coolant is used and the electrode's temperature is read on the main control panel. This manual mode typically is used for the brief coagulation of the access tract as the electrode is withdrawn. The power is increased until the temperature reading indicates immediate coagulation (usually targeting near or above 80°C), and then the electrode is pulled back through the normal tissues. Before complete removal from the body, the power is turned off. In addition to tract coagulation, manual mode without cooling can be used to perform RFA of tumors in which both time and temperature are provided as feedback to the operator.

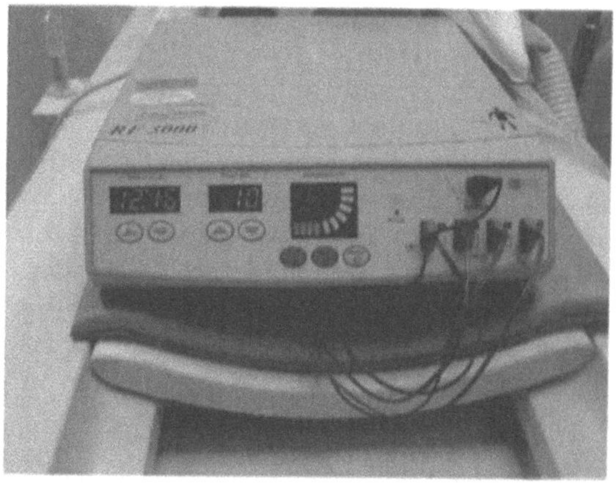

FIGURE 7.4. Boston Scientific Corporation–Oncology RF generator. The main control panel displays the elapsed time, power, and tissue impedance. With this device, the power is manually increased stepwise over time. The end point for tissue ablation is a marked rise in impedance above baseline, e.g., to 467 ohms from a baseline of 50 at 12 minutes as seen in the figure. The power automatically ramps down when the end point is achieved. (Photo printed with permission from Boston Scientific Corporation.)

Boston Scientific

The LeVeen needle electrode (Boston Scientific Corporation–Oncology, Natick, MA) is an array-type electrode. It consists of a 14-gauge bevel-tipped cannula (12, 15, or 25 cm long) fixed to a handle. Within the cannula are the individual elements of the array that are deployed from the tip into tissue by a driving mechanism in the handle. The electrode is shown in Figure 7.3. On deployment, the tines of the array splay radially out and arch back, each in a semicircular fashion, forming an umbrella-like pattern. Each tine serves as a separate noninsulated element of the electrode. The array diameters can be selected (2, 3, 3.5, 4 or 5 cm) to match the tumor volume. The electrode is powered and controlled by the RF 3000 generator shown in Figure 7.4 that operates at a frequency of 460 kHz and provides up to 200 W of power (2). As with most of the RF systems under discussion, the electrical circuit is completed with the attachment of four return electrodes (grounding pads) to the patient.

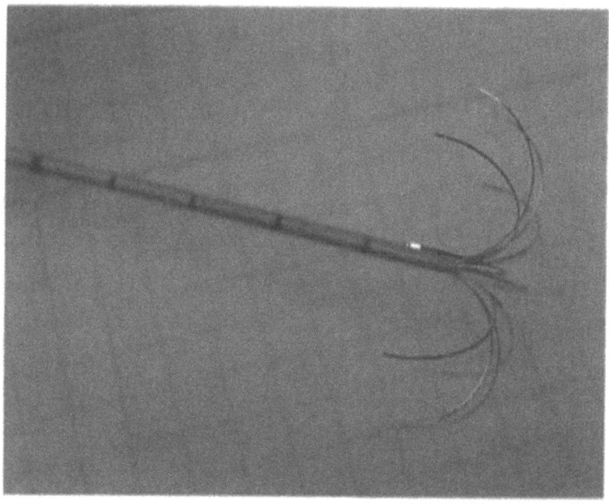

FIGURE 7.3. Boston Scientific Corporation–Oncology array-type RF electrode. The deployed array of multiple noninsulated tines establishes an extended source of RF in tissue, here 4 cm in diameter. The electrode is initially placed into tissue with the tines withdrawn into the cannula. (Photo printed with permission from Boston Scientific Corporation.)

The main control panel of the generator has primary displays for time, power, and impedance. There are also control keypads for adjusting the power, setting a time duration, starting, stopping, and resetting the system. On powering up the generator, there is a series of quick self-checks leaving it in a ready mode. When the start button is pressed, it enters into an operating mode. A small blue light on the panel and an audible tone serve as indicators that RF energy is being delivered. The operator sets the power to a starting value (e.g., 50 W for a 3.5-cm array). Per the manufacturer's operating instructions this is increased manually over time to a preestablished maximum value (i.e., by 10 W per minute to a 100 W limit).

The signature feature of the system is its *impedance feedback mechanism.* The electrode's geometry and the incremental power-adjustment algorithm allow tissue impedance to serve as an end point for the ablation. With this device, the rise in impedance is due to tissue coagulation and desiccation around the array. No measure of temperature is provided by this device. While the time is marked by the user, it serves as a guide for each power increase and does not dictate the duration of the ablation. Overall, the impedance changes little, if at all, from its initial value when the electrode is activated. Generally, after many minutes, the impedance rises substantially and rapidly (i.e., by tens and then by hundreds of ohms in less than a minute). This is known casually as "roll-off", and the power automatically drops to near zero. Figure 7.4 shows the system at the end of an ablation. Notably, the manufacturer's instructions call for a second phase of treatment after roll-off ("booster"). Without a change in electrode location, the generator is activated again at 70% power, until a repeat roll-off is achieved.

RITA

The RFA system of RITA Medical Systems, Inc. (Mountain View, CA) is composed of the model 1500X RF generator and the StarBurst XL and XLi electrodes. The salient features of the system are: (a) the applicator is an array-type electrode, (b) one mode of operation allows temperatures at multiple sites of the array to be monitored, and (c) the XLi version provides for the infusion of hypertonic saline through select elements of the array. The device operates at 460kHz and up to 100W (3).

The StarBurst XL electrode is composed of a 14-gauge trocar (10, 15, 25cm long) attached to a handle. The device is introduced into the patient with the tines of the array retracted within the cannula. When properly situated in tissue, a mechanism on the user end of the handle deploys the tines. The nine tines splay forward and radially out from the tip. The array is intended to provide a 3- to 5-cm-diameter volume of ablation; a smaller 15-gauge seven-tine version provides 2- to 3-cm-diameter ablations. Each array includes tines containing thermocouples by which tip temperatures are continuously measured. The nine-tine array has five thermocouples.

The XLi version of the electrode provides saline infusion into the tissue during RF ablation. The XLi electrode is shown in Figure 7.5. This feature is intended to provide for larger ablations (up to 7cm) using the introduction of saline in the tissue as an extended source for the RF current deposition due to its conductivity. The slow flow of saline is controlled by a separate syringe pump and control unit.

The main control panel of the RITA model 1500X includes readouts and controls for temperature, power, and impedance, as shown in Figure 7.6. Prominently featured on the panel are the displays for the probes' thermocouples

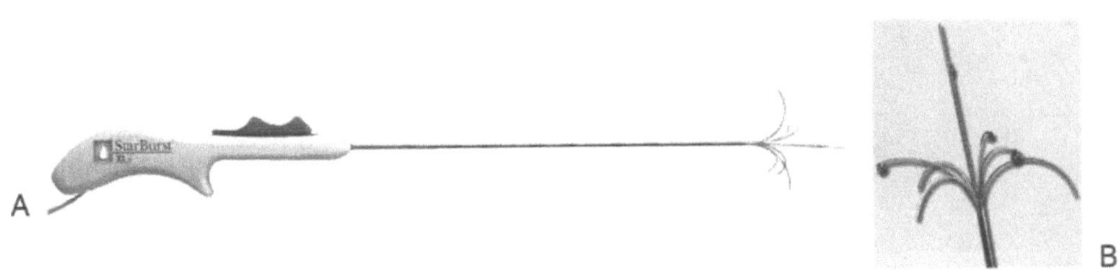

FIGURE 7.5. RITA Medical Systems, Inc. array-type RF electrode. These array-type electrodes (A) include thermocouples in a number of the tines by which separate temperature measurements are obtained for ablation control. Also, in the XLi version of the device, saline can be infused into the tissue from the central tine (B) to provide an extended RF source for larger ablation volumes. The Xli Electrode shown is intended to create 7cm diameter lesions. (Photos courtesy of RITA Medical Systems, Inc.)

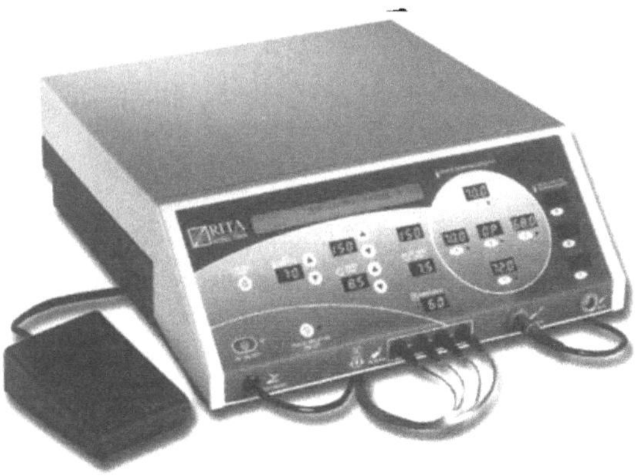

FIGURE 7.6. RITA Medical Systems, Inc. RF generator. The main control panel displays user-defined settings for the target tissue temperature, power, and time. Feedback to the user includes the actual RF power being delivered, the elapsed time, and tissue impedance. Up to eight thermocouple measurements to assess the temperature at the tines of the array (up to four) and at separate locations targeted with added needle-thermocouples can be displayed. In the figure, as an example, the device controls power to give average temperature readings of 70°C in four tines of an array. Temperature and time serve as the end points for ablation. (Photo courtesy of RITA Medical Systems, Inc.)

by which up to five temperatures can be monitored. A signature mode of operation for the device is its *automatic temperature control mode*. In this mode, a target temperature is chosen. The electrode's power is controlled by an internal computer algorithm whereby it increases the power until the thermocouples' readings average the set temperature (i.e., 90°C). The power is then adjusted automatically to maintain this temperature. A timer counts from the time this temperature is reached. The end point for the ablation is a 10-minute duration at the set temperature. Additional temperature information can be gained by using add-on, nonarray needle thermocouples that can be monitored; there are three extra readouts on the main control panel for this purpose. In addition to a temperature control based on the average of temperature values observed, the device can operate in a highest or lowest set-temperature mode to keep temperatures below or above some prescribed value, respectively.

Alternatively, the system can be run in a mode that allows the user to manually control the power output to the electrode. This can serve as a technique for volume ablation of tissue, or this can provide for coagulation along the electrode's tract as it is withdrawn from tissue. The latter is accomplished by heat emission from a noninsulated portion of the cannula's tip with the tines undeployed. The company recently developed a flexible trocar shaft for improved entry and monitoring for CT-guided ablations.

Berchtold

The Berchtold HiTT electrode (Berchtold, GmbH, Tuttlingen, Germany) is a needle-type electrode designed to provide saline infusion (4). That company identifies this method as *high-frequency induced thermo-treatment* (HiTT). Saline infusion is used to provide additional thermal and electrical conductivity in the tissue to enhance the thermal effect, that is, to provide large ablation volumes up to 5 cm in diameter. The saline is not intended to provide cooling for the electrode. A series of microholes have been drilled in the tip of the probe to deliver the saline. The HiTT electrodes are manufactured with active lengths of 1, 1.5, and 2 cm. These are 1.2 to 2.0 mm in diameter, and range from 10 to 20 cm long. A sample electrode is shown in Figure 7.7.

The Elektrotom HiTT 106 generator operates at a frequency of 375 kHz and provides power up to 60 W. It is shown in Figure 7.8 along with the fluid pump used to control the flow of saline. The generator's main control panel displays the temperature, flow rate (mL/hr), power, energy, impedance, and elapsed time. For automatic control of the power output, the device can be run in either *impedance control* or *temperature control mode*. The temperature control mode can operate on readings from the temperature sensor in the electrode, or from a separate temperature sensor that can be placed into the tissue for a reading remote from the electrode. A separate manual mode provides the operator with control over the power for coagulation of the electrode's tract on removal from the site of ablation. The infusion pump can

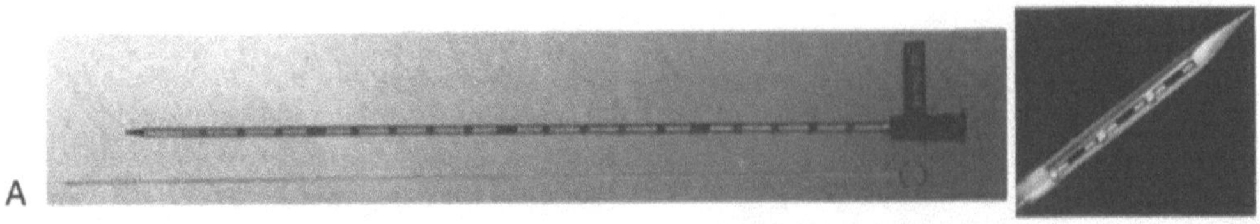

FIGURE 7.7. Berchtold GmbH & Co. needle-type electrode (A). Microholes along the tip of the electrode (B) allow saline infusion into tissue to provide an extended RF source for enhancement of the RF ablation. (Photos courtesy of Berchtold GmbH & Co.)

be controlled manually, as well as automatically. In automatic mode, the flow depends on the power setting of the unit at the outset of ablation.

Celon

The Celon ProSurge applicators (Celon AG Medical Instruments, Berlin, Germany) are needle-type RF electrodes. These differ from the above-mentioned RFA devices in that they are bipolar electrodes (5). In the bipolar configuration, instead of an electrical circuit established from the needle-electrode through tissue to the grounding pads, both electrode elements are situated at the needle tip. RF current flows between these elements and thus only in the vicinity of the device's tip. No grounding pads are used with this device. Celon electrodes are available in a range of styles for a variety of ablation procedures. They have active lengths ranging from 9mm to 3cm, shaft lengths from 10 to 120cm (the latter for endoscopic use), and diameters range from 1.3 to 1.8mm. The ProSurge line of electrodes for interstitial volume ablation is internally cooled (used in conjunction with a coolant pump), and intended to provide ablations 2cm wide with the length depending on the choice of active length (1.7–3.0cm) of the device. These are 1.8mm in diameter, and 10, 15, or 20cm long. A sample Celon ProSurge electrode is shown in Figure 7.9.

The CelonLab PRECISION generator is shown in Figure 7.10. The unit operates at 470 kHz. The power available from the unit (range 1–25W) is relatively low due to the efficiency of the bipolar system. The main control panel features readouts of power, time, and impedance. The system runs in an *impedance control mode*. An initial power is set, impedance is monitored, and an acoustic display provides an audible tone at a frequency that increases in proportion to tissue impedance. The ablation end point is reached when the tone changes to a pulsed tone, indicating that the optimum impedance has been reached.

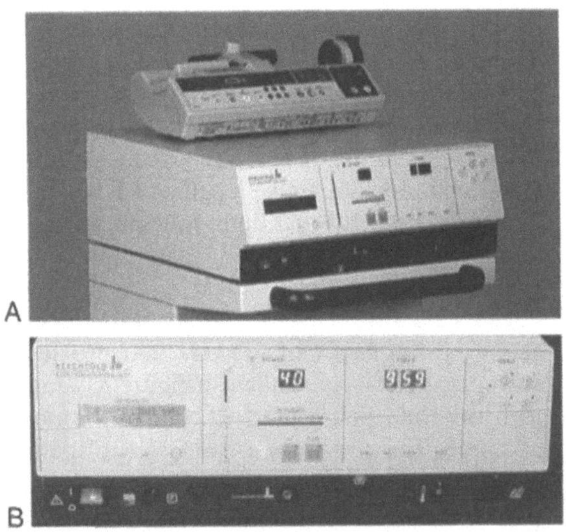

FIGURE 7.8. Berchtold GmbH & Co. RF generator and infusion pump. Saline is delivered to the RF electrode for infusion into tissue by the pump sitting atop the RF generator (A). The main control panel of the generator displays temperature, flow rate of the saline, power, and time (B). The system can be operated in either an impedance control or temperature control mode, whereby feedback to the user would be impedance in the tissue, or time and temperature, respectively. (Photos courtesy of Berchtold GmbH & Co.)

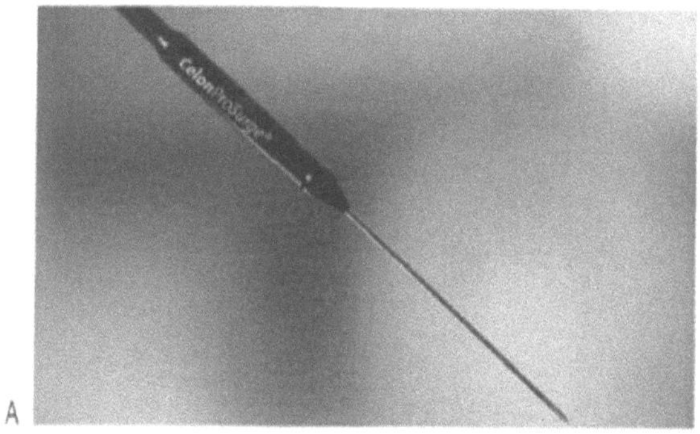

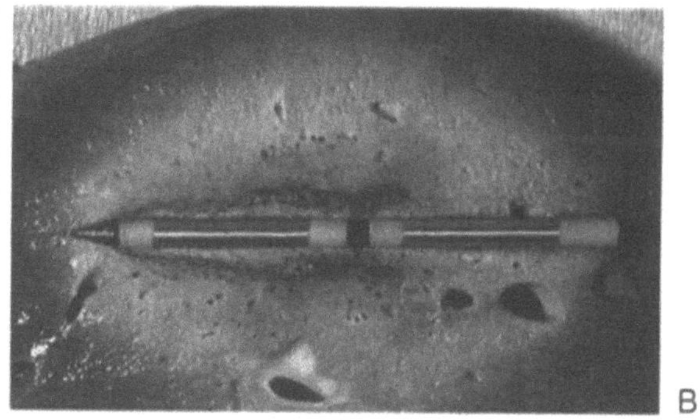

FIGURE 7.9. Celon AG Medical Instruments needle-type RF electrode. This bipolar device (A) includes both positive and negative electrode elements at the tip (B). Electrical current flows between these elements and generates resistive heating that results in tissue coagulation. No grounding pads are connected to the patient. An internal, closed-loop flow of water can be used to cool the tip to reduce tissue char that can impede RF current flow. (Photos printed with permission from Celon AG Medical Instruments.)

Cryoablation Systems

Medical systems designed for cryoablation of tumors utilize applicators of various geometries that are placed in contact with tissue to subject cells to freezing at lethal temperatures. For interstitial therapy, the probes are needle-like, designed to penetrate tissue. Each cryoprobe is incorporated into a handle that is in turn tethered to the main component of the system for the cryogenic medium to pass into the probe.

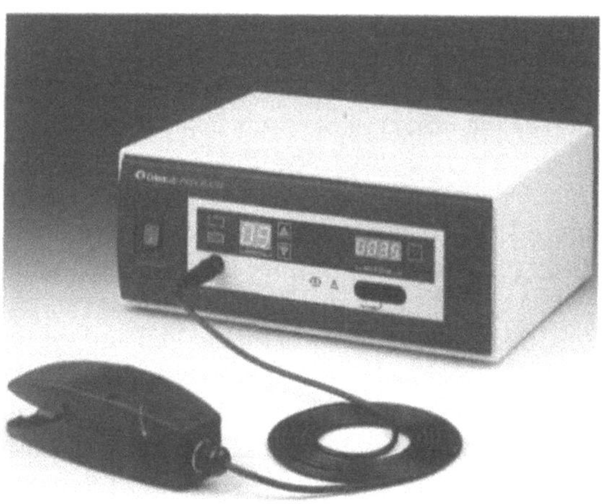

FIGURE 7.10. Celon AG Medical Instruments RF generator. The main control panel displays the power output by the device and the elapsed time. It operates in an impedance control mode. An audible tone provides the user with an indication that the tissue impedance has markedly increased, indicating complete ablation around the tip. (Photo printed with permission from Celon AG Medical Instruments.)

Contemporary systems freeze tissue using an argon gas–based cryogenic technique to achieve low temperatures. High-pressure argon gas is driven through a very thin tube situated inside the probe, and oriented coaxially to the probe's outer hull. Gas exits through a small aperture at the end of the tube near the probe's tip. The argon gas returns to the system in a closed loop. No gas is deposited into the tissue. Thus, the argon gas undergoes a change from a high pressure of approximately 3000 psi (pounds per square inch) to a relatively low 200 psi. In accordance with the Joule-Thompson effect, this results in a decrease in argon's temperature to freezing values (as low as −180°C). The use of a gas as the cryogen enables the design and manufacture of relatively small probes and allows for the use and control of multiple probes simultaneously.

These gas-based systems take advantage of the markedly different behavior of gaseous helium. Under essentially the same conditions as for argon above, due to its different physical properties, high-pressure helium undergoes an increase in temperature on passing through the aperture. Thus, while passing argon through the probe provides freezing temperatures, passing helium enables the probe to be heated. This allows for quick freezing and thawing by the argon and helium, respectively. This can be used for immediate control of the freezing process, as well as for the quick release of the probe from frozen tissue. The latter assists in the repositioning of probes to treat multiple sites during a procedure.

Galil

The CryoHit ablation system (Galil Medical, Westbury, NY) is gas-based and uses argon and helium as described above (6). While cryoprobes are available for direct surface contact (having rounded hemispherical tips or flat ends), a needle-type design also is available for interstitial use. The latter probes are sized at 1.5, 2.4, and 3.2 mm in diameter with lengths ranging from 17 to 40 cm. A probe is shown in Figure 7.11. The CryoHit system is shown in Figure 7.12. The system is not a tabletop device, but rather is a free-standing wheeled unit. Notably, it must be located so as to be able to connect to tanks that provide gases during the procedure. Up to seven probes can be used simultaneously with the system.

The main control panel is accessed through a standard computer monitor with operations controlled by a keyboard and touch-pad mouse. The software provides a menu of screens for the user to enter information or observe treatment parameters. Included are screens for preprocedural entries, one of which allows for clinical data such as the physician's name, patient name, hospital record number, sex, date of birth, and history to be recorded. The *Targets Setup* screen includes choices for the target temperatures for all primary modes of operation for each cryoprobe: freeze, thaw, and stick. Typical choices are −180°C for freezing and +35°C for thawing. The additional stick mode (typically −20°C) is used to provide a limited freeze to the probe, whereby the probe attaches to the immediate surrounding tissue, and prevents migration of the probe while other probes are placed.

The primary interface during the procedure is the *General Operations* screen shown in Figure 7.12. It shows the temperature readings of the probes during the freezing and thawing processes and the elapsed times. Probes can be individually controlled via this screen and set to stick, freeze, thaw, or off (inactive, no gas flow). Target values can be modified during ablation to control individual probes. Temperature and time provide the primary feedback to the user. Treatments are composed of a timed freeze (usually 15 minutes) with a thaw; some practitioners use a repeat freeze after the thaw.

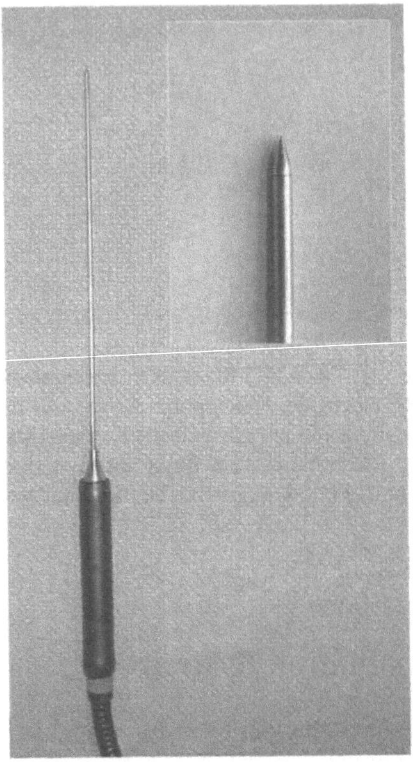

FIGURE 7.11. Galil Medical needle-type cryoablation probe. The figure shows a 2.4-mm-diameter probe designed for percutaneous tumor ablation. High-pressure argon gas flows in a closed loop to the probe tip (inset) where it undergoes a thermodynamic process and generates freezing temperatures in tissue. Alternatively, helium gas can be used, whereby the tissue can be warmed and thawed.

Endocare

The CRYOcare system (Endocare, Inc., Irvine, CA) for cryoablation is also an argon/helium-

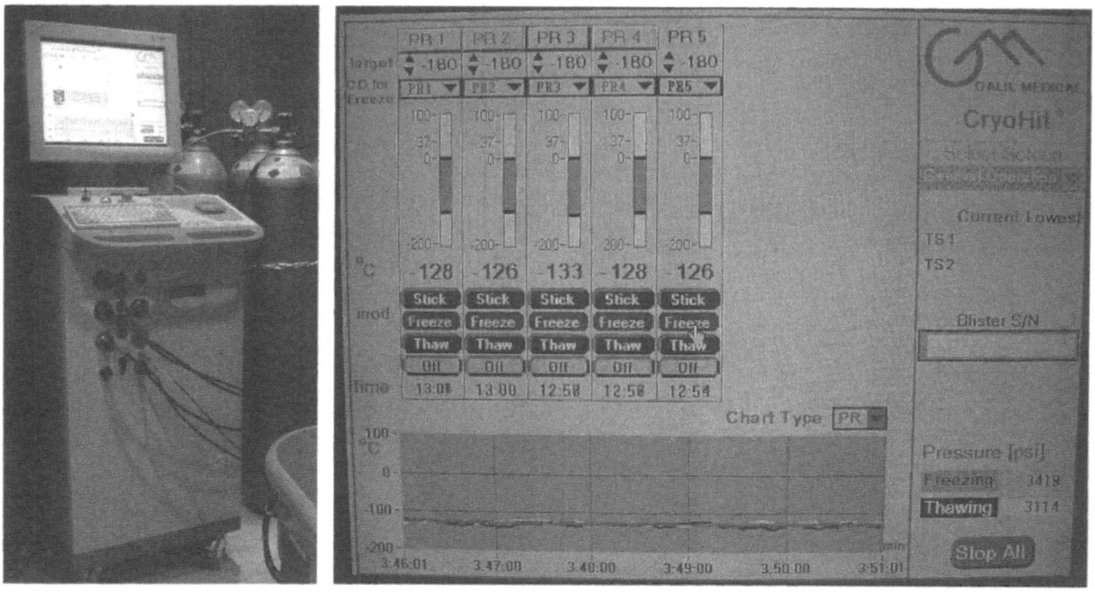

A B

FIGURE 7.12. Galil Medical cryoablation system. The system (A) requires connections to tanks and reservoirs of argon and helium gases. For each of up to seven probes, the main control console (B) displays the selected target temperature, the actual temperature, and the elapsed time. Each can be controlled independently. The display also indicates the status of each probe (stick, freeze, thaw, off). Here, a five-probe freeze is ongoing and viewed after approximately 13 minutes with a temperature average of –128°C.

based system. Probes are available with diameters of 2 to 8mm, a range intended to cover both percutaneous and open surgical procedures (i.e., prostate and liver ablation, respectively). An example of these needle-type probes is shown in Figure 7.13. The four-probe cryoablation system is shown in Figure 7.14; an eight-probe system also is available.

The main control panel is displayed on a computer monitor. Multiple probes can be operated simultaneously with individual control. The status of each probe is displayed, and indicates whether the probe is in stick, freeze, thaw, or off mode. The panel displays each tip's temperature and elapsed time at a given status. Duration and depth of the freeze serve as feedback to the physician. The default setting for stick mode is –10°C, and thaw is +40°C; typical temperatures recorded during the freeze cycle are between –130° and –150°C.

The freeze temperature can be adjusted by modifying the duty cycle of the argon gas, referring to the time over which gas is sent to the

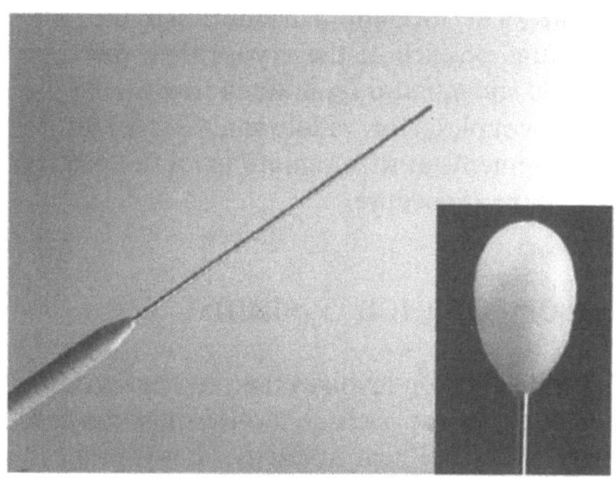

FIGURE 7.13. Endocare, Inc. needle-type cryoablation probe. Argon and helium gases are used to provide freezing and thawing of the ablation probe. Utilizing gases for temperature control allows for quick reversal of freezing to control ablation, and for release of the probe from frozen tissue for repositioning. A sample in vitro freeze demonstrates the ice ball formed at the probe tip (inset). (Photos courtesy of Endocare, Inc.)

A 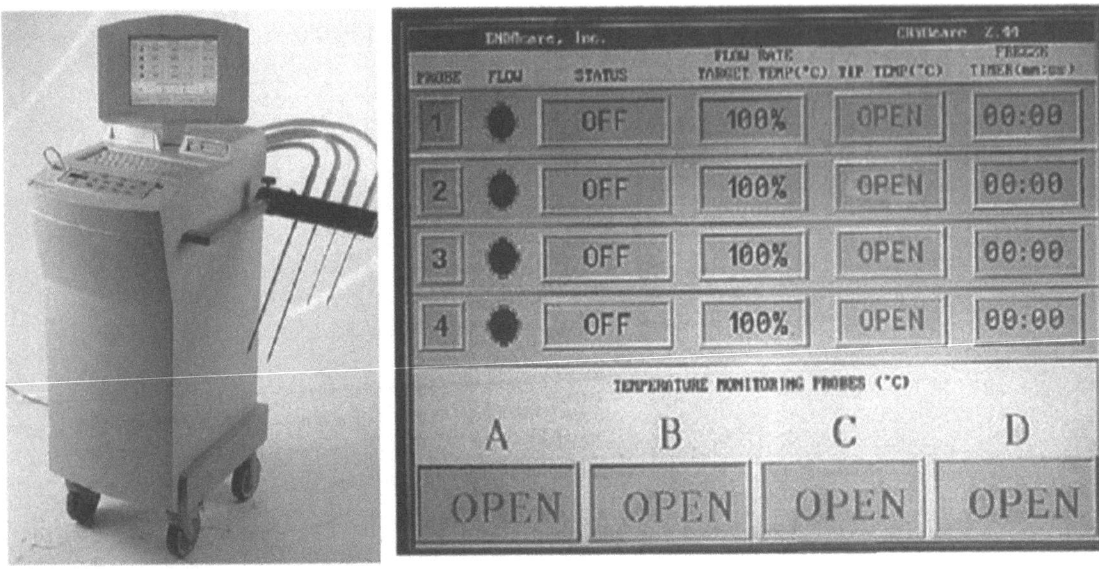 B

FIGURE 7.14. Endocare, Inc. cryoablation system. The system (A) supports the use of multiple probes simultaneously. For each probe, the main control console (B) displays the probe's status (off, stick, freeze, thaw), the flow duty cycle, target temperature, actual tip temperature, and the elapsed time. In the figure, probes are disconnected and read as "open", whereas connected probes would be active and display values. Temperature and time are selected to effect an ablation. (Photos courtesy of Endocare, Inc.)

probe. A duty cycle of 50% would adjust the flow of gas to be on-then-off half the time, respectively, allowing the physician to control the rate of ice formation. In addition to the temperatures of each of the cryoprobes, the user can add and monitor separate individual needle thermocouples for additional temperature measurements at sites remote from the probes during the procedure.

Laser Ablation Systems

Thermal ablation involves the physical properties of the tissue such as the thermal conductivity and the heat capacity. Laser-induced ablation also relies on the optical properties of the tissue (including absorption and scattering), coupled with the characteristics of the laser light (including wavelength, energy, power). A medical laser system provides a strong reproducible source of monochromatic light that can be delivered in a controlled fashion. Ablation techniques either use lenses to focus light to either a broad or a pinpoint beam, or use contact applicators. Contact tips touch tissue and are used for thermal resection (laser scalpel) or interstitial coagulation in situ. Interstitial laser ablation can be done with a simple bare fiber optic inserted into the tissue. A more contemporary interstitial approach uses an extended light source, the diffusing tip. It acts as a cylindrical light source whereby light is emitted radially along the end of the tip to provide a volume of ablation larger than that of the simple bare fiber. These fibers may be placed in catheters that have a closed-loop coolant flow to prevent charring and optimize light penetration into the tissue. Usually, the laser light is in the near infrared portion of the electromagnetic spectrum.

PhotoMedex

The PhotoMedex diffuser (PhotoMedex, formerly SLT, Montgomeryville, PA) is an optical fiber that includes a light diffusing segment (active diffusing portion) that ranges from 1 to 4 cm. The diffusing tip is shown in Figure 7.15. The fiber's overall length is either 3.5 or 12 m.

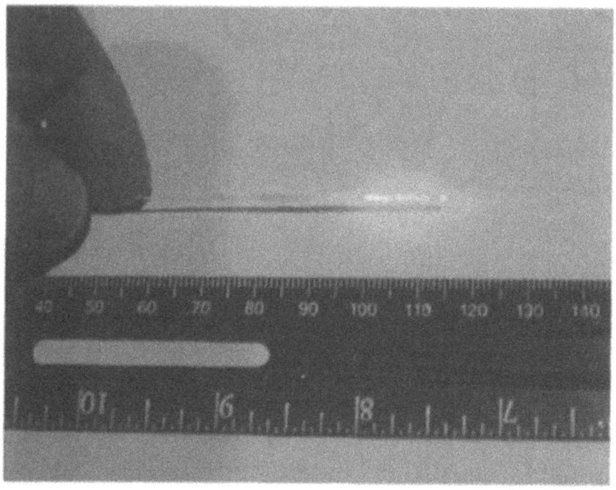

FIGURE 7.15. PhotoMedex (formerly SLT) laser fiber. This 1.5-cm diffusing tip provides an extended light source for tissue ablation. The fiber disperses light radially out along the final length of the tip. The fiber is placed into tissue itself within a catheter for added mechanical support and penetration. The catheters can be cooled by a closed-loop flow of water to prevent tissue char that can impede the penetration of near infrared light into tissue. (Photo printed with permission from PhotoMedex.)

It is intended for tissue coagulation with wavelengths of light from 980 to 1064 nanometers (nm). The power delivered to the fiber must be less than 2 W per cm (maximum 6 W), that is, no more than 4 W to a 2-cm tip or 6 W to a 3-cm or 4-cm tip. Since the fiber's tip is both blunt and flexible, it is used in conjunction with a more rigid catheter that is designed for penetration into tissue. This interstitial cooling catheter, available from Somatex, Inc., is available in a version that can be cooled with flowing water (~22°C); this allows up to 12 W per centimeter to create larger lesions.

The PhotoMedex CL MD/220 100 W medical laser system is based on a neodymium: yttrium-aluminum-garnet (Nd: YAG) continuous laser emitting at 1064 nm, and is shown in Figure 7.16 (8). It is a free-standing system that is internally air cooled; it can deliver up to 100 W (other CL MD series versions provide 25, 40, and 60 W). The primary displays of the main control panel (also shown in Fig. 7.16) show the laser power and exposure duration. The laser can be run in

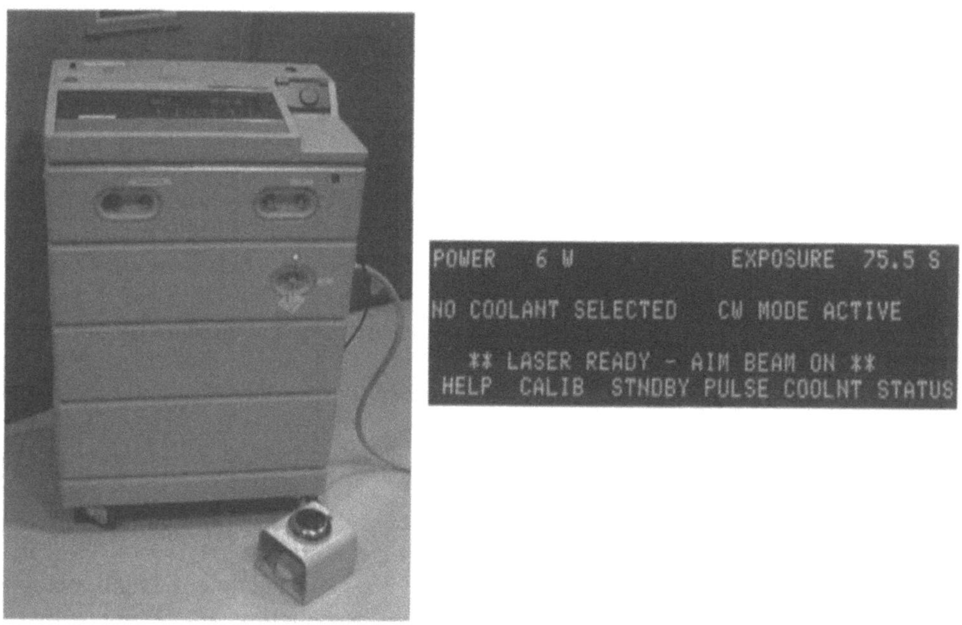

A

B

FIGURE 7.16. PhotoMedex (formerly SLT) laser system (A). This is a neodymium: yttrium-aluminum-garnet (Nd: YAG) laser operating at 1064 nm. For interstitial thermal ablation with the laser, the primary elements of the display on the main control panel (B) are the power delivered to the tissue and the duration of the exposure. In the figure, 6 W of power have been delivered over 75.5 seconds. (Photo printed with permission from PhotoMedex.)

a continuous wave (CW) mode or pulsed model; the CW mode delivers power continuously with the press of a foot pedal; the pulsed mode provides a shuttering of the light in set limited exposures from 0.1 to 90 seconds.

Microwave Ablation Systems

Microwave (MW) ablation systems radiate electromagnetic radiation into tissue where it is absorbed and transformed into heat to thermally coagulate the target. The applicator is an antenna that emits in the microwave region of the electromagnetic spectrum. The antenna provides a complete electrical circuit at the tip, and thus there is no requirement for grounding pads to be placed on the patient.

Azwell

The Microtaze AZM-520 (Azwell, Inc., Osaka, Japan) MW ablation system operates at a frequency of 2450MHz, and provides power output up to 110W (9). The probes (antennae) are available in a variety of designs for use in open, percutaneous, laparoscopic, and endoscopic procedures. An example of the tip of a probe for interstitial use is shown in Figure 7.17. The probe tips are needle-like to traverse tissues for deep applications; they range from 1.6 to 2mm in diameter with overall lengths

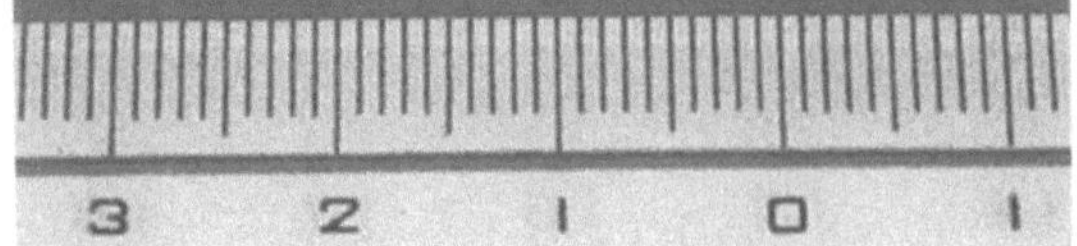

FIGURE 7.17. Alfresa Pharma Corp. needle-type microwave antenna. The tip of the microwave probe designed for interstitial use is needle-like for tissue penetration, and ranges between 1.6 and 2mm in diameter. (Photo printed with permission from Alfresa Pharma Corp.)

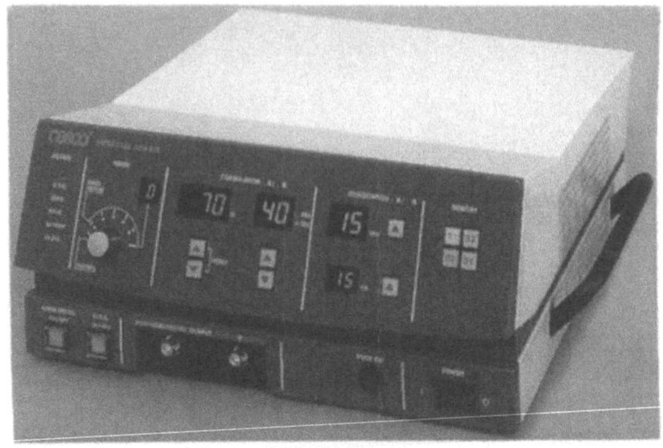

FIGURE 7.18. Alfresa Pharma Corp. microwave generator. The main control panel displays the user-selected parameters for the ablation. These include the output power, exposure duration, and the dissociation parameters mentioned in the text. Here, the ablation cycle is set for a duration of 40 seconds at 70W with a dissociation current of 15mA lasting 15 seconds. Also, the generator can power two probes simultaneously. (Photo printed with permission from Alfresa Pharma Corp.)

ranging between 15 and 25cm. It is possible to activate two antennae simultaneously for added tumor coverage during a single application of energy.

The main control panel of the AZM-520 is shown in Figure 7.18. It is divided into sections: coagulation, dissociation, mode, and memory. The primary intraprocedural controls are through the power setting and the duration of exposure, both of which are displayed in the coagulation section of the panel. Power output and duration can be adjusted. Separately, the system provides the dissociation feature, which establishes a polarity on the antenna that is intended to electrically attract water molecules to the probe to induce tissue hydration to reduce unwanted tissue adherence to the probe. The dissociation current and cycle time are set by the user. Separately, a selection between the normal and auto-repeat modes is made. The normal mode establishes a preset cycle of coagulation and dissociation with a press of the control foot switch; the application of energy ceases when the switch is released. The auto-repeat mode repeats a number of cycles of preselected outputs without having to maintain pressure on the foot switch. Values for ablation settings can be saved in the memory via buttons in the memory section. Sample settings are 70W power, 40-second duration, and 15 seconds at 15mA dissociation current.

Vivant

The VivaWave microwave generator (Vivant Medical, Mountain View, CA) operates at a source frequency of 915MHz (10). It can provide up to 60W of power. The VivaWave is used in conjunction with Vivant's VivaTip or VivaRing probes. These are shown in Figure 7.19. The VivaTip is a 14G needle-type antenna that can be inserted directly into tissue. It can be used as a single probe, or, it can be used in a configuration together with 2 other probes simultaneously. The multiple probe configuration is aligned by a handheld template for keeping the three probes at a fixed distance from one another. This is intended to optimize the volume of ablation to the target volume. The user can select from three choices for interprobe distance. The VivaRing is an array-type device for microwave delivery to tissue. The array is established in tissue after the insertion and positioning of three 14G cannulae; these cannulae are held together at a fixed distance from each other by a common handle to which they are affixed. Through each cannula is extended a stylette that curves into a 3- (or 4-) cm circle on deployment. Each stylette is actually the antenna for the microwave deposition. The three circular stylettes together define a sphere that encompasses the tissue to be treated.

The control panel for the VivaWave generator is shown in Figure 7.20. The primary feedback from the system to the user is a visual display of the elapsed time at a given power. The power output is set by the user for a given energy deposition—it can be adjusted up to 60W in increments of 5W. There is also a pair of control buttons and a display for setting the duration of exposure from 0–30min in 1min increments. Cable connections are made on the front of the device. The front panel provides a visual cue (light), and there is an audible tone heard when energy is sent through the probe.

Focused Ultrasound Systems

Focused ultrasound (FUS) ablation of soft tissue is distinct from the techniques described above in that it is a noninvasive transcutaneous application of energy used to create volumes of ablation. Thus, it does not use a probe as an

A

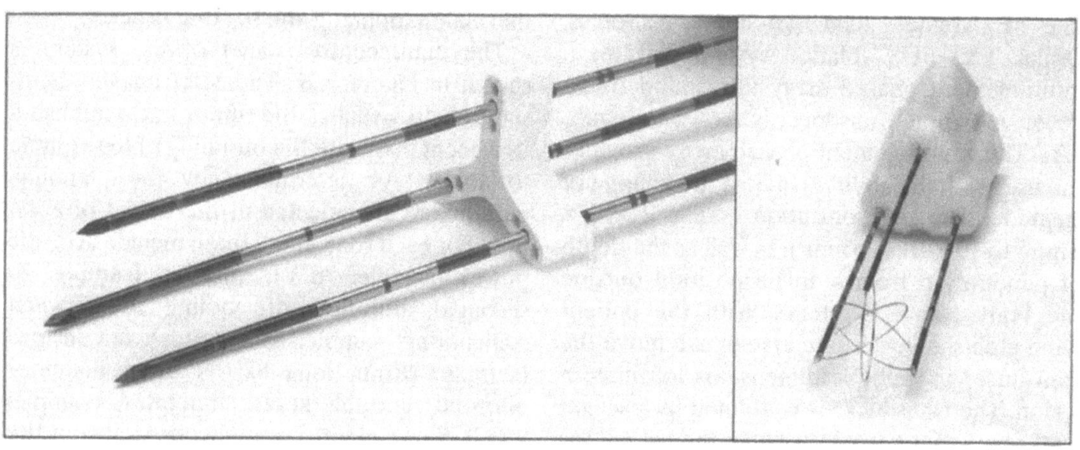

B

Figure 7.19. Vivant Medical needle-type VivaTip microwave probe in a multi-probe configuration (A) and the array-type VivaRing Atom microwave probe (B). The VivaTip is designed for direct penetration through tissue and can be used individually or with additional probes, as shown, for larger ablation volumes. The VivaRing provides an array of antennae that is deployed interstitially and intended to encircle the volume to be ablated. (Photo courtesy of Vivant Medical, Inc.)

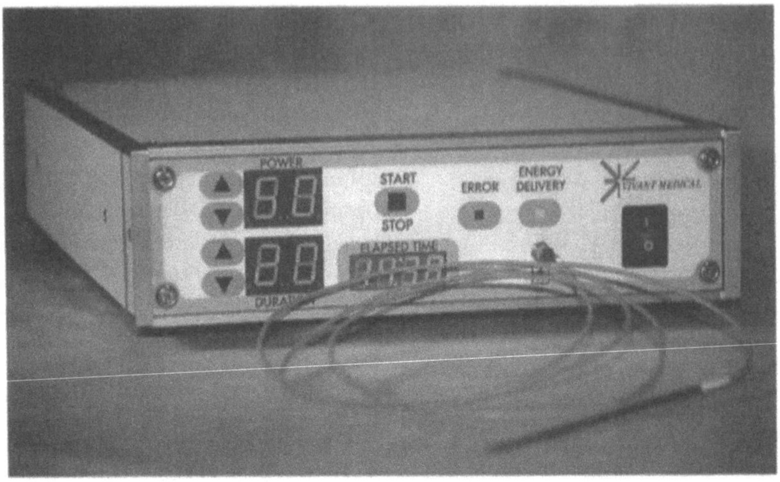

FIGURE 7.20. Vivant Medical VivaWave microwave generator. The main control panel allows the user to adjust power (up to 60W) and duration (up to 30min) for the ablation. Multiple needle-probes or the array-type probes require multiple generators. The primary feedback to the user is the display of the elapsed time during energy deposition. (Photo courtesy of Vivant Medical, Inc.)

applicator, but rather uses a transducer placed in contact with the skin. Also, FUS is based on tissue heating by the transmission and absorption of high-frequency ultrasonic waves instead of electromagnetic energy. The user ablates a tumor by covering the targeted volume with multiple abutting ellipsoids of coagulation.

InSightec-TxSonics

The ExAblate 2000 (InSightec-TxSonics, Dallas, TX) FUS ablation system features a multi-element phased array ultrasound transducer. A sample transducer is shown in Figure 7.21. This multi-element phased array provides the user with the ability to adjust the volume of treated tissue per sonication (range $2 \times 2 \times 4\,mm^3$ to $10 \times 10 \times 35\,mm^3$), as well as the depth of penetration from a single position outside the body (range 5–20cm). With the patient lying atop the device, the system can move the transducer in multiple dimensions to ablate a lesion. The transducer is contained in a sealed water-bath that is in contact with the patient for effective transmission of the ultrasound waves into tissue. The operating frequency is centered on approximately 1.61MHz.

The transducer is incorporated into a modified magnetic resonance imaging (MRI) table also shown in Figure 7.21. Up to this point in this chapter, there has been no discussion of specific radiologic imaging techniques to plan or monitor therapy (again, the chapter is an overview of the *operation* of each of the systems). However, MRI is integral to the operation of the ExAblate 2000 system. At all stages of the ablation process, MRI (a) offers soft tissue visualization for pre- and postprocedural assessment, and (b) provides quantitative thermal mapping of the heating process.

The main control panel of the system is shown in Figure 7.22. The MRI images themselves help visualize the tumor and establish a treatment plan with the outlining of the volume to ablate. As determined by the planning, parameters are selected at the outset of ablation. For each sonication, these include acoustic power (sample: 70W), duration (sample: 20 seconds); duration of cooling in between sonications (sample: 85 seconds); dimensions (sample: 28mm long axis × 6mm diameter ellipsoid), and the target temperature (sample: 85°C). Subsequently, spatial coordinates of the sonications consistent with the plan are identified. During the procedure, feedback to the user includes the average temperature achieved in each sonication, the number of sonications performed, the number remaining, and the total

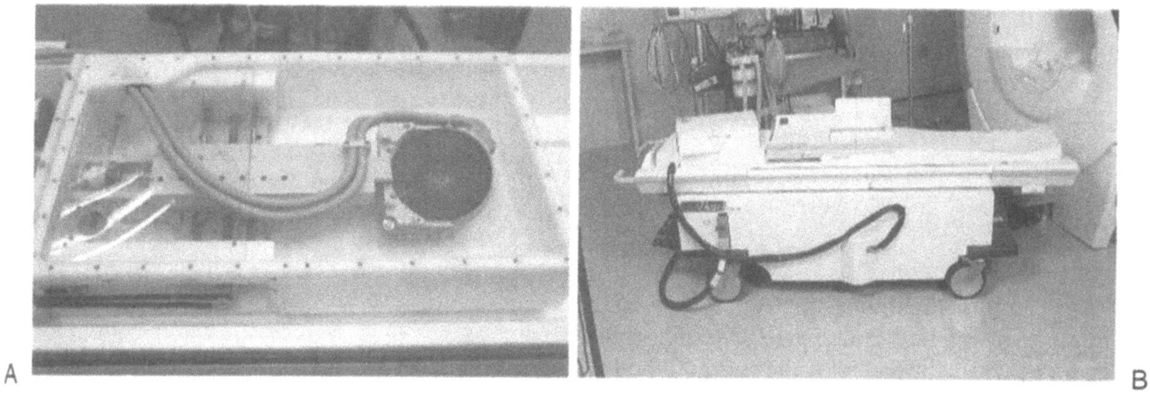

FIGURE 7.21. InSightec ultrasound transducer. A multi-element phased array transducer (A) is integrated into an MRI table (B). The patient is placed atop the table and the location of the transducer can be adjusted to target tissue at a depth, with individual sonications. Multiple overlapping sonications are used to ablate a targeted volume. (Photos printed with permission from InSightec.)

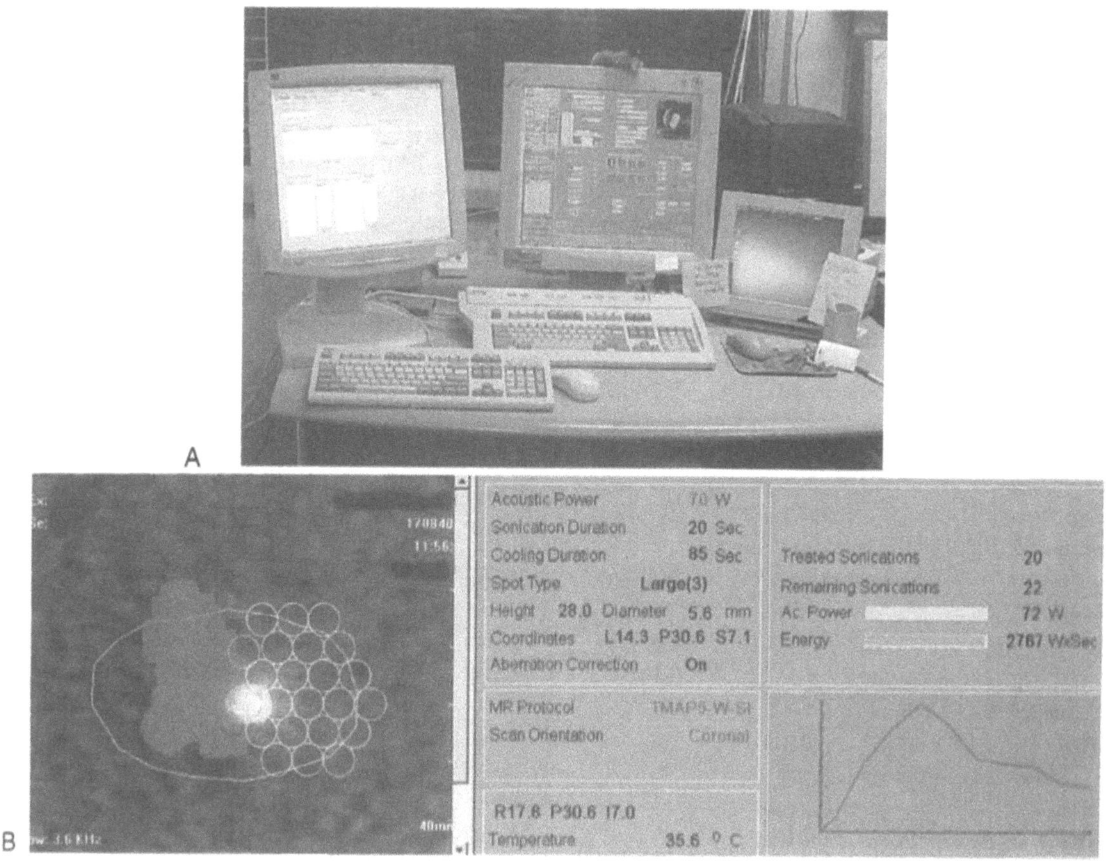

FIGURE 7.22. InSightec console. The main control console for the ablation system (A) resides to the left of the MRI scanner console (A). Salient features of the ablation and monitoring are shown in the sample screen (B). Here, an ovoid outline of a target in one MRI scan plane is seen. Individual sonications are recorded (circles) as the energy is deposited into tissue. A cross-hair indicates the location of the current sonication. In this case, 70 W of focused energy are delivered for 20 seconds; the tissue is allowed to cool for 85 seconds before the next sonication. (Photos printed with permission from InSightec.)

energy delivered to tissue. Further, superimposed on the MRI images is a cumulative visual record of the ablation associated with each sonication for comparison with the original treatment plan.

Conclusion

This chapter highlights the operation of a number of medical devices for thermal ablation. It reveals the scope of the thermal modalities available to physicians to induce tissue necrosis: from heating at +100°C to a −180°C freeze; from passing an electrical current to depositing invisible photons; from manipulating the placement of an antenna into tissue to the remote sonication of a tumor from a computer console. Ten ablation systems have been reviewed. Readers should consider these systems as representative of the ablation mechanisms, and interested individuals are encouraged to investigate each for themselves and to understand the principles behind the devices to better assess their use and implementation.

References

1. Instructions for Use 921-91-003 Rev. B. and 460-92-001 Rev. F. Radionics, Burlington, MA.
2. Instructions for Use. Boston Scientific Corporation—Oncology, Natick, MA.
3. User's Guide and Service manual Ref 160-102025, RITA Medical Systems, Mountain View, CA.
4. http://hittmethod.com, Berchtold, GmbH, Tuttlingen, Germany.
5. User's Manual. Ref: 991.027 and 991.0287/2002. Celon AG Medical Instruments, Berlin, Germany.
6. Operator's Manual. Galil Medical, Westbury, NY.
7. http://www.endocare.com, Endocare, Inc., Irvine, CA.
8. Operations and Maintenance Manual for the CL MD Series Laser. PN 0800-0370. Rev. 5.11/94. PhotoMedex *formerly* SLT, Montgomeryville, PA.
9. Operation Manual Microtaze AZM-520, Azwell, Inc. Osaka, Japan.
10. VivaWave Microcoagulation System User Manual, PN0339 Rev C, Vivant Medical, Mountain View, CA.
11. Personal communications. InSightec-TxSonics, Dallas, TX.

Section III
Imaging for Tumor Ablation

8
Intraoperative Ultrasound-Guided Procedures

Robert A. Kane

While the continuous development and improvements in tumor ablation techniques and equipment have made the percutaneous nonsurgical approach ever more successful, even for larger lesions, there is still a need for ablative treatments in the operating room. In some practices, based on local referral patterns, the surgical approach to tumor ablation may be predominant, either via laparoscopy or open laparotomy. In other settings, additional tumor sites may be encountered during a planned surgical excision that can be efficiently treated intraoperatively with a variety of ablative approaches. Finally, some techniques, such as cryoablation, may be best performed intraoperatively, particularly when treating large tumors with 5- to 10-mm diameter cryoprobes. Therefore, a review of intraoperative ultrasound (IOUS) scanning and guidance techniques for ablation is appropriate. This chapter discusses the optimal approach to intraoperative and laparoscopic ultrasound (LUS) scanning techniques, equipment, technical preparations, and methods for guidance of interventional techniques. Since most of the intraoperative tumor ablations involve lesions in the liver, we focus the discussion on hepatic ultrasonography and guidance.

Equipment

All of the major ultrasound manufacturers have specifically designed probes for open intraoperative ultrasound uses (Fig. 8.1). These probes tend to be smaller than conventional abdominal ultrasound probes. Since the probe can be positioned directly on the target organ, higher scanning frequencies can be utilized successfully as there is much less attenuation of the sound beam than when scanning through the skin and subcutaneous fat and other intervening tissues. The probes designed for intraoperative abdominal use are linear, curvilinear, or phased array electronic probes that have the capacity both for gray scale imaging as well as spectral and color Doppler scanning. Some manufacturers offer probes with a choice of multiple frequencies (5–7.5 MHz), while others utilize broadband technology to display a range of frequencies from near to far field, and for abdominal uses ranging from 3 up to 10–12 MHz.

Because of the sophisticated electronics and the encasing plastic housing and rubber membranes over the transducer, heat sterilization via autoclaving is not possible. Some of the earliest intraoperative probes were designed for direct sterilization using techniques such as ethylene oxide gas sterilization or prolonged immersion in glutaraldehyde. However, other manufacturers prohibited gas sterilization because of concerns of possible damage to the transducer. In addition, with heightened environmental concerns more recently, many hospitals and operating suites no longer allow the use of such agents as ethylene oxide or glutaraldehyde. Therefore, the method of choice for maintaining sterilization in the operative field is the use of specifically designed sterile

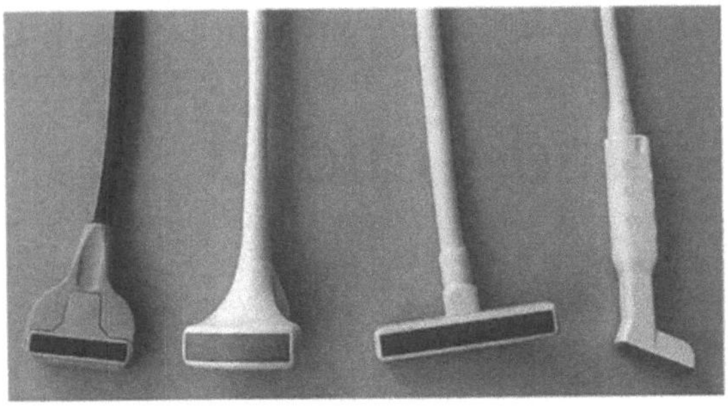

Figure 8.1. Intraoperative ultrasound (IOUS) probes. Various linear and curvilinear, end-fire, and side-fire probes are available for intraoperative use. The side-viewing probes are most optimal for imaging the liver.

probe covers that are individually manufactured to fit snugly over the specific size and shape of the intraoperative ultrasound probe. Acoustic coupling is required between the probe and the probe cover, which is most optimally accomplished by using sterile gel or possibly sterile saline. A snug fit must be maintained over the transducer surface so that no air bubbles are present between the transducer and the target organ, since these will cause artifacts due to acoustic shadowing. Most of the probe covers also are manufactured complete with a long sterile sleeve that can extend over the electronic cord to connect the transducer to the ultrasound scanner console (1).

Several, but not all ultrasound companies also manufacture laparoscopic ultrasound probes that are designed to fit through a standard 10- to 11-mm laparoscopy port. These are either linear or curvilinear transducers. They are approximately 2 to 4cm in length and are mounted on a 30- to 40-cm-long shaft. The very first of these systems was entirely rigid, but this proved impractical, since good contact could not be maintained easily on the curved surfaces of the abdominal organs. Currently available systems offer flexibility of the scanning tip, with systems similar to those used on endoscopes (Fig. 8.2). These systems allow either two-way flexion and extension maneuverability or four-way maneuverability, including left and right deflection, as well as flexion and extension (2). As with open abdominal ultrasound probes, pulsed Doppler and color flow imaging are available, and the systems also offer either multiple frequencies or broadband technology. Covers for laparoscopic probes require a long, thin, sterile sheath that must be applied tightly to the shaft of the laparoscopic probe to fit easily through the laparoscopic port without tearing. Once again, acoustic coupling

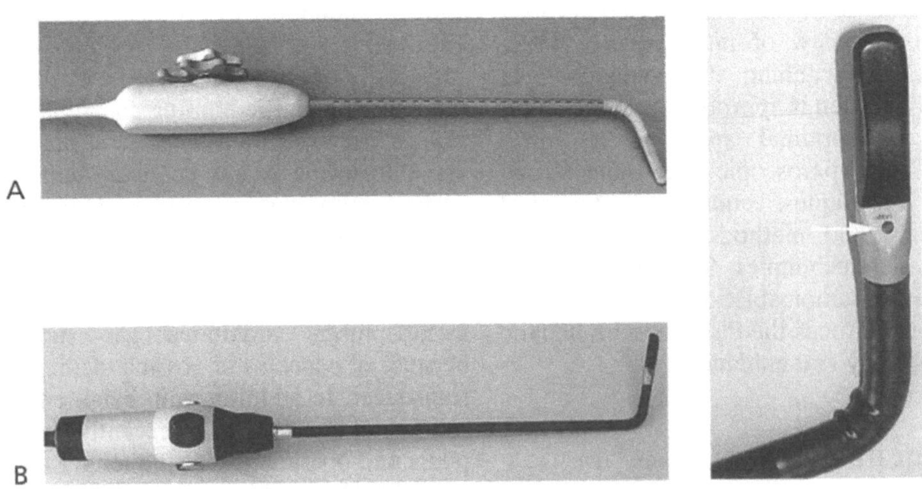

Figure 8.2. Laparoscopic ultrasound (LUS) probes. (A) Linear array probe in flexion. (B) Curved array probe demonstrating left deflection. (C) Close-up of curved array probe demonstrating the biopsy port (arrow).

is required at the transducer interface, usually accomplished by placing sterile saline in the sheath prior to insertion of the probe (1).

Scanning Technique

While it is essential to provide acoustic coupling between the surface of the transducer and the overlying sterile sheath using either sterile gel or sterile saline, the natural moisture within the body cavity is usually sufficient for good acoustic coupling between the ultrasound probe and the liver or other intraabdominal organs. If the surfaces are somewhat dry, sterile saline can be applied over the organ surface to improve acoustic coupling. For maximal detection of occult liver lesions, a systematic approach to scanning the liver should be followed carefully (3). We prefer to scan from the anterior surface of the liver that is relatively smooth, rather than the deep surface, which has numerous fissures and undulations, and may present difficulties in maintaining good contact with the liver. Side-viewing probes are preferable to allow scanning of the entire liver surface. Our scanning convention is to begin with the cephalad-lateral aspect of the left lobe (segment II). The probe is positioned in a transverse orientation and scans are performed slowly in a cephalocaudad direction until the caudal edge of the liver is reached. This maneuver is then repeated by moving the probe toward the right by the width of the transducer and repeating a cephalocaudad sweep. In this fashion, moving left to right, the entire liver can be scanned with approximately five to eight cephalocaudad sweeps, taking approximately 5 minutes for a complete scan (4). Each successive series of sweeps should slightly overlap the preceding one to ensure coverage of the entire liver.

The optimal frequency for liver imaging is 5 MHz, since the attenuation of soft tissue in the liver may be too great at higher frequencies, thereby compromising imaging of the deep portions of the liver. With fatty infiltration, even at 5 MHz, complete penetration may be a problem, but if a lower frequency option is not available, satisfactory images of the deep liver can be obtained either by increasing compression of the anterior liver and placing the focal zones more deeply in the liver, or by scanning from the lateral or deep liver surfaces when necessary.

Using laparoscopic ultrasound, the technical challenges to obtaining a complete scan of the liver are greater. Often, the laparoscopic ultrasound probe must be exchanged with the laparoscope, and scans must be obtained from more than one port site (2). Typically, a midline or periumbilical port may provide good access to the left lateral segment, but the falciform ligament may impede positioning of the probe on the right side of the liver. In other patients, a periumbilical or midline port may provide better access to the right lobe, with associated difficulties scanning to the left of the falciform ligament. A right subcostal port may be helpful to image the right lobe; care must be taken that this port is not placed too close to the tip of the right lobe to leave room to maneuver the probe over the anterior surface of the liver. As with open intraoperative scanning, a consistent, planned approach to scanning the liver is important to obtain a complete study. Our approach is to begin either to the right or left of the falciform ligament and fan the probe across the dome of the liver from the medial to lateral position, and then withdraw the probe 2 to 4 cm (the length of the probe surface) and repeat the scans again from medial to lateral, withdrawing and scanning until the entire liver has been imaged from cephalad to caudal margins. This is much more tedious and time-consuming than with open intraoperative scanning, since the probe lengths are substantially smaller for laparoscopic ultrasound systems. Consequently, a complete scan of the liver using the laparoscopic approach takes at least 10 to 15 minutes to accomplish.

Numerous studies have demonstrated the superiority of intraoperative and laparoscopic ultrasound imaging over preoperative imaging studies for maximal liver lesion detection (Fig. 8.3). The spatial resolution is capable of depicting cystic structures as small as 1 to 3 mm and solid nodules as small as 3 to 5 mm. Studies have demonstrated improved liver lesion detection of 20% to 30%, compared to standard computed tomography (CT) and magnetic resonance (MR) techniques (5,6), and increased detection of 10% to 15% compared to CT arterial portography (7). More recently, development of multidetector CT scanning, as well as improvements in MR technology resulting in decreasing scan speeds have markedly improved detection of small liver lesions, particularly with multiphase contrast-enhanced scans. There are no recent studies to compare the efficacy of intraoperative imaging to these latest high-speed scanning techniques, and, undoubtedly, fewer additional lesions will probably be detected by intraoperative scanning, but some additional lesions will still be detected and may be highly influential on the selection of appropriate intraoperative therapies (Fig. 8.4). Therefore, a compulsive systematic assessment of the entire liver is still of considerable importance. In fact, detection of additional unsuspected lesions often is an event that results in a tumor ablation technique being undertaken in the operating room either instead of, or in addition to, the planned surgical tumor resection (8).

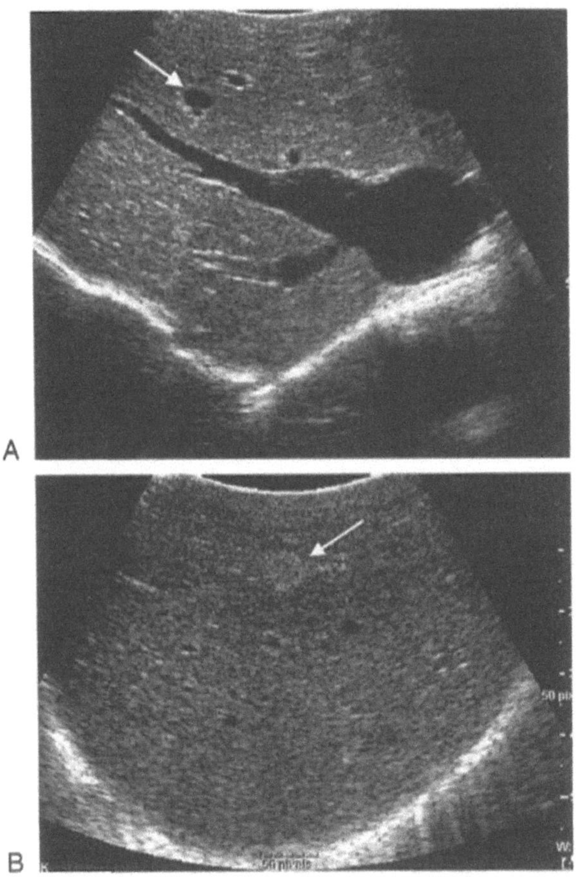

FIGURE 8.3. IOUS liver in a patient with breast metastases. (A) A 3-mm hepatic cyst (arrow). (B) A 6-mm echogenic metastasis (arrow), not seen on preoperative imaging. Three additional metastases were identified at IOUS.

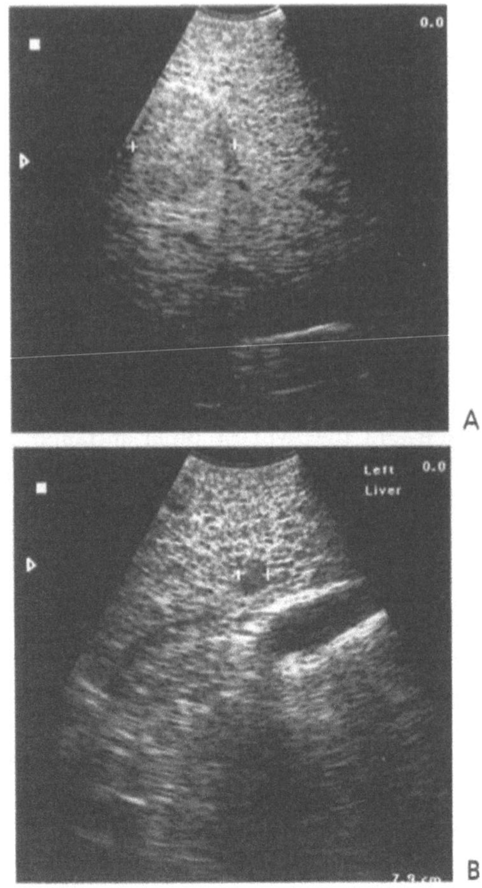

FIGURE 8.4. LUS images in a patient with hepatocellular carcinoma (HCC). (A) A 2.5-cm HCC in a cirrhotic liver. (B) Unsuspected 5.6-mm HCC nodule. Two unsuspected nodules were identified at LUS, not seen on preoperative imaging.

Ultrasound Guidance Techniques

If additional unsuspected lesions are encountered during scanning, ultrasound-guided biopsy and immediate frozen section analysis of the biopsy can be performed to confirm the presence of additional tumor sites. At open intraoperative ultrasonography, this can be readily performed using the free-hand technique (9). The lesion is positioned under the ultrasound probe and a needle is advanced along the midline of the long axis of the transducer, such that the entire length of the needle can be imaged. This allows precise changes in angulation of the needle that can be placed accurately within 1 to 2mm of the target. We utilize automated 18-gauge core biopsy needles to obtain intraoperative biopsies. Occasionally, a lesion may be so deeply seated that the free-hand technique is difficult. Fixed electronic biopsy guides are not available for most intraoperative ultrasound probes, but there is an alternative solution that we have used successfully for deep, difficult needle placements. This technique utilizes an end-fire endorectal prostate probe covered with a sterile sheath (Fig. 8.5). Over this sheath, a sterile biopsy guide can be positioned and a precise electronic depiction of the path of the biopsy needle can then be utilized for accurate needle positioning (Fig. 8.6), even at 15cm depth.

Biopsy guidance during laparoscopic ultrasound imaging is considerably more difficult and problematic. Most laparoscopic ultrasound systems lack electronic biopsy guidance systems, although there is one system that allows passage of a biopsy guide through the length of the laparoscopic ultrasound probe (Fig. 8.2C), but this is a somewhat cumbersome device to use, and it is expensive.

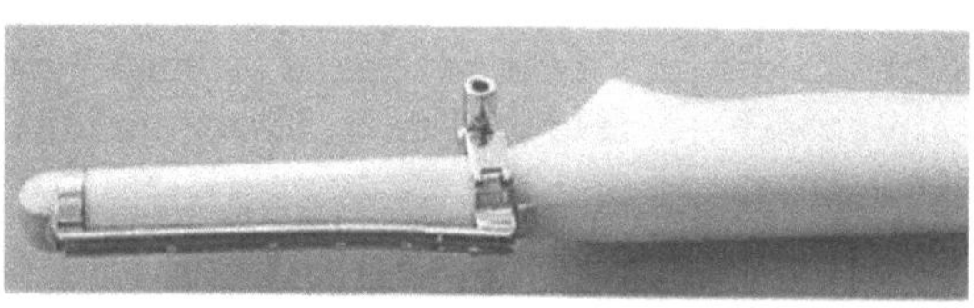

FIGURE 8.5. Curvilinear endoluminal probe with biopsy guide. The biopsy needle or ablation probe can be positioned in the trough of the biopsy guide for precise intraoperative placement.

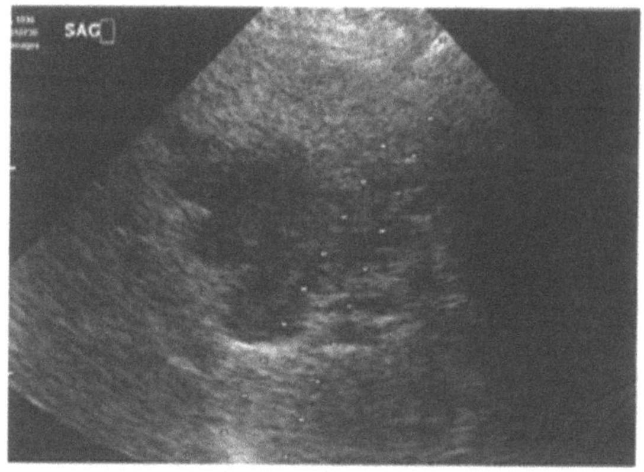

FIGURE 8.6. Electronic biopsy guidance. The hypoechoic tumor is positioned within the electronic cursors, which can be used to guide placement of biopsy needles or ablation devices.

An alternative approach to laparoscopic ultrasound-guided biopsy is to puncture through the anterior abdominal wall, using a long laparoscopic biopsy needle, and then position the needle immediately adjacent to the laparoscopic ultrasound transducer, using the real-time images to adjust the angulation and depth of the biopsy needle (2). This approach is feasible with lesions that are of moderate size and not too deeply placed within the liver. However, attempting to biopsy small, unsuspected lesions detected during laparoscopic ultrasound can be quite difficult, since these additional lesions tend to be quite small, usually less than 1 to 2cm in size.

The same techniques used to biopsy liver lesions are also used to accurately place needles and probes for tumor ablation (10). With alcohol ablation or hyperthermia techniques such as radiofrequency, microwave, and laser ablation, the size of the needles and probes approximates 16 to 21 gauge, and hence free-hand ultrasound guidance is quite feasible and accurate (Fig. 8.7). Once again, utilizing an end-fire prostate-type probe with an electronic biopsy guidance system is useful for accurate placement of probes and needles into small, deeply situated lesions.

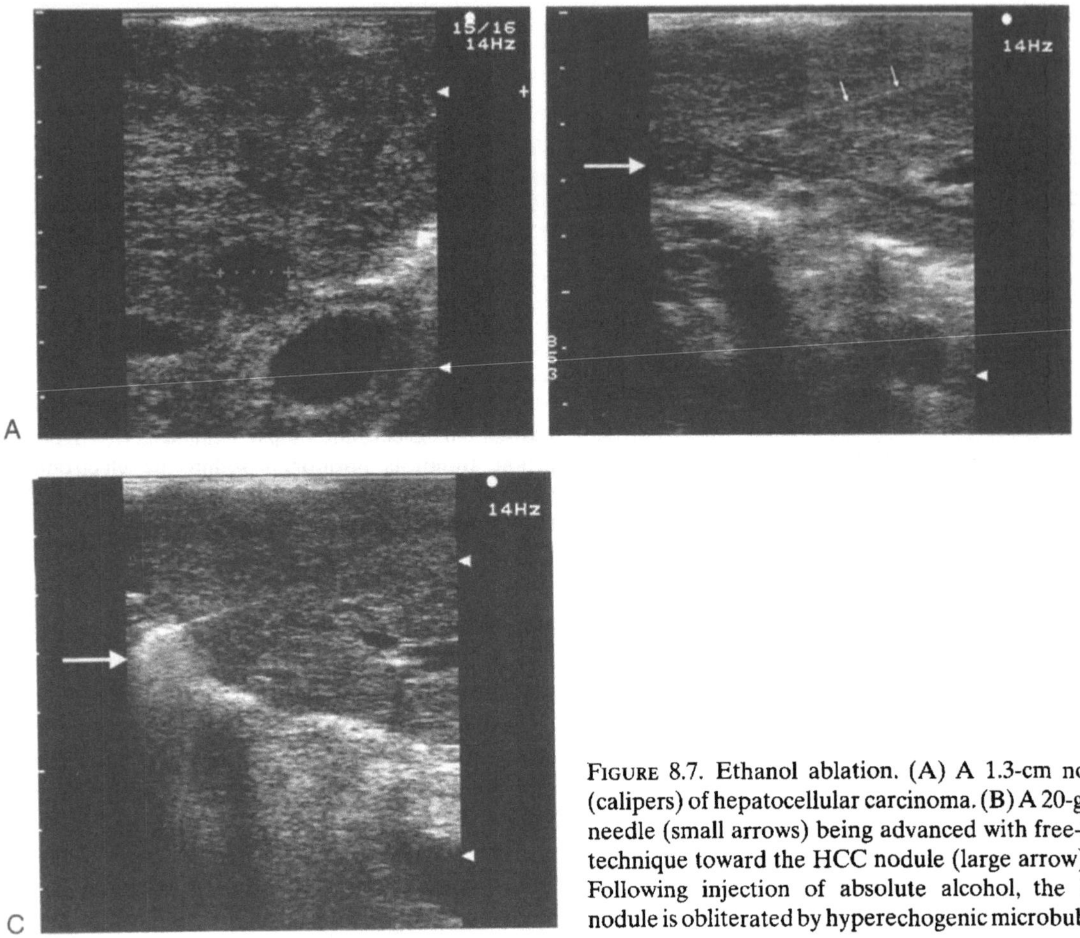

FIGURE 8.7. Ethanol ablation. (A) A 1.3-cm nodule (calipers) of hepatocellular carcinoma. (B) A 20-gauge needle (small arrows) being advanced with free-hand technique toward the HCC nodule (large arrow). (C) Following injection of absolute alcohol, the HCC nodule is obliterated by hyperechogenic microbubbles.

For cryoablation, the size of the cryoprobes tends to be somewhat larger, ranging from 3 to 5 mm and even 10 mm in diameter. These larger probes are more difficult to place under direct real-time guidance. If the lesion is sufficiently large, the probes can be placed manually with intermittent ultrasound imaging to confirm accurate placement, or alter the course and depth of penetration as needed (11). Another approach is to use smaller, 18-gauge needles for precise placement, and then place the larger cryoprobe alongside the guiding needle in tandem, or by the Seldinger technique, using an 18-gauge needle, guidewires, and dilators (12). Whatever method is used, precise placement is essential to ensure adequate freezing of the entire lesion and the contiguous liver.

For all intraoperative or laparoscopic ablation techniques, ultrasound is imperative to ensure proper placement of the probes or needles, as well as to monitor the actual ablation procedure. For optimal therapeutic efficacy, it is essential that the ablation margin extends beyond the borders of the tumor into the surrounding normal liver parenchyma. Ideally, one seeks to create a 1-cm margin of normal liver around all borders of the tumor (13) to minimize local recurrence due to inadequately lethal temperatures at the periphery of the mass.

With cryoablation, the iceball is sharply defined and precisely imaged as an echogenic curvilinear freeze front, behind which there is complete acoustic shadowing. Studies have established that within a few millimeters of this visible freeze front, lethally cold temperatures will have produced complete necrosis (14). The difficulty encountered in cryoablation is that only the advancing half of the freeze front can be imaged while the deep portion is obscured by acoustic shadowing. Consequently, for complete monitoring of the cryoablation, images must be obtained from the deep surface as well as the superficial surface whenever possible. In this fashion, the freeze front can be observed to extend through the tumor into the surrounding liver, and the freezing time can be extended as long as required for complete tumor treatment (Fig. 8.8). The limitation occurs when the freeze front extends to one of the liver surfaces, in which case images can be obtained only from the opposite surface, and hence a complete sonographic assessment may not be attainable.

There are also limitations in monitoring the various hyperthermic ablation techniques as well as injection of absolute alcohol, acetic acid, or other fluid, such as heated saline. Once again, the goal is to extend the ablation margin into the surrounding liver on all sides of the tumor. However, these techniques usually produce microbubbles within the ablated tissue soon after treatment has begun (15). These microbubbles cause acoustic shadowing along the deep surface and result in considerable ultrasound scatter at the superficial and lateral margins of the tumor, resulting in difficulty in precise definition of the ablation front. As with cryoablation, imaging from the opposing deep surface may help to overcome the acoustic shadowing, as long as the treated area does not extend to the deep surface.

One of the limitations of both hyperthermic and cryoablation techniques occurs with tumors that are contiguous to large arterial or venous structures. The flowing blood in these

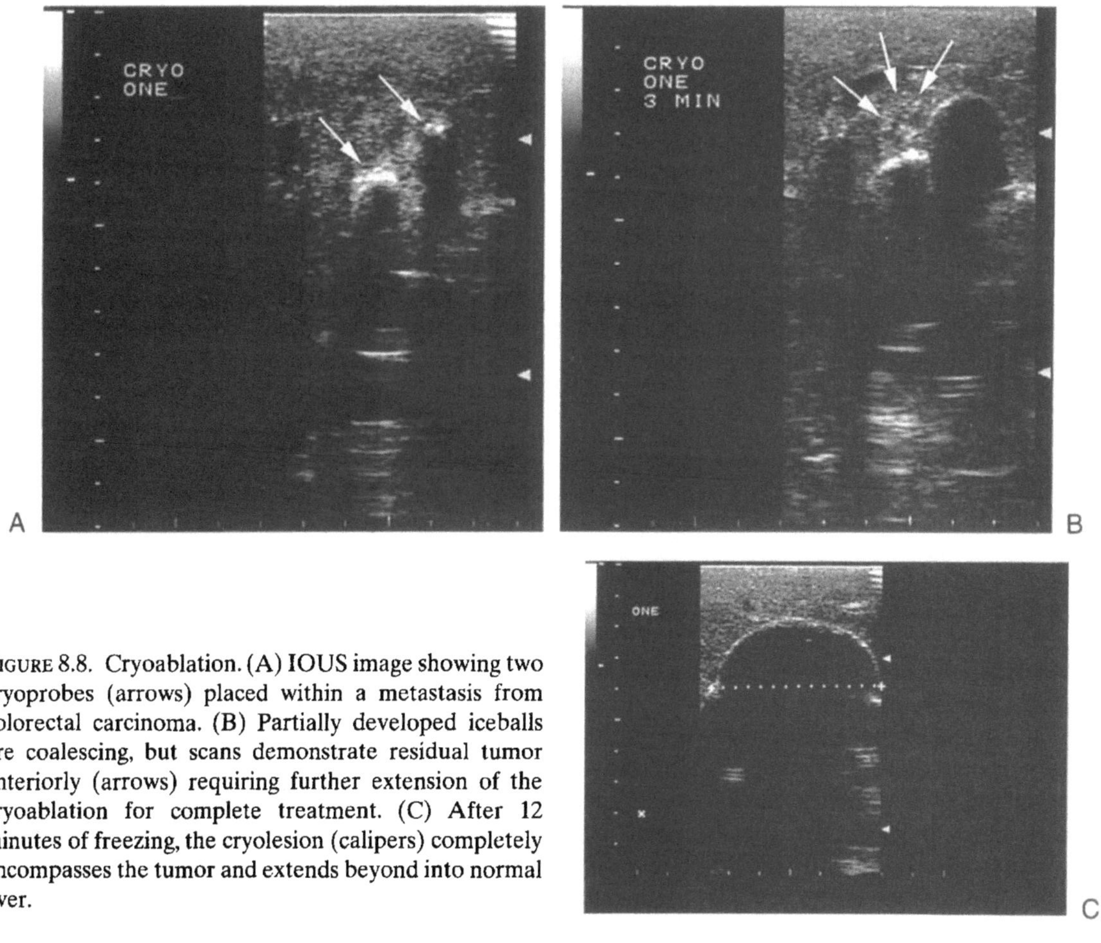

FIGURE 8.8. Cryoablation. (A) IOUS image showing two cryoprobes (arrows) placed within a metastasis from colorectal carcinoma. (B) Partially developed iceballs are coalescing, but scans demonstrate residual tumor anteriorly (arrows) requiring further extension of the cryoablation for complete treatment. (C) After 12 minutes of freezing, the cryolesion (calipers) completely encompasses the tumor and extends beyond into normal liver.

TABLE 8.1. Advantages and disadvantages of the intraoperative and percutaneous approaches to tumor ablation.

Approach	Advantages	Disadvantages
Intraoperative	IOUS for maximal lesion detection Safety—avoidance of bowel, gallbladder, heart, lung Safety—control of bleeding Pringle maneuver to decrease heat sink effect Easy access to tumor sites with open surgery	General anesthesia Surgical recovery time at least 1–3 days in hospital Monitoring of ablation margins may be less precise Limited access to some tumor sites with laparoscopic approach Expensive—1–2 hours of operating room time
Percutaneous	Local anesthesia/conscious sedation Short recovery time—same day discharge More accurate monitoring of ablation margins with contrast-enhanced CT, MRI, or US Repeat treatments feasible Less expensive	Less complete lesion detection Avoidance of critical structures (bowel, gallbladder, heart, lung) can present problems Difficult to access some lesions Cannot restrict blood flow to decrease heat sink effect Possible tumor seeding of percutaneous access tract

IOUS, intraoperative ultrasound.

large vessels can dilute and carry off sufficient heat or cold to cause the temperatures in the contiguous portion of tumor to remain in the sublethal zone. This is probably a frequent cause of local failure of various ablation techniques. In the intraoperative approach to liver tumor ablation, a Pringle maneuver can be performed by placing an atraumatic occlusive clamp across the vascular pedicle to the liver, thereby restricting hepatic arterial and portal venous inflow. The effects of this maneuver can be assessed by intraoperative ultrasonography, particularly using color flow imaging to demonstrate the reduction of blood flow.

Conclusion

There are advantages and disadvantages to both the intraoperative and percutaneous approaches to tumor ablation (16–18) (Table 8.1). However, at least in the liver, for which we have the most extensive experience and survival data, all of the approaches to tumor treatment, including surgical resection, are relatively ineffective over time. The most successful surgical series have shown approximately 30% five-year survival, and a significant portion of those five-year survivors are alive with recurrent disease. Actuarial survival results from various ablation procedures appear to be showing comparable results (17–19). Therefore, it is reasonable to suggest that percutaneous techniques for tumor ablation in the liver are preferable to intraoperative approaches in general.

The most mature survival data are for surgical resection of liver tumors. The experience with the various ablation techniques is not as mature, nor have there been sufficient prospective randomized trials comparing resection to various forms of tumor ablation (16,20). For this reason, there will still be a demand for intraoperative approaches to tumor ablation, particularly when unexpected findings are encountered at the time of a planned surgical resection.

References

1. Sammons LG, Kane RA. Technical aspects of intraoperative ultrasound. In: Kane RA, ed. Intraoperative, Laparoscopic, and Endoluminal Ultrasound. Philadelphia: Churchill Livingstone/Saunders, 1999:1–11.
2. Kane RA. Laparoscopic ultrasound. In: Kane RA, ed. Intraoperative, Laparoscopic, and Endoluminal Ultrasound. Philadelphia: Churchill Livingstone/Saunders, 1999:90–105.

3. Kane RA. Intra-operative ultrasound. In: Meire HB, Cosgrove DO, Dewbury KC, Farrant P, eds. Clinical Ultrasound: A Comprehensive Text: Abdominal and General Ultrasound. 2nd ed. London; Churchill Livingstone, 2001:143–164.
4. Kruskal JB, Kane RA. Intraoperative ultrasound of the liver. In: Kane RA, ed. Intraoperative, Laparoscopic, and Endoluminal Ultrasound. Philadelphia: Churchill Livingstone/Saunders, 1999:40–67.
5. Machi J, Isomoto H, Kurohiji T, et al. Accuracy of intraoperative ultrasound in diagnosing liver metastases from colorectal cancer: evaluation with postoperative follow-up results. World J Surg 1991;15:551–556.
6. Clarke MP, Kane RA, Steele GD, et al. Prospective comparison of preoperative imaging and intraoperative ultrasonography in the detection of liver tumors. Surgery 1989;106:849–855.
7. Soyer P, Levesque M, Elias D, Zeitoun G, Roche A. Detection of liver metastases from colorectal cancer: comparison of intraoperative US and CT during arterial portography. Radiology 1992;183:541–544.
8. Kane RA, Hughes LA, Cua EJ, et al. The impact of intraoperative ultrasonography on surgery for liver neoplasms. J Ultrasound Med 1994;13:1–6.
9. Lee RA. Kane RA, Lantz EJ, Charboneau JW. Intraoperative and laparoscopic sonography of the abdomen. In: Rumack CM, Wilson SR, Charboneau JW, eds. Diagnostic Ultrasound, vol 1. St. Louis: Mosby, 1998:671–699.
10. Patterson EJ, Scudamore CH, Buczkowski AK, Owen DA, Nagy AG. Radiofrequency ablation in surgery. Surg Technol Int 1997;6:69–75.
11. McPhee MD, Kane RA. Cryosurgery for hepatic tumor ablation. Semin Intervent Radiol 1997;14:285–293.
12. Littrup PJ, Lee FT, Rajan D, Meetze K, Weaver D. Hepatic cryotherapy: state-of-the-art techniques and future developments. Ultrasound Q 1998;14(3):171–188.
13. Ravikumar TS, Kane RA, Cady B, et al. A 5-year study of cryosurgery in the treatment of liver tumors. Arch Surg 1991;126:1520–1523.
14. Onik G, Kane RA, Steele G, et al. Monitoring hepatic cryosurgery with sonography. AJR 1986;147:665–669.
15. DeSanctis JT, Goldberg SN, Mueller PR. Percutaneous treatment of hepatic neoplasms: a review of current techniques. Semin Intervent Radiol 1997;14(3):255–284.
16. Simonetti RG, Liberati A, Angiolini C, Pagliaro L. Treatment of hepatocellular carcinoma: a systematic review of randomized controlled trials. Ann Oncol 1997;8:117–136.
17. Livraghi T, Bolondi L, Buscarini L, et al., and the Italian Cooperative HCC Study Group. No treatment, resection and ethanol injection in hepatocellular carcinoma: a retrospective analysis of survival in 391 patients with cirrhosis. J Hepatol 1995;22:522–526.
18. Korpan NN. Hepatic cryosurgery for liver metastases: long-term follow-up. Ann Surg 1997;225:193–201.
19. Goldberg SN, Lazzaroni S, Meloni F, et al. Hepatocellular carcinoma: Radio-frequency ablation of medium and large lesions. Radiology 2000;214:761–768.
20. Rush BJ, Koneru B. Locoregional techniques in the treatment of hepatic tumors. J Surg Oncol 1997;64:259–261.

9
Computed Tomography Imaging for Tumor Ablation

Thierry de Baère

Computed tomography (CT) affords the best visualization of all organs in the body, simultaneously depicting air, soft tissue, and bones on the same scan. This ability makes CT an ideal imaging modality for tissue ablation, as it enables the physician to target any type of organ accurately and to avoid inadvertently puncturing others along the needle path. However, in the past, as the duration of image acquisition and reconstruction was long with CT, this time-consuming aspect appeared inconvenient for tissue ablation. Recent improvements in computerized data management have transformed CT into almost a real-time imaging technique, and even more recently, the advent of multislice CT has made imaging of a volume in a single acquisition feasible, thereby improving the scope of CT guidance for tissue ablation. CT can now be used throughout tissue ablation for guidance, monitoring, and follow-up.

Image guidance is critical when ablating a tumor, because accurate positioning of the ablation instrument in the targeted tumor is a key factor for treatment efficacy. Moreover, accurate guidance avoids nontargeted structures or organs located close to or in the path of the tumor.

Image monitoring is also important. Ablation should be tailored to the tumor target volume to avoid incomplete treatment, recurrence, and the need for re-treatment. Injury to neighboring tissue and collateral damage also can be evaluated in real time.

Follow-up imaging is mandatory after tumor ablation because monitoring techniques and current ablation systems are unable to confirm complete tumor eradication at the time of treatment. The treated organ, therefore, requires follow-up imaging to ascertain whether ablation of the targeted tumor was efficient, as well as to detect new tumors and treatment complications.

Image Guidance

Indications

The first step in the ablation procedure is to guide the ablation instrument (the probe, the needle, the fiber, the electrode) toward the targeted tumor. Imaging used for guidance should clearly depict the ablation instrument and the targeted tumor, so that the instrument is positioned accurately within the tumor. Computed tomography is mandatory for guidance when it is the only technique capable of imaging the targeted tumor. Such is the case for most lung and bone tumors, given that fluoroscopic guidance is not accurate enough, and that interventional magnetic resonance (MR) is far from commonplace today. Such is also the case for some soft organ tumors that are not well defined by ultrasound (US). Computed tomography can be useful when the tumor is depicted by US, but is virtually inaccessible for puncture with US on account of the location, or because gas or bones obstruct the imaging window or needle tract. For example, tumors that are seated high in the liver are sometimes inaccessible to puncture under US, whereas CT guidance allows access via the transthoracic route, which is impossible with US guidance due to air in the lung that obstructs the imaging window. Computed tomography is also preferred when a safe pathway to the targeted tumor cannot be imaged with US, for example, when a hollow organ containing air is very close. Finally, combining CT and US guidance sometimes can be useful. Computed tomography can be used to guide the ablation instrument toward the targeted organ along a safe tract that cannot be easily depicted with US, and once the organ has been reached, US can then be used to guide the instrument in real time into an ill-defined tumor on CT.

When tumor visualization and accessibility for puncture are equivalent under both US and CT guidance, the technique of choice is that preferred by the operator or according to the availability of the equipment. In clinical practice today, most liver tumors are treated under US guidance because this technique is widely available, the cost is low, angulation possibilities are virtually limitless, and real-time guidance is achievable. Today, with the advent of almost real-time CT, often called CT fluoroscopy (fluoro-CT), the time required for needle insertion during ablation is short, thus overcoming the previous drawback with CT. A comparative study on a phantom demonstrated no significant differences between US and fluoro-CT in the time needed to guide a biopsy; helical CT guidance was threefold longer (1).

Technique

Some technical requirements need to be emphasized. The gantry must be large enough to allow the passage of the instrument that has been partially inserted in the patient. As some handles on the instruments are quite long, a handle-less guiding trocar needle or a flexible device may facilitate placement in the tumor. For practical and sterility reasons, a TV screen is mandatory inside the CT room. It is also useful to have a footswitch to use to direct and release the table, and to be able to perform CT acquisition inside the room. To minimize radiation to the patient and to the physician, the dose and time must be limited. The quality of the image needed for guidance is not the same as that needed for diagnostic purposes, and usually is not as good.

Scanning time should be as short as possible for image reconstruction. Consequently, almost real-time CT imaging, or fluoro-CT, is now preferred. Continuous fluoro-CT with systems able to produce at least eight images per second with a reconstruction time of less than 0.2 second allows almost real-time guidance. This has been demonstrated to shorten the duration of the puncture procedure, and to improve the accuracy of tumor targeting, demonstrated by an increase in the sensitivity and the negative predictive value when used for biopsy (2).

If imaging time is maintained at a minimum, and certain precautions such as milliampere reduction for scans to evaluate needle position, fluoro-CT does not increase the dose to the patient or the physician (3). However, one of the drawbacks of real-time fluoro-CT is that the needle is handled by the physician while x-rays are being delivered, and this increases the radiation received by the physician's hands that are in, or close to, the imaging field. Special needle holders have been designed so that the physician can guide the needle while keeping his/her hands away from the x-ray beam (4,5). To further minimize radiation delivered to the patient and the physician, the "quick-check" technique can be used. This technique uses brief single-section fluoro-CT imaging that is repeated whenever the needle is advanced, but unlike real-time fluoro-CT, the needle is advanced without real-time imaging. The quick-check technique is accurate and rapid for guiding the needle to the target (6). In practice, the quick-check technique is adequate for the majority of cases. Continuous fluoro-CT probably should be reserved for difficult cases, for example, in moving structures, or when the access for the target is narrow, or finally for the actual puncture when the instrument is penetrating the targeted tumor.

Multislice CT is even more user friendly for puncturing under CT guidance, as it offers one or two center rows to image the needle course, and two lateral ones to ensure that the instrument does not overstep the track in the upper or lower imaging planes. The most recent multislice CT unit with up to 16 rows provides rapid three-dimensional (3D) volumetric imaging to such an extent that it may be possible in the near future to guide the needle in all planes with the help of real-time reconstruction. However, this type of software is not capable of providing oblique multiplanar imaging in real-time as yet. This is why, even today, a perpendicular approach is always preferred when possible, because it is the simplest. If an angled approach is used, it allows the entire puncture tract and needle to be imaged in one slice (7).

In practice, the procedure for inserting the ablation instrument begins with a detailed CT examination of the region. The patient is placed in the most favorable position for access to the entry point. Treatment of a limb tumor may require a different degree of rotation. Securing the limb with tape or straps can be useful during treatment of bone tumors, because the force required for drilling can cause extremity movement that can be bothersome on subsequent CT scans. Next, the level of the targeted slice is highlighted with a laser marker light, and the entry point is marked on the skin. A metallic marker can be used to delineate the entry point precisely. The anticipated angle of the path and depth of the target are determined according to this entry point using the electronic calipers on the CT console.

Once these parameters have been defined, it is often useful to stick a short, small-caliber needle in this entry point that can be used for local anesthesia if needed. This needle confirms that the entry point and tract angulation are accurate on the subsequent CT scan, before insertion of the ablation instrument using the tandem technique. Then, while the clinician is advancing the instrument, CT imaging can be obtained at regular intervals to verify the depth and direction of the incoming instrument, and this depends on the rapidity of image acquisition and reconstruction. Real-time fluoro-CT or quick-check imaging can be used, as discussed above. A distal shadow due to a partial-volume effect allows the physician to distinguish the tip of the instrument, but one should always image a slice above and another below the tool to ensure that the tip is not overstepping the reference slice.

With conventional CT guidance, only tumors visualized without injection of contrast medium were punctured, because the time necessary to perform the puncture was longer than the duration of enhancement. Nowadays, with fluoro-CT, a tumor can be punctured during transient enhancement, as described in the literature for tumors enhancing from 50 to 130 seconds (8,9). The target lesion should be in the scan plane to do so. This scan plane and delayed imaging should be determined according to temporal measurement of delay times, based on the previous diagnostic CT examination. The physician should be ready, standing at the side of the patient clothed in a sterile garment in front of the gantry, poised for the puncture.

When the puncture cannot be performed within gantry angulation possibilities, it will be less accurate and more time-consuming. In the past, the only alternative was to use the triangulation technique in such situations. Today, guidance with a laser goniometer (10) or electromagnetic virtual targeting systems (11) can be extremely helpful as they heighten accuracy and shorten the duration of the procedure and the number of needle passes. However, the remaining disadvantage of these out-of-plane techniques is the nonvisualization of the complete needle on a single image. Electromagnetic targeting systems are composed of a computer that is first loaded with a set of reference CT scans obtained immediately before puncturing the tumor, and the patient is maintained immobile thereafter. This set of CT scans encompasses the target and the entry point when an out-of-plane puncture is needed, or provides a single reference slice when an in-plane puncture is to be performed. The target and the entry point are then marked with calipers on the screen of the targeting system. Before actually inserting the needle, a virtual needle path can be visualized on the set of CT scans, and multiplanar reconstruction can be performed in any direction and angulation. Once this viewing has demonstrated that no vital structures would be violated, the puncture can be performed following the direction indicated on the screen of the guiding system. During the puncture, an electromagnetic sensor placed on the proximal needle, close to the needle hub or instrument handle, allows (with the help of algorithms similar to those used in global positioning systems) accurate localization of the needle tip in real time, as well as the route chosen by the physician, both of which are superimposed over the reference set of previously loaded images (Fig. 9.1). The electromagnetic targeting system has a built-in respiratory phase monitoring system that allows the needle to be inserted during the same phase of the respiratory cycle as that during which reference images were acquired. As the position of the needle tip and its future route and position are a "straight projection" of the direction of the proximal part of the needle, great care should be taken not to bend the needle, as this will lead to incorrect projection of the position of needle tip and future path. Using a small-gauge needle with a bevel can be problematic, since the needle tract may become curved. Rotating the needle while advancing it has been described to minimize possible curving and deviation.

The laser goniometer is a laser light unit that can be either attached to the gantry or be separate from it. Angulate coordinates, determined on the CT unit from previously acquired slices, are calculated. Then the laser beam is angulated according to these coordinates, and focused on the entry point on the patient's skin. The direction of the needle is kept within the laser beam, demonstrating the desired angle while advancing the needle for the puncture. The greatest contribution of such a system occurs when performing double angulation punctures within the limits of gantry angulation (10,12).

As thermal ablation instruments are relatively large in caliber, the best option is to access the target organ without traversing any other structure. When the window for safe access to the target organ is quite narrow, or even virtual, the physician can inject a large volume of saline to widen the path artificially by enlarging the anatomic space between two organs. This technique has been reported for biopsy in the mediastinum (13,14), the retroperitoneum (15), and the pelvis (16). For this technique, first, a small (often 22 gauge), caliber needle is inserted as deeply as possible in the narrow tract chosen for insertion. Then, saline is manually injected slowly to enlarge the tract and move the untargeted organ away. The needle is then advanced further and the injection is repeated until a large-enough area is created for insertion of the ablation instrument. Usually 10 to 30 mL of saline are used, but up to 60 mL may be required.

In high-seated liver tumors that are inaccessible under US, access using CT often is diffi-

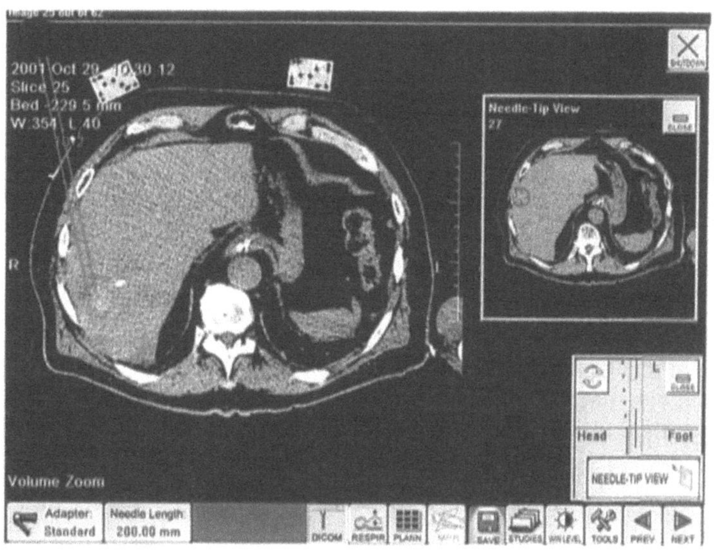

FIGURE 9.1. View of the screen of an electromagnetic targeting system. The circle on the right frame represents the location of the needle tip. The parallel lines on the left frame represent the future needle path; the distance to the target is also shown. Note the two respiratory sensors on the anterior abdominal wall used to monitor the respiratory cycle. (Courtesy of Dr. Afshin Gangi.)

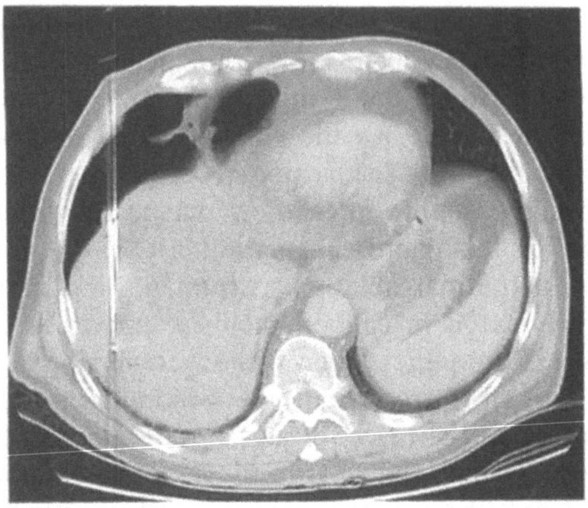

FIGURE 9.2. Computed tomography (CT) scan depicts insertion of a cool-tip cluster radiofrequency (RF) needle in a very high-seated segment VII liver metastasis via an air-filled right pleural cavity. The large right pneumothorax has been induced to avoid piercing the lung. This pneumothorax will be expelled after transpleurodiaphragmatic RF ablation.

cult or impossible via a transhepatic route as well. Transpulmonary access has been described for ethanol injection in hepatocellular carcinomas, but pneumothoraces occur in 30% of the cases and require a chest tube in 7% (17). Even if some ablative techniques, such as radiofrequency (RF), are used in the lung, in our opinion it is safer to try and avoid collateral lung damage. When transpleural access is needed, we first induce a pneumothorax to retract the lung toward its hilum. A path for the ablation instruments is thus created in a pleural cavity that is transiently devoid of lung parenchyma and filled with iatrogenic air (Fig. 9.2). The pneumothorax is induced with an epidural needle by maintaining positive pressure on the piston of an air-filled syringe during the puncture in a similar manner to an epidural injection. When the needle tip reaches the pleural space, the decrease in resistance will allow a few milliliters of air to be injected. CT is then used to check that the needle is positioned correctly and that air has been injected in the right location. Then, the amount of air needed to move the lung away from the future needle path is aspirated through a filter, and manually injected into the pleural cavity. Usually, 100 to 400 mL of air are enough to clear the lung from the needle path. Finally, the lung is separated from the diaphragm; then the liver can be accessed through the air-filled pleural space while avoiding injury to the lung, and reproducing, in a manner akin to the surgical transpleurodiaphragmatic access described by surgeons, an efficient way of treating tumors of the dome of the liver (18). At the end of the ablation procedure, the needle is exchanged over a 0.035-inch wire for a 5-French side-hole catheter to remove air from the pneumothorax, and to expel it through a three-way stopcock.

Treating tumors in proximity to organs that are sensitive to heat or cold can cause collateral damage to these organs. Such complications have been reported to occur in the colon, stomach, and gallbladder when treating liver tumors, and to nerve roots when bone tumors are treated with RF. Clearly, the simplest way to avoid such collateral damage is not to treat tumors that are less than 1 cm from sensitive organs. Another option is to refer the patient for a preoperative or laparoscopic ablation procedure during which the untargeted organ will be manually moved away from the targeted organ. Finally, when a percutaneous approach is required, one can try to move the tumor away from the untargeted organ. A thin needle can be inserted in the narrow or virtual space between the two organs for this purpose, and then a few milliliters of air or saline (a test amount) are injected. Once injection in the targeted space has been confirmed, a larger amount of air/saline can be used. This technique can be used, for example, in the peritoneum in an attempt to widen the space between a peripheral liver tumor and a sensitive organ such as the colon or stomach (Fig. 9.3). In this setting, CT imaging provides a unique and accurate view of any structure, as well as the injected air or saline.

Positioning of the ablation instrument in relation to the tumor under CT guidance is akin to placing the needle in a biopsy procedure. However, a major difference between ablation and biopsy is that sampling in the latter can be performed practically anywhere in the tumor

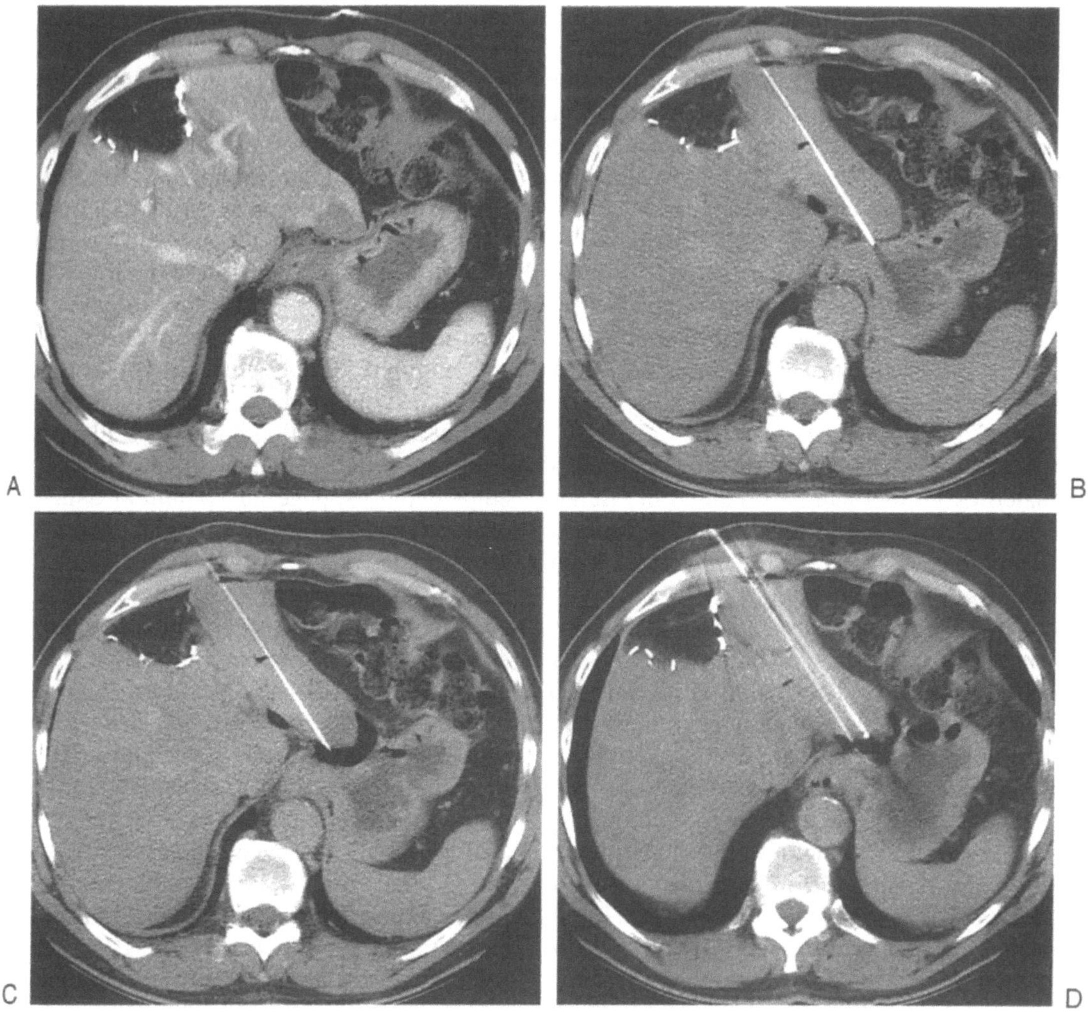

FIGURE 9.3. (A) A CT scan shows a segment I liver metastasis abutting on the gastric wall, which developed after liver surgery. (B) The tip of a 22-gauge Chiba needle, inserted via a transhepatic route under CT guidance, is located in the narrow space between the stomach and segment I of the liver. (C) Ten milliliters of air have been manually injected through the needle, allowing the gastric wall to be moved away from the subcapsular metastasis in segment I. (D) A cool-tip RF needle is placed in the metastasis in segment I and thermal ablation can be performed without collateral damage to the stomach. (Courtesy of Dr. Philippe Brunner.)

provided a necrotic center, if present, is avoided. During ablation therapy, the active tip of the probe must be positioned in a precise location inside the targeted tumor. Most of the time the ablation site should be in the center of the tumor so that the entire lesion is destroyed, along with a rim of healthy tissue. Entering the tumor only once without completely traversing it with the tip of the needle is of paramount importance. Multiple punctures can lead to tumor cell spillage and seeding. This is also pertinent when expandable multiple-array needles are used for RF ablation; being in the right location is critical to avoid repeated deployment of the hook-shaped inner electrodes, as this is likely to promote tumor seeding.

Accurate positioning of the ablation instrument in relation to the tumor usually is evaluated on axial images without contrast injection. In some instances, contrast injection can be useful, particularly when the contrast between the tumor and the surrounding liver is low. Thin control scans should be used, because although thick scans make it easier to visualize the lesion, they are less accurate to judge the probe position in relation to the target. Moreover, it has been demonstrated that the use of multiplanar reformation in the coronal and sagittal planes statistically improves the accuracy of instrument placement. In 44% of cases, instrument repositioning was required under imaging guidance in the axial plane (19).

When tumors are larger than the volume of ablated tissue that can be obtained in one application, overlapping ablation is needed to attempt to destroy the tumor completely. When such overlapping ablations are needed, CT probably has an edge over ultrasound for monitoring. The overriding advantage is that the probe position is easier to visualize with CT than with US after changes caused by previous ablations. Indeed, the slight decrease in Hounsfield units (HU) exhibited by the thermal lesions on CT (see Image Monitoring, below) does not impede subsequent instrument placement at all, and can even be useful for guidance. The second advantage is that CT multiplanar reconstruction can probably help to position the probes equidistantly in any direction, and that would be ideal placement. In contrast, postablation US imaging demonstrates either hyperechoic or hypoechoic tissue changes, but always with posterior shadowing that impedes visualization of the tumor or needle. Subsequent probe placement is difficult, and inevitably inaccurate, even if the basic recommendation to treat the deepest part of the tumor first is followed. Whatever the guidance system used, it should be borne in mind that if overlapping deliveries are to be performed, six deliveries will only increase the diameter of the thermal lesion by 25% (20), and the efficacy of local ablation decreases rapidly when the size of the target increases (21).

Liver tumors should be punctured via the shortest route possible, avoiding large vessels, and, of course, the liver hilum, as well as the gallbladder. However, when tumors are subcapsular, it is always preferable to first traverse healthy liver parenchyma to avoid bleeding and tract seeding. Indeed, tumor seeding along the needle tract has been reported to occur particularly after treatment of subcapsular hepatocellular carcinomas. Treating the tract with cauterization is a potential option to try to minimize such seeding and bleeding. *A word of warning*: Treatment of the liver capsule is always painful and thus requires deep sedation.

Computed tomography guidance is often used for bone tumors because of the high quality of visualization it provides. Planning an entry point perpendicular to the bone surface helps avoid slippage and potential damage to other organs. Drilling the cortical bone is often required to reach a deep-seated lesion. For example, a safe anatomic entrance is sometimes via the normal cortex on the opposite side. After drilling, a sheath or a guiding needle can be useful to exchange the drill for the ablation instrument. It is therefore advisable to use a drill needle that is at least one gauge larger than the ablation tool. If the external metallic sheath of the drill system is used to guide the ablative tool for RF or microwave ablation, one should retract the sheath a few centimeters before power deposition to avoid contact between the active part of the probe and the metallic sheath; this contact could cause burns along the track and must be avoided (Fig. 9.4). A plastic sheath is preferred for cryotherapy to avoid freezing of the track.

Osteoid osteoma is a good indication for ablation. Laser and RF have both been reported to be effective to treat osteoid osteomas (22–24). More sophisticated and larger caliber devices such as cooled or expandable multiple-array needles are not required for osteoid osteomas, as the target is small and a single bare laser fiber or a single RF needle is sufficient. On the other hand, in the case of large osteolytic bone tumors, good results have been demonstrated with the expandable multiple-array needle probe for treatment of pain in cases refractory to standard management with analgesics and radiation therapy (25). When used to manage pain, this particular needle is usually chosen to target the margin of

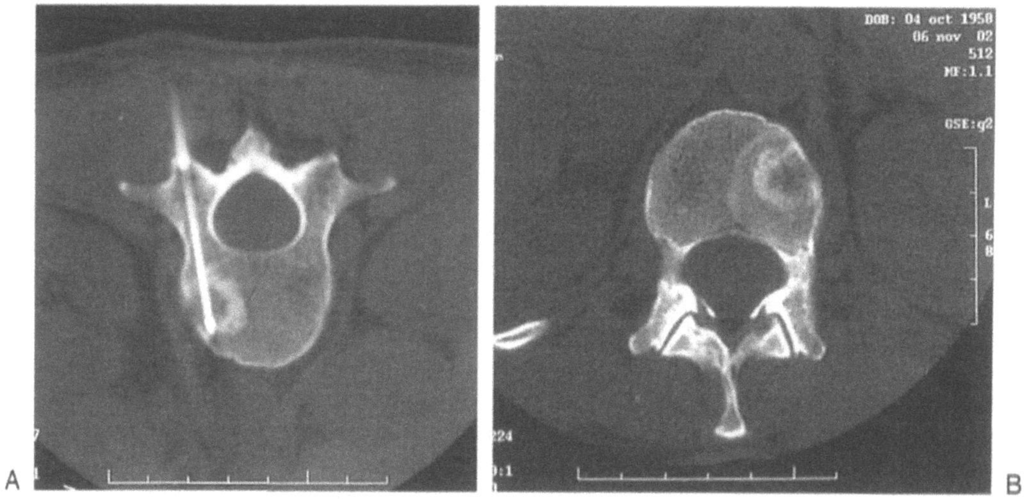

FIGURE 9.4. (A) A CT scan of second lumbar vertebral body lytic metastasis from breast cancer, which has been accessed via a transpedicular approach. A single cool-tip RF needle has been inserted through the metallic sheath of the drill needle. A few centimeters of the sheath have been retracted, up to the level of the cortical bones, to avoid contact between the metallic sheath and noninsulated distal part of the needle. (B) Two months after RF delivery, CT scan shows a rim of hyperattenuating tissue, seemingly delimiting the external borders of the ablated area.

metastases that involve bones with the objective of treating the soft tissue–bone interface, especially when the entire tumor volume cannot be destroyed because the metastases are large. It is straightforward to achieve such targeting under CT guidance, and is important because sensory nerve fibers involving the bone periosteum and cortex can be destroyed to inhibit pain transmission. The expandable multiple-array RF needle is difficult to deploy when dealing with large osteoblastic bone tumors. Nonexpandable probes are preferred in this situation.

When treating lung tumors, the needle path should traverse the shortest length of aerated lung parenchyma, avoiding fissures and minimizing the number of passes through the pleural surfaces. Transgression of fissures and pleural surfaces increases the incidences of pneumothoraces (26). Furthermore, trying to insert a needle as perpendicular as possible to the pleura also appears to be important in averting the risk of pneumothorax (27). Whatever the ablation technique used, it is recommended that only one lung be treated at a time to avoid life-threatening complications that can occur in cases of bilateral adverse events such as massive hemorrhage (28) or pneumothorax. Notwithstanding, several tumors can be treated on one side during the same session. Using an expandable needle for lung RF ablation may be an advantage, as this type of needle will not slip out of the tumor in case of a massive pneumothorax that can push the target tumor away from the needle. The physician should be ready to insert a chest tube if a significant pneumothorax occurs. Computed tomography imaging is useful for chest tube placement if a postablation pneumothorax occurs while the patient is still on the CT table. We usually try to manually expel the pneumothorax by inserting a 5-French side-hole catheter in the air-filled pleural cavity under CT guidance. This catheter is connected to a 50-mL syringe via a three-way stopcock; air is drawn from the pneumothorax into the syringe and then expelled. Larger caliber chest tubes are used only in cases of recurrent pneumothorax.

Image Monitoring

As no imaging technique is capable of confirming cell death with 100% accuracy, there is no way of knowing whether the tumor has been completely destroyed at the time of treatment. Image monitoring of the ablation procedure rarely examines the extent of treatment directly. Only MR thermometry directly evaluates the extent of heat or cold. All the other imaging techniques simply image changes that are indirect consequences of treatment. These modifications do not correspond exactly to the extent of the ablated volume, nor to certain cell death within the volume. In the liver, for example, US monitoring depicts a hyperechoic area induced by the formation of gas after RF, laser, or microwave ablation; US demonstrates a hypoechoic iceball after cryotherapy, and hyperechoic changes after alcohol injection. The consequences of treatment depicted by MR imaging are areas of hypointense signal following cryotherapy and RF, and/or devascularized tissue that any ablative technique can produce.

Most of the data and experience with CT monitoring of tissue ablation are related to RF ablation. RF ablation in the liver was well described in an animal study by Cha et al (29), in which CT was performed immediately and 2 and 8 minutes after treatment. Unenhanced CT scans 2 minutes after RF showed a 14-HU decrease in ablated tissue compared to healthy liver, and this difference increased to 22 HU at 8 minutes. After cryotherapy, frozen tissue also was described as a well-demarcated region of lower attenuation than normal liver (30).

After hyperthermia or cryoablation, the postablation hypoattenuating area on CT often contains several small gas bubbles of various sizes that are irregularly distributed in the ablated tissue. After injection of contrast medium, the differences between RF-ablated tissue and healthy liver increase to 55 HU, with improved conspicuity and edge detection. CT was found to correlate better than US with the real volume of ablated liver tissue measured at pathologic examination (29,31); the peripheral rim of enhancement that corresponds to an inflammatory reaction is not taken into account for the measurement of ablated tissue. Ultrasound slightly underestimated the true size of ablated tissue. Better correlation with the pathologic study also has been reported for CT monitoring versus intraoperative US in the kidney (32).

As enhanced CT provides a more clear-cut delineation of the ablated area than unenhanced CT, enhanced CT is performed at the end of the treatment to try to best determine the extent of coagulation. The goal of ablation is to obtain an unenhanced area that is at least as large as the tumor, and ideally a few millimeters larger. Of course, if the targeted tumor exhibits high enhancement before ablation, disappearance of this enhancement must be achieved. If tumor enhancement persists, CT allows retargeting of residual foci during the same treatment session. As the amount of contrast medium that can be injected is limited and enhancement is less intense after subsequent injections, enhanced imaging cannot be repeated at will. The use of contrast medium at CT optimally is left for the final evaluation.

During chemical ablation, CT is able to image the spatial diffusion of the injected liquid. Alcohol is slightly hypoattenuating, but any toxic liquid or gel can be transformed into a hyperattenuating substance by adding contrast medium to the therapeutic compound, as reported for alcohol (33,34) or chemotherapeutic drugs (35). Once again, although imaging is capable of depicting the diffusion of the toxic agent, it cannot predict the efficacy of the treatment. Here again, injection of contrast medium can help to evaluate the extent of coagulation necrosis by imaging the unenhanced area; conversely, an area of the tumor with persistent enhancement can be subsequently targeted for retreatment, as reported for alcohol therapy of hepatocellular carcinomas (HCCs) (4).

Computed tomography monitoring of thermal ablation in bone or kidney tumors delineates roughly the same features as described previously in the liver. The formation of gas bubbles at irregularly distributed points within the ablated lesion is common. If the tumor is initially highly enhanced, this enhancement disappears if treatment is efficient; otherwise there is a small decrease in density.

In the lung, RF ablation causes lung tissue to became more dense in the ablated area (Fig. 9.5). This is akin to alveolar consolidation, and is often very faint during the course of treatment. It becomes more intense and slightly more extensive during the following hours and days (see Follow-Up Imaging, below). Although it is unclear whether these CT imaging changes

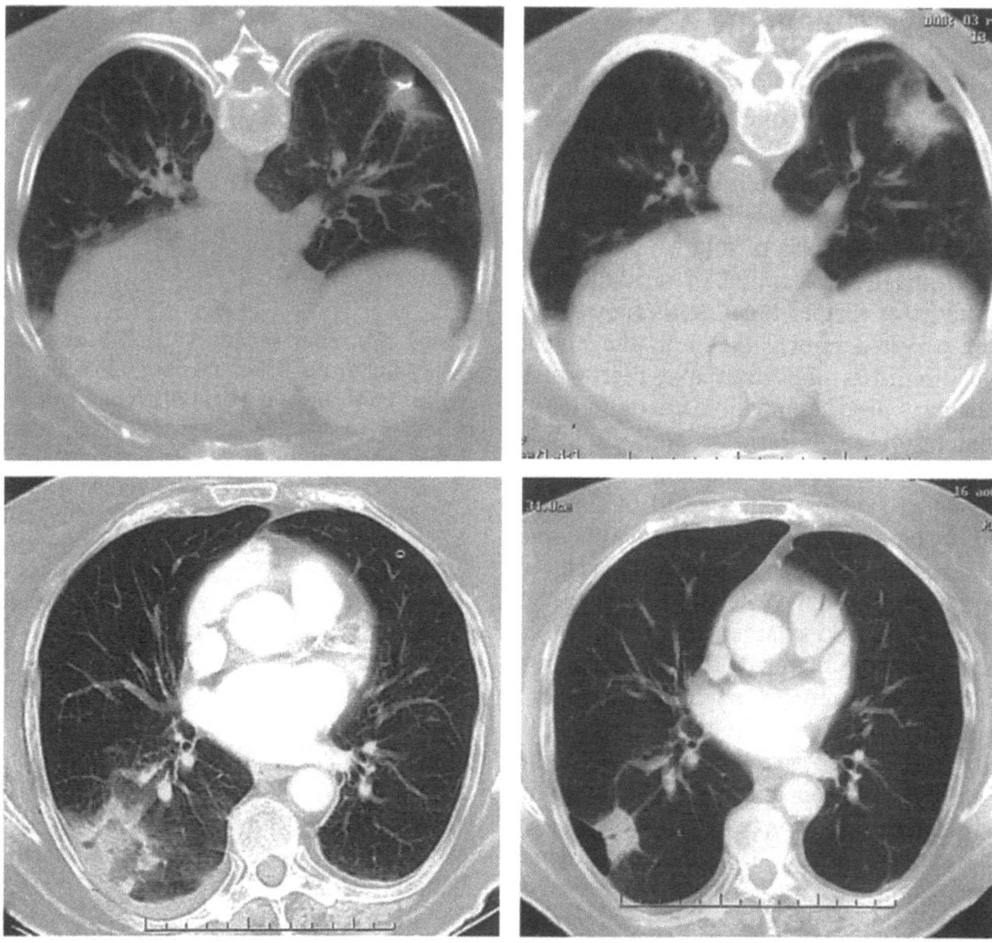

A B C D

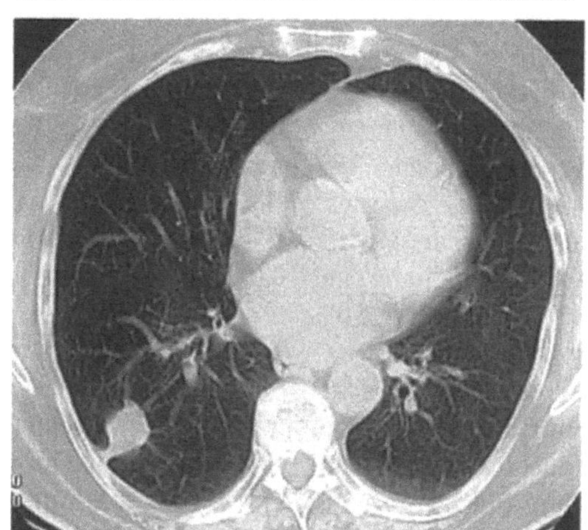

E

FIGURE 9.5. (A) Prone CT scan of the lungs shows an expandable RF needle inserted in a 17-mm lung metastasis from colon cancer. Note the small pneumothorax, which will not necessitate any aspiration or drainage. (B) Lung tissue consolidation around the treated tumor can be seen after 17 minutes of RF ablation. (C) One day later, the post-RF alveolar condensation has increased in size and density. There is a little pleural effusion. (D) Two months later, there is retraction and increased density of the thermally destroyed area. (E) Four months after treatment, the scar is even smaller.

really represent coagulation necrosis, this area of density is helpful when attempts are made to shape the thermal lesion so that it is equivalent to the tumor size.

Follow-Up Imaging

As stated earlier, there is no way of affirming that a tumor has been completely ablated during the procedure itself. Consequently, follow-up imaging is crucial to determine treatment efficiency, or, on the contrary, local failure of ablation. When failure occurs, follow-up imaging is used to image the location of residual tumor accurately for further ablative therapy. As the tumor size is a critical factor in the efficacy of ablation, it is important that regrowth be unveiled as early as possible to optimize retreatment of small lesions. Thus, follow-up imaging should be performed at regular intervals and over a long period of time, because incomplete ablation often leaves small undetectable tumor foci that will be visible on delayed imaging only when the residual cells have grown to form a larger tumor (Fig. 9.6).

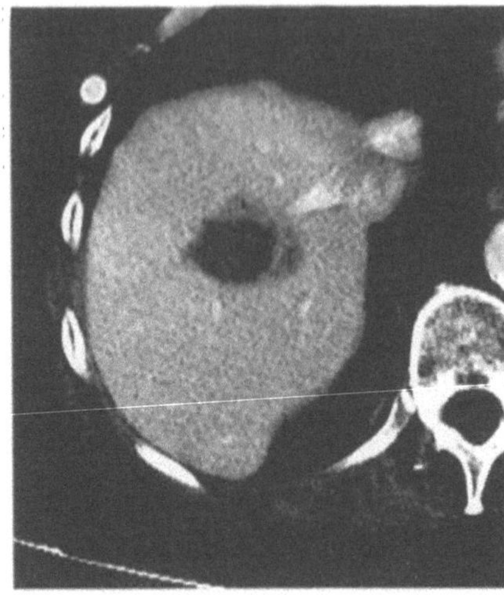

FIGURE 9.6. Four months after RF ablation of a metastasis from colon cancer, CT scan shows a hypoattenuating unenhanced round area corresponding to ablated tissue. The heterogeneously enhanced curviform area at the anteromedial border of the scar, in contact with the middle hepatic vein, has appeared since the previous CT scan performed 2 months earlier. This is tumor regrowth from residual unablated foci. This incomplete ablation has probably been promoted by heat sink induced by the neighboring large hepatic vein.

As the aim of ablation is to generate an area of necrosis, the diameter of which is larger or at least equivalent to that of the tumor. Ideally, the destroyed tissue or "scar" should be larger than the treated lesion, encompassing the tumor and safety margins. If treatment is successful, this scar will decrease in size, albeit slowly. Indeed, in our experience with mostly colon cancer metastases in the liver, 66% of successfully treated tumors decreased in size during 12 months of imaging follow-up. The decrease in the product of the two largest dimensions of the scar attained a mean of 15% (range 10–30%) at 6 months, and 35% (range 15–90%) at 12 months (36). A series of 43 hepatocellular carcinomas treated with RF showed a decrease in the immediate postablation scar volume of 21% at 1 month, 50% at 4 months, 65% at 7 months, and 89% at 16 months. This slow decrease in the scar volume has also been reported after cryotherapy (30). Ethanol-induced necrosis seems to decrease in size more often and faster, with reports of a diminution of size in all treated tumors that attained a mean of 45% at 6 months and 63% at 12 months (37).

World Health Organization (WHO) criteria or Response Evaluation Criteria in Solid Tumors (RECIST) criteria (38,39) cannot be applied to assess response to ablative therapies, at least not early during the posttreatment period. By these criteria, anticancer treatment is based on a decrease in tumor size, which is not really applicable to ablation. Other methods are needed to assess the efficacy of ablative treatment. Today, there is no clear consensus about which imaging techniques are the most appropriate for follow-up after ablation and various imaging techniques are used from one study to another. However, the criteria most commonly used to assess this efficacy on CT, MR, or US imaging is the absence of tissue enhancement, probably while awaiting functional imaging (positron emission tomography [PET] scanning).

Liver

Enhanced CT and MR imaging are at present considered the most useful modalities to assess thermal ablation efficacy in the liver. Preliminary reports suggest that the size of the nonenhancing region after RF visualized at CT and MR imaging corresponded to within 2mm of the size of the necrosis measured histologically (40–42) or with cryotherapy (43).

When RF therapy is successful, a hypoattenuating well-demarcated, round or oval scar is depicted on CT. Areas of higher attenuation can be found within the thermally ablated area after RF, microwave, laser, or cryotherapy, corresponding to hemorrhage. The thermally ablated area does not enhance after injection of contrast medium.

Two particular postthermoablation imaging patterns must be underscored. The first is the presence of wedge-shaped areas of contrast enhancement abutting on the RF scar seen in 12% of patients in the arterial phase on CT (Fig. 9.7) (36). These wedge-shaped areas of contrast enhancement are probably due to perfusion disorders, such as small-vessel thrombosis and arterioportal fistulas induced by ablation. The second pattern found after any type of ablation is a thin peripheral rim of enhancement, usually measuring less than 2mm in width, which is often seen surrounding the radiofrequency scars (Fig. 9.8). This rim is due to inflammatory and granulation tissue with profuse neovascularization found after most ablative techniques, as that described in an experimental model after focused US (44) or cryotherapy (43), as well as in clinical practice after RF (36,40,45). This rim has been described less commonly in hepatocellular carcinoma treated with alcohol injection (46,47) and in hepatic metastases treated with laser-induced thermotherapy (48,49). The inflammatory rim decreases with time. We found this rim in 24% and 18% of RF-treated tumors, respectively, on MR and CT at 2 months, in 4% on MR at 4 months, and in 2% on MR at 9 months (36). Others have reported this rim in 89% of CT studies after RF treatment within 1 month, in 56% between 1 and 3 months, and in 22% between 3 to 6 months (45).

Residual active tumor foci depicted on CT usually are found at the periphery of the RF-induced lesion, and can appear as a nodule or

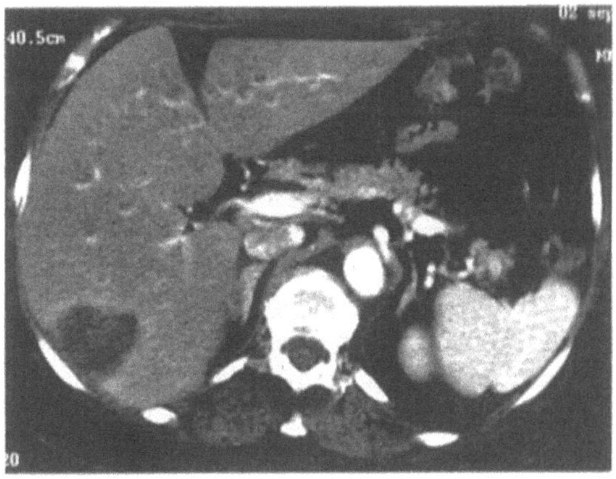

FIGURE 9.8. A CT scan 2 months after RF ablation of a subcaspsular metastasis shows a thin peripheral rim of enhancement corresponding to inflammatory tissue.

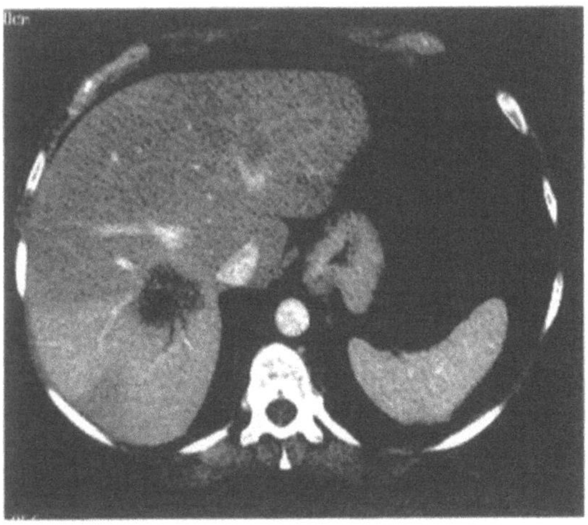

FIGURE 9.7. Two months after RF ablation of a breast cancer metastasis, the scar is not enhanced. There is a large wedge-shaped perfusion disorder demonstrating early and heavy enhancement of the parenchyma in segment VII. Note the faint dilation of the biliary tract at the periphery of the scar, imaged as periportal hypoattenuatting linear structures.

local thickening of the peripheral rim. More rarely, an increase in the size of the treated area signifies incomplete treatment. This increase in size, also called the halo pattern of recurrence, is found more frequently in recurrent metastases than with HCC (50).

Foci of active tumor exhibit hypo- or hyperattenuation on CT, and HCC's usually demonstrate contrast enhancement during the arterial phase. In contrast, metastases remain mostly hypovascular, and sometimes demonstrate low-grade enhancement at their periphery on imaging of the portal phase. The arterial phase image is therefore best to detect recurrent HCC, while the portal phase image is best to depict recurrent colorectal metastases. Due to the heat sink effect encountered during thermal ablation with RF, considerable attention should be paid to scars located in the vicinity of large vessels where incomplete treatment is seen more frequently (42,51).

A major question is when postablation imaging follow-up should be initiated and how regularly it should be repeated. It is difficult to appraise results soon after treatment because of the peripheral inflammatory rim that enhances and can be misinterpreted as residual tumor, or small foci of remnant tumor embedded in this rim that may be overlooked. These are reasons why the first imaging studies are usually performed 1 to 3 months after RF, and then repeated every 2 or 3 months. Repeat imaging eventually will demonstrate regrowth of small foci of unablated tumor that remain in the scar, but were too small to be detected earlier. However, for most authors, including Solbiati et al (52), who reported 77% occurring before 6 months, and 96% depicted by 1 year, the likelihood of such local regrowth after 12 months is low (36,53). This signifies that after 1 year, the main aim of follow-up imaging is to search for new hepatic tumors rather than local recurrences.

In most studies, CT and MR are used variably to assess the efficacy of RF treatment. We compared CT and MR in our early experience in RF of liver tumors, imaging every 2 months with both CT and MR (36). Incomplete treatment was depicted in nine cases. At 2 months of follow-up, CT revealed four local failures and MR found eight. However, equivalent imaging results were obtained at 4 months with both imaging techniques, which revealed eight of nine incomplete treatments, with the ninth being discovered at 6 months. T2-weighted images were the most reliable sequences, due to good contrast between the hypointense scar and the mildly hyperintense residual tumor. However, caution should be exercised when distinguishing the mildly hyperintense signal indicative of residual tumor from the heavily hyperintense, fluid-like appearance of liquid necrosis.

Contrast-enhanced harmonic power Doppler US, compared to CT, appears to be useful to demonstrate local relapse after RF treatment. The technique demonstrated a sensitivity of 90% to 98%, a specificity of 100%, and 98% accuracy, in detecting local recurrence 3 to 7 days after RF ablation of hypervascular HCC's (54,55). However, this technique is much less efficient in detecting residual tumor after treatment of colorectal metastases. Among 75% of tumors that showed enhancement before treatment, only 50% of the post-RF local relapses were seen the day after treatment (52).

Imaging of complications is an important reason for follow-up imaging, and CT has a major role to play in this context. One of the more common complications after ablation therapy is an abscess in the liver after RF (56,57), and to a lesser extent after cryotherapy (58). This complication seems to be much more frequent in patients who have a bilioenteric anastomosis. These abscesses typically have been reported after an interval that ranges from 8 days to 5 months (51,56,57). Clinical symptoms may be mild, so imaging plays a major role in their depiction. They usually appear as a gas-containing mass that has developed in the ablated bed. They usually can be drained under CT guidance. However, small gas bubbles are nearly always imaged during ablation either with hyperthermia or cryotherapy, and they can persist for several days. In our experience with RF ablation, all the ablated areas containing gas after 2 weeks always were aspiration-proven abscesses. However, gas bubbles have been described in the liver several weeks after cryotherapy without a related infection (30). Biliary tract dilation upstream from an ablated area is common, and found in 8% of follow-up imaging in our hands (Fig. 9.7). This condition was always clinically asymptomatic in our experience, as no tumors were targeted for ablation close to the liver hilum.

Lung

One or 2 days after RF ablation, CT imaging depicts an increase in the size and density of the blurred parenchyma surrounding the treated tumor, compared to that imaged immediately after the ablation procedure (Fig. 9.5). This increase in the size of the ablated lesion varies considerably among patients. It can be up to 5 to 10mm and usually is concentric, but can cover a complete lung segment with a blurred outline, unless the border is sharply defined by the neighboring fissure. A small pleural effusion is nearly always seen during the early post-treatment period. After 1 to 2 months, this large and blurred area of consolidation shrinks, and forms a scar with a sharper border and higher tissue density. This scar usually continues to be slightly larger than the targeted tumor. If the treatment is successful, the scar will continue to shrink, but slower than during the first 2 months, akin to that reported for liver (Fig. 9.5).

Using contrast-enhanced CT to assess the efficacy of lung RF ablation has yet to be evaluated, but probably depends on the type of enhancement of the tumor before treatment. Late complications are rare. Early and midterm complications are mostly pleural effusions and pneumothoraces. Hemorrhage is unusual in the lung parenchyma even though minor hemoptysis is common from 1 to 10 days after the procedure. One case of major hemorrhage has been reported (28), and avoiding major vessels during the puncture may be a way to avert such complications. Finally, sepsis may appear as segmental or lobar consolidation on imaging that represents a pneumonia. In cases of long-lasting fever, CT should be used to search for an abscess at the ablation site that generally appears as a partially air-filled cavity instead of the usual scar tissue.

Bones

Computed tomography imaging after ablation of bone tumors demonstrates late changes. After ablation of an osteoid osteoma, healing of the ablated area usually takes more than 1 year. As a small volume is treated, usually with a bare laser fiber or a single RF needle, no changes are usually found in the bone surrounding the ablated lesion; however, early pain relief (usually in less than a week), is the best sign that therapy has been effective.

In the case of malignant bone tumors, late signs of efficacy are a shrunken ablated lesion and healing of bone destruction. No enhancement in ablated areas signifies the absence of viable tumor, as in other organs. Furthermore, after a few weeks, CT often shows a rim of hyperattenuating bone tissue that outlines the external borders of the ablated area (Fig. 9.4), although the true explanation for this appearance remains obscure. Spontaneous high bone density prohibits the study of rim contrast enhancement with CT. However, on MR, this rim appears as low signal on T1-weighted images, and high signal on T2-weighted images. Enhanced signal occurs after injection of gadolinium. These imaging patterns are similar to those of the inflammatory rim described in the liver after all types of ablative therapy, and therefore confirm the hypothesis that this is the external border of the ablated area.

Kidney

The size and enhancement criteria used to assess treatment efficacy in the liver with CT are also valid for kidney tumors after ablation. However, stranding of the perirenal fat, usually roughly parallel to the ablated area is an additional feature that evolves on sequential follow-up CT scans into a more organized rim of hyperattenuating tissue, seemingly delineating the external borders of the ablated area (Fig. 9.9) (59,60). Wedge-shaped nonenhancing areas in the kidney adjacent to the ablated lesion are seen on more than half of the follow-up CT images performed at 2 months. They are probably due to peripheral renal infarcts after coagulation of small arterial feeding branches. A

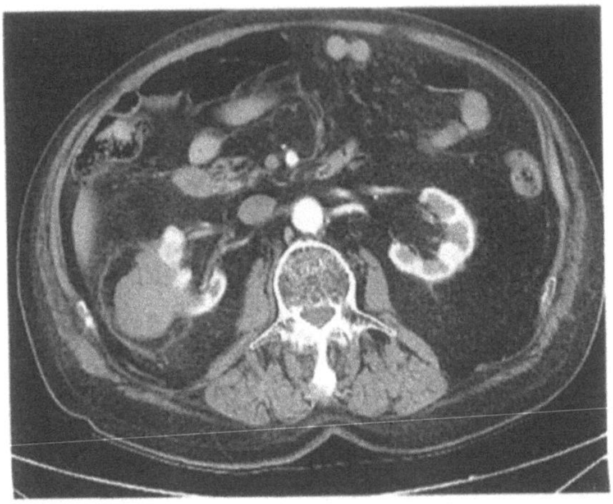

FIGURE 9.9. Follow-up CT scan obtained 8 months after RF ablation of an exophytic renal carcinoma. The unenhanced scar is composed of ablated tumor and a few millimeters of enhanced renal parenchyma adjacent to its inner limit. There is a thin rim of hyperattenuating tissue in the perirenal/peritumorous fat, a few millimeters from the ablated area.

small amount of peri- or pararenal blood is seen in 10% to 40% of ablated renal lesions, but it always disappears on the first follow-up CT at 1 or 2 months (59,60).

References

1. Sheafor DH, Paulson EK, Kliewer MA, DeLong DM, Nelson RC. Comparison of sonographic and CT guidance techniques: does CT fluoroscopy decrease procedure time? AJR 2000;174: 939–942.
2. Kirchner J, Kickuth R, Laufer U, Schilling EM, Adams S, Liermann D. CT fluoroscopy-assisted puncture of thoracic and abdominal masses: a randomized trial. Clin Radiol 2002;57:188–192.
3. Teeuwisse WM, Geleijns J, Broerse JJ, Obermann WR, van Persijn van Meerten EL. Patient and staff dose during CT guided biopsy, drainage and coagulation. Br J Radiol 2001;74: 720–726.
4. Takayasu K, Muramatsu Y, Asai S, Kobayashi T. CT fluoroscopy-assisted needle puncture and ethanol injection for hepatocellular carcinoma: a preliminary study. AJR 1999;173:1219–1224.
5. Kato R, Katada K, Anno H, Suzuki S, Ida Y, Koga S. Radiation dosimetry at CT fluoroscopy: physician's hand dose and development of needle holders. Radiology 1996;201:576–578.
6. Paulson EK, Sheafor DH, Enterline DS, et al. CT fluoroscopy-guided interventional procedures: techniques and radiation dose to radiologists. Radiology 2001;220:161–167.
7. Yueh N, Halvorsen RA Jr, Letourneau JG, Crass JR. Gantry tilt technique for CT-guided biopsy and drainage. J Comput Assist Tomogr 1989;13: 182–184.
8. Kirchner J, Kickuth R, Walz MV, et al. CTF-guided puncture of an unenhanced isodense liver lesion during continuous intravenous injection of contrast medium. Cardiovasc Intervent Radiol 1999;22:528–530.
9. Schweiger GD, Brown BP, Pelsang RE, Dhadha RS, Barloon TJ, Wang G. CT fluoroscopy: technique and utility in guiding biopsies of transiently enhancing hepatic masses. Abdom Imaging 2000;25:81–85.
10. Jacobi V, Thalhammer A, Kirchner J. Value of a laser guidance system for CT interventions: a phantom study. Eur Radiol 1999;9:137–140.
11. Holzknecht N, Helmberger T, Schoepf UJ, et al. [Evaluation of an electromagnetic virtual target system (CT-guide) for CT-guided interventions]. Rofo Fortschr Geb Rontgenstr Neuen Bildgeb Verfahr 2001;173:612–618.
12. Pereles FS, Baker M, Baldwin R, Krupinski E, Unger EC. Accuracy of CT biopsy: laser guidance versus conventional freehand techniques. Acad Radiol 1998;5:766–770.
13. Goodacre BW, Savage C, Zwischenberger JB, Wittich GR, vanSonnenberg E. Salinoma window technique for mediastinal lymph node biopsy. Ann Thorac Surg 2002;74:276–277.
14. Langen HJ, Klose KC, Keulers P, Adam G, Jochims M, Gunther RW. Artificial widening of the mediastinum to gain access for extrapleural biopsy: clinical results. Radiology 1995;196:703–706.
15. Karampekios S, Hatjidakis AA, Drositis J, et al. Artificial paravertebral widening for percutaneous CT-guided adrenal biopsy. J Comput Assist Tomogr 1998;22:308–310.
16. Shah H, Harris VJ, Konig CW, et al. Saline injection into the perirectal space to assist transgluteal drainage of deep pelvic abscesses. J Vasc Interv Radiol 1997;8:119–121.
17. Shibata T, Iimuro Y, Yamamoto Y, et al. CT-guided transthoracic percutaneous ethanol injection for hepatocellular carcinoma not detectable with US. Radiology 2002;223:115–120.
18. Elias D, de Baere T, Goharin A, Lasser P, Roche A. Transpleurodiaphragmatic radiofrequency thermoablation of a liver metastasis. J Am Coll Surg 2000;191:683–685.

19. Antoch G, Kuehl H, Vogt F, Debatin J, Stattaus J. Value of CT volume imaging for optimal placement of radiofrequency ablation probes in liver lesions. J Vasc Interv Radiol 2002;13:1155–1161.
20. Dodd GD III, Frank MS, Aribandi M, Chopra S, Chintapalli KN. Radiofrequency thermal ablation: computer analysis of the size of the thermal injury created by overlapping ablations. AJR 2001;177:777–782.
21. Livraghi T, Goldberg SN, Lazzaroni S, et al. Hepatocellular carcinoma: radio-frequency ablation of medium and large lesions. Radiology 2000;214:761–768.
22. Gangi A, Dietemann JL, Gasser B, et al. Interstitial laser photocoagulation of osteoid osteomas with use of CT guidance. Radiology 1997; 203:843–848.
23. Rosenthal DI. Percutaneous radiofrequency treatment of osteoid osteomas. Semin Musculoskelet Radiol 1997;1:265–272.
24. Rosenthal DI, Hornicek FJ, Wolfe MW, Jennings LC, Gebhardt MC, Mankin HJ. Percutaneous radiofrequency coagulation of osteoid osteoma compared with operative treatment. J Bone Joint Surg [Am] 1998;80:815–821.
25. Callstrom MR, Charboneau JW, Goetz MP, et al. Painful metastases involving bone: feasibility of percutaneous CT- and US-guided radiofrequency ablation. Radiology 2002;224:87–97.
26. Haramati LB, Aviram G. What constitutes effective management of pneumothorax after CT-guided needle biopsy of the lung? Chest 2002; 121:1013–1015.
27. Saji H, Nakamura H, Tsuchida T, et al. The incidence and the risk of pneumothorax and chest tube placement after percutaneous CT-guided lung biopsy: the angle of the needle trajectory is a novel predictor. Chest 2002;121:1521–1526.
28. Vaughn C, Mychaskiw G, II, Sewell P, et al. Massive hemorrhage during radiofrequency ablation of a pulmonary neoplasm. Anesth Analg 2002;94:1149–1151.
29. Cha CH, Lee FT Jr, Gurney JM, et al. CT versus sonography for monitoring radiofrequency ablation in a porcine liver. AJR 2000;175:705–711.
30. McLoughlin RF, Saliken JF, McKinnon G, Wiseman D, Temple W. CT of the liver after cryotherapy of hepatic metastases: imaging findings. AJR 1995;165:329–332.
31. Raman SS, Lu DS, Vodopich DJ, Sayre J, Lassman C. Creation of radiofrequency lesions in a porcine model: correlation with sonography, CT, and histopathology. AJR 2000;175:1253–1258.
32. Crowley JD, Shelton J, Iverson AJ, Burton MP, Dalrymple NC, Bishoff JT. Laparoscopic and computed tomography-guided percutaneous radiofrequency ablation of renal tissue: acute and chronic effects in an animal model. Urology 2001;57:976–980.
33. Hamuro M, Kaminou T, Nakamura K, et al. Percutaneous ethanol injection under CT fluoroscopy for hypervascular hepatocellular carcinoma following transcatheter arterial embolization. Hepatogastroenterology 2002;49: 752–757.
34. Ueda K, Ohkawara T, Minami M, et al. [Non-real-time computed tomography-guided percutaneous ethanol injection therapy for hepatocellular carcinoma undetectable by ultrasonography]. Gan To Kagaku Ryoho 1998;25: 1254–1258.
35. Farres M, de Baere T, Lagrange C, et al. Percutaneous mitoxantrone injection for primary and secondary liver tumors: preliminary results. Cardiovasc Intervent Radiol 1998;21:399–403.
36. Dromain C, de Baere T, Elias D, et al. Hepatic tumors treated with percutaneous radiofrequency ablation: CT and MR imaging follow-up. Radiology 2002;223:255–262.
37. Ebara M, Kita K, Sigiura YM, et al. Therapeutic effect of percutaneous ethanol injection on small hepatocellular carcinoma: evaluation with CT. Radiology 1995;195:371–377.
38. Miller AB, Hoogstraten B, Staquet M, Winkler A. Reporting results of cancer treatment. Cancer 1981;47:207–214.
39. Padhani AR, Ollivier L, Shibata T, et al. The RECIST (Response Evaluation Criteria in Solid Tumors) criteria: implications for diagnostic radiologists. Br J Radiol 2001;74:983–986.
40. Goldberg SN, Gazelle GS, Compton CC, Mueller PR, Tanabe KK. Treatment of intrahepatic malignancy with radiofrequency ablation: radiologic-pathologic correlation. Cancer 2000;88: 2452–2463.
41. Morimoto M, Sugimori K, Shirato K, et al. Treatment of hepatocellular carcinoma with radiofrequency ablation: radiologic-histologic correlation during follow-up periods. Hepatology 2002;35:1467–1475.
42. Solbiati L, Livraghi T, Goldberg SN, et al. Percutaneous radio-frequency ablation of hepatic metastases from colorectal cancer: long-term results in 117 patients. Radiology 2001;221: 159–166.
43. Kuszyk BS, Boitnott JK, Choti MA, et al. Local tumor recurrence following hepatic cryoablation: radiologic-histopathologic correlation in a rabbit model. Radiology 2000;217:477–486.

44. Rowland I, Rivens I, Chen L, et al. MRI study of hepatic tumours following high intensity focused ultrasound. Br J Radiol 1997;70:144–153.
45. Tsuda M, Majima K, Yamada T, Saitou H, Ishibashi T, Takahashi S. Hepatocellular carcinoma after radiofrequency ablation therapy: dynamic CT evaluation of treatment. Clin Imaging 2001;25:409–415.
46. Ito K, Honjo K, Fujita T, Awaya H, Matsumoto T, Matsunaga N. Enhanced MR imaging of the liver after ethanol treatment of hepatocellular carcinoma: evaluation of areas of hyperperfusion adjacent to the tumor. AJR 1995;164:1413–1417.
47. Sironi S, De Cobelli F, Livraghi T, et al. Small hepatocellular carcinoma treated with percutaneous ethanol injection: unenhanced and gadolinium-enhanced MR imaging follow-up. Radiology 1994;192:407–412.
48. Amin Z, Donald JJ, Masters A, et al. Hepatic metastases: interstitial laser photocoagulation with real-time US monitoring and dynamic evaluation of treatment. Radiology 1993;187:339–347.
49. Vogl T, Muller P, Hammersting R, et al. Malignant liver tumors treated with MR imaging-guided laser-induced technique: technique and prospective results. Radiology 1995;196:257–265.
50. Chopra S, Dodd GD III, Chintapalli KN, Leyendecker JR, Karahan OI, Rhim H. Tumor recurrence after radiofrequency thermal ablation of hepatic tumors: spectrum of findings on dual-phase contrast-enhanced CT. AJR 2001; 177:381–387.
51. de Baere T, Elias D, Dromain C, et al. Radiofrequency ablation of 100 hepatic metastases with a mean follow-up of more than 1 year. AJR 2000;175:1619–1625.
52. Solbiati L, Goldberg S, Ierace T, Dellanoce M, Livraghi T, Gazelle S. Radio-frequency ablation of hepatic metastases: post procedural assessment with US microbubble contrast agent—early experience. Radiology 1999;211:643–649.
53. Curley SA, Izzo F, Ellis LM, Vauthey JN, Vallone P. Radiofrequency ablation of hepatocellular cancer in 110 patients with cirrhosis. Ann Surg 2000;232:381–391.
54. Cioni D, Lencioni R, Rossi S, et al. Radiofrequency thermal ablation of hepatocellular carcinoma: using contrast-enhanced harmonic power Doppler sonography to assess treatment outcome. AJR 2001;177:783–788.
55. Meloni MF, Goldberg SN, Livraghi T, et al. Hepatocellular carcinoma treated with radiofrequency ablation: comparison of pulse inversion contrast-enhanced harmonic sonography, contrast-enhanced power Doppler sonography, and helical CT. AJR 2001;177:375–380.
56. Wood TF, Rose DM, Chung M, Allegra DP, Foshag LJ, Bilchik AJ. Radiofrequency ablation of 231 unresectable hepatic tumors: indications, limitations, and complications. Ann Surg Oncol 2000;7:593–600.
57. Zagoria RJ, Chen MY, Shen P, Levine EA. Complications from radiofrequency ablation of liver metastases. Am Surg 2002;68:204–209.
58. Bilchik AJ, Wood TF, Allegra D, et al. Cryosurgical ablation and radiofrequency ablation for unresectable hepatic malignant neoplasms: a proposed algorithm. Arch Surg 2000;135:657–662; discussion 662–664.
59. de Baere T, Kuoch V, Smayra T, et al. Radiofrequency ablation of renal cell carcinoma: preliminary experience. J Urol 2002;167:1961–1964.
60. Gervais D, O'Neill M, Arellano R, McGovern R, McDougal W, Mueller P. Peritumoral CT changes associated with radiofrequency ablation of focal renal lesions: description, incidence, and significance (abst.). Radiology 2001;221(P): 180.

10
Positron Emission Tomography Imaging for Tumor Ablation

Annick D. Van den Abbeele, David A. Israel, Stanislav Lechpammer, and Ramsey D. Badawi

Nuclear Oncology and FDG-PET

Nuclear medicine imaging involves the injection or ingestion of radioactive pharmaceuticals known as radiotracers, each designed to track a particular physiologic or pathophysiologic process. In contrast to conventional radiologic imaging such as x-ray computed tomography (CT) and magnetic resonance imaging (MRI), which map out anatomic structure and depend on changes in morphology or size for determination of pathology, nuclear medicine imaging provides information on the metabolic *function* of the investigated organ or tissue.

Fluorine-18-fluoro-2-deoxy-D-glucose (FDG) is a glucose analog labeled with the positron emitter fluorine 18. Positron emission tomography (PET) with FDG (FDG-PET) is a whole-body, functional imaging technique that measures glucose metabolism. Malignancies can be detected in resulting images due to their higher rates of glucose transport compared to normal tissue (1–4). Most common types of malignancies, including cancers of the lung, breast, esophagus, colon, head and neck, and thyroid, as well as lymphomas and melanomas show increased FDG uptake (1,4–16).

The Centers for Medicaid and Medicare Services (CMS) have recognized the utility of FDG-PET in the management of patients with cancer and have approved reimbursements in all of the aforementioned indications (17). Positron emission tomography scanning has now found widespread applications in the diagnosis, staging, and restaging of these and other malignancies and has been shown to be as reliable and accurate as conventional imaging modalities including CT and MRI, or even moreso (6,18–40). Owing substantially to PET scanning, nuclear oncology has become an integral part of the multidisciplinary clinical management of patients with cancer in many institutions (41). Today, nuclear oncology is one of the most dynamic and rapidly growing areas of contemporary nuclear medicine.

The evolving roles of noninvasive PET imaging reported in the monitoring of response to therapy, and as a predictor of response to therapy and survival (21,42–62) place FDG-PET in an optimal position to evaluate response to tumor ablation procedures.

Principles of PET Imaging

The radionuclides used for the creation of labeled radiotracers for PET imaging are positron emitters, as opposed to the single photon emitters used in conventional nuclear medicine imaging. Positrons do not penetrate human tissue very far (0–2 mm) before combining with electrons and undergoing annihilation reactions. In such a reaction, a positron and an electron are converted into two 511-keV annihilation photons, emitted at very nearly 180 degrees to each other. PET cameras usually consist of rings of detectors that surround the patient. When two annihilation photons are detected within a certain (~6–12 ns) time frame by detectors in these rings, a radioactive decay is deemed to have occurred along the line joining the two detectors involved. In this way, information regarding the location of radioactivity within the patient can be obtained. Reconstruction of this information yields tomographic images estimating the radiotracer concentration within the patient.

The radionuclides used for clinical PET imaging possess relatively short half-lives (approximately between 2 minutes and 2 hours), and most are produced by a cyclotron. The most widely used radionuclide in clinical PET applications is fluorine 18, which has a half-life of 109.8 minutes. This half-life is sufficient to allow outsourcing of radiotracer production to off-site commercial manufacturing facilities.

Modern dedicated whole-body PET scanners generate images with a spatial resolution on the order of 7 mm, and lesions of that size and smaller demonstrate a diminished density of counts compared to larger lesions having the same biologic characteristics. Lesions below 7 mm in size, therefore, may not be detectable. If the imaging is done using a dual-headed nuclear medicine imaging camera, the smallest detectable lesion will be even larger (around 15 mm).

FDG-PET Pharmacokinetics

FDG is transported into metabolically active cells by normal glucose transporter mechanisms. Once in the cell, FDG is phosphorylated by hexokinase to FDG-6-phosphate in the same way that glucose is phosphorylated to glucose-6-phosphate, but as opposed to glucose-6-phosphate, FDG-6-phosphate does not undergo further metabolism within the cell. Since FDG-6-phosphate cannot easily cross the cell membrane, and since the dephosphorylation by glucose-6-phosphatase is a relatively slow process in comparison to that of glucose-6-phosphate, FDG-6-phosphate remains effectively trapped within the cell. The resulting buildup of radiotracer within viable tissue is further potentiated in malignant cells, which often have enhanced glucose transport at the cell surface, more intense hexokinase activity, and reduced glucose-6-phosphatase activity.

Patient Preparation and Normal Biodistribution of FDG

Patients are asked to fast for 4 to 6 hours prior to the injection of FDG to maintain low serum glucose and endogenous insulin levels. Patients are also asked to refrain from exercise 24 hours prior to the study to minimize striated muscle uptake. A normoglycemic status aids in minimizing competition between circulating glucose and FDG at the cellular level, which maximizes tumor-to-background ratio and results in optimal lesion detection. However, compliance with these prescanning instructions may be challenging in diabetic patients, particularly those who are insulin-dependent and whose disease is poorly controlled. If a patient is diabetic and insulin-dependent, the injection of FDG is performed approximately 4 hours after the last insulin injection. A hyperinsulinemic state favors preferential uptake of FDG by striated muscles and increases the likelihood of a false-negative study. Patients with normal blood glucose control also may have a suboptimal study if they do not fast prior to the scan.

Intense tracer uptake in muscle and fat is sometimes seen in the neck, paraspinal, pectoral, and shoulder regions, particularly in young patients. This uptake may be ameliorated or reduced with the oral administration of benzodiazepine anxiolytics prior to the injection of the tracer.

The brain cortex, basal ganglia, and thalami typically show high FDG uptake. Myocardial uptake is variable, and the fasting state assists in reducing the myocardial uptake of FDG. Bowel uptake is also variable, but bowel preparations typically are not used in routine clinical practice since the procedure is similar to that used for colonoscopy preparation and may be too demanding for oncologic patients. Low to mild diffuse uptake of FDG is usually seen throughout the liver and splenic parenchyma. Focal uptake of higher intensity than the surrounding parenchyma should raise the suspicion for the presence of disease. Of note, attenuation correction artifacts also may mimic lesions, particularly in the liver. Analysis of the non–attenuated-corrected images will help differentiate an image artifact from a true lesion.

Focal FDG uptake does not necessarily translate to neoplastic involvement, particularly if the level of uptake is mild to moderate, since nonmalignant conditions such as infectious and inflammatory conditions can demonstrate FDG avidity (63–65). These conditions include pyogenic abscesses, tuberculosis, coccidioidomycosis, aspergillosis, histoplasmosis, sarcoidosis, postradiation inflammatory changes, and postoperative wound healing (4). In this context, inflammatory changes secondary to local tumor ablation procedures such as cryoablation, radiofrequency ablation, and ethanol injection may also lead to false-positive FDG uptake (discussed later in this chapter).

The strength of PET scanning relies on its high negative predictive value. If there is no FDG uptake within a lesion that is at least 7 mm or greater in size, it is most likely not malignant. Exceptions to this rule include carcinoid tumor, bronchioloalveolar carcinoma, some renal cell cancers, prostate cancer, hepatocellular carcinoma, and cancers with myxoid features. These cancers may exhibit low or no FDG uptake (4,66–78).

PET Imaging: Methodology

In the longitudinal evaluation of patients with FDG-PET, attention should be paid to strict adherence to protocol details such as adequate fasting, glycemic status, time of imaging, acquisition and quantitation techniques, and minimization of subcutaneous dose infiltration. These are important factors to consider because differences in glycemic or insulin levels may significantly alter the biodistribution of FDG. Dose extravasation can result in significant image artifacts, which may impair quantification accuracy and may result in nonpathologic focal uptake in the lymphatic system, which may be difficult to distinguish from malignancy.

Several methods are available for evaluating therapeutic response using FDG-PET (79–81). The simplest method is visual assessment of tumor uptake by comparing FDG activity in tumor lesions with normal surrounding tissues and organs. This is a purely qualitative approach, which is unavoidably subjective and does not allow for detection of subtle changes in tumor uptake. A more precise method is measurement of a tumor-to-background (i.e., normal tissue) ratio (TBR). This is a semiquantitative method, and has some limitations. For example, even with a constant ^{18}F-FDG uptake within the tumor, TBR values could falsely change due to variations in the surrounding normal tissue activity caused by changes in glucose level, time of scanning, or therapeutic effect.

Today, the most widely accepted semiquantitative method for assessment of treatment response by PET is the standardized uptake value (SUV), which is defined as the ratio of FDG concentration in the tumor to the mean value in the whole body (injected dose divided by patient weight in kilograms) (82–84). This value has an advantage over TBR in that no measurement of normal tissue is required. However, SUV also may be significantly affected by changes in glucose level, time delay between injection and scanning, or therapy effect. Changes in SUV of less than 25% between scans are not normally considered to be significant (81,85).

Interventional Radiology and PET: Clinical Considerations

Assessment of the therapeutic outcomes of interventional radiology procedures is classically based on bidimensional changes in a lesion size, density, and enhancement changes on CT, or signal enhancement characteristics on MRI before and after the treatment. However, such anatomic assessments have limitations in cases in which residual masses often are seen during and after treatment, for example in lymphomas. In these cases, differentiation between residual viable tumor tissue and scar tissue is often limited based on anatomic imaging (e.g., CT, MRI) modalities alone. In these circumstances, functional imaging demonstrates useful complementarity to anatomic imaging and can help in determining appropriate levels of cancer treatment in patients. Since FDG-PET scanning can reliably detect the presence of viable tumor within residual masses that are 7 mm or greater in size, it can help to differentiate residual/recurrent tumor from posttherapeutic inflammatory changes or scar.

The basic prerequisite for use of FDG-PET in the evaluation of therapeutic response is the demonstration of FDG avidity within the lesion of interest (i.e., malignancy) prior to treatment. Therefore, the usual protocol for use of FDG-PET in therapeutic evaluation should include a baseline scan obtained before the interventional procedure and follow-up scan(s) performed after completion of the therapeutic procedure. The timing of the follow-up scan depends on several factors, including the nature of the treated lesion, the type of the applied therapeutic modality, and the findings of other imaging modalities. The use of FDG-PET in the assessment of tumor ablation in various cancers is discussed later in this chapter.

Combined Multimodality Imaging

As much as FDG-PET can be helpful in the assessment of the viability of a lesion of interest, the absence of detailed anatomic information can lead to diagnostic dilemmas in the evaluation of complex anatomic regions. In practice, interpretation is performed by visually correlating the PET scans with high-quality anatomic images provided by CT or magnetic resonance (MR) scans (86).

Functional-morphologic correlation may be assisted by digital image fusion of independently performed PET and CT images. Results of several studies have shown the superior clinical value of digitally fused images in patients with brain, lung, and abdominal tumors and for radiation therapy planning (87,88). Such digitally fused images are reported to be particularly helpful to anatomically localize pathologic FDG uptake in retroperitoneal masses and abdominal or pelvic wall lesions (88). Registration errors, however, occur because of difficulties in proper patient repositioning when imaging with the second modality.

In an attempt to avoid these errors, integrated systems capable of sequentially acquiring both PET and CT data in a single imaging session have been designed (89–91). The first such system was developed at the University of Pittsburgh and consisted of a spiral CT scanner integrated with a rotating partial-ring PET scanner. Today, combined PET/CT scanners are available from multiple vendors and will likely dominate the market for PET systems in the near future. Image fusion obtained on the current generation of integrated scanners is less prone to error due to body positioning, but some inaccuracies still exist due to, for example, differences in respiratory chest movement between fast CT and slower PET acquisitions, or patient motion and bowel activity distribution over the course of the two scans (92–95).

Nevertheless, early experiences gathered on a wide range of malignancies including lung, colorectal, head and neck, and ovarian cancer, as well as lymphoma and melanoma, have been very positive (96–98). Integrated diagnostic systems will add value in providing not only a more accurate diagnosis and localization of the hypermetabolic focus seen on PET (88,99,100), but also in allowing PET/CT-guided interventions such as aspiration biopsy for lesion characterization or transcatheter tumor chemoembolization, radiofrequency, and other ablation techniques.

Preliminary Clinical Experience with FDG-PET in Tumor Ablation in Our Practice

Over the past several years, FDG-PET imaging has become widely used in the diagnosis and staging of a variety of malignant tumors and as a tool for follow-up of these tumors to assess the response to treatment and disease progression. This section discusses our clinical experience with the use of FDG-PET imaging for follow-up in patients undergoing tumor ablation.

At our institution, patients referred for tumor ablation are imaged before and after ablation by standard anatomic methods, usually by MRI, often supplemented by CT. Occasionally, only CT imaging is used if MRI is not feasible. As FDG-PET imaging has become more commonly used, many of these patients have had pre- and/or postprocedure PET scans. Of approximately 160 ablation procedures done since we began performing PET scans, 21 patients undergoing these procedures have had FDG-PET scans both before and after their ablation procedures. All 21 patients had standard anatomic imaging before and after their procedures, so we have a basis for qualitative comparison of the information provided by anatomic and functional imaging in ablation cases. The following discussion is based on clinical interpretations, in which the imaging scan readers had access to any and all clinical information, including the results of other imaging techniques, and is intended to illustrate the clinical possibilities and some of the potential pitfalls of FDG-PET imaging in the context of tumor ablation.

Colorectal Cancer

The largest subgroup of these patients, nine of the 21, had colorectal cancer. Six of these patients had metastatic disease to the liver that was the target for ablation. One patient had adrenal and lung metastases in addition to liver metastases. The remaining two patients had pelvic masses, which were the target lesions. One patient study in our group of colorectal cancer patients was limited by a hyperglycemic state.

Typically in this disease setting, the preprocedure MRI and PET scans were in agreement regarding the disease in the target lesion(s). All of the intended target lesions were detectable by both modalities. Other metastatic lesions, some definite and some questionable, were detected on the preprocedure studies in four of these patients by PET and in two by MRI. It should be noted that the standard clinical oncologic PET protocol in our Department calls for imaging the whole body from the base of the skull to the proximal thighs. The preprocedure MRI tends to scan a more restricted region (e.g., liver only, pelvis only), and for that reason can be expected to be less effective for staging.

Preprocedure PET can provide valuable staging information. The discovery of previously undetected metastatic sites in a patient with an apparent solitary focus may modify the plans for ablation, or at least alter the nature of the preprocedure counseling of the patient. The postablation follow-up studies are of clinical interest for assessing the effectiveness of the procedure in destroying the tumor, for evaluating the presence of residual or recurrent disease, and for assessing interval change in other known sites, or development of new disease sites (Fig. 10.1) (101,102).

In five of these nine patients, both follow-up PET and MRI demonstrated recurrent disease at the ablation site. In another three of these nine patients, follow-up PET and MRI showed no evidence of recurrence at the ablation site, although in one the follow-up PET showed extensive new metastatic disease elsewhere in liver, nodes, skeleton, and lungs. Finally, in one of these nine colorectal cancer patients, a postprocedure PET 3 months posttherapy detected mildly increased uptake at the site of one of the ablated lesions, which was indeterminate for either inflammatory or residual disease. However, subsequent PET scans showed further resolution of tracer uptake at this site in spite of documenting definite progression of disease elsewhere. Thus, FDG tracer uptake is not specific for tumor, and intense tracer uptake can be seen at sites of inflammation, which may occur at postablation sites.

Lung Cancer

Six of the 21 patients who underwent ablation with both pre- and postprocedure PET imaging had lung cancer of various types. Three of these had metastatic lesions to the liver that were the target lesions for ablation, while the others had lung or chest-wall lesions that were not amenable to surgery. In all of these cases, the

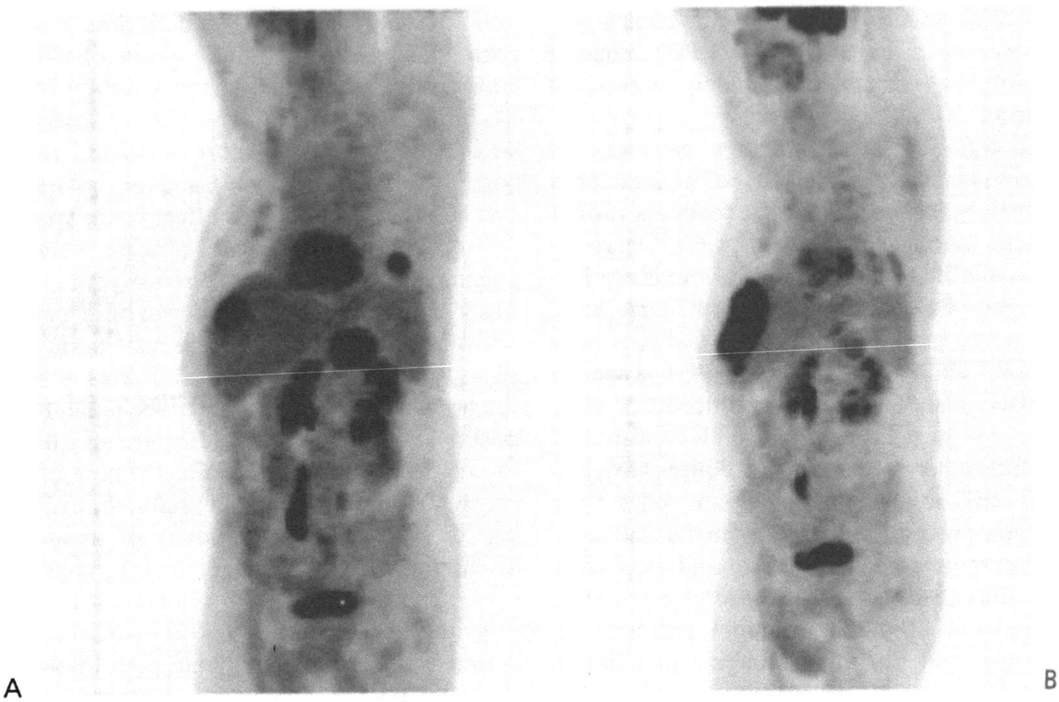

FIGURE 10.1. Colon cancer metastatic to liver, lung, and left adrenal. Left anterior oblique (LAO) projection images (MIP). (A) Preprocedure study. Metastases are seen in the right lobe of the liver, left lung base, and left adrenal. Note physiologic tracer excretion in kidneys, right ureter, and bladder. (B) Postprocedure study. The left lung and adrenal lesions show posttherapeutic inflammatory changes, although residual tumor cannot be excluded. The metastatic disease to the liver has progressed. A new small focus that projects just below the heart is a new metastasis located in the right lung base.

target lesion was detected preprocedure by both anatomic and functional imaging.

In one patient with squamous cell lung cancer metastatic to liver, initial and follow-up PET scans identified a hilar nodal metastasis that was not seen on the liver MRI. In another patient with non–small-cell lung cancer with several metastases to liver, the postprocedure PET and MRI both showed residual lesions. The PET result was interpreted as showing posttherapeutic inflammation at a treated site, while the MRI scan was interpreted as showing residual disease. However, a subsequent repeat PET scan confirmed disease progression at this site. In a third patient with lung cancer, a single 5-cm liver metastasis was identified and treated. The PET obtained 3 months after the procedure showed only slight interval decrease in tracer uptake in the lesion, and was consistent with residual tumor. The MRI appearance was concordant, suggesting recurrent or residual tumor.

There were three patients with lung primaries in whom the target lesion for ablation was in the chest. One of these patients had a lung tumor seen on both initial MR and PET. The repeat PET 1 month after the procedure showed residual disease at the ablation site and also a new metastasis in the pelvis, which was not, of course, seen on the postprocedure chest CT. Another patient had non–small-cell lung cancer with a large right apical mass with chest wall invasion, and a right hilar mass, both of which were evident on the preprocedure PET and chest MRI, and were consistent with neoplasm by PET. This patient was not a candidate for surgery, and radiofrequency ablation of the lung mass was undertaken with palliative intent. A postprocedure PET at 6 weeks demonstrated a central photopenic region at the site of the ablation, with a rim of surrounding increased FDG uptake. The latter appearance could have been caused either by residual tumor at the boundaries of the treated region, or alternately by postprocedure inflammatory change, although the former explanation was favored. A subsequent follow-up CT obtained 5 weeks after the PET did demonstrate interval increase in the size of the mass, confirming progression of the tumor.

The differential diagnosis of residual tumor versus inflammatory changes at a site of increased or residual FDG uptake may be challenging in the early postprocedure phase since posttherapeutic inflammatory changes also can cause increased uptake of tracer particularly soon after therapy. This phenomenon has been described during radiation therapy (4,45,103–106). Since qualitative readings of PET scans can be reader-dependent, training and experience in PET imaging interpretation help nuclear medicine physicians and radiologists become familiar with the various patterns of inflammatory versus tumoral uptake. Dual time point FDG-PET imaging at 45 to 70 minutes and at approximately 90 minutes postinjection of the tracer also has been proposed to help in the differentiation of benign from malignant disease (107,108). Continuous increase in SUV was seen in malignant lesions, while SUVs of benign lesions or inflammation decreased over time, or remained stable. Follow-up scans 4 to 6 weeks or later after the procedure also can be helpful since inflammatory changes may continue to resolve with time after the procedure, assuming that the postprocedure course is not complicated by infection or other unusual circumstances. However, long-term residual uptake has been observed, particularly after proton therapy (106).

The last patient in our study population had lung cancer, with a large left lung lesion visible on CT and PET. Follow-up PET, about 1 month after the ablation, showed a photopenic defect with mild increased uptake at the rim thought to be inflammatory and two distinct small intense foci, which could be residual disease (Fig. 10.2). Follow-up CT performed 2 months later showed treatment changes in the main lesion, but an interval increase in a separate nodule anterior to the main lesion, suggesting recurrent disease.

Other Tumors

Ovarian Cancer

One patient had ovarian cancer metastatic to the abdomen, pelvis, and liver surface that was detected by PET, although two small liver lesions seen on CT (less than 1 cm) were not visualized on PET, probably because of the small size of the lesions.

In this patient, the preprocedure MRI showed at least four metastatic lesions to the liver. The patient underwent radiofrequency/ethanol ablation of two of these lesions for symptomatic relief. The postprocedure MRI showed treatment effect in some of the lesions, and growth of nontreated lesions. A postprocedure PET performed 5 months later showed interval complete resolution of one treated lesion, residual disease at another, and interval development of a new lesion in Morison's pouch.

Cholangiocarcinoma

In a patient with cholangiocarcinoma, a preprocedure MRI showed a 16-cm central hepatic mass with vascular encasement. The initial PET showed a large central liver lesion with central photopenia, and possible bone lesions were detected.

Larger tumors often have a shell-like appearance on PET, with relative photopenia centrally. Reasons for this observation could include central necrosis of the tumor, with a lack of viable cells in the photopenic regions, or relatively poor blood supply and tracer delivery to these regions. This fact can somewhat complicate the interpretation of a tumor ablation case, in which the therapy is applied to the center of the lesion, which in a big lesion may have shown little tracer uptake to begin with.

In the case of this patient, the follow-up MRI at 1 week postprocedure showed no change in the appearance of the tumor; PET at 5 weeks showed a larger region of central photopenia in the tumor, but peripheral tracer uptake. This was interpreted as showing partial response to the ablation therapy.

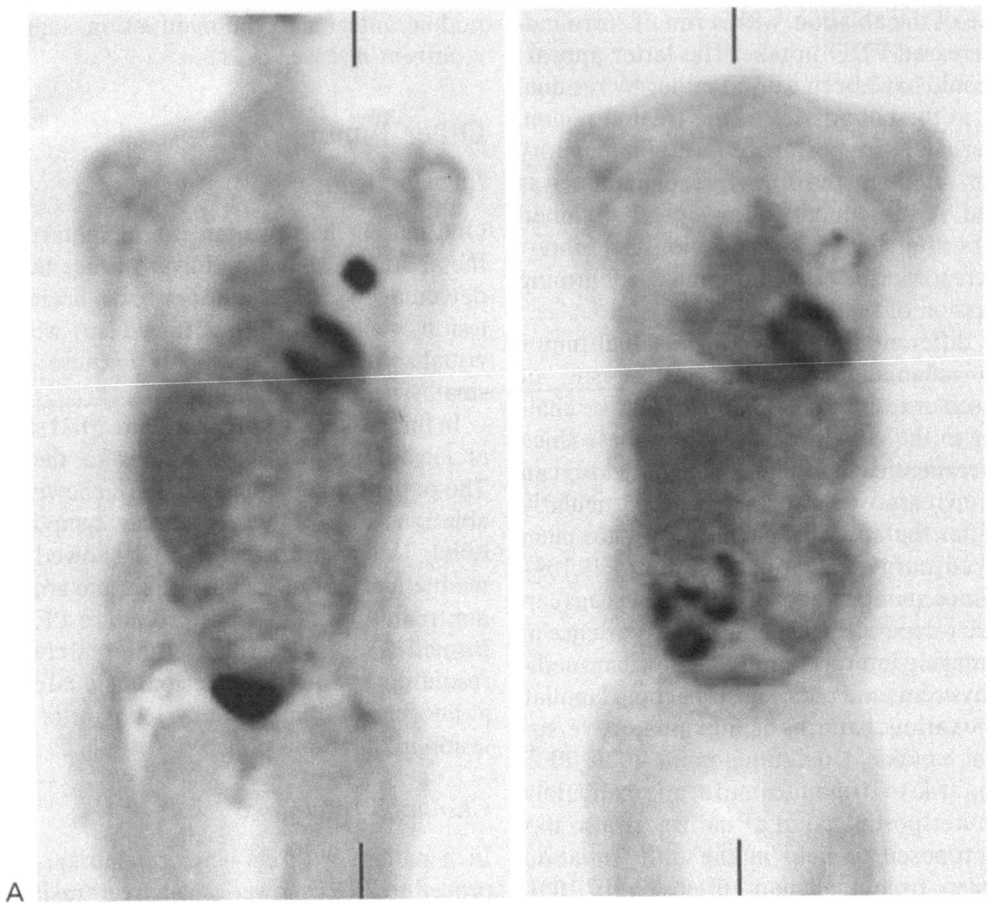

FIGURE 10.2. (A) Preprocedure study. A single coronal image showing an intensely FDG-avid non–small-cell lung tumor in the left lung. Note the right hip prosthesis. (B) Postprocedure study at 1 month. A single coronal image through the treated lesion shows central photopenia in the lesion, with surrounding mild uptake consistent with postprocedure inflammatory changes and a slightly more intense focus at the upper margin, suspicious for residual disease.

Gastric Cancer

One patient had gastric cancer metastatic to the gastrohepatic ligament and the retroperitoneum around both the celiac axis and superior mesenteric artery. These lesions were visible on both MRI and PET prior to the procedure. A PET obtained 2 months after the procedure demonstrated central photopenia in the ablated lesion, but otherwise interval progression of disease. An MRI obtained after another 3 months showed overall improvement. However, according to the report of that study, some nonablated sites improved as well. Following the procedure, the patient had been started on new chemotherapy, which most likely was responsible for the improvement in all lesions.

Gastrointestinal Stromal Tumor (GIST)

One patient with GIST had multiple metastatic liver and abdominal lesions that were progressing on therapy. A preprocedure PET showed recurrence of GIST in previously treated locations in the right lobe of the liver, with a possible new lesion in the left lobe despite ongoing therapy with imatinib mesylate (Gleevec). A postprocedure PET done 6 weeks later showed interval resolution of the increased uptake in the treated lesions, and no definite evidence of metabolically active tumor. A CT performed at 6 weeks provided confirmatory evidence that the treated lesions showed no recurrence.

Tumors with Variable FDG Avidity

Renal Cell Carcinoma

Not all tumor types show increased avidity for FDG, so FDG-PET cannot be used to follow such cases if there is no FDG avidity within the tumor site in the baseline scan. For example, one patient with a history of metastatic ovarian cancer had a large left renal mass, presumably metastatic, for which ablation was being considered. The preprocedure PET demonstrated the multiple FDG-avid metastatic foci of ovarian cancer in the abdomen, but no focal increased uptake in the large renal lesion. A subsequent biopsy showed the renal mass to be a renal cell carcinoma.

Some primary renal cell carcinomas can be negative on FDG-PET (69), but others are not, and a baseline FDG-PET is helpful to determine if PET could be useful or not. In this particular case, FDG-PET was a valuable tool to assess the patient's ovarian cancer, but not for the second renal cell primary.

Hepatocellular Carcinoma

Hepatocellular carcinoma (HCC) is a tumor with variable avidity for FDG (74–77). One patient had a known 2.7-cm HCC in the inferior posterior segment of the right lobe. This lesion was seen on the MRI, but was not detected on the PET done the next day. Again, baseline PET may help determine if this modality might be useful in the follow-up of these patients.

Conclusion

Interventional radiology techniques typically represent the least invasive definitive diagnostic or therapeutic options available for patients with cancer. These techniques are usually performed at a lower cost and with less associated morbidity than other interventions. Radiologic assessment of bidimensional changes in tumor size is still largely considered a "gold standard" for the evaluation of therapeutic response in such patients. However, there is rapidly increasing evidence that functional imaging with FDG-PET has a significant advantage in the evaluation of response to therapy, particularly in the evaluation of residual masses.

Acknowledgment

The authors gratefully acknowledge the valuable assistance of Clay H. Holdsworth, Ph.D., and Richard J. Tetrault, CNMT, for their assistance in reviewing this chapter.

References

1. Maisey MN, Wahl RL, Barrington SF. Atlas of Clinical Positron Emission Tomography. London: Arnold, 1999:346.
2. Brown RS, Wahl RL. Overexpression of Glut-1 glucose transporter in human breast cancer. An immunohistochemical study. Cancer 1993; 72(10):2979–2985.
3. Brown RS, et al. Expression of hexokinase II and Glut-1 in untreated human breast cancer. Nucl Med Biol 2002;29(4):443–453.
4. Wieler H, Coleman R. PET in Clinical Oncology. Darmstadt: Steinkopff Verlag, 2000:422.
5. Gambhir SS, Shepherd JE, Shah BD, et al. Analytical decision model for the cost-effective management of solitary pulmonary nodules. J Clin Oncol 1998;16(6):2113–2125.
6. Gambhir SS, Czernin J, Schwimmer J, Silverman DH, Coleman RE, Phelps ME. A tabulated summary of the FDG PET literature. J Nucl Med 2001;42(5 suppl):1S–93S.
7. Huebner RH, Park KC, Shepherd JE, et al. A meta-analysis of the literature for whole-body FDG PET detection of recurrent colorectal cancer. J Nucl Med 2000;41(7):1177–1189.
8. Kubik-Huch RA, Dorffler W, von Schulthess GK, et al. Value of (18F)-FDG positron emission tomography, computed tomography, and magnetic resonance imaging in diagnosing primary and recurrent ovarian carcinoma. Eur Radiol 2000;10(5):761–767.
9. Meta J, Seltzer M, Schiepers C, et al. Impact of 18F-FDG PET on managing patients with col-

orectal cancer: the referring physician's perspective. J Nucl Med 2001;42(4):586–590.
10. Park KC, Schwimmer J, Shepherd JE, et al. Decision analysis for the cost-effective management of recurrent colorectal cancer. Ann Surg 2001;233(3):310–319.
11. Park KC, Schwimmer J, Gambhir SS. Decision analysis for the cost-effective management of recurrent colorectal cancer. Ann Surg 2002; 235(2):309–310; author reply 10.
12. Schwimmer J, Essner R, Patel A, et al. A review of the literature for whole-body FDG PET in the management of patients with melanoma. Q J Nucl Med 2000;44(2):153–167.
13. Scott WJ, Shepherd J, Gambhir SS. Cost-effectiveness of FDG-PET for staging non-small cell lung cancer: a decision analysis. Ann Thorac Surg 1998;66(6):1876–1883; discussion 83–85.
14. Seltzer MA, Yap CS, Silverman DH, et al. The impact of PET on the management of lung cancer: the referring physician's perspective. J Nucl Med 2002;43(6):752–756.
15. Wu D, Gambhir SS. Positron emission tomography in diagnosis and management of invasive breast cancer: current status and future perspectives. Clin Breast Cancer 2003;4(suppl1): S55–S63.
16. Yap CS, Seltzer MA, Schiepers C, et al. Impact of whole-body 18F-FDG PET on staging and managing patients with breast cancer: the referring physician's perspective. J Nucl Med 2001;42(9):1334–1337.
17. Services DOHH. Coverage and related claims processing requirements for positron emission tomography (PET) scans. Program Memorandum Intermediaries/Carriers. CMS-Pub. 60AB (AB-02-065). 2002:1–4.
18. Kinkel K, Lu Y, Both M, Warren RS, Thoeni RF. Detection of hepatic metastases from cancers of the gastrointestinal tract by using noninvasive imaging methods (US, CT, MR imaging, PET): a meta-analysis. Radiology 2002;224(3): 748–756.
19. Jerusalem G, Beguin Y, Fassotte MF, et al. Whole-body positron emission tomography using 18F-fluorodeoxyglucose for posttreatment evaluation in Hodgkin's disease and non-Hodgkin's lymphoma has higher diagnostic and prognostic value than classical computed tomography scan imaging. Blood 1999;94(2): 429–433.
20. Dittmann H, Sokler M, Kollmannsberger C, et al. Comparison of 18FDG-PET with CT scans in the evaluation of patients with residual and recurrent Hodgkin's lymphoma. Oncol Rep 2001;8(6):1393–1399.
21. Mikhaeel NG, Timothy AR, O'Doherty MJ, Hain S, Maisey MN. 18-FDG-PET as a prognostic indicator in the treatment of aggressive non-Hodgkin's lymphoma—comparison with CT. Leuk Lymphoma 2000;39(5–6):543–553.
22. Pieterman RM, van Putten JW, Meuzelaar JJ, et al. Preoperative staging of non-small-cell lung cancer with positron-emission tomography. N Engl J Med 2000;343(4):254–261.
23. Berman CG, Clark RA. Positron emission tomography in initial staging and diagnosis of persistent or recurrent disease. Curr Opin Oncol 2000;12(2):132–137.
24. Lowe VJ, Fletcher JW, Gobar L, et al. Prospective investigation of positron emission tomography in lung nodules. J Clin Oncol 1998;16(3): 1075–1084.
25. Lowe VJ, Naunheim KS. Positron emission tomography in lung cancer. Ann Thorac Surg 1998;65(6):1821–1829.
26. Lowe VJ, Naunheim KS. Current role of positron emission tomography in thoracic oncology. Thorax 1998;53(8):703–712.
27. Delbeke D. Oncological applications of FDG PET imaging: brain tumors, colorectal cancer, lymphoma and melanoma. J Nucl Med 1999; 40(4):591–603.
28. Delbeke D. Oncological applications of FDG PET imaging. J Nucl Med 1999;40(10):1706–1715.
29. Erasmus JJ, McAdams HP, Connolly JE. Solitary pulmonary nodules: part II. Evaluation of the indeterminate nodule. Radiographics 2000;20(1):59–66.
30. Erasmus JJ, Connolly JE, McAdams HP, Roggli VL. Solitary pulmonary nodules: part I. Morphologic evaluation for differentiation of benign and malignant lesions. Radiographics 2000;20(1):43–58.
31. Coleman RE. PET in lung cancer. J Nucl Med 1999;40(5):814–820.
32. Erasmus JJ, McAdams HP, Patz EF, Jr. Non-small cell lung cancer: FDG-PET imaging. J Thorac Imaging 1999;14(4):247–256.
33. Rinne D, Baum RP, Hor G, Kaufmann R. Primary staging and follow-up of high risk melanoma patients with whole-body 18F-fluorodeoxyglucose positron emission tomography: results of a prospective study of 100 patients. Cancer 1998;82(9):1664–1671.

34. Lowe VJ, Boyd JH, Dunphy FR, et al. Surveillance for recurrent head and neck cancer using positron emission tomography. J Clin Oncol 2000;18(3):651–658.
35. Skehan SJ, Brown AL, Thompson M, Young JE, Coates G, Nahmias C. Imaging features of primary and recurrent esophageal cancer at FDG PET. Radiographics 2000;20(3):713–723.
36. Luketich JD, Friedman DM, Weigel TL, et al. Evaluation of distant metastases in esophageal cancer: 100 consecutive positron emission tomography scans. Ann Thorac Surg 1999;68(4): 1133–1136; discussion 1136–1137.
37. Zimmer LA, McCook B, Meltzer C, et al. Combined positron emission tomography/computed tomography imaging of recurrent thyroid cancer. Otolaryngol Head Neck Surg 2003; 128(2):178–184.
38. Frilling A, Tecklenborg K, Gorges R, Weber F, Clausen M, Broelsch EC. Preoperative diagnostic value of [(18)F] fluorodeoxyglucose positron emission tomography in patients with radioiodine-negative recurrent well-differentiated thyroid carcinoma. Ann Surg 2001;234(6): 804–811.
39. Helal BO, Merlet P, Toubert ME, et al. Clinical impact of (18)F-FDG PET in thyroid carcinoma patients with elevated thyroglobulin levels and negative (131)I scanning results after therapy. J Nucl Med 2001;42(10):1464–1469.
40. Yeo JS, Chung JK, SO Y, et al. F-18-fluorodeoxyglucose positron emission tomography as a presurgical evaluation modality for I-131 scan-negative thyroid carcinoma patients with local recurrence in cervical lymph nodes. Head Neck 2001;23(2):94–103.
41. Hustinx R, Benard F, Alavi A. Whole-body FDG-PET imaging in the management of patients with cancer. Semin Nucl Med 2002; 32(1):35–46.
42. Bassa P, Kim EE, Inoue T, et al. Evaluation of preoperative chemotherapy using PET with fluorine-18-fluorodeoxyglucose in breast cancer. J Nucl Med 1996;37(6):931–938.
43. Berlangieri SU, Brizel DM, Scher RL, et al. Pilot study of positron emission tomography in patients with advanced head and neck cancer receiving radiotherapy and chemotherapy. Head Neck 1994;16(4):340–346.
44. Findlay M, Young H, Cunningham D, et al. Noninvasive monitoring of tumor metabolism using fluorodeoxyglucose and positron emission tomography in colorectal cancer liver metastases: correlation with tumor response to fluorouracil. J Clin Oncol 1996;14(3):700–708.
45. Haberkorn U, Strauss LG, Dimitrakopoulou A, et al. PET studies of fluorodeoxyglucose metabolism in patients with recurrent colorectal tumors receiving radiotherapy. J Nucl Med 1991;32(8):1485–1490.
46. Ichiya Y, Kuwabara Y, Otsuka M, et al. Assessment of response to cancer therapy using fluorine-18-fluorodeoxyglucose and positron emission tomography. J Nucl Med 1991;32(9): 1655–1660.
47. Okazumi S, Isono K, Enomoto K, et al. Evaluation of liver tumors using fluorine-18-fluorodeoxyglucose PET: characterization of tumor and assessment of effect of treatment. J Nucl Med 1992;33(3):333–339.
48. Reisser C, Haberkorn U, Dimitrakopoulou-Strauss A, Seifert E, Strauss LG. Chemotherapeutic management of head and neck malignancies with positron emission tomography. Arch Otolaryngol Head Neck Surg 1995;121(3):272–276.
49. Wahl RL, Zasadny K, Helvie M, Hutchins GD, Weber B, Cody R. Metabolic monitoring of breast cancer chemohormonotherapy using positron emission tomography: initial evaluation. J Clin Oncol 1993;11(11):2101–2111.
50. Schulte M, Brecht-Krauss D, Werner M, et al. Evaluation of neoadjuvant therapy response of osteogenic sarcoma using FDG PET. J Nucl Med 1999;40(10):1637–1643.
51. Minn H, Lapela M, Klemi PJ, et al. Prediction of survival with fluorine-18-fluoro-deoxyglucose and PET in head and neck cancer. J Nucl Med 1997;38(12):1907–1911.
52. Allal AS, Dulguerov P, Allaoua M, et al. Standardized uptake value of 2-[(18)F] fluoro-2-deoxy-D-glucose in predicting outcome in head and neck carcinomas treated by radiotherapy with or without chemotherapy. J Clin Oncol 2002;20(5):1398–1404.
53. Eary JF, Krohn KA. Positron emission tomography: imaging tumor response. Eur J Nucl Med 2000;27(12):1737–1739.
54. Folpe AL, Lyles RH, Sprouse JT, Conrad EU, III, Eary JF. (F-18) fluorodeoxyglucose positron emission tomography as a predictor of pathologic grade and other prognostic variables in bone and soft tissue sarcoma. Clin Cancer Res 2000;6(4):1279–1287.
55. Wong RJ, Lin DT, Schoder H, et al. Diagnostic and prognostic value of [(18)F]fluorodeoxyglu-

cose positron emission tomography for recurrent head and neck squamous cell carcinoma. J Clin Oncol 2002;20(20):4199–4208.
56. Spaepen K, Mortelmans L. Evaluation of treatment response in patients with lymphoma using [18F]FDG-PET: differences between non-Hodgkin's lymphoma and Hodgkin's disease. Q J Nucl Med 2001;45(3):269–273.
57. Spaepen K, Stroobants S, Dupont P, et al. Can positron emission tomography with [(18)F]-fluorodeoxyglucose after first-line treatment distinguish Hodgkin's disease patients who need additional therapy from others in whom additional therapy would mean avoidable toxicity? Br J Haematol 2001;115(2): 272–278.
58. Spaepen K, Stroobants S, Dupont P, et al. Prognostic value of positron emission tomography (PET) with fluorine-18 fluorodeoxyglucose ([18F]FDG) after first-line chemotherapy in non-Hodgkin's lymphoma: is [18F]FDG-PET a valid alternative to conventional diagnostic methods? J Clin Oncol 2001;19(2):414–419.
59. Jerusalem G, Warland V, Najjar F, et al. Whole-body 18F-FDG PET for the evaluation of patients with Hodgkin's disease and non-Hodgkin's lymphoma. Nucl Med Commun 1999;20(1):13–20.
60. Naumann R, Vaic A, Beuthien-Baumann B, et al. Prognostic value of positron emission tomography in the evaluation of post-treatment residual mass in patients with Hodgkin's disease and non-Hodgkin's lymphoma. Br J Haematol 2001;115(4):793–800.
61. de Wit M, Bohuslavizki KH, Buchert R, Bumann D, Clausen M, Hossfeld DK. 18FDG-PET following treatment as valid predictor for disease-free survival in Hodgkin's lymphoma. Ann Oncol 2001;12(1):29–37.
62. Becherer A, Mitterbauer M, Jaeger U, et al. Positron emission tomography with [18F]2-fluoro-D-2-deoxyglucose (FDG-PET) predicts relapse of malignant lymphoma after high-dose therapy with stem cell transplantation. Leukemia 2002;16(2):260–267.
63. Bakheet SM, Saleem M, Powe J, Al-Amro A, Larsson SG, Mahassin Z. F-18 fluorodeoxyglucose chest uptake in lung inflammation and infection. Clin Nucl Med 2000;25(4):273–278.
64. Wolf G, Aigner RM, Schwarz T. Pathologic uptake in F-18 FDG positron emission tomography of the residuals of a surgically removed needle abscess. Clin Nucl Med 2002;27(6):439–440.
65. Yoon SN, Park CH, Kim MK, Hwang KH, Kim S. False-positive F-18 FDG gamma camera positron emission tomographic imaging resulting from inflammation of an anterior mediastinal mass in a patient with non-Hodgkin's lymphoma. Clin Nucl Med 2001;26(5):461–462.
66. Erasmus JJ, McAdams HP, Patz EF, Jr., Coleman RE, Ahuja V, Goodman PC. Evaluation of primary pulmonary carcinoid tumors using FDG PET. AJR Roentgenol 1998;170(5): 1369–1373.
67. Rege SD, Hoh CK, Glaspy JA, et al. Imaging of pulmonary mass lesions with whole-body positron emission tomography and fluorodeoxyglucose. Cancer 1993;72(1):82–90.
68. Hoh CK, Seltzer MA, Franklin J, deKernion JB, Phelps ME, Belldegrun A. Positron emission tomography in urological oncology. J Urol 1998;159(2):347–356.
69. Miyakita H, Tokunaga M, Onda H, et al. Significance of 18F-fluorodeoxyglucose positron emission tomography (FDG-PET) for detection of renal cell carcinoma and immunohistochemical glucose transporter 1 (GLUT-1) expression in cancer. Int J Urol 2002;9(1):15–18.
70. Hofer C, Kubler H, Hartung R, Breul J, Avril N. Diagnosis and monitoring of urological tumors using positron emission tomography. Eur Urol 2001;40(5):481–487.
71. Effert PJ, Bares R, Handt S, Wolff JM, Bull U, Jakse G. Metabolic imaging of untreated prostate cancer by positron emission tomography with 18-fluorine-labeled deoxyglucose. J Urol 1996;155(3):994–998.
72. Hofer C, Laubenbacher C, Block T, Breul J, Hartung R, Schwaiger M. Fluorine-18-fluorodeoxyglucose positron emission tomography is useless for the detection of local recurrence after radical prostatectomy. Eur Urol 1999; 36(1):31–35.
73. Seltzer MA, Barbaric Z, Belldegrun A, et al. Comparison of helical computerized tomography, positron emission tomography and monoclonal antibody scans for evaluation of lymph node metastases in patients with prostate specific antigen relapse after treatment for localized prostate cancer. J Urol 1999;162(4):1322–1328.
74. Dimitrakopoulou-Strauss A, Gutzler F, Strauss LG, et al. [PET studies with C-11 ethanol in intratumoral therapy of hepatocellular carcinomas]. Radiologe 1996;36(9):744–749.
75. Wudel LJ, Jr., Delbeke D, Morris D, et al. The role of [18F]fluorodeoxyglucose positron emis-

sion tomography imaging in the evaluation of hepatocellular carcinoma. Am Surg 2003;69(2): 117–124, discussion 24–26.
76. Iwata Y, Shiomi S, Sasaki N, et al. Clinical usefulness of positron emission tomography with fluorine-18-fluorodeoxyglucose in the diagnosis of liver tumors. Ann Nucl Med 2000;14(2):121–126.
77. Schroder O, Trojan J, Zeuzem S, Baum RP. [Limited value of fluorine-18-fluorodeoxyglucose PET for the differential diagnosis of focal liver lesions in patients with chronic hepatitis C virus infection]. Nuklearmedizin 1998;37(8): 279–285.
78. Schwarzbach MH, Dimitrakopoulou-Strauss A, Mechtersheimer G, et al. Assessment of soft tissue lesions suspicious for liposarcoma by F18-deoxyglucose (FDG) positron emission tomography (PET). Anticancer Res 2001;21(5): 3609–3614.
79. Hoekstra CJ, Paglianiti I, Hoekstra OS, et al. Monitoring response to therapy in cancer using [18F]-2-fluoro-2-deoxy-D-glucose and positron emission tomography: an overview of different analytical methods. Eur J Nucl Med 2000;27(6): 731–743.
80. Weber WA, Ziegler SI, Thodtmann R, Hanauske AR, Schwaiger M. Reproducibility of metabolic measurements in malignant tumors using FDG PET. J Nucl Med 1999; 40(11):1771–1777.
81. Young H, Baum R, Cremerius U, et al. Measurement of clinical and subclinical tumour response using [18F]-fluorodeoxyglucose and positron emission tomography: review and 1999 EORTC recommendations. European Organization for Research and Treatment of Cancer (EORTC) PET Study Group. Eur J Cancer 1999;35(13):1773–1782.
82. Ahuja V, Coleman RE, Herndon J, Patz EF, Jr. The prognostic significance of fluorodeoxyglucose positron emission tomography imaging for patients with nonsmall cell lung carcinoma. Cancer 1998;83(5):918–924.
83. Schelling M, Avril N, Nahrig J, et al. Positron emission tomography using [(18)F]Fluorodeoxyglucose for monitoring primary chemotherapy in breast cancer. J Clin Oncol 2000;18(8): 1689–1695.
84. Saunders CA, Dussek JE, O'Doherty MJ, Maisey MN. Evaluation of fluorine-18-fluorodeoxyglucose whole body positron emission tomography imaging in the staging of lung cancer. Ann Thorac Surg 1999;67(3):790–797.
85. Hallett WA, Marsden PK, Cronin BF, O'Doherty MJ. Effect of corrections for blood glucose and body size on [18F]FDG PET standardised uptake values in lung cancer. Eur J Nucl Med 2001;28(7):919–922.
86. Zimny M, Wildberger JE, Cremerius U, et al. [Combined image interpretation of computed tomography and hybrid PET in head and neck cancer.] Nuklearmedizin 2002;41(1):14–21.
87. Caldwell CB, Mah K, Ung YC, et al. Observer variation in contouring gross tumor volume in patients with poorly defined non-small-cell lung tumors on CT: the impact of 18FDG-hybrid PET fusion. Int J Radiat Oncol Biol Phys 2001;51(4):923–931.
88. Schaffler GJ, Groell R, Schoellnast H, et al. Digital image fusion of CT and PET data sets—clinical value in abdominal/pelvic malignancies. J Comput Assist Tomogr 2000;24(4):644–647.
89. Beyer T, Townsend DW, Brun T, et al. A combined PET/CT scanner for clinical oncology. J Nucl Med 2000;41(8):1369–1379.
90. Townsend DW, Cherry SR. Combining anatomy and function: the path to true image fusion. Eur Radiol 2001;11(10):1968–1974.
91. Cook GJ, Ott RJ. Dual-modality imaging. Eur Radiol 2001;11(10):1857–1858.
92. Osman MM, Cohade C, Nakamoto Y, Marshall LT, Leal JP, Wahl RL. Clinically significant inaccurate localization of lesions with PET/CT: frequency in 300 patients. J Nucl Med 2003;44(2): 240–243.
93. Osman MM, Cohade C, Nakamoto Y, Wahl RL. Respiratory motion artifacts on PET emission images obtained using CT attenuation correction on PET-CT. Eur J Nucl Med Mol Imaging 2003;30(4):603–606.
94. Beyer T, Antoch G, Blodgett T, Freudenberg LF, Akhurst T, Mueller S. Dual-modality PET/CT imaging: the effect of respiratory motion on combined image quality in clinical oncology. Eur J Nucl Med Mol Imaging 2003;30(4):588–596.
95. Nakamoto Y, Tatsumi M, Cohade C, Osman M, Marshall LT, Wahl RL. Accuracy of image fusion of normal upper abdominal organs visualized with PET/CT. Eur J Nucl Med Mol Imaging 2003;30(4):597–602.
96. Israel O, Keidar Z, Iosilevsky G, Bettman L, Sachs J, Frenkel A. The fusion of anatomic and physiologic imaging in the management of patients with cancer. Semin Nucl Med 2001;31(3):191–205.

97. Martinelli M, Townsend D, Meltzer C, Villemagne VV. 7. Survey of Results of Whole Body Imaging Using the PET/CT at the University of Pittsburgh Medical Center PET Facility. Clin Positron Imaging 2000;3(4):161.
98. D'Amico TA, Wong TZ, Harpole DH, Brown SD, Coleman RE. Impact of computed tomography-positron emission tomography fusion in staging patients with thoracic malignancies. Ann Thorac Surg 2002;74(1):160–163; discussion 3.
99. Charron M, Beyer T, Bohnen NN, et al. Image analysis in patients with cancer studied with a combined PET and CT scanner. Clin Nucl Med 2000;25(11):905–910.
100. Hany TF, Steinert HC, Goerres GW, Buck A, von Schulthess GK. PET diagnostic accuracy: improvement with in-line PET-CT system: initial results. Radiology 2002;225(2):575–581.
101. Langenhoff BS, Oyen WJ, Jager GJ, et al. Efficacy of fluorine-18-deoxyglucose positron emission tomography in detecting tumor recurrence after local ablative therapy for liver metastases: a prospective study. J Clin Oncol 2002;20(22): 4453–4458.
102. Anderson GS, Brinkmann F, Soulen MC, Alavi A, Zhuang H. FDG positron emission tomography in the surveillance of hepatic tumors treated with radiofrequency ablation. Clin Nucl Med 2003;28(3):192–197.
103. Hautzel H, Muller-Gartner HW. Early changes in fluorine-18-FDG uptake during radiotherapy. J Nucl Med 1997;38(9):1384–1386.
104. Engenhart R, Kimmig B, Hover KH, Strauss LG, Lorenz WJ, Wannenmacher M. [Photon-neutron therapy for recurrent colorectal cancer—follow up and preliminary results.] Strahlenther Onkol 1990;166(1):95–98.
105. Higashi K, Clavo AC, Wahl RL. In vitro assessment of 2-fluoro-2-deoxy-D-glucose, L-methionine and thymidine as agents to monitor the early response of a human adenocarcinoma cell line to radiotherapy. J Nucl Med 1993;34(5): 773–779.
106. Fischman AJ, Thornton AF, Frosch MP, Swearinger B, Gonzalez RG, Alpert NM. FDG hypermetabolism associated with inflammatory necrotic changes following radiation of meningioma. J Nucl Med 1997;38(7):1027–1029.
107. Zhuang H, Pourdehnad M, Lambright ES, et al. Dual time point 18F-FDG PET imaging for differentiating malignant from inflammatory processes. J Nucl Med 2001;42(9):1412–1417.
108. Hustinx R, Smith RJ, Benard F, et al. Dual time point fluorine-18 fluorodeoxyglucose positron emission tomography: a potential method to differentiate malignancy from inflammation and normal tissue in the head and neck. Eur J Nucl Med 1999;26(10):1345–1348.

11
Ultrasound Imaging in Tumor Ablation

Massimo Tonolini and Luigi Solbiati

Diagnostic imaging plays a key role in all steps of radiofrequency (RF) tumor ablation:

1. Detection of lesions and selection of patients for treatment;
2. Targeting of lesions and guidance of the procedure;
3. Immediate assessment of treatment result;
4. Long-term follow-up.

Conventional, unenhanced ultrasound (US) is utilized worldwide for screening of liver disease, but variable sensitivity and well-known drawbacks limit its role in the staging of liver tumors. Furthermore, sonography represents the most commonly used imaging modality for the guidance of percutaneous ablative treatments owing to its availability, rapidity, and ease of use. Differentiation of induced necrosis from viable tumor is not possible with baseline and color Doppler sonography, and therefore the immediate and long-term assessment of therapeutic result is usually accomplished by contrast-enhanced helical computed tomography (CT) and magnetic resonance (MR).

In our experience the use of contrast-enhanced ultrasound (CEUS) represents a significant improvement over conventional US in each of the above-mentioned steps and has proven useful to achieve optimal patient management and treatment results (1).

Detection of Lesions and Selection of Patients

A wide range of treatment options currently is available for both primary and metastatic liver tumors. Therefore, timely detection and accurate quantification of neoplastic involvement at the time of diagnosis or during the course of the disease allows optimal patient management and treatment selection and ultimately may result in prolonged survival and possible cure.

Adequate local tumor control is feasible by percutaneous RF ablation provided that correct indications are observed. In most institutions patients with chronic hepatitis or cirrhosis without functional liver decompensation, portal thrombosis, or extrahepatic tumor spread may undergo RF of one to four or five dysplastic lesions or hepatocellular carcinoma foci, each not exceeding 4 to 4.5 cm; hepatomas larger than 5 cm usually are treated by means of combined therapies (transarterial chemoembolization, ethanol injection, RF) (2–4). Effective ablation of liver metastases requires the creation of a 0.5- to 1-cm "safety margin" of ablated peritumoral liver tissue to destroy microscopic infiltrating tumor and therefore limit the incidence of local recurrence. In patients with previous radical treatment for colorectal, breast, or other primary tumors, RF treatment is feasible when up to five liver metastases are present, each one not exceeding 4 cm in size (5–10).

Cross-sectional imaging modalities such as multiphasic contrast-enhanced helical CT and dynamic gadolinium-enhanced MR represent the mainstay for staging hepatic and extrahepatic neoplastic involvement. The use of hepatobiliary and reticuloendothelial-specific MR contrast agents may be helpful in selected patients to maximize lesion detection (11,12).

The "gold standard" for detection of focal liver lesions undoubtedly is by intraoperative ultrasound (IOUS). Unenhanced, B-mode ultrasound is cheap, fast, and widely available; therefore it is commonly used for screening of focal lesions in patients with chronic liver disease or with a history of cancer. Liver metastases display an extremely varied sonographic appearance, even within the same patient, as well as during the course of therapy (13).

The sensitivity of US depends on the operator's experience and available equipment, acoustic window from the patient's body habitus, bowel gas distention, and enlargement and inhomogeneity of the liver parenchyma due to steatosis, fibrosis, chronic liver disease and postchemotherapeutic changes.

The rate of detection of hepatic metastases with unenhanced ultrasound is lower than that of CT and MR; the reported accuracy ranges from 63% to 85%. The sensitivity of US is particularly poor for smaller focal lesions (less than 1 cm). Moreover, only limited characterization of focal liver lesions is possible with baseline US (13). To overcome the limitations of conventional US and increase the detection of focal lesions for accurate disease staging, CEUS has proved to be a valuable tool (1,13).

The recent development of contrast-specific ultrasound software systems by the major ultrasound companies (systems for *pulse inversion, phase inversion, contrast-tuned imaging, coherent contrast imaging, contrast pulse sequencing*, etc.), all based on the principle of wideband harmonic sonography that displays microbubble enhancement in gray scale with optimal contrast and spatial resolution, facilitated the evaluation of the microcirculation. This prompted the evolution of CEUS from vascular imaging to tissue perfusion imaging (14).

Many authors used CEUS examination in the late liver-specific phase, 2 to 5 minutes after the administration of an air-based first-generation contrast agent such as Levovist. Malignant tumors appear as hypoechoic defects in the brightly enhanced liver parenchyma achieving both an increase in lesion conspicuity, particularly for subcentimeter lesions, and better characterization of lesions as malignant. Improvement in sensitivity for the detection of individual metastases was reported to be from 63–71% to 87–91%. Still, the examination has limited value in the deepest portions of the liver and in patients with an unsatisfactory sonographic window (15–18).

Second-generation microbubble contrast agents such as SonoVue (sulfur hexafluoride) have higher harmonic emission capabilities and prolonged longevity. Their use, coupled with very low acoustic power (mechanical index values 0.1–0.2) that limits microbubble destruction, allows a continuous-mode CEUS examination. Signals from stationary tissues are canceled and only harmonic frequencies generated by microbubbles are visualized. This imaging modality enables the display of both macro- and microcirculation. The enhancement is displayed in real time over the arterial, early/full portal, and delayed phases. Motion or color blooming artifacts characteristic of color and power Doppler sonography are not present. Although SonoVue has no live-specific accumulation, significant enhancement persists in the liver parenchyma 4 to 5 minutes after the injection (1).

In our experience continuous-mode CEUS can significantly improve the accuracy of ultrasound for the detection, characterization, and staging of liver tumors, reaching very high sensitivity for the detection of both hyper- and hypovascular liver malignancies. In particular, in cancer patients increased conspicuity for small hypovascular metastases with detection of satellite and additional previously invisible lesions, leads to a modification in the therapeutic approach with exclusion of treatment in 25% of patients.

Given these capabilities of CEUS, before performing ablative therapies in our institution our diagnostic workup includes laboratory tests and tumor markers along with conventional and contrast-enhanced US. At least one cross-sectional imaging modality (CT and/or MRI) performed no more than 1 week prior to the therapeutic session also is obtained.

Targeting of Lesions and Guidance of RF Ablation Treatment

In consideration of its advantages, including nearly universal availability, portability, ease of use, and low cost, US represents the modality of choice for the guidance of percutaneous interventional procedures. Quick and convenient real-time visualization of electrode positioning is a characteristic feature of sonography, whereas the same procedure may be cumbersome in CT and MR environments.

In our institution pretreatment CEUS examination is repeated as the initial step of the RF ablation session during the induction of anesthesia, to reproduce mapping of lesions as shown on CT/MRI examinations. Images or movie clips are again digitally stored to be compared with immediate postablation study.

Continuous-mode CEUS allows real-time targeting of lesions, which means precise needle insertion performed during the specific phase of maximum lesion conspicuity. In the arterial phase for highly vascularized lesions such as hepatocellular carcinoma (HCC) and hypervascular metastases, and in the portal or equilibrium phases for hypovascular lesions such as colorectal and breast cancer metastases is when needle insertion is optimally performed.

Real-time guidance of needle positioning during CEUS does not significantly prolong the total duration of the RF ablation session. In our opinion, this approach is considered mandatory for the following indications:

1. Small HCCs detected by CT/MR but not visible with unenhanced US against an inhomogeneous cirrhotic liver parenchyma; these lesions may be reached only during the transient arterial phase of CEUS, in which they appear as hyperenhancing foci (19) (Fig. 11.1);
2. Small, usually subcentimeter hypovascular metastases, barely or not perceptible with unenhanced US, but clearly evident as focal hypoenhancing nodules in the portal or late phase of CEUS (Fig. 11.2);
3. Areas of residual untreated or locally recurrent tumor, both primary and metastatic; unenhanced US can almost never differentiate between coagulation necrosis and viable tumor, but the difference is usually straightforward during CEUS in which viable tumor displays its native, characteristic enhancement pattern and coagulation necrosis is avascular (see Fig. 11.4A–C).

Assessment of Treatment Results

Local treatment of neoplastic liver lesions with the application of RF ablation induces the formation of coagulation necrosis. Obtaining adequate necrosis, and therefore effective tumor eradication, may be limited by the inhomogeneity of heat deposition and by the cooling effect of blood flow (20).

During the treatment, a progressively increasing hyperechogenic "cloud" that corresponds to gas microbubble formation and tissue vaporization appears around the distal probe and may persist for some minutes. B-mode sonographic findings observed during and after RF energy application (mostly the diameter of the hyperechoic region) represent only a rough estimate of the extent of induced coagulation necrosis and therefore are not useful to reliably assess treatment completeness (20,21). Similarly, color-flow and power Doppler US are unreliable to evaluate the adequacy of therapy of HCCs treated with RF ablation. Furthermore, additional repositioning of electrodes may be hindered by the hyperechoic focus.

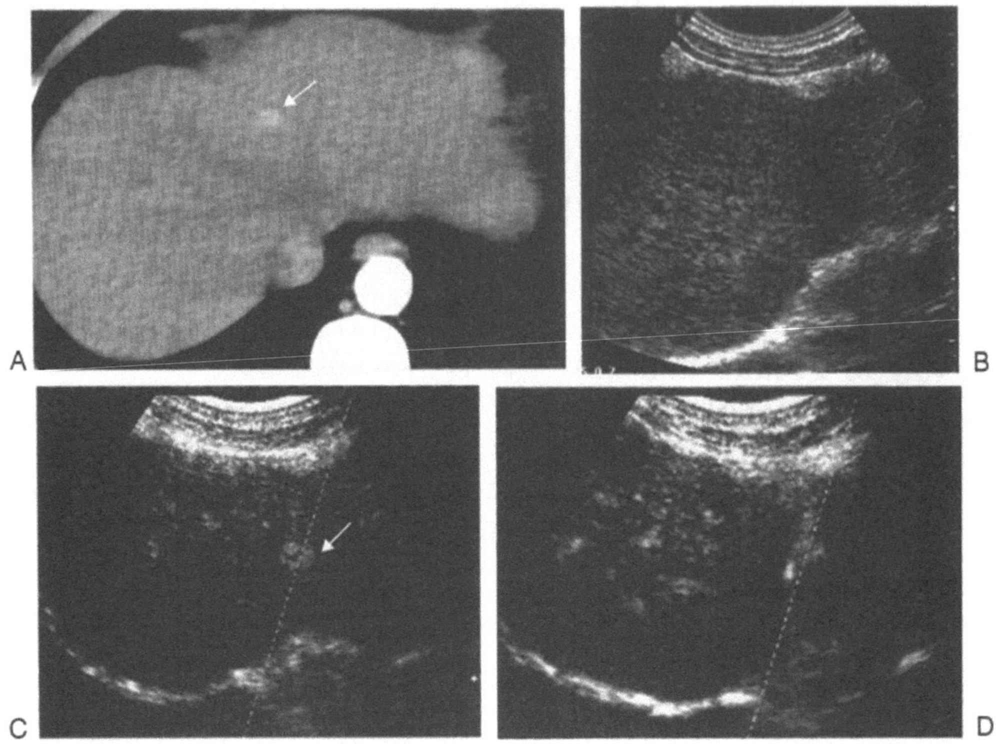

FIGURE 11.1. Tiny (9mm) hepatocellular carcinoma (HCC) detected with contrast-enhanced helical computed tomography (CT) in arterial phase at segment 4 (A), in patient with additional two larger HCCs in the right lobe. During the same ablation session all three HCCs are scheduled for treatment, but B-mode sonography (B) does not detect the smallest HCC. After bolus injection of 2.4mL of SonoVue, the lesion is clearly visible (arrow) (C) and the cool tip needle for RF ablation (Radionics, Burlington, VT) is inserted into the target during the arterial phase of enhanced sonography (D) with clear real-time control of the procedure.

The assessment of the size of the induced coagulation necrosis and therefore of the completeness of the tumor ablation usually is accomplished for both hepatoma and metastatic lesions by means of contrast-enhanced helical CT or MRI. Being practically unfeasible when ablations are performed in the interventional US room, biphasic CT (or less frequently dynamic MRI) is performed on the first day or within 1 week after the RF ablation session and compared with baseline examinations to differentiate between treated regions and residual viable tumor that requires additional treatment (20). Findings with both modalities can predict the extent of coagulation area to within 2 to 3mm, as a radiologic-pathologic correlation demonstrated in experimental and clinical studies (22). Imaging features on immediate posttreatment CT/MR examinations, along with patterns of complete and partial necrosis, are discussed elsewhere in this book.

Most reported series demonstrate a high rate of apparently complete tumor necrosis on initial postablation evaluation. However, local recurrences occur frequently and result from a lack of complete ablation (19,23). Incomplete tumor necrosis determines the need for additional treatment sessions with more patient discomfort and increased costs.

Furthermore, delayed retreatment often is technically difficult owing to the unreliable discrimination of active tumor from coagulation necrosis with unenhanced sonography against an inhomogeneous liver parenchyma

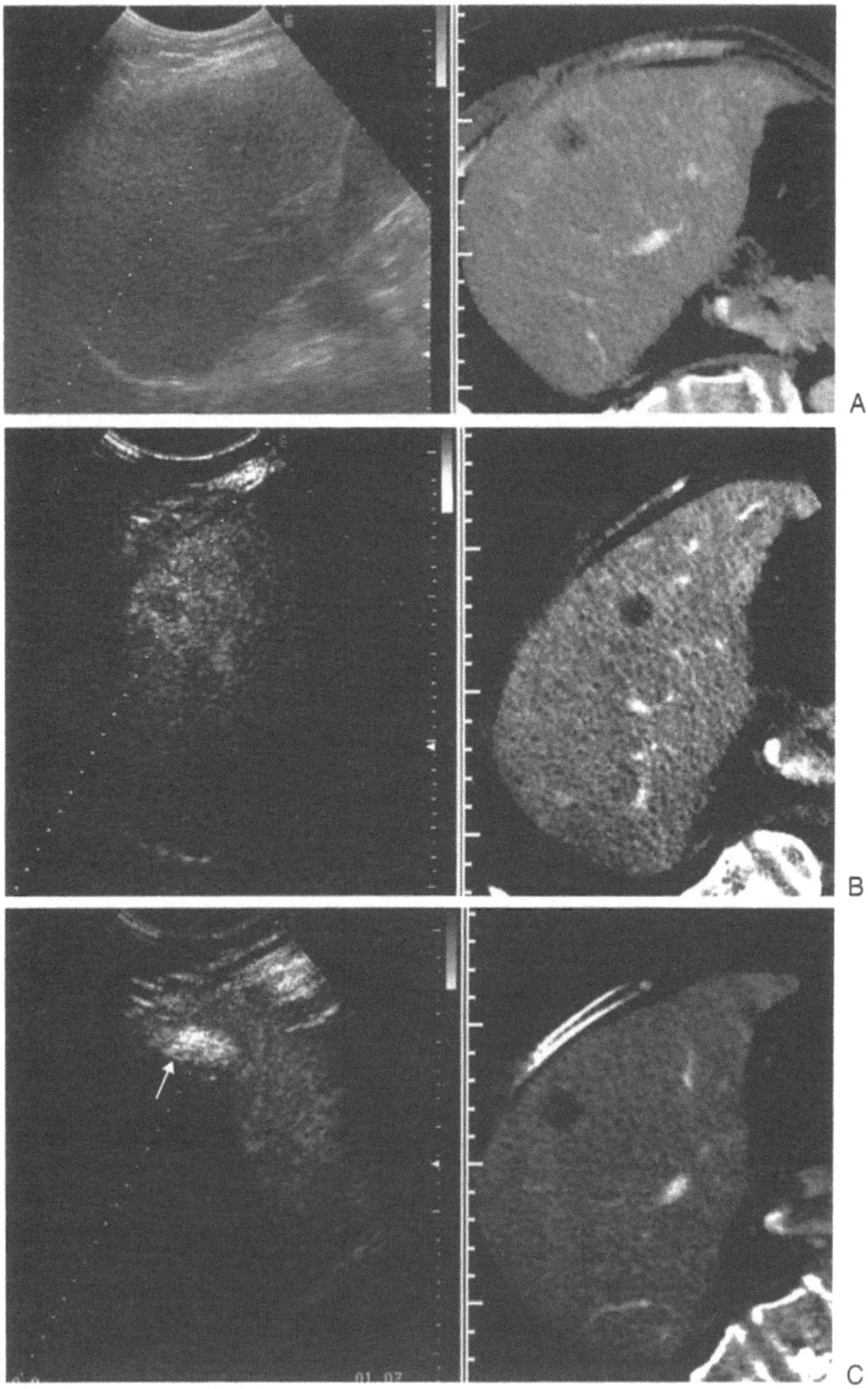

FIGURE 11.2. An 1.8-cm liver metastases from colorectal carcinoma at segment 8. The ablation procedure is performed using a multimodality navigator system, which allows the simultaneous visualization of helical CT (performed earlier) and B-mode sonography. Both real-time ultrasound (US) and CT move simultaneously with excellent spatial correspondence. However, the metastasis is not seen with B-mode sonography (A). (B) After bolus administration of 2.4mL of SonoVue, the lesion is clearly demarcated as a hypovascular area, corresponding to the CT pattern (on the right). This allows targeting the lesion with the cool-tip electrode in real time during the portal enhancement phase (C) (arrow).

because of chronic liver disease, steatosis, and presence of previous treated areas. Effective targeting of residual tumor foci is often impossible and re-treatment has a higher rate of failure (19,24).

Therefore, imaging strategies that enable rapid assessment of the extent of tissue destruction induced by thermal ablation are desirable. Since the ablative treatment leads to the disruption of tumor vascularity, the demonstration of disappearance of any previously visualized vascular enhancement inside and at the periphery of the tumor by means of contrast-enhanced imaging methods is the hallmark of complete treatment of a focal liver tumor (25).

Since the introduction of first-generation ultrasound contrast agents, the use of microbubbles allowed better depiction of microcirculation and parenchymal blood flow compared with conventional color and power Doppler. Initial experiences with enhanced color and power Doppler imaging addressed the evaluation of response of HCC to interventional treatments including RF ablation. Better differentiation between perfused and nonperfused tissue and accurate detection of persistent viable HCC after ablation, compared with conventional color and power Doppler has been reported (26,27). Similarly, our group demonstrated that enhanced color/power Doppler sonography could detect residual tumor immediately after RF ablation of liver metastases, prompting repeat treatment sessions in some cases (28).

More recently, CEUS has been employed to reveal residual enhancement after ablation. CEUS has demonstrated agreement and comparable accuracy to helical CT, the latter adopted as the "gold standard" after different treatment modalities (RF, PEI, TACE) for HCC (29,30). Meloni et al (31) reported an increase in sensitivity from 9.3% with contrast-enhanced power Doppler to 23.3% with pulse inversion CEUS for the detection of residual HCC after RF ablation.

In our protocol, immediate postablation evaluation using continuous-mode CEUS is performed 5 to 10 minutes after the assumed completion of the RF session with the patient still under general anesthesia. We use a second-generation contrast agent (SonoVue; Bracco; Milan, Italy) (Figs. 11.3 and 11.4). Comparison of immediate postablation images with stored preablation scans is essential. As visible on contrast-enhanced CT and MRI, a thin and uniform enhancing rim corresponding to reactive hyperemia may surround the periphery of the necrotic area.

Residual viable tumor, usually located at the periphery of a lesion, maintains the enhancement behavior characteristic of native lesions visualized on pretreatment studies. Partial necrosis of HCC may be diagnosed when a portion of the original lesion still has hypervascular enhancement in the arterial phase (Fig. 11.5). Residual untreated hypovascular metastases sometimes appear indistinguishable from necrosis in the portal and equilibrium phases; with CEUS, evaluation of the early phase is important since viable tumor shows weak but perceptible enhancement (25).

If even questionable residual tumor foci with enhancement or vascular supply are depicted, we perform immediate CEUS-guided targeted re-treatment. The treatment session ends only when complete avascularity is demonstrated. In our experience this approach greatly simplifies patient management and reduces costs by decreasing both the number of RF procedures and follow-up examinations.

In the study period 2000 to 2002 at our institution no residual tumor was detected with CEUS in 176 of 199 liver malignancies treated; of these, CT depicted residual foci in only four cases (specificity 97.7%) all of which were very small (0.8–1.7 cm). In the remaining 23 tumors, single or multiple (1.0–2.2 cm) residual viable tumor portions were visible and immediately submitted to additional RF application in the same session until no further residual enhancement was detectable. In only two cases a 1.2- to 1.9-cm residual tumor was demonstrated by CT. The routine adoption of CEUS (as the only technical improvement) achieved a final result of a decrease of partial necrosis from 16.1% to a 5.1% rate in 429 hepatocellular and metastatic treated lesions.

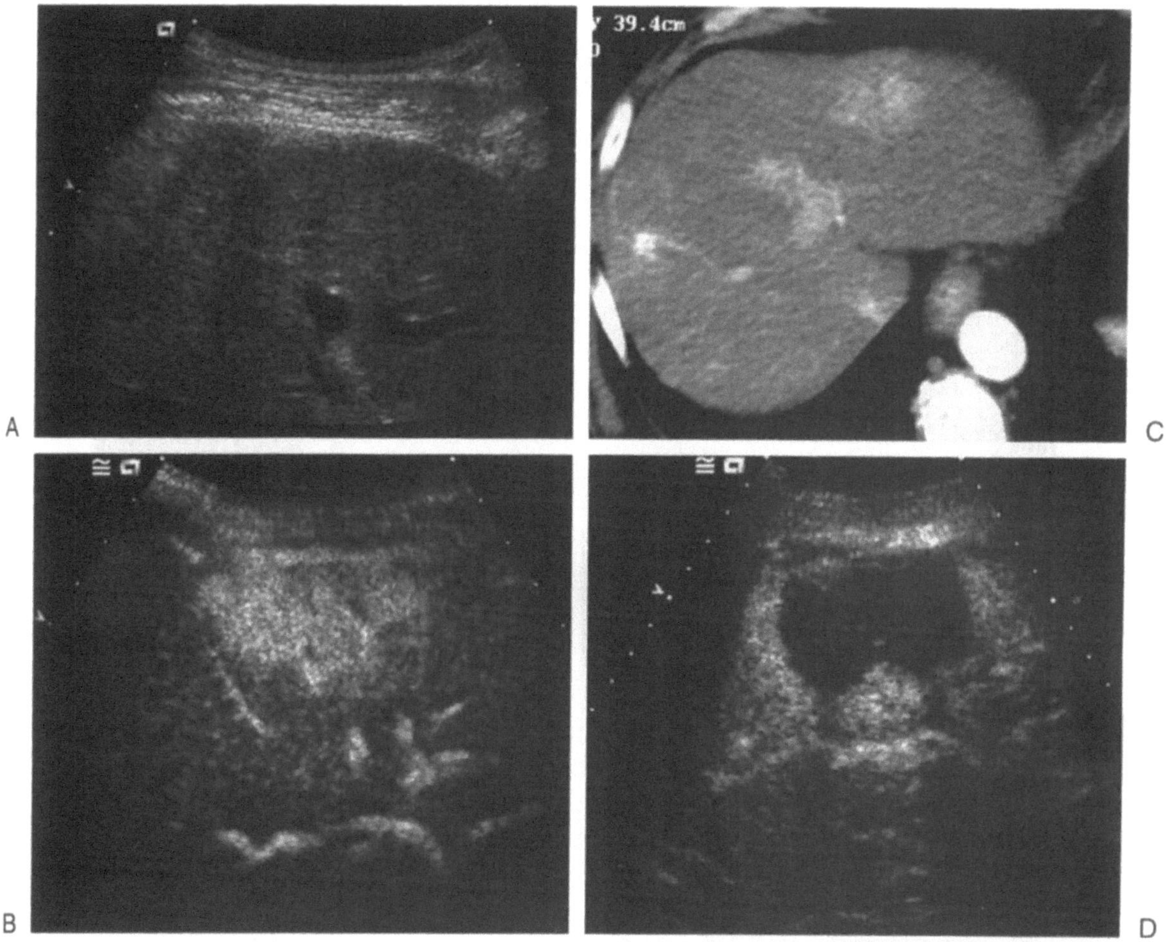

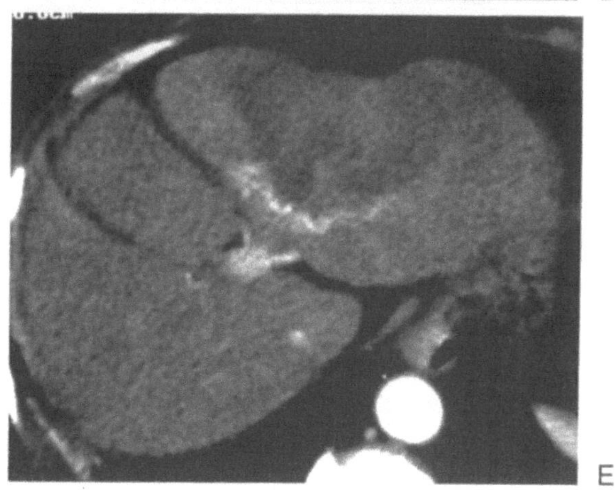

FIGURE 11.3. Hepatocellular carcinoma at segment 4 in a cirrhotic patient. The 3.5-cm lesion is poorly visualized with B-mode sonography (A), but clearly detected with contrast-enhanced ultrasound (CEUS) (B) and contrast-enhanced CT (C) as a hypervascular tumor. Ten minutes after completing ablation, CEUS is repeated and shows a hypovascular area of coagulative necrosis (D) with peripheral extralesional hyperemic halo due to postablative hyperemia. The size of the necrotic area is larger than the original HCC, suggesting complete ablation. (E) Contrast-enhanced CT confirms the result of CEUS (complete ablation).

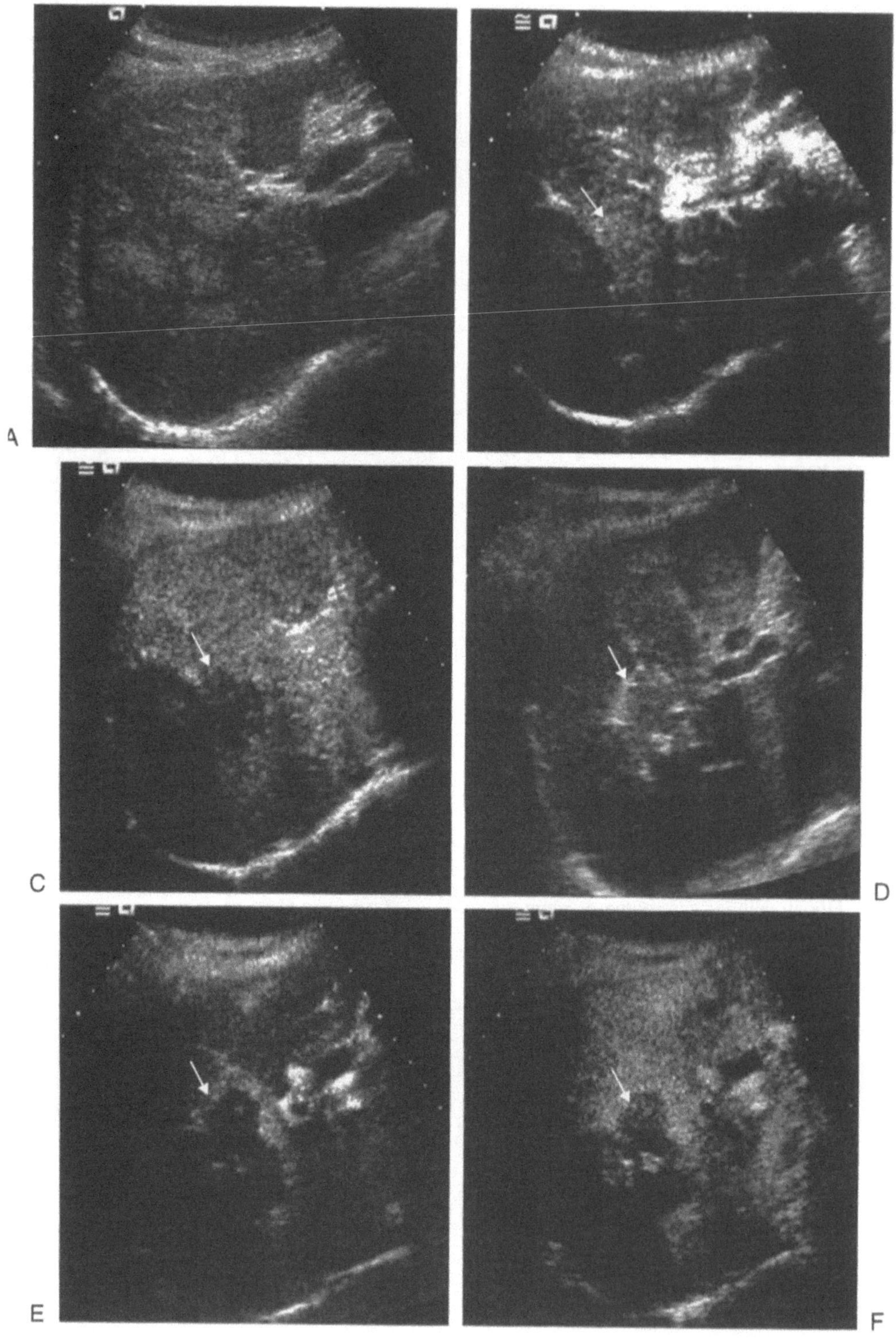

FIGURE 11.4.

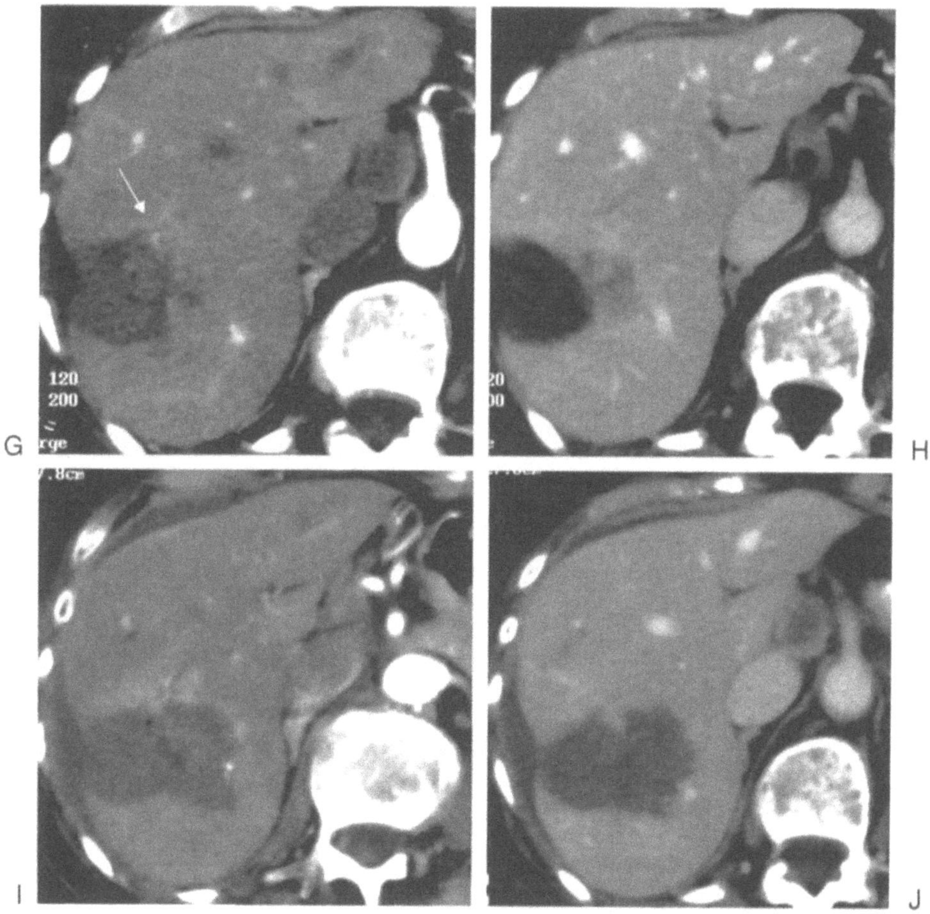

FIGURE 11.4. (*continued*) In a patient treated with percutaneous cool-tip RF ablation 2 years ago for a large colorectal metastases at segment 8, the serum level of carcinoembryonic antigen (CEA) increased. B-mode unenhanced sonography shows a large mass at segment 8, but cannot differentiate the necrotic area from previous ablation from local recurrence (A). After bolus injection of SonoVue, the larger lateral portion of the mass remains avascular in both arterial (B) and portal (C) phase, while the smaller medial portion (arrows) appears hypervascular in arterial phase (B) and hypovascular in portal phase (C) and therefore corresponds to local recurrence. Under real-time guidance with enhanced sonography the recurrence is treated with cool-tip needle RF ablation (arrow) with gas formation in the area of treatment (D). Seven minutes after removing the RF electrode, a second study with SonoVue is performed and the recurrence appears avascular in both arterial (E) and portal (F) phase, suggesting complete treatment. The excellent correlation of enhanced sonography and contrast-enhanced helical CT is clearly appreciable; a previous necrotic area and local recurrence are shown in the arterial and portal phases before ablation (G,H) and at 24 hours following ablation (I,J).

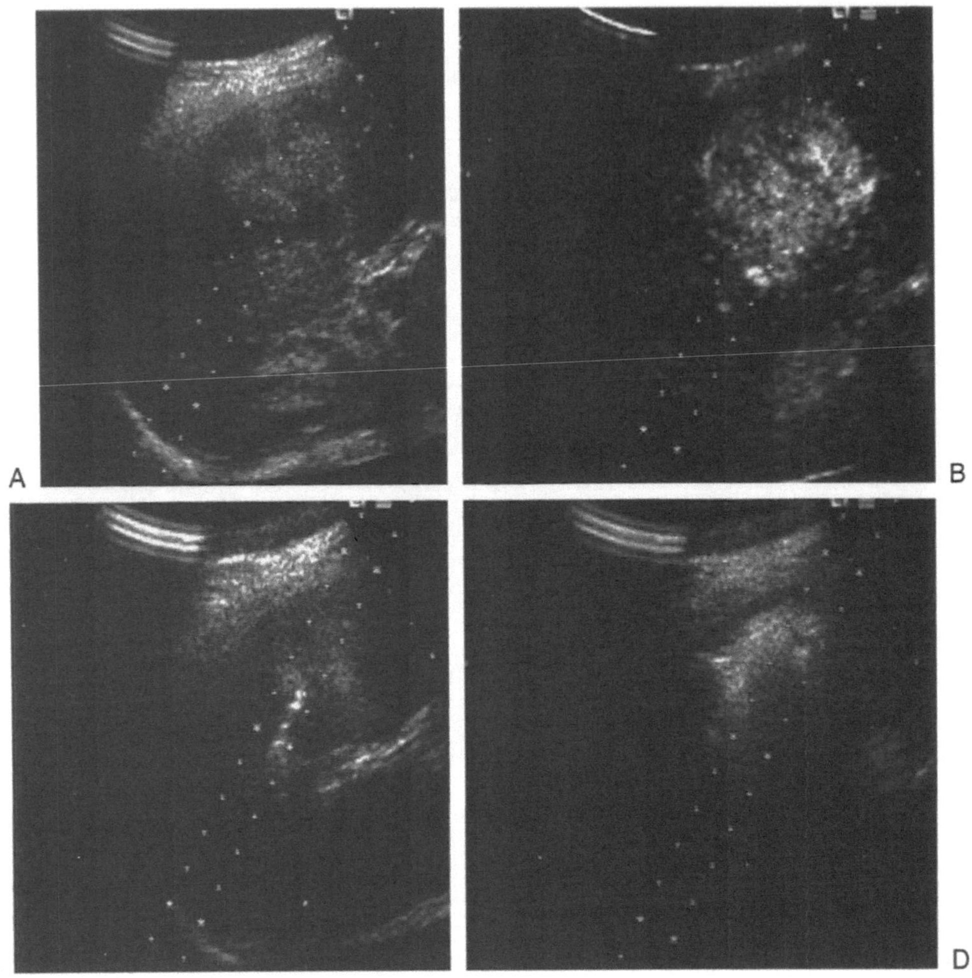

FIGURE 11.5. Contrast-enhanced sonography performed during the ablation session can help to achieve complete treatment and thus avoid the need for local re-treatment. A large (5-cm) HCC is seen in the right lobe before ablation with B-mode sonography (A) and SonoVue-enhanced sonography in arterial phase (B). After precise targeting with RF electrode (arrow) (C), apparently optimal treatment is performed, with formation of a wide diffusion of gas (D). However, SonoVue-enhanced sonography is repeated 6 minutes after withdrawing the electrode and clearly shows that only a small central portion of the mass is actually avascular (E). Therefore, immediate new insertion of an RF electrode is performed under the guidance of enhanced sonography. As a result, complete devascularization of the mass is demonstrated with further administration of microbubbles at the end of ablation (F) and confirmed with contrast-enhanced helical CT in arterial phase at 24 hours (G).

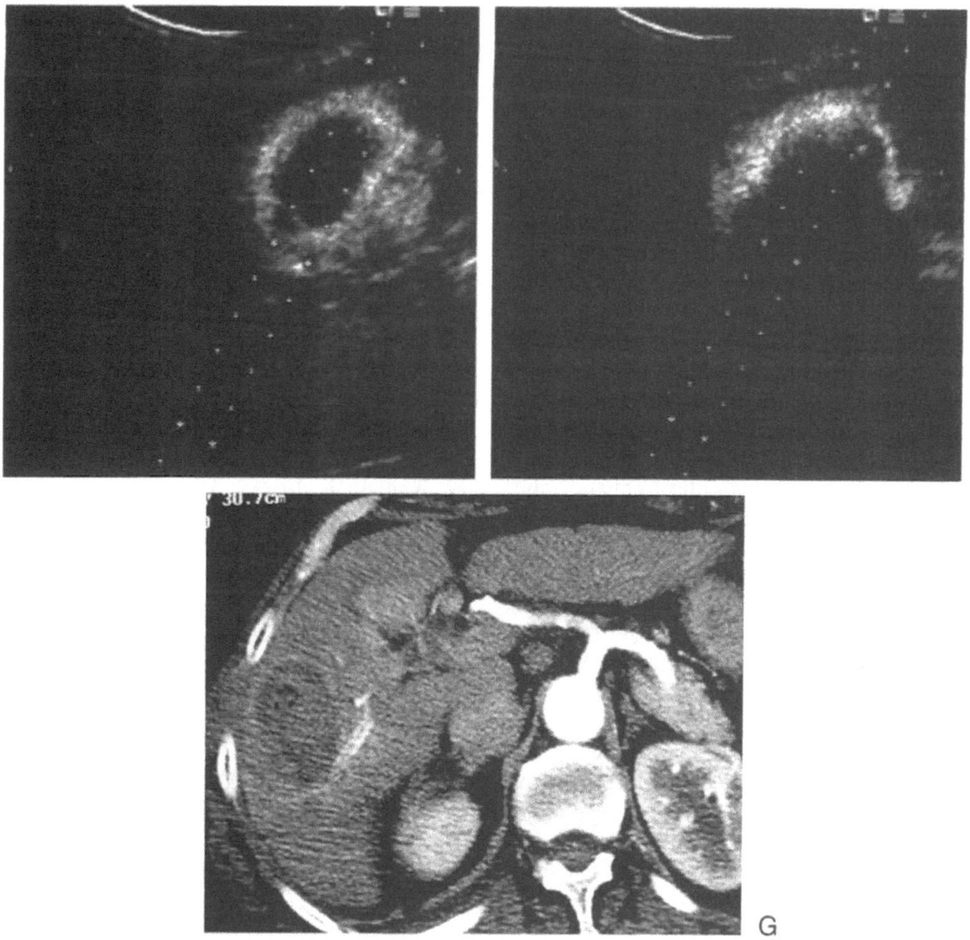

FIGURE 11.5. (*continued*)

Long-Term Follow-Up

Contrast-enhanced helical CT and, in some institutions, dynamic gadolinium-enhanced MRI are the mainstays for imaging follow-up of treated patients and the detection of local, remote intrahepatic and extrahepatic disease relapse (32–35). Recently, the use of functional imaging with fluorine-18-fluoro-2-deoxy-D-glucose (FDG) proved superior to cross-sectional studies (36).

At our institution serum tumor markers are correlated with biphasic helical CT obtained every 3 to 4 months in the long-term follow-up of patients treated for both primary and metastatic liver malignancies. Continuous-mode CEUS has proved to be of value to confirm or exclude possible or suspicious local recurrences and metachronous new lesions detected by cross-sectional imaging and to assess the possibility of their CEUS-guided retreatment.

References

1. Solbiati L, Tonolini M, Cova L, Goldberg SN. The role of contrast-enhanced ultrasound in the detection of focal liver lesions. Eur Radiol 2001; 11(Suppl 3):E15–E26.
2. Livraghi T, Goldberg SN, Lazzaroni S, Meloni F, Solbiati L, Gazelle GS. Small hepatocellular carcinoma: treatment with radiofrequency ablation

versus ethanol injection. Radiology 1999;210: 655–661.
3. Livraghi T, Goldberg SN, Lazzaroni S, et al. Hepatocellular carcinoma: radiofrequency ablation of medium and large lesions. Radiology 2000;214:761–768.
4. Buscarini L, Buscarini E, Di Stasi M, Vallisa D, Quaretti P, Rocca A. Percutaneous radiofrequency ablation of small hepatocellular carcinoma: long-term results. Eur Radiol 2001;11: 914–992.
5. Solbiati L, Ierace T, Goldberg SN, et al. Percutaneous US-guided radiofrequency tissue ablation of liver metastases: treatment and follow-up in 16 patients. Radiology 1997;202:195–203.
6. Solbiati L, Goldberg SN, Ierace T, et al. Hepatic metastases: percutaneous radio-frequency ablation with cooled-tip electrodes. Radiology 1997; 205:367–373.
7. Solbiati L, Livraghi T, Goldberg SN, et al. Percutaneous radiofrequency ablation of hepatic metastases from colorectal cancer: long-term results in 117 patients. Radiology 2001;221: 159–166.
8. Livraghi T, Goldberg SN, Solbiati L, Meloni F, Ierace T, Gazelle GS. Percutaneous radiofrequency ablation of liver metastases from breast cancer: initial experience in 24 patients. Radiology 2001;220:145–149.
9. De Baere T, Elias D, Dromain C, et al. Radiofrequency ablation of 100 hepatic metastases with a mean follow-up of more than 1 year. AJR 2000; 175:1619.
10. Solbiati L, Ierace T, Tonolini M, et al. Radiofrequency thermal ablation of hepatic metastases. Eur J Ultrasound 2001;13:149–158.
11. Sica GT, Ji H, Ros PR. CT and MR imaging of hepatic metastases. AJR 2000;174:691–698.
12. Valls C, Andia E, Sanchez A, et al. Hepatic metastases from colorectal cancer: preoperative detection and assessment of resectability with helical CT. Radiology 2001;218:55–60.
13. Harvey CJ, Albrecht T. Ultrasound of focal liver lesions. Eur Radiol 2001;11:1578–1593.
14. Lencioni R, Cioni D, Bartolozzi C. Tissue harmonic and contrast-specific imaging: back to gray scale in ultrasound. Eur Radiol 2002;12: 151–165.
15. Harvey CJ, Blomley MJK, Eckersley RJ, et al. Hepatic malignancies: improved detection with pulse-inversion US in the late phase of enhancement with SHU 508A—early experience. Radiology 2000;216:903–908.
16. Albrecht T, Hoffmann CW, Schmitz SA, et al. Phase-inversion sonography during the liver specific late phase of contrast enhancement: improved detection of liver metastases. AJR 2001;176:1191–1198.
17. Quaia E, Bertolotto M, Forgacs B, et al. Detection of liver metastases by pulse inversion harmonic imaging during Levovist late phase: comparison with conventional ultrasound and helical CT in 160 patients. Eur Radiol 2003;13: 475–483.
18. Albrecht T, Blomley MJK, Burns PN, et al. Improved detection of hepatic metastases with pulse-inversion US during the liver-specific phase of SHU 508A: multicenter study. Radiology 2003;227:361–370.
19. Numata K, Isozaki T, Ozawa Y, et al. Percutaneous ablation therapy guided by contrast-enhanced sonography for patients with hepatocellular carcinoma. AJR 2003;180:143–149.
20. Goldberg SN, Gazelle GS, Mueller PR. Thermal ablation therapy for focal malignancy. A unified approach to underlying principles, techniques, and diagnostic imaging guidance. AJR 2000;174: 323–331.
21. Leyendecker JR, Dodd GD, Halff GA, et al. Sonographically observed echogenic response during intraoperative radiofrequency ablation of cirrhotic livers: pathologic correlation. AJR 2002;178:1147–1151.
22. Goldberg SN, Gazelle GS, Compton CC, Mueller PR, Tanabe KK. Treatment of intrahepatic malignancy with radiofrequency ablation: radiologic-pathologic correlation. Cancer 2000;88: 2452–2463.
23. Chopra S, Dodd GD III, Chintapalli KN, Leyendecker JR, Karahan OI, Rhim H. Tumor recurrence after radiofrequency thermal ablation of hepatic tumors: spectrum of findings on dual-phase contrast-enhanced CT. AJR 2001; 177:381–387.
24. De Baere T, Elias D, Dromain C, et al. Radiofrequency ablation of 100 hepatic metastases with a mean follow-up of more than 1 year. AJR 2000;175(6):1619–1625.
25. Rhim H, Goldberg SN, Dodd GD III, et al. Essential techniques for successful radiofrequency thermal ablation of malignant hepatic tumors. Radiographics 2001;21:S17–S31.
26. Choi D, Lim HK, Kim SH, et al. Hepatocellular carcinoma treated with percutaneous radiofrequency ablation: usefulness of power Doppler

US with a microbubble contrast agent in evaluation therapeutic response-preliminary study. Radiology 2000;217:558–563.
27. Cioni D, Lencioni R, Rossi S, et al. Radiofrequency thermal ablation of hepatocellular carcinoma: using contrast-enhanced harmonic power Doppler sonography to assess treatment outcome. AJR 2001;177:783–788.
28. Solbiati L, Goldberg SN, Ierace T, Della Noce M, Livraghi T, Gazelle GS. Radio-frequency ablation of hepatic metastases: postprocedural assessment with a US microbubble contrast agent—early experience. Radiology 1999;211: 643–649.
29. Ding H, Kudo M, Onda H, et al. Evaluation of posttreatment response of hepatocellular carcinoma with contrast-enhanced coded phase-inversion harmonic US. Comparison with dynamic CT. Radiology 2001;221(3):712–730.
30. Numata K, Tanaka K, Kiba T, et al. Using contrast-enhanced sonography to assess the effectiveness of transcatheter arterial embolization for hepatocellular carcinoma. AJR 2001;176: 1199–1205.
31. Meloni MF, Goldberg SN, Livraghi T, et al. Hepatocellular carcinoma treated with radiofrequency ablation. Comparision of pulse inversion contrast-enhanced harmonic sonography, contrast-enhanced power Doppler sonography and helical CT. AJR 2001;177:375–380.
32. Choi H, Loyer EM, DuBrow RA, et al. Radiofrequency ablation of liver tumors: assessment of therapeutic response and complications. Radiographics 2001;21:S41–S54.
33. Catalano O, Lobianco R, Esposito M, et al. Hepatocellular carcinoma recurrence after percutaneous ablation therapy: helical CT patterns. Abdom Imaging 2001;26:375–383.
34. Dromain C, De Baere T, Elias D, et al. Hepatic tumors treated with percutaneous radiofrequency ablation: CT and MR imaging follow-up. Radiology 2002;223:255–262.
35. Sironi S, Livraghi T, Meloni F, et al. Small hepatocellular carcinoma treated with percutaneous RF ablation: MR imaging follow-up. AJR 1999; 173:1225–1229.
36. Anderson GS, Brinkmann F, Soulen MC, et al. FDG position emission tomography in the surveillance of hepatic tumors treated with radiofrequency ablation. Clin Nucl Med 2003;28: 192–197.

12 Magnetic Resonance Imaging Guidance for Tumor Ablation

Koenraad J. Mortele, Stuart G. Silverman, Vito Cantisani, Kemal Tuncali, Sridhar Shankar, and Eric vanSonnenberg

Since the late 1980s, magnetic resonance imaging (MRI) has been added to ultrasound (US) and computed tomography (CT) as a cross-sectional imaging tool that can be used to guide the interventional diagnosis and treatment of a variety of disorders. Due to its superior soft tissue contrast, multiplanar capabilities, lack of ionizing radiation, and, most importantly, ability to image tissue function and temperatures, MRI has been suggested as the ideal tool to guide minimally invasive therapies (1,2). Nevertheless, when the concept of percutaneous MRI-guided tumor ablation was first introduced, restricted patient access and limited spatial and temporal resolution with conventional high- and mid-field MRI systems limited its widespread use. Technical advances in both open-configuration magnet design and the development of fast gradient-echo pulse sequences have contributed substantially to an increasing interest in MRI-guided interventions (1,2). As a consequence, percutaneous tumor ablations now can be performed under real-time MRI guidance.

This chapter discusses the rationale for using MRI to plan, guide, monitor, and control percutaneous tumor ablations; reviews the history and development of open-configuration MRI systems and how they can be used to guide percutaneous interventions; highlights the unique principles and issues of designing and implementing an interventional MRI suite; and discusses the current status of MRI-guided tumor ablation trials that use a variety of ablative agents in several organ systems, including the abdomen, pelvis, breast, and musculoskeletal system.

Interventional Guidance: Modality Comparison

Role of Imaging in Image-Guided Therapy

All image-guided percutaneous tumor ablations require five processes: (a) planning, (b) targeting, (c) monitoring, (d) controlling, and (e) assessing. Planning is done before the procedure and determines whether the intervention is appropriate, and how the lesion can be best approached. This also includes a decision regarding which image guidance modality best accomplishes the requirements for this task. The first step in the procedure is targeting the lesion, typically with a biopsy needle or therapy probe. For this, accurate depiction of the tumor and surrounding anatomy is critical. All of the instruments used to perform the procedure should be visible so that adjustments can be made as the lesion is targeted. Real-time, interactive, and multiplanar imaging are helpful in targeting. For example, real-time imaging allows the operator to obtain instantaneous feedback of image information that can be used to make adjustments. A procedure that is interactive allows the operator to make adjustments in the course or trajectory of the needle and immediately assess the effects of those adjustments. Visualizing the tumor and instrument in multiple planes gives the operator a three-dimensional (3D) understanding of the target. Being able to monitor the ablation and the tissue changes are other critical components of image-guided ablation. Monitoring should depict the location and extent of ablative effects and allow the operator to differentiate treated from untreated tumor, and affected from unaffected normal tissue. Similarly, the ability to control the changes induced by the procedure or the ability to change the amount and location of the ablation intraprocedurally is important. Monitoring and controlling are essential components of image guidance because it is not always possible to predict accurately the size and shape of an ablative lesion. Only with imaging can an ablation protocol be optimized to cover a tumor maximally, while minimizing effects in normal tissues. Finally, following the procedure, imaging is used to assess the extent of ablative changes, the completeness of the ablation, and complications.

Image-Guided Ablations: Magnetic Resonance Imaging Advantages

Given these five critical components of image-guided ablations, each guidance modality has inherent benefits and disadvantages. Planning requires visualization of the lesion and the surrounding anatomy, and a survey of the rest of the target organ for additional lesions. In clinical practice, MRI is often not needed because US and CT demonstrate most lesions. However, MRI is a sensitive technique for imaging and can be helpful in surveying for other sites of disease. Ultrasound and CT are commonly used for targeting also, but MRI-guidance may be indicated in patients with lesions that either are not visualized by US and CT (e.g., breast and prostate cancers), or are visible by CT and MRI but not with US and require angling the needle, such as a liver lesion beneath the hepatic dome or an adrenal gland mass (Fig. 12.1). In such cases, using CT guidance, if the pleural space and lung are avoided, lesions in the upper abdomen can be reached by either angling the gantry or angling the needle using the triangulation method. The triangulation method is limited in that it does not allow direct visualization of the entire needle tract in one image (3). Although US can be used to image in multiple planes, the path of the needle tract may be obscured by bony structures such as the ribs or air from interposed bowel loops (3).

Magnetic resonance imaging–guided interventions depend on the ability of the interventional radiologist to position a needle probe under MRI guidance into a relatively small target within the body. Therefore, research and development of MRI-guided biopsy techniques have been an important and fundamental aspect of the beginning of interventional MR. Mueller et al (4) first described the use of an MR-compatible needle and showed that after US-guided placement, both the liver lesion and the needle could be viewed using a conventional MRI system. Silverman et al (5) reported the first MRI-guided biopsy wherein the entire procedure was performed under MRI guidance. This technique employed a 0.5-T vertically open configuration MRI system specifically designed to guide radiologic intervention and surgery (Signa SP; GE Medical Systems; Milwaukee, WI). In addition to being open, the system contained two important features: (a) images were displayed to the operator inside the room on two MR-compatible monitors mounted above the field, that allowed ongoing review of images during procedures; (b) the system contained an integrated optical localizer and tracker, which allowed interactive control of the biopsy needle. Subsequently, Frahm et al (6) and Lu et al (7) each reported MRI-guided biopsy using a 0.2-T horizontally open configuration MRI system in which free-hand techniques using fast gradient-echo sequences were utilized. Fast gradient-echo sequences were used successfully to guide liver biopsies in closed magnet systems (8,9).

Similarly, although transrectal ultrasound (TRUS) is useful in the vast majority of prostate gland biopsies, MRI may be used in patients: in whom the serum prostate specific antigen (PSA) is elevated and rising despite a negative TRUS biopsy, in whom the lesion is visible only with MRI imaging, or in whom the rectum is absent (e.g., post–abdominoperineal resection) and thus TRUS-guided biopsy is not

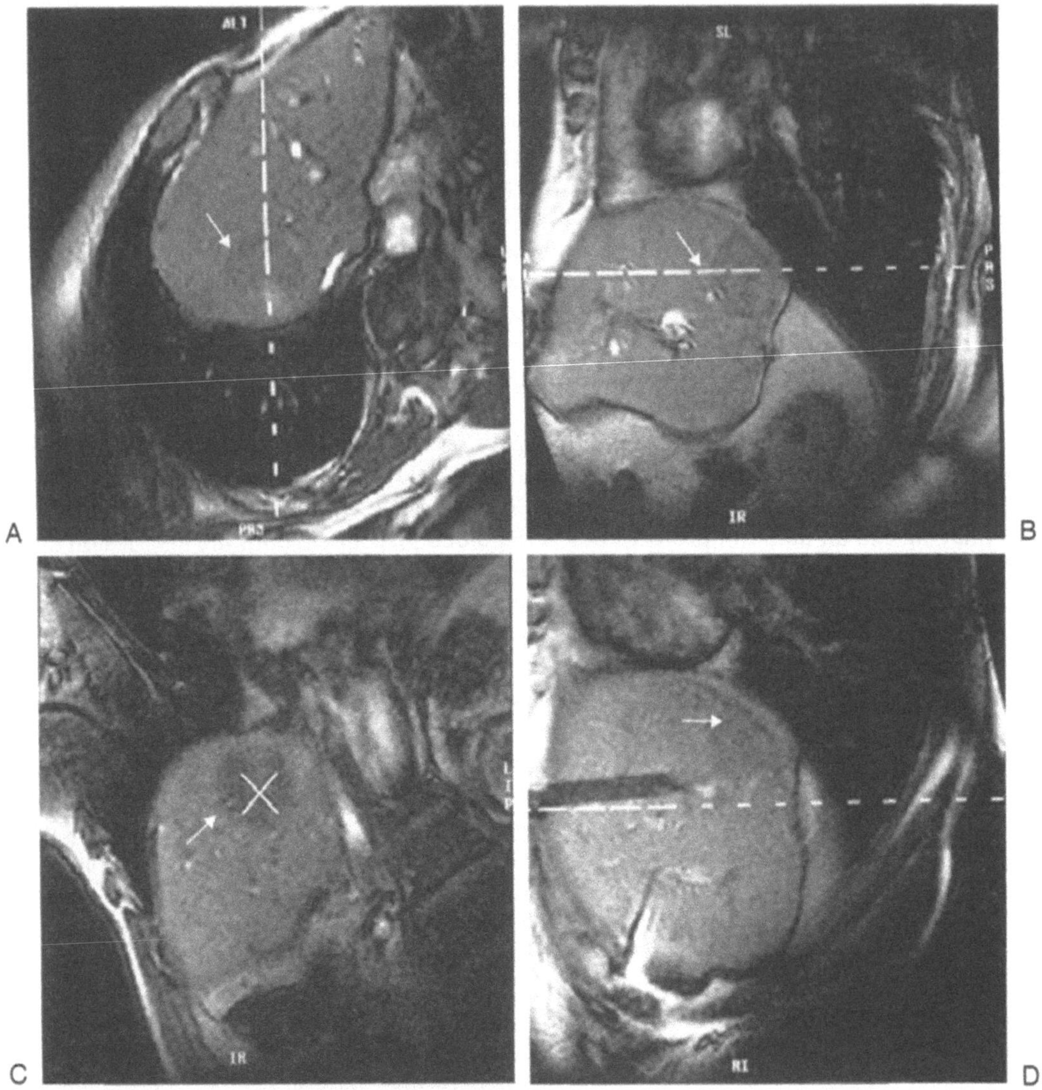

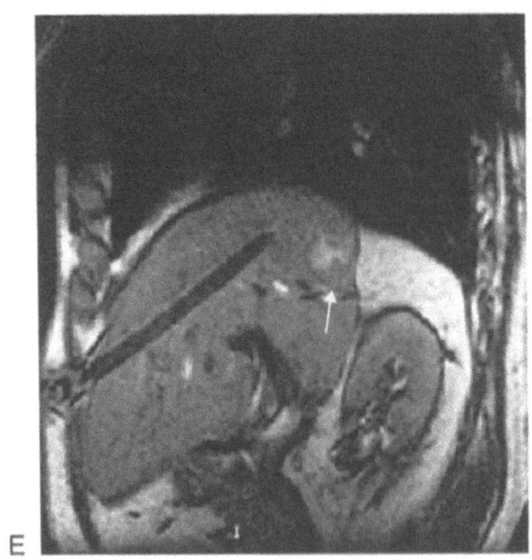

FIGURE 12.1. Magnetic resonance imaging (MRI)-guided percutaneous biopsy of hepatic metastasis of gastrointestinal stromal tumor (GIST). (A–C) Axial, sagittal, and coronal gradient-echo T1-weighted images obtained with the open MR scanner during the procedure planning show the expected trajectory of the needle using the optical tracking system. The lesion (arrow) is located in segment 8 beneath the diaphragm. (D,E) Oblique sagittal and coronal gradient-echo T1-weighted images show the presence of a fine biopsy needle (22-gauge) at the edge of the mass.

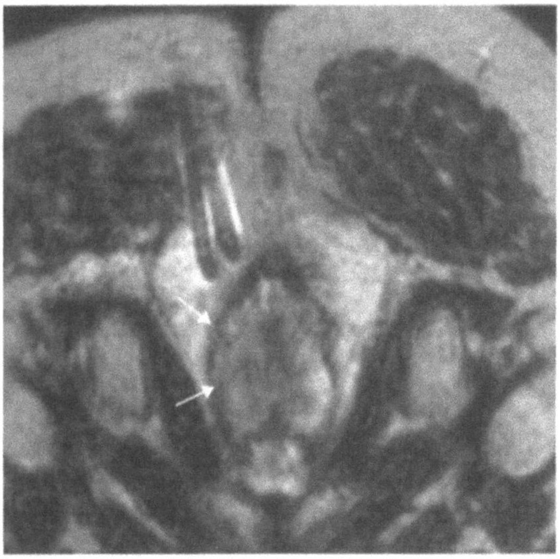

FIGURE 12.2. MRI-guided percutaneous transgluteal biopsy of adenocarcinoma in the prostate gland in a patient post–abdominoperineal resection for rectal cancer. Axial TSE T2-weighted image obtained with the open MR scanner during the procedure shows two biopsy needles targeting the low signal intensity areas (arrows) in the apex of the prostate.

possible. The first group is quite numerous and includes anxious men who are facing rising PSA levels with no diagnosis. Magnetic resonance imaging–guided prostate gland biopsy may be done either in a closed bore system using a transgluteal approach, or in an open system using a transrectal or transperineal approach (Fig. 12.2) (10).

Because studies have shown that MRI is both sensitive and specific for the detection of breast cancer, MRI has been used to biopsy the breast (11,12); MRI is needed because many lesions are not seen at x-ray mammography. Targeting is achieved either using template guidance at high-field closed systems (13) or freehand, with open systems (14). Although interventions are feasible with closed MRI systems, they can be cumbersome as the patient needs to be moved out of the magnet bore to manipulate the instruments, and, therefore, the procedure is only intermittently imaged. As a consequence, since most structures move with respiration, targeting may be difficult. Generally, open systems offer improved patient access during the procedure compared with closed systems.

There are many ways in which an interventional device can be tracked during a procedure using MR guidance. Most procedures reported to date are performed using passive tracking in which imaging is used to follow the needle. In passive tracking, the needle or probe is visualized by the signal void created by the needle's magnetic susceptibility artifact. The needle can be seen as long as the imaging plane includes it. The frequency with which the needle is seen is determined by how fast the images are acquired, reconstructed, and shown to the operator during the procedure (15,16). Some open interventional MR systems, by using an optical tracking system, automatically image the device (e.g., a needle) because it is attached to a probe whose position is sensed by the optical tracker. As the probe is moved, its position is sensed, and the scan plane is changed. Other methods of localization include active tip tracking, mechanical sensors, and radiofrequency (RF) localizers (17–20). Active tip-tracking is achieved by embedding a miniature RF coil in the tip of a needle or therapy probe. This allows active intraprocedural identification of the spatial position of the tip. The most important advantages of active tracking over passive tracking are its high temporal resolution and the option to use the three-dimensional coordinates to steer the scan plane (17–20).

Although MRI can be used to plan an ablation and target a tumor, its ability to monitor (and thus control) ablations is its greatest advantage (21). Through MR monitoring, thermal lesion size and configuration can be directly controlled by the interventionalist and adjusted during the procedure. There has been intense interest in developing noninvasive methods of monitoring temperature distributions in vivo, since the biologic efficacy of thermal-ablation techniques is strongly dependent on achieving desired temperatures in all parts of the tumor. Temperature-sensitive MR sequences have been developed to enable accurate online monitoring of heat deposition (22–24). Three-dimensional mapping of temperature changes with MRI are based on relaxation time T1, diffusion coefficient (D), or proton resonance frequency (PRF) of tissue water. Temperature-sensitive contrast agents also may be used (25,26). Among these methods of MRI-based temperature mapping, the PRF-based method is the preferred choice for many applications at mid- and high field (≥1 T), because of its sensitivity and linear relation with temperature, and near-independence with respect to tissue type. The PRF methods utilize RF-spoiled gradient-echo imaging methods to measure the phase change in resonance that results from the temperature-dependent change in resonance frequency. When field homogeneity is poor due to small ferromagnetic parts in the needle, or at low field strengths (≤0.5 T), diffusion and T1-based methods may provide better results. Temperature-sensitive contrast agents may be particularly suitable when absolute thermoregulation is desired, for example, when an indication exists for exceeding a certain temperature threshold (26).

History and Development of Interventional MRI

Interventional MRI Systems

Open Systems

In the mid- to late 1980s, open-configuration MRI systems were developed primarily for the purpose of combating claustrophobia and aiding the MRI of pediatric patients. Forward-thinking interventional radiologists, however, used these open MRI systems to gain access to patients to perform a variety of interventions (27–29). As a consequence, interventional MRI systems were developed that provided guidance systems integrated with open configuration MRI systems that allowed intervention and surgery to occur simultaneously with imaging (28,29). Open-configuration MRI scanners are now produced by most major MRI manufacturers. In general, access to the patient may be achieved via a horizontally open system (of which there are many—Magnetom Open System; Siemens Medical Solutions; Erlangen, Germany, is one) or a vertically open system (e.g., Signa SP; General Electric Medical Systems; Milwaukee, WI). Most of these systems are either low or midfield in magnet strength. The gradient performance of these systems is good and ranges typically between 10 and 15 mT/m, providing sufficient image quality for guiding tumor ablations (30–32).

Closed Systems

Interventional MRI-guided procedures also may be performed using conventional MR systems (22). Closed systems, operating at higher field strengths, provide better image quality by means of a higher signal-to-noise ratio. However, patient access is limited and instrument manipulations are performed when the patient is outside the magnet, or when using a system with a flared opening, with the operator leaning in. Some lesions, however, may be visualized only using a conventional closed MRI system and not with an open MRI system of lower field strength. MRI-guided procedures in both closed and open systems may not be possible in large patients because the space within the magnet bore typically is restricted.

Interventional MRI Suites

An MR-compatible environment is needed to support an interventional MR scanner (2). Important principles of installing an interventional MR scanner relate to issues of siting, patient care, and MR-compatible instrumentation (1). Siting an interventional MR scanner must take into account essential issues related to MRI scanners: magnetic shielding, RF shielding, floor loading, vibration, acoustic dampening, and cryogen venting and storage. Factors related to siting the scanner in an interventional suite or operating room also need to be considered: control of air quality/flow, humidity, temperature, zoned lighting, the inclusion of scrub sinks, restricted and semirestricted areas, and ports for suction, gases, and therapy devices.

Issues related to patient care include the ability of all operators to have access to the patient for the purpose of performing the procedure, observing and monitoring the patient, and administering drugs and/or anesthesia. Emergency therapy must be able to be performed. Emergency treatment can be performed inside the procedure room with MR-compatible devices, such as airways and intravenous tubing. Cardiac defibrillators are not MR-compatible. Therefore, to treat ventricular fibrillation, either the magnet needs to be quenched or the patient brought out of the room.

Another important point is that silent myocardial ischemia cannot be detected in an MR environment (33,34). Therefore, before undergoing interventional MRI procedures, all patients need to be screened for coronary artery disease and a risk/benefit assessment made as to whether the procedure should be performed using MRI guidance. Magnetic resonance imaging–guided procedures should be performed only in patients for whom the benefit of performing the procedure is greater than the risk of not detecting silent myocardial ischemia. Just as patients need to be screened before undergoing an MRI examination, physicians also need to be screened in the same fashion. The interventional MR room needs to be surrounded by a checkpoint at the 5-gauss line, which is typically, depending on the field system and parameters of the system, 1 m outside the procedure room.

MRI Compatible Instruments

All instruments used in the interventional MR procedure room must be MR-compatible. A device is MR compatible if it can be used in the scanner room during the procedure safely and without adversely affecting the device itself or the procedure for which it is being used (1,2). Magnetic resonance compatibility includes issues related to ferromagnetism, electric interference, image distortion, and device heating from RF energy (Table 12.1). Interventional and surgical instruments may cause artifacts, which lead to image distortion. The size of the artifacts depends mainly on the following factors: the size of the instrument, the orientation of the instrument to the main magnetic field, the imaging sequence used, and the orientation of the frequency-encoding gradient (35). The amount of artifact in an MR image increases with instrument size and increasing angle of the instrument to the main magnetic field B_O (1).

Once a major obstacle, MR-compatible instrumentation now is developed such that a

TABLE 12.1. Overview of magnetic resonance (MR) compatibility.

Factor	Effect	Example	Solution
Ferromagnetic attraction	Object moves/rotates to align with magnet; may endanger occupants	Most conventional surgical instruments	Change instrument materials
Electrical interference			
Device on MR scanner	Low signal-to-noise ratio, stripes, zippers, bright spots	Almost anything with electrical plug, ferromagnetic, and an interference hazard	Provide RF shielding device; remove the electronics to remote location
MR scanner on device	Magnetic field/RF interferes with device often with subtle effects	Computer discs, video displays	Provide remote electronics; use liquid crystal displays
Image distortion by devices	Image artifacts, spatial distortions	Signal void around needle	Move devices out of image field of view; match materials to tissue susceptibility; break up eddy current paths
Device heating from RF energy (in or out of patient)	Patient burns from RF inductive heating of device and from contact with patient	Pulse oximeter wire, ECG wire	Use nonconductive materials (e.g., fiberoptics); keep antennae length to a minimum; inspect for patient/device grounding paths

ECG, electrocardiogram; RF, radiofrequency.

variety of procedures can be performed (1). An array of basic interventional and surgical instruments including needles, scissors, elevators, forceps, and blades have been manufactured for use during both interventions and surgery (36). MR-compatible monitors and anesthesia delivery systems are used to monitor patients safely. Therapy delivery systems such as electrocautery, laser, RF, and cryotherapy, discussed in further detail below, also are available for use during MRI-guided interventions.

Percutaneous MRI-Guided Tumor Ablation

Concomitant with the development of open-configuration MR systems and interventional MRI, there has been worldwide interest in the use of imaging to guide percutaneous ablation of liver tumors using both vascular and direct percutaneous approaches (37). Successes in the focal therapy of both hepatocellular carcinoma (HCC) and metastatic colorectal cancer to the liver have been the major driving force in developing image-guided percutaneous tumor ablation. It has led to the research of percutaneous tumor ablation in organs elsewhere in the body, including the kidney, bone, soft tissue, breast, and lung. The rationale for percutaneous tumor ablation research is to develop a less invasive, repeatable, and effective method that will allow more patients, including nonsurgical candidates, to be treated (38).

Many ablative agents have been investigated. In general, these agents result in tumor cell death using either thermal-based energy (e.g., heat or cold) or chemical agents such as ethanol. Thermal agents include lasers, RF, and microwaves, all of which heat tissue, and cryotherapy, which freezes tissue (39–42).

Cryotherapy

Cryotherapy is defined as therapeutic tissue destruction in situ by freezing. Once administered predominantly through "open" surgical means, it was known mostly by the term *cryosurgery* (43–48). Now, cryotherapy can be performed percutaneously, without the use of surgical techniques and therefore the term *cryotherapy* is more appropriate. *Cryoablation* and *cryodestruction* refer to processes that occur during cryotherapy.

Cryotherapy is one of the oldest methods of tissue destruction known to mankind. It was used even during the times of Hippocrates to control hemorrhage. In the 20th century and currently, cryotherapy has been used for a variety of cancer treatments in the brain, head and neck, breast, and more recently, in the liver and prostate gland. Cryotherapy destroys tissue mainly by cellular dehydration, cell membrane rupture, and vascular stasis. Cell death occurs typically at –30° to –40°C, and is dependent on several factors including tissue type, freezing and thawing rate, duration, and depth of freezing (49,50). Cryotherapy is a time-tested, effective ablation technique. It is not dose-limited, blood loss is minimal, and, perhaps more importantly, it is amenable to imaging. Tissue effects can be seen with US, CT, and MRI. Furthermore, lesions produced by cryotherapy are sharply marginated and depict the zone of tissue necrosis accurately (49,50).

The liver and prostate gland have been the most common sites in which cryotherapy has been used (Fig. 12.3). In the liver, it has been used in patients with HCC or metastases who are unable to undergo hepatic resection (39,43). In the operating room, US is used for lesion detection, for guidance of cryosurgical probe placement, and monitoring of the freezing process (44). Ultrasound depicts the effects of freezing in real time and accurately demonstrates the zone of necrosis that is subsequently produced (45). However, US is limited by its inability to image beyond the proximal edge of the iceball because the energy is reflected at this front edge. As a result, the tumor may not be completely visualized during the treatment, and thus it may be incompletely treated. The relatively small surgical incisions used during minimally invasive liver surgery also may limit the ability of US to image lesions completely (46). Although liver cryosurgery with intraoperative ultrasound guidance has been used in many centers for more than a decade, the overall survival in patients with metastatic

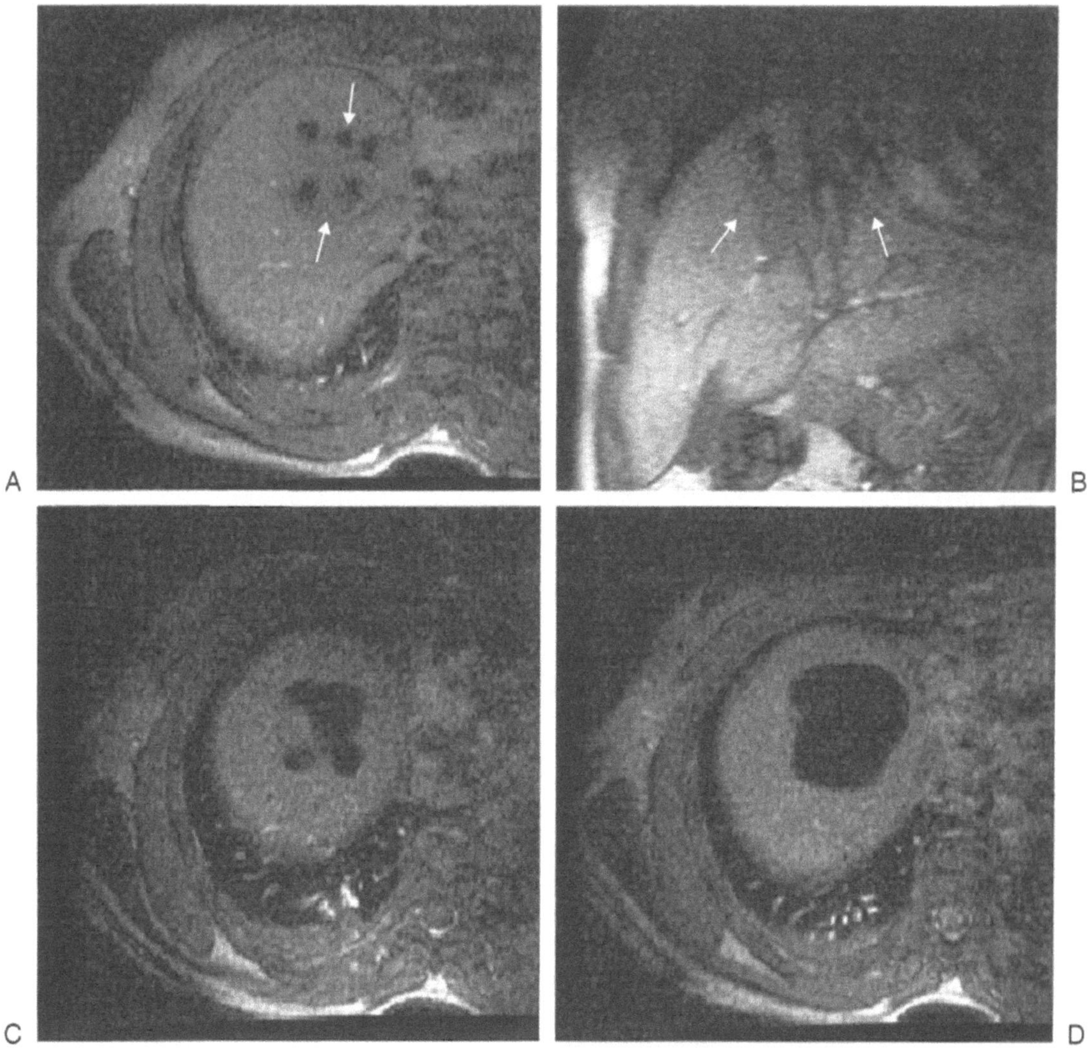

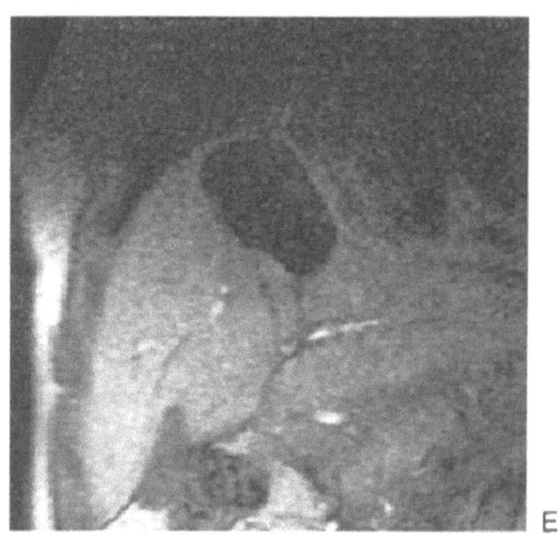

FIGURE 12.3. MRI-guided cryoablation of liver metastasis. (A,B) Intraprocedural axial and coronal SPGR images show location of five cryoprobes within the lesion (arrows) located in segment 8 of the liver. (C–E) Axial and coronal SPGR T1-weighted MR images obtained during cryotherapy with five cryoprobes show enlargement of the iceball.

colorectal carcinoma has not been significantly different from that which is achieved using conventional surgical techniques (47). Nevertheless, cryosurgery is used for surgically unresectable disease, and because more normal liver can be preserved than with surgical resection.

While cryotherapy has been recognized as a useful ablative agent in the treatment of malignant liver lesions, it was considered a "surgical only" option because of the necessity for large probes. Recently, there has been the development of cryoneedles (as small as 18-gauge needles) that can be placed percutaneously. Tacke et al (36) reported on the use of a novel MRI-compatible probe in animals using a 1.5-T magnet in the rabbit liver.

Magnetic resonance imaging–guided cryotherapy holds significant promise for several reasons. First, the short T2 relaxation time of ice results in excellent visualization of the iceball or cryolesion, which, using either T1- or T2-weighted sequences, is represented as a signal void (48,49). Using a variety of pulse sequences, excellent contrast between the iceball and tumor can be achieved in either a multiplanar or a three-dimensional format. This results in the accurate depiction of the entire iceball and its relationship in all dimensions with the treated tumor (48,49). As with ultrasound, the size of the iceball or cryolesion visualized with MRI correlated closely with necrosis. Silverman et al (31) described a method for cryoablating tumors percutaneously under MRI guidance. Using an optical tracking system, cryoneedles were placed, and liver tumors were ablated during two freeze cycles. Using repetitive multiplanar T1-weighted fast spin echo (FSE) or T1-weighted spin echo (SE) images, MRI was used to monitor progress of the treatment, whether the lesion was adequately covered, and to be sure vital structures were avoided. Consistent with the results of animal studies, intraprocedural appearance of iceballs correlated well with postprocedural estimates of necrosis (31).

Percutaneous cryotherapy of renal tumors has been performed successfully using MRI guidance (Fig. 12.4) (51). Indications for percutaneous tumor ablation (PTA) of renal tumors include elderly patients, patients with comorbidity that increases the risks of nephrectomy, and conditions that warrant a nephron-sparing procedure, such as solitary kidneys, multiple tumors, or renal insufficiency.

Percutaneous MRI guided cryoablation of soft tissue and bone lesions has been performed as well. Most patients are poor surgical candidates and they are referred for palliation or local tumor or pain control. A common indication for soft tissue cryoablation is presacral recurrence of anorectal cancer following abdominoperineal resection (APR) (Fig. 12.5). Other situations in which cryoablation has proven to be helpful include treatment of soft tissue sarcomas, vascular malformations, and metastatic lesions (52,53).

The rationale for MRI-guided cryotherapy is summarized as follows: (a) freezing is an effective ablative technique and can be monitored well with MRI; (b) MRI, like US, is near real time and multiplanar; (c) unlike US, it can depict the entire iceball and surrounding structures, and the iceball can be discriminated from tumor during the procedure; (d) unlike heating, the margins of necrosis following cryoablation are sharp and unambiguous, and the MR assessments correlate well with necrosis. Visualizing ablative changes intraprocedurally obviates 24-hour follow-up MRI or CT. Although tumor ablation with ethanol injection, RF, and interstitial laser therapy also may be performed with imaging guidance, the amount of tissue change demonstrated at US and CT during these therapies is limited, variable, and does not accurately reflect the zone of necrosis (54).

Ethanol Ablation

Ethanol was one of the first ablative agents used percutaneously. It is relatively easy to use, inexpensive, and effective in ablating tissues. Percutaneous injection of absolute ethanol is an established form of therapy for treatment of small HCCs in many parts of the world (42). Alcohol causes tissue necrosis predominantly by cellular dehydration and vascular thrombosis. Two characteristics of HCC make it amenable to alcohol injection therapy (42): (a) it is a well-vascularized, soft tumor so that ethanol easily diffuses within it; (b) it is frequently encapsulated, which prevents ethanol from

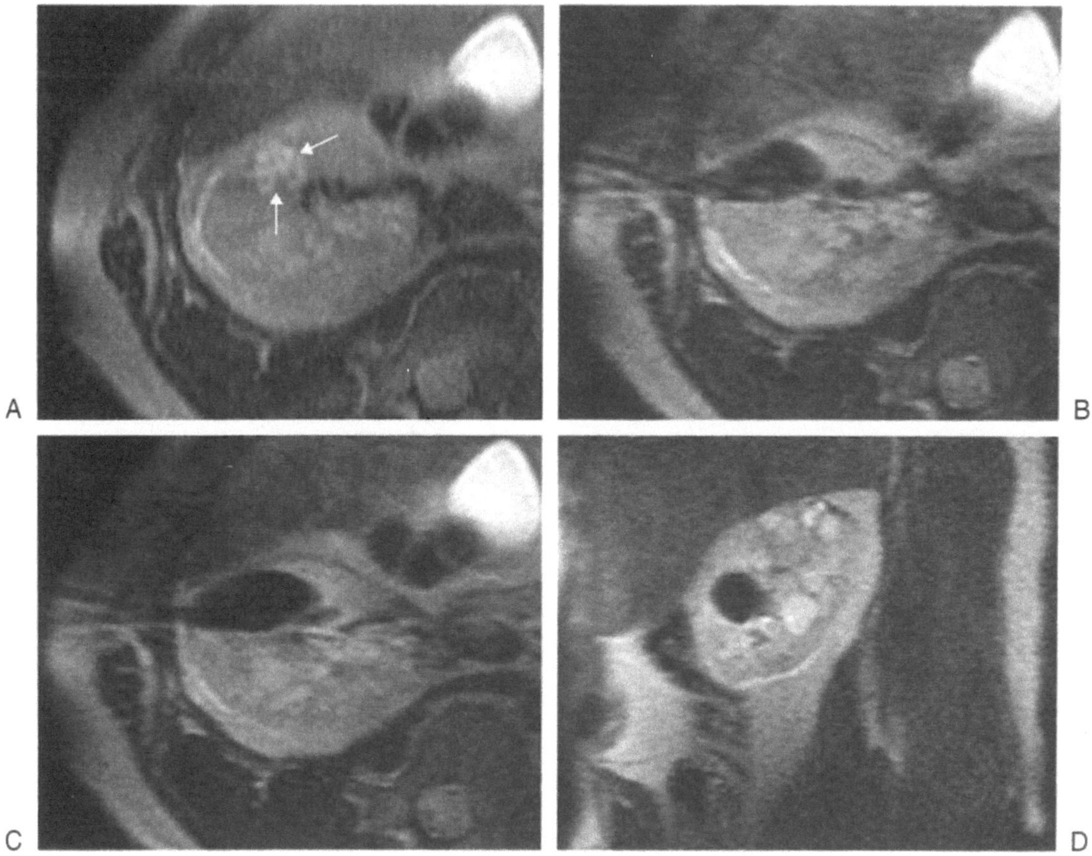

FIGURE 12.4. MRI-guided cryoablation of renal cell carcinoma (RCC) in the right kidney in a patient post left nephrectomy. (A) Axial fast spin echo (FSE) T2-weighted MR image shows hyperintense appearance of the renal mass (arrows) in the interpolar region of the right kidney. (B–D) Intraprocedural oblique axial and coronal TSE T2-weighted images show location of three cryoprobes within the lesion and enlargement of the iceball.

escaping. Metastatic tumors typically are not soft or encapsulated, and therefore alcohol is not as useful in the treatment of metastatic liver disease.

Ultrasound and CT have been used successfully in the guidance for alcohol and, as such, MRI has not been used widely. But MRI may be helpful in the guidance of percutaneous injection of alcohol into lesions that are not viewed by ultrasound or CT. In addition, MR monitoring of ethanol diffusion may be useful (7,55). Lu et al (7) reported on the use of MRI in the treatment of hepatic lesions in anesthetized pigs. Their study showed that ethanol appeared hypointense on T2-weighted images. They postulated that if ethanol was injected into HCCs under MRI guidance, it could be distinguished easily from T2-hyperintense tumor during treatment. Shinmoto et al (55) showed that a water-suppressed T2-weighted rapid acquisition with relaxation enhancement (RARE) sequence could be used to differentiate alcohol from long T2 water components of tumor and edema. The future of MRI-guided alcohol ablation is uncertain, and will probably be dictated by the relative benefits of alcohol as an ablative agent in the treatment of liver tumors.

Laser Ablation

Bown (56) described interstitial hyperthermia via laser technology with the insertion of a light-conducting quartz-fiber into a tumor in

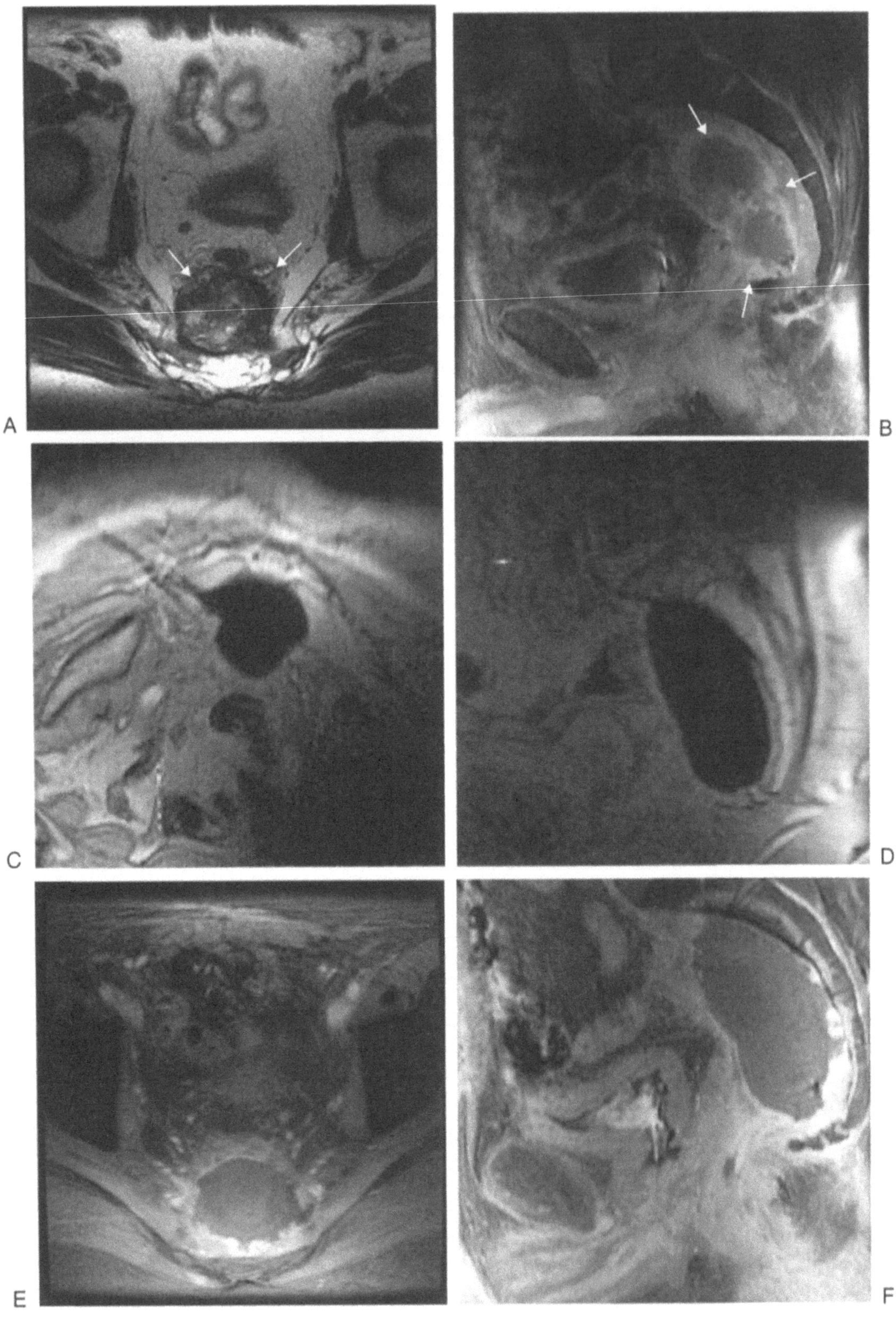
A
B
C
D
E
F

1983. In 1989 Steger et al (57) described interstitial laser photocoagulation (ILP) for metastatic liver lesions in two patients. Since then, lasers have been used to deliver localized, controlled heat deposition in multiple organs. Laser energy can be delivered using different materials such as a neodymium:yttrium-aluminum-garnet (Nd:YAG), carbon dioxide, and argon via tiny fiberoptics that are small enough to be inserted coaxially through an 18-gauge needle (58). Laser light is converted into heat in the target area, resulting in coagulative necrosis, secondary degeneration and atrophy, and tumor shrinkage with minimal damage to surrounding structures (58).

Early clinical trials using US and CT guidance were encouraging, with up to 82% of treated lesions achieving greater than 50% tumor necrosis (59–61). However, the "zone of kill" achieved with a single fiberoptic was limited, requiring multiple fibers and several sessions to treat most liver tumors. Diffusing tip fibers, loaded into small catheters, produce larger kill zones. To date, the largest experience with MRI-guided laser ablation of tumors has been reported by Vogl et al (22); using an Nd:YAG laser, 932 liver tumors were treated in 335 patients. Computed tomography was used to guide the placement of the catheters. Then, the patient was moved to a closed MR system so that the thermal changes during laser deposition could be observed. The local tumor control rate was 71% in the first 100 patients, 79% in the following 75 patients, and 97% at 6 months in the remaining patients who were treated with a cooled power-laser-ablation system. The study demonstrated feasibility and utility of monitoring tissue destruction using MRI.

Law and Regan (30) reported their experience with MRI-guided laser ablation of symptomatic uterine fibroids in 30 outpatients. The procedure was well-tolerated by all but one patient. Three months after the ablation, the treated fibroid volume decreased in size by a mean of 37.5% (range 25% to 49%). At 6 month follow-up, all patients were asymptomatic and none required further medical or surgical treatments for the fibroids.

Laser energy delivered through a stereotactically guided needle also has been used to ablate small breast cancers (62,63). New technical developments, such as robotic systems that allow the coordinates of a lesion to be approached in a high magnetic field, make a combination of breast biopsy and subsequent laser treatment feasible (63).

Radiofrequency Ablation (RFA)

Percutaneous radiofrequency electrocautery is a thermal ablation technique that causes local tissue destruction by inducing ionic agitation. This results in heat deposition within the tissue. Nearly immediate coagulation necrosis is induced at temperatures between 60° and 100°C. At higher temperatures tissue vaporizes and carbonizes. Thus, an essential objective of RF ablations is to achieve and maintain temperatures between 50° and 100°C throughout the entire target volume for at least 4 to 6 minutes (64).

Although this approach was used neurosurgically for over three decades, Rossi et al (65) reported its first use in 13 patients with small HCCs who were treated with ultrasound-guided percutaneous RF ablation. Subsequently, Livraghi et al (66) reported using RFA for metastatic liver tumors. Typically, one or more 18- to 21-gauge RF probes are placed using image-guidance into the lesion. Complete ablation of lesions measuring 2 to 4 cm can be

FIGURE 12.5. MRI-guided cryoablation of rectal cancer recurrence in a patient post–abdominoperineal resection. (A) Axial FSE T2-weighted MR image shows heterogeneous hyperintense mass (arrows) in the presacral area. (B) Gadolinium-enhanced sagittal SPGR T1-weighted MR image shows predominant peripheral enhancement of the mass. (C,D) Intraprocedural axial and sagittal SPGR T1-weighted images show cryoprobes within the lesion and enlargement of the iceball. (E,F): Gadolinium-enhanced axial and sagittal SPGR T1-weighted MR images obtained 3 months after the cryotherapy show subtotal necrosis of the recurrent rectal cancer.

achieved (67). New RF probes designs are now available, which include multipronged arrays, internally cooled electrodes, clustered electrodes, and saline-cooled electrodes. These advances increase the lesion diameter that can be treated (64).

Because of the interference of RF ablation with MRI, multiple strategies have been attempted to allow MRI to monitor RF ablations in real time. Lewin et al (67) reported on the first human clinical series of MRI-guided RF ablation of abdominal masses. Although RF needle electrodes were placed under MR guidance, when MRI was performed the generator was turned off during imaging, then ablated regions were re-imaged after each session. Using an open configuration MRI system (Magnetom Open; Siemens Medical Solutions; Erlangen, Germany), a 50- to 200-W RF generator (Radionics, Inc.; Burlington, MA), and prototype MR-compatible 17- × 2-mm shielded electrodes with a 1- to 3-cm exposed tip, 11 tumors were treated in seven patients for a total of 13 ablations. There was no significant morbidity. Four patients showed stable or decreasing tumor on average follow-up of 152 days. Short-tau inversion recovery (STIR) T2-weighted sequences were used in between ablations for monitoring with RF. This study showed that MRI-guided RF ablation of abdominal masses was feasible. Intraprocedural monitoring with MRI, in which imaging occurs during the treatment, may be possible with a recently developed switching mechanism that briefly interrupts RF deposition during the sampling for imaging pulse sequences. Ablation duration of a particular lesion is then determined by MRI.

Focused Ultrasound Surgery

Focused ultrasound surgery (FUS), or high-intensity focused ultrasound, is the therapeutic heat destruction of tissues using US energy that is focused on a target deep in the body (68–70). Ultrasound beams can be focused and controlled for energy delivery deep into the body without affecting superficial structures. The US beam interacts with tissue at the target volume through two mechanisms. First, the temperature is elevated due to energy absorption from the sonic waves, resulting in different degrees of thermal damage. Second, there is the phenomenon of transient or inertial cavitation.

Focused ultrasound surgery has two major advantages: it is less invasive than percutaneous treatment, as it requires no skin puncture; and the ablative effect is not limited by the geometry of a probe. Focused ultrasound surgery ablates a small focal spot-like zone of necrosis. Using a series of FUS ablations, an ablation zone can be achieved that is of virtually any desired shape. Focused ultrasound surgery can be targeted to more complicated lesion geometries by arranging the multiple sonications to conform to the target shape. Recently, Wu et al (71) reported their experience in the investigation of the pathologic changes of HCCs after FUS treatment. They examined the surgical specimens of six patients previously treated with FUS 5 to 18 days earlier, and confirmed that complete necrosis of the tumors was achieved.

Focused ultrasound surgery is limited in that it can be applied only in areas where there is no intervening bone or air between the ultrasound probe and target lesion. However, techniques are now being developed to traverse bone (72). Also, current FUS systems are designed for fixed targets, and therefore applications in the upper abdomen in which the targets move with respiration are difficult. However, just as US is used today to image the liver and kidney, FUS may be used to treat liver and kidney tumors in the future.

Uterine fibroids have been one of the first major areas of clinical application of FUS using MR guidance (73). Preliminary experience with MRI-guided ultrasound surgery has shown that MRI-guided FUS is feasible for local treatment of leiomyomas (Fig. 12.6) (73). The advantage of using MRI to guide this form of therapy is that not only is it excellent for depicting fibroids, but also it allows direct, continuous real-time monitoring of the effect. It ensures that a therapeutic thermal dose has been delivered to the target. If, for example, those changes are not achieved, repeated sonications in the same area will be possible. Other areas in which FUS is currently under investigation are the

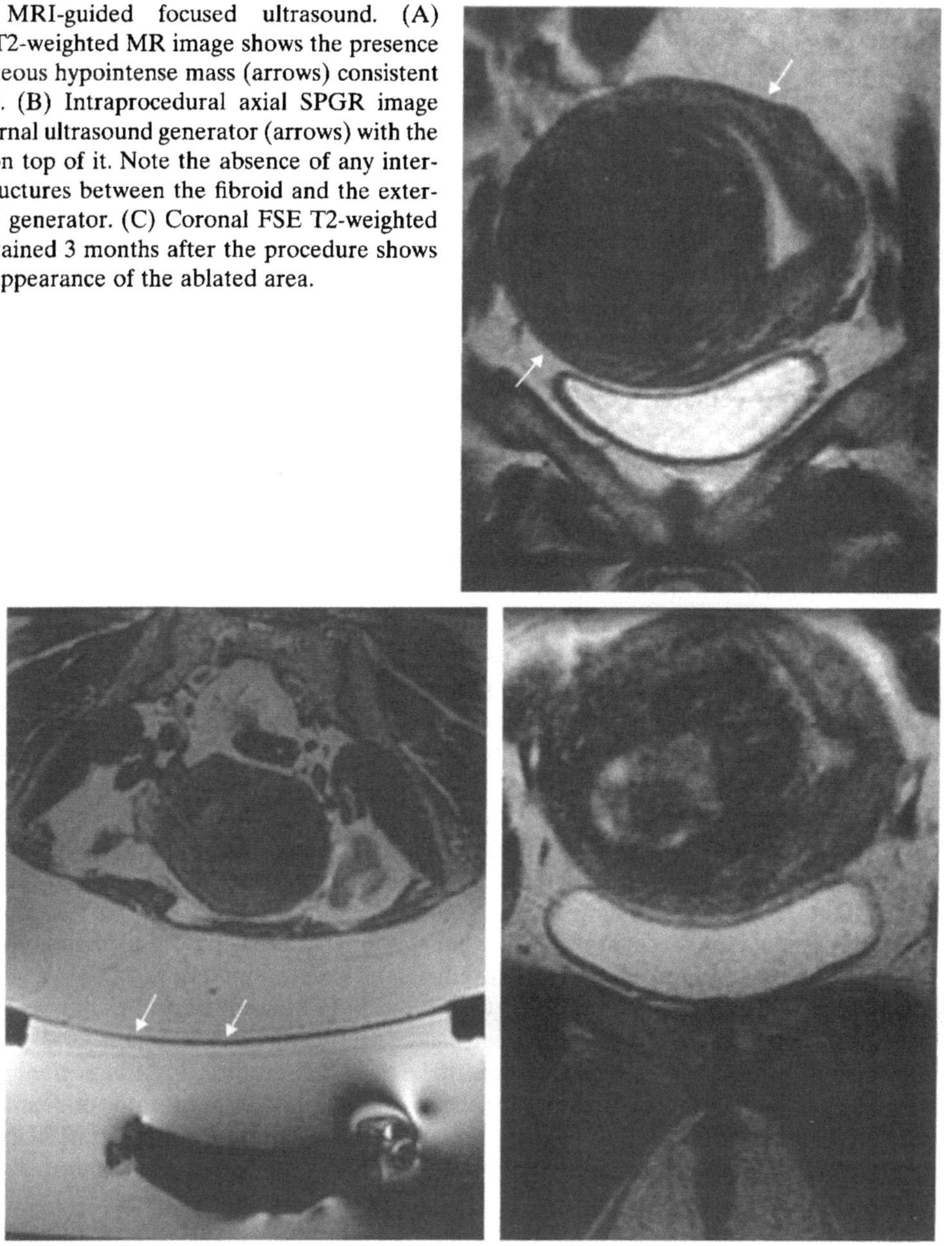

A

B

C

FIGURE 12.6. MRI-guided focused ultrasound. (A) Coronal TSE T2-weighted MR image shows the presence of a heterogeneous hypointense mass (arrows) consistent with a fibroid. (B) Intraprocedural axial SPGR image shows the external ultrasound generator (arrows) with the patient lying on top of it. Note the absence of any interfering vital structures between the fibroid and the external ultrasound generator. (C) Coronal FSE T2-weighted MR image obtained 3 months after the procedure shows hyperintense appearance of the ablated area.

treatment of breast fibroadenomas and breast cancer (72).

Brachytherapy

Prostate cancer is the second leading cause of cancer death in American men (74). Treatment options for localized prostate cancer include radical prostatectomy, cryotherapy, external beam radiation therapy, and interstitial radiation therapy (brachytherapy). The latter involves the placement of radiation seeds transperineally. When performed using US guidance, it is a desirable treatment because it is an outpatient procedure with low morbidity and low cost relative to other treatment options

(75). However, ultrasound is limited in its ability to define the margins of the prostate gland, urethra, and rectum and in its guidance of the intended radiation dose to selected portions of the gland.

Magnetic resonance imaging defines the prostate gland anatomy and the extent of prostate cancer better than ultrasound (76). Therefore, it can be used to improve both radiation dosimetry planning and radiation seed placement (Fig. 12.7). With the patient under general anesthesia, in the lithotomy position and the bladder catheterized, MRI of the prostate gland is first performed using a surface coil. Then, the prostate, urethra, and rectum are manually contoured on axial T2-weighted images. Using special computer software, prostate gland volumes and the desired radiation dose to each portion of the gland are calculated. These dosimetric calculations determine both the number of needles and number of radiation seeds required to ablate the peripheral gland that contains the cancer. Then, I-125 radiation seeds, loaded into 18-gauge needles, are placed into the prostate gland at predetermined depths at locations defined by the dosimetric plan. The ability to place the seeds precisely is aided both by real-time MRI that views the advancing needles and a Plexiglas template that contains rows and columns of holes at 5-mm intervals. This template is attached to a rectal obturator, which keeps the template at a fixed position abutting the perineum. It also serves to straighten the anorectal junction, and to delineate the rectal wall. Multiplanar MRI is used to confirm accurate placement of each needle before each seed is deposited.

The feasibility and safety of MRI-guided prostate brachytherapy have been demonstrated previously (77). In this initial report, all patients were implanted successfully without complication and all patients received 95% or more of the ideal radiation dose, a significant improvement over the 85% reported with US-guided methods. In a more recent update (78), a minimum of 89% coverage of the tumor volume was achieved, while maintaining the prostatic urethra and the anterior rectal wall below tolerance levels. Whether MRI-guided prostate brachytherapy improves survival and cancer control measures (e.g., PSA measurements) remains to be established.

Microwave Thermocoagulation

Microwave (thermo)coagulation is another minimally invasive therapy that has been developed for the local ablation of tumors. It also destroys tumor by creating a hyperthermic injury. Several studies have shown the feasibility of MR-guided microwave therapy in the treatment of liver tumors (79,80). Morikawa et al (79) reported their results in 30 patients with liver tumors. All procedures could be successfully carried out without complications, and the therapeutic effects were deemed satisfactory. Using a notched filter, MRI could be performed without electromagnetic interference during the ablation.

Conclusions

Magnetic resonance imaging guidance for tumor ablation, although still in its early stages of development, is generally gaining acceptance as the field expands to include tumors in deep and difficult locations. For example, although a small nonperipheral liver tumor may be fully and safely ablated with US or CT guidance, a large tumor abutting the heart or colon requires meticulous image guidance and monitoring. Therefore, MRI is needed. Overall, the ability of MRI to monitor real-time changes in tissue temperature suggests MRI as the optimal method for monitoring tumor ablation using thermal-based energies. The advantages of diagnostic MRI throughout the body, with its superior ability to detect and characterize lesions and depict anatomy, support its use in planning ablations and assessing outcomes.

While the feasibility of MRI-guided tumor ablations has been demonstrated, it is hoped that future clinical trials will demonstrate the added value of MRI and precisely define when MRI should be used instead of US or CT. Undoubtedly, as the field evolves, more applications will be introduced, and the advantages of MRI should become more apparent.

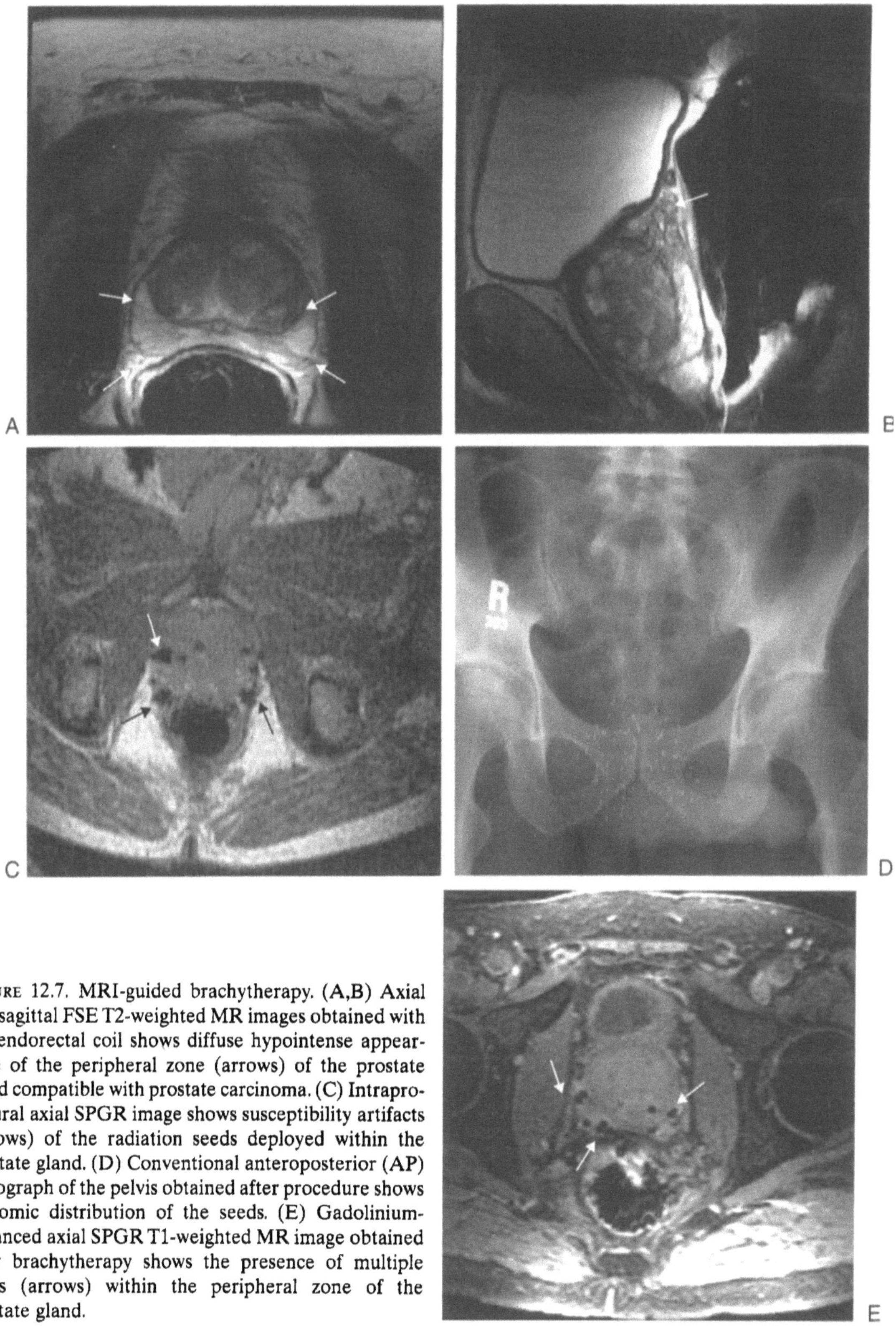

FIGURE 12.7. MRI-guided brachytherapy. (A,B) Axial and sagittal FSE T2-weighted MR images obtained with the endorectal coil shows diffuse hypointense appearance of the peripheral zone (arrows) of the prostate gland compatible with prostate carcinoma. (C) Intraprocedural axial SPGR image shows susceptibility artifacts (arrows) of the radiation seeds deployed within the prostate gland. (D) Conventional anteroposterior (AP) radiograph of the pelvis obtained after procedure shows anatomic distribution of the seeds. (E) Gadolinium-enhanced axial SPGR T1-weighted MR image obtained after brachytherapy shows the presence of multiple seeds (arrows) within the peripheral zone of the prostate gland.

References

1. Silverman SG, Jolesz FA, Newman RW, et al. Design and implementation of an interventional MR imaging suite. AJR 1997;168:1465–1471.
2. Jolesz FA, Silverman SG. Interventional magnetic resonance therapy. Semin Intervent Radiol 1995;12:20–27.
3. Lu DSK, Lee H, Farahani K, Sinha S, Lufkin R. Biopsy of hepatic dome lesions: semi-real-time coronal MR guidance technique. AJR 1997;168: 737–739.
4. Mueller PR, Stark DD, Simeone JF, et al. MR-guided aspiration biopsy: needle design and clinical trials. Radiology 1986;161:605–609.
5. Silverman SG, Collick BD, Figueira MR, et al. Interactive biopsy in an open configuration MRI system. Radiology 1995;197:175–181.
6. Frahm VC, Gehl HB, Robberg WA. Technique or MR-guided core biopsy of abdominal masses using an open low-field scanner: feasibility and first clinical results. Fortschr Rontgenstr 1996; 164:1:62–67.
7. Lu DSK, Sinha S, Lucas J, Farahani K, Lufkin R, Lewin K. MR-guided percutaneus ethanol ablation of liver tissue in a .2-T open MR system: preliminary study in porcine model. J Magn Reson Imaging 1997;7:303–308.
8. Mahfouz AE, Rahmouni A, Zylbersztejn C, Mathieu D. MR-guided biopsy using ultrafast T1- and T2-weighted reordered turbo fast low-angle shot sequences: feasibility and preliminary clinical applications. AJR 1996;167:167–169.
9. Duerk JL, Lewin JS, Wendt M, Petersilge C. Remember true-FISP? A high SNR, near 1-second imaging method for T2-like contrast interventional MRI at 0.2T. J Magn Reson Imaging 1998;8:203–208.
10. Papanicolaou N, Eisenberg PJ, Silverman SG, McNicholas MM, Althausen AF. Prostatic biopsy after proctocolectomy: a transgluteal, CT-guided approach. AJR 1996;166:1332–1334.
11. Kneeshaw PJ, Turnbull LW, Drew PJ. Current applications and future direction of MR mammography. Br J Cancer 2003;13:4–10.
12. Hlawatsch A, Teifke A, Schmidt M, Thelen M. Preoperative assessment of breast cancer: sonography versus MR imaging. AJR 2002;179: 1493–1501.
13. Pflleiderer SO, Reichenbach JR, Azhari, et al. A manipulator system for 14-gauge large core breast biopsies inside a high-field whole-body MR scanner. J Magn Reson Imaging 2003;17: 493–498.
14. Daniel BL. Intraprocedural magnetic resonance imaging-guided interventions in the breast. Top Magn Reson Imaging 2000;11:184–190.
15. Dumoulin CL, Souza P, Darrow RD. Real time position monitoring of invasive devices using magnetic resonance imaging. Magn Reson Med 1993;29:411–415.
16. Göhnde SC, Pfammatter T, Steiner P, Erhart P, Romanowski BJ. MR-guided cholecystectomy: assessment of biplanar, real-time needle tracking in three pigs. Cardiovasc Intervent Radiol 1997; 20:295–299.
17. Leung DA, Debatin JF, Wildermuth S, et al. Intravascular MR tracking catheter: preliminary experimental evaluation. AJR 164:1265–1270.
18. Wendt M, Busch M, Wetzler R, et al. Shifted rotated keyhole imaging and active tip-tracking for interventional procedure guidance. J Magn Reson Imaging 1998;8:251–258.
19. Glovinski A, Adam G, Buecker A, et al. Catheter visualization using locally induced actively controlled field inhomogeneities. Magn Reson Med 1997;38:251–258.
20. Glowinski A, Kürsch J, Adam G, et al. Device visualization for interventional MRI using local magnetic fields: basic theory and its application to catheter visualization. IEEE Trans Med Imaging 1998;17:786–793.
21. Vogl TJ, Mack MG, Muller PK, Straub R, Engelmann, Eichler K. Interventional MR: interstitial therapy. Eur Radiol 1999;9:1479–1487.
22. Vogl TJ, Mack MG, Straub R et al. Magnetic resonance imaging–guided abdominal interventional radiology: laser induced thermotherapy of liver metastasis. Endoscopy 1997;29(6):577–583.
23. Dickinson RJ, Hall AS, Hind AJ, Young IR. Measurement of changes in tissue temperature using MR imaging. J Comput Assist Tomogr 1986;10: 468–472.
24. Kettenbach J, Silverman SG, Hata N, et al. Monitoring and visualization for MR-guided laser ablations in an open MR system. J Magn Reson Imaging 1998;8:933–943.
25. Fosshelm S, Ilyasov K, Wiggen U, et al. Paramagnetic liposomes as thermosensitive probes for MRI in vitro feasibility studies. In: Proceedings of the ISMRM Annual Meeting. Philadelphia: ISMRM, 1999:725.
26. Bartholet A, Goudemant J, Laurent S, et al. Spin transition molecular materials: intelligent contrast agents for magnetic resonance thermometry. In: Proceedings of the ISMRM Annual Meeting. ISMRM, 2000;138.

27. Mueller PR, Stark DD, Simeone JF, et al. Clinical use of a nonferromagnetic needle for magnetic resonance-guided biopsy. Gastrointest Radiol 1989;14:61–64.
28. Schenck JF, Jolesz FA, Roemer PB, et al. Superconducting open configuration MR imaging system for image-guided therapy. Radiology 1995;195:805–814.
29. Gronemeyer DH, Kaufman L, Rothschild P, et al. New possibilities and aspects of low-field magnetic resonance tomography. Radiol Diagn 1989;30:519–527.
30. Law P, Regan L. Interstitial thermo-ablation under MRI guidance for the treatment of fibroids. Curr Opin Obstet Gynecol 2000;12: 277–282.
31. Silverman SG, Tuncali K, Adams DF, et al. MR imaging-guided percutaneous cryotherapy of liver tumors: initial experience. Radiology 2000; 217:657–664.
32. Lewin JS, Connell CF, Duerek JL, et al. Interactive MRI-guided radiofrequency interstitial thermal ablation of abdominal tumors: clinical trial for evaluation of safety and feasibility. J Magn Reson Imaging 1998;8:40–47.
33. Shellock FG, Kanal E. Magnetic Resonance: Bioeffects, Safety, and Patient Management. New York: Raven, 1994:61–69.
34. Hughes CW, Bell C. Anesthesia equipment in remote hospital locations. In: Ehrenwerth J, Eisenkraft JB, eds. Anesthesia Equipment: Principles and Applications. St. Louis: Mosby, 1993: 565–587.
35. Lewin JS, Duerk JL, Jain JR, et al. Needle localization in MR guided biopsy and aspiration: effect of field strength, sequence design, and magnetic field orientation. AJR 1996;166:1337–1345.
36. Tacke J, Adam G, Speetzen R, et al. MR-guided interstitial cryotherapy of the liver with a novel, nitrogen-cooled cryoprobe. Magn Reson Med 1998;39:354–360.
37. D'Agostino HB, Solinas A. Percutaneous ablation therapy for hepatocellular carcinomas. AJR 1995;164:1165–1167.
38. Steele G Jr, Ravikumar TS. Resection of hepatic metastases from colorectal cancer: biologic perspectives. Ann Surg 1989;210:127–138.
39. Crews KA, Kuhn JA, McCarty TM, et al. Cryosurgical ablation of hepatic tumors. Am J Surg 1997;114:614–618.
40. Gazelle GS, Goldberg SN, Solbiati L, Livraghi T. Tumor ablation with radio-frequency energy. Radiology 2000;217:633–646.
41. Vogl TJ, Müller PK, Hammerrstingl R, Weinhold N, Felix R. Malignant liver tumors treated with imaging guided laser induced thermotherapy, technique and prospective results. Radiology 1995;196:257–265.
42. Livraghi T, Vettori C, Lazzaroni S, et al. Liver metastases: results of percutaneous ethanol injection in 14 patients. Radiology 1991;179:709–712.
43. Wong WS, Patel SC, Cruz FS, et al. Cryosurgery as a treatment for advanced stage hepatocellular carcinoma. Cancer 1998;82(7):1268–1278.
44. Brewer WH, Austin RS, Capps GW, et al. Intraoperative monitoring and postoperative imaging of hepatic cryosurgery. Semin Surg Oncol 1998; 14:129–155.
45. Weber SM, Lee FT, Warner TF, Chosy SG, Mahvi DM. Hepatic cryoablation: US monitoring of extent of necrosis in normal pig liver. Radiology 1998;207:73–77.
46. Lee FT, Mahve DM, Chosy SG, et al. Hepatic cryosurgery with intraoperative US guidance. Radiology 1997;202:624–632.
47. Steele G Jr. Cryoablation in hepatic surgery. Semin Liver Dis 1994;14:120–125.
48. Gilbert JC, Rubinsky B, Roos MS, Wong STS, Brennan KM. MR-monitored cryosurgery in rabbit brain. Magn Reson Imaging 1993;11: 1155–1164.
49. Matsumoto R, Oshio K, Jolesz FA. Monitoring of laser and freezing-induced ablation in the liver with T1-weighted MR imaging. J Magn Reson Imaging 1993;3:770–776.
50. Silverman SG, Tuncali K, Adams DF, et al. Percutaneous MR imaging-guided cryotherapy of liver metastases. Suppl Radiol 1999;213:122.
51. Shingleton BW, Sewell PE. Percutaneous tumor ablation with magnetic resonance imaging guidance. J Urol 2001;165:773–776.
52. vanSonnenberg E, Hadjipavlou A, Chaljub G, Nolsöe C, Ko E. Therapeutic cryotherapy guided by MRI and ultrasound for vascular malformations in erector muscles of the back. Minim Invasive Ther Allied Technol 1997;6:343–348.
53. Menendez LR, Tan MS, Kiyabu MT, Chawla SP. Cryosurgical ablation of soft tissue sarcomas: a phase I trial of feasibility and safety. Cancer 1999;86:50–57.
54. Goldberg SN, Gazelle GS, Mueller PR. Thermal ablation therapy for focal malignancy: a unified approach to underlying principles, techniques, and diagnostic imaging guidance. AJR 2000;174: 323–331.
55. Shinmoto H, Mulkern RV, Oshio SG, et al. MR appearance and spectral features of injected ethanol in the liver: implication for fast MR-guided percutaneous ethanol injection therapy. J Comput Assist Tomo 1997;21:82–88.

56. Bown SG. Phototherapy of tumors. World J Surg 1983;7:700–709.
57. Steger AC, Lees WR, Walmsley K, Brown SG. Interstitial laser hyperthermia: a new approach to local destruction of tumours. BMJ 1989;299: 362–365.
58. Amin Z, Bown SG, Lees WR. Liver tumor ablation by interstitial laser photocoagulation review of experimental and clinical studies. Semin Intervent Radiol 1993;10:88–100.
59. Amin Z, Bown SG, Lees WR. Local treatment of colorectal liver metastases: a comparison of interstitial laser photocoagulation (ILP) and percutaneous alcohol injection (PAI). Clin Radiol 1993;48:166–171.
60. Amin Z, Buonaccorsi G, Mills T, et al. Interstitial laser photocoagulation: evaluation of a 1320 nm Nd-Yag and an 805 nm diode laser: the significance of charring the fibre tip. Lasers Med Sci 1993;8:113–120.
61. Amin Z, Donald J, Masters A, et al. Hepatic metastases: interstitial laser photocoagulation with real-time US monitoring and dynamic CT evaluation treatment. Radiology 1993;187:339–347.
62. Dowlatshahi K, Francescatti DS, Bloom KJ. Laser therapy for small breast cancers. Am J Surg 2002;184:359–363.
63. Kaiser WA, Fisher H, Vagner J, Selig M. Robotic system for biopsy and treatment of breast lesions in a high-field whole-body magnetic resonance tomography unit. Invest Radiol 2000;35:513–519.
64. Goldberg SN, Gazelle GS, Dawson S, Rittman W, Mueller PR, Rosenthal DI. Tissue ablation with radiofrequency: effect of probe size, gauge, duration, and temperature on lesion volume. Acad Radiol 1995;2:399–404.
65. Rossi S, Fornari F, Buscarini L. Percutaneous ultrasound-guided radiofrequency electrocautery for the treatment of small hepatocellular carcinoma. J Intervent Radiol 1993;8:97–103.
66. Livraghi T, Goldberg S, Monti F, et al. Saline-enhanced radiofrequency tissue ablation in the treatment of liver metastases. Radiology 1997; 202:205–210.
67. Lewin JS, Connell CF, Duerek JL, et al. Interactive MRI-guided radiofrequency interstitial thermal ablation of abdominal tumors: clinical trial for evaluation of safety and feasibility. J Magn Reson Imaging 1998;8:40–47.
68. Hynynen K. Damainou CA, Colucci Y, et al. MR monitoring of focused ultrasonic surgery of renal cortex: experimental and simulation studies. J Magn Reson Imaging 1995;5:259–266.
69. Yang R, Reilly CR, Rescorla FJ, et al. High-intensity focused ultrasound in the treatment of experimental liver cancer. Arch Surg 1991;126: 1002–1010.
70. Yang R, Sanghvi NT, Rescorla FJ, et al. Extracorporeal liver ablation using sonography-guided high-intensity focused ultrasound. Invest Radiol 1992;27:796–803.
71. Wu F, Wang Z, Chen W. Pathological study of extracorporeally ablated hepatocellular carcinoma with high-intensity focused ultrasound. Zhonghua Zhong Liu Za Zhi 2001;23:237–239.
72. Hynynen K, Darkazanli A, Unger E, Schenck JF. MRI-guided noninvasive ultrasound surgery. Med Phys 1992;20:107–116.
73. Tempany CM, Stewart EA, McDermodt N, Quade BJ, Jolesz FA, Hynynen K. MR imaging-guided focused ultrasound surgery of uterine leiomyomas: a feasibility study. Radiology 2003; 226:897–905.
74. Wingo PA, Landio S, Reis LAG. An adjustment to the 1997 estimate for new prostate cancer cases. CA Cancer J Clin 1997;47:239–242.
75. Prestidge BR, Prete JJ, Bucholtz TA, et al. A survey of current clinical practice of permanent prostate brachytherapy in the United States. Int J Radiat Oncol Biol Phys 1998;40:461–465.
76. Seltzer SE, Getty DJ, Tempany CM, et al. Staging prostate cancer with MR imaging: a combined radiologist-computer system. Radiology 1997; 202:219–226.
77. D'Amico AV, Cormack R, Tempany CMC, et al. Real time magnetic resonance image guided interstitial brachytherapy in the treatment of selected patients with clinically localized prostate cancer. Int J Radiat Oncol Biol Phys 1998;42:507–515.
78. D'Amico A, Cormack R, Kumar S, Tempany CM. Real-time magnetic resonance imaging-guided brachytherapy in the treatment of selected patients with clinically localized prostate cancer. J Endourol 2000;14:367–370.
79. Morikawa S, Inubushi T, Kurumi, et al. MR-guided microwave thermocoagulation therapy of liver tumors: initial clinical experiences using a 0.5 T open MR system. J Magn Reson Imaging 2002;16:576–583.
80. Naka S, Kurumi Y, Shimizu, et al. Tumor ablation with MRI navigation: a novel method of microwave coagulation therapy for hepatic tumour. Gan To Kagaku Ryoho 2001;28:1591–1594.

13 Magnetic Resonance Imaging Guidance of Radiofrequency Thermal Ablation for Cancer Treatment

Daniel T. Boll, Jonathan S. Lewin, Sherif G. Nour, and Elmar M. Merkle

Recent trends in the care of cancer patients emphasize minimizing invasiveness while improving the effectiveness of treatment by utilizing medical resources in a cost-effective manner. This has been evident in the emerging and steadily evolving utilization of interventional radiology over the past quarter century.

Minimally invasive interventions performed by interventional radiologists cover applications ranging from straightforward diagnostic procedures, such as biopsy and aspiration, to a more complicated array of palliative as well as therapeutic procedures, such as tumor embolization, biliary and hollow viscus stenting, percutaneous gastrostomy, celiac plexus nerve blocks, inferior vena cava filter application, and percutaneous image-guided brachytherapy. While the range of anatomic sites amenable to minimally invasive intervention steadily increases, oncologic therapy also has advanced rapidly; minimally invasive intervention, therefore, has assumed a competitive role beyond the conventional therapeutic chain of surgery–radiotherapy–chemotherapy. Numerous exciting developments in cancer treatment have evolved and include gene therapy (1,2), targeted drug delivery (3,4), control of angiogenesis (5), and the delivery of various forms of thermal energy for tumor ablation, such as radiofrequency (RF), laser (6), focused ultrasound (7), microwave (8), and cryotherapy (9).

These developments are expected to profit from the substantial contributions of magnetic resonance imaging (MRI), based on its high soft tissue contrast, vascular conspicuity, thermo- and ligand-sensitive sequences, multiplanar imaging capabilities, and lack of radiation exposure. These factors make MRI an ideal modality for planning, guiding, monitoring, and evaluating cancer treatment procedures. This chapter highlights the current utility and future directions of interventional MRI for use with radiofrequency energy in multiple anatomic regions.

General Principles

Radiofrequency Thermal Ablation

Interstitial RF thermal ablation therapy is an attractive treatment option for numerous reasons. This modality has a long and successful history as it has been utilized in stereotactic neurosurgical procedures for more than 30 years (10). Neurosurgical indications for this form of therapy historically have included cordotomy, pallidotomy, leukotomy, and thalamotomy for the treatment of intractable pain and involuntary movement disorders (11–14). Based on data from our site and others, complications resulting from RF ablation are uncommon as coagulation effects of the heating process contribute to a very low incidence of hemorrhage in the central nervous system (15,16) and abdomen (17,18).

Reproducible tissue destruction has been observed in a variety of anatomic structures. Furthermore, both human and animal studies have shown that thermal lesion shape and size can be controlled through electrode design, as well as the duration and magnitude of the energy delivered (19,20). The feasibility of controlling energy deposition and allowing gradual tissue heating while performing RF ablations is demonstrated by a thermistor placed in the electrode tip (15). Thermistors continuously monitor tissue temperature, while impedance measurements provide another parameter related to tissue changes at the ablation site.

Unlike radiation therapy but like other thermal ablative therapies, interstitial RF thermal ablation can be repeated numerous times without concern for the cumulative dose.

The efficacy and safety of RF thermal ablation procedures are demonstrated by the wide variety of benign and malignant conditions for which they can be utilized. The vast majority of reports describe RF thermal ablation treatments for liver (21–23) and kidney (24–26) tumors, while other target organs in the trunk include the pancreas (27), prostate (28,29), breast (30), spleen (31), and lung (32).

Magnetic Resonance Imaging Guidance of Radiofrequency Thermal Ablation Therapy

Much of the excitement about expanding the therapeutic uses of RF energy beyond the neurosurgical, cardiac, and direct intraoperative fields, is engendered by the advancements in imaging technology. The ability to perform thermal treatment of cancer percutaneously under direct image guidance has advanced RF ablation as a minimally invasive option to surgery that is more suitable for the large sector of poor operative candidates.

The primary principle of image guidance for ablation electrode-based thermal treatment is to secure safe and precise electrode advancement into the targeted abnormality, and the subsequent monitoring of the growth and morphology of thermally induced coagulative necrosis from the RF energy. The process of image guidance for minimally invasive therapeutic procedures such as RF thermal ablation can be subdivided into a planning and guidance phase prior to performing the therapy, as well as a treatment and evaluation phase during and after the ablation.

The initial *planning phase* is essential because the ideal electrode trajectory during the actual procedure is often significantly different from that suggested on the preprocedure imaging data due to the frequent shift of anatomic structures when using modified patient positions during the treatment. Therefore, only preprocedural visualization of the spatial relationships of the anatomic structures, localization of the pathology itself, identification of even the smallest blood vessels for vascular road-mapping, and the appearance of other tumor foci or the accumulation of ascites in the final procedural patient position allow realistic planning of the optimal ablation electrode trajectory (Fig. 13.1A,B).

The subsequent *guidance phase* emphasizes that temporal and spatial resolutions are competing objectives in interventional MRI. Continuous visualization, characterized by automated sequential acquisition, reconstruction, and in-room display of multiple image data sets of highly sensitive anatomic entities, such as blood vessels and neural structures, allows safe and fast interventional device advancement and final probe placement, while sparing vital abdominal structures, such as the gallbladder, bowel loops, and the renal pelvis. Once the RF electrode is delivered successfully into the targeted tumor and the interventionalist is satisfied with the electrode position, the deployment of RF energy can be instituted confidently (Fig. 13.1C).

The *treatment phase* represents the greatest challenge for any visualization modality. The transformation of unique tissue characteristics such as density, water and protein content, temperature, as well as fluid vaporization, microbubble, and gas formation, can be imaged by various devices. However, the correlation of these phenomena with thermal lesion size and expected coagulative necrosis is based on complex estimations.

In the early phase of our clinical series, when nonperfused ablation electrodes were used, interstitial RF thermal ablation was performed at an electrode tip temperature of 90° ± 2°C. Using this electrode design, lesion length is

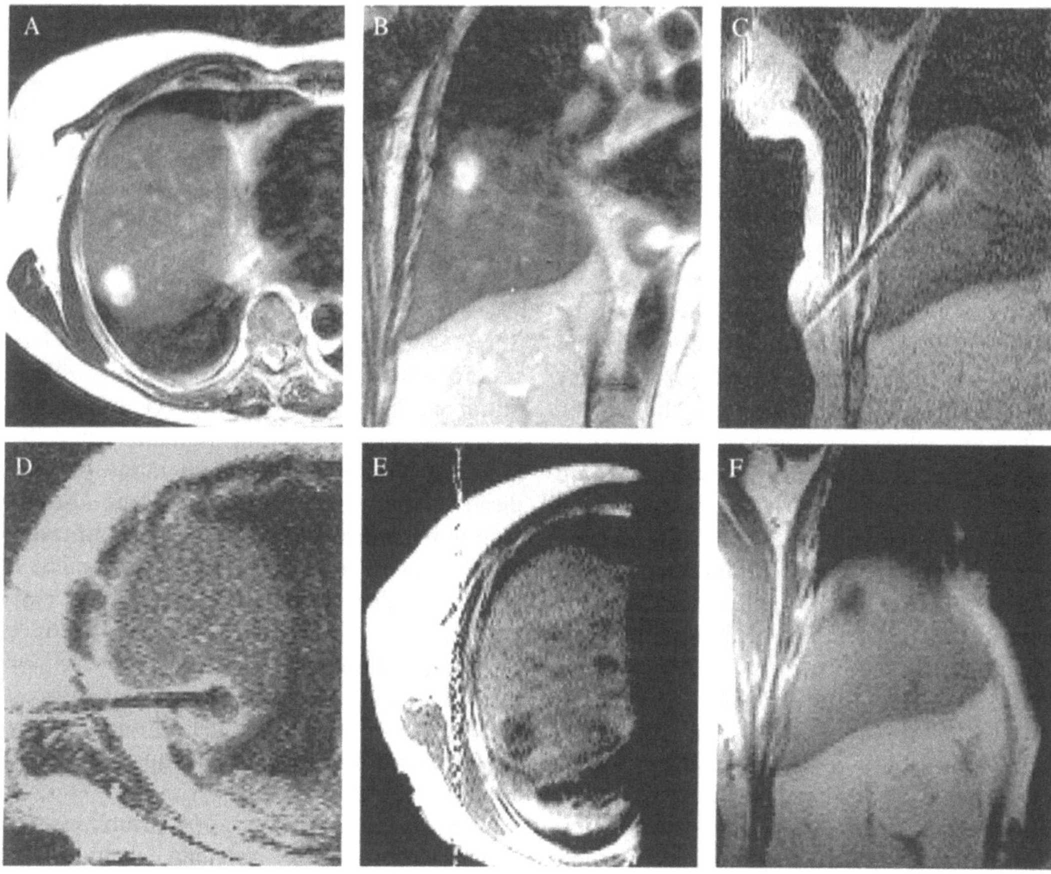

FIGURE 13.1. Hepatic dome metastasis. Transverse (A) and coronal (B) turbo spin echo T2-weighted images of the abdomen demonstrate hyperintense metastasis in the posterior dome of the right lobe of the liver. (C) Turbo spin echo T2-weighted coronal image along the course of the MR-compatible radiofrequency (RF) electrode demonstrates the electrode positioned within the tumor. (D) Oblique axial-sagittal turbo spin echo T2-weighted sequence noting the effects of interstitial RF thermal ablation as the marked hypointensity developed around the active distal 3cm of the electrode, surrounded by a rim of hyperintensity reflecting edema and hyperemia. Transverse (E) coronal (F) contrast-enhanced T1-weighted images following interstitial RF thermal ablation demonstrate hypointensity corresponding to avascular area of tumor necrosis. This approximates the volume of the originally identified tumor, along with a small margin of surrounding normal parenchyma.

dependent on the exposed conductive tip length, and lesion diameter is limited to approximately 2cm (33,34). The limitation to achieving larger lesion diameters is thought to be due to carbonization at the electrode and tissue interface, which in turn impairs and finally leads to the cessation of energy transfer.

With the water-cooled electrode concept, a roller pump is used to circulate chilled water inside channels within the electrode to cool the tip to 10° to 20°C, thereby preventing charring and carbonization at the electrode–tissue interface. This allows energy delivery to regions more distant from the electrode source (35,36). Single ablations can be performed with this electrode design that would formerly have required multiple ablations with intervening electrode repositioning using a standard RF electrode. To maximize the area of necrosis, we usually use a combination of the cool-tip electrode with pulsed application of RF energy during which brief periods of current interruption are triggered automatically when tissue impedance rises beyond a preset threshold. Again, the intention is to prevent tissue charring, carbonization, and cavitation, all of which lead to cessation of RF current deposition. The ablation time usually ranges from 6 to 20 minutes at each electrode location prior to electrode repositioning for total ablation of larger tumors (37,38).

At the conclusion of ablation sessions using cool-tip electrode designs, a second application of RF energy at the same electrode position may be necessary without cooling, once the desired margins are achieved, to destroy the area adjacent to the cooled electrode. A practical method to test the necessity for such additional RF applications is to continue measuring the RF electrode tip temperature for 2 minutes after the RF power has been turned off. We reablate the center of the annulus-shaped thermal lesion if its temperature falls below 60°C before the 2 minutes have elapsed (Fig. 13.1D).

After the ablation, during the *evaluation phase*, high-resolution postprocedure scanning is performed for the final evaluation of thermal lesion size and morphology and to exclude possible complications in neighboring anatomic regions. Subsequently, patients at our institution are observed overnight before being discharged the following morning. According to this thermal ablation protocol, we bring the patient back for follow-up imaging at 2 weeks, and then again at 3 months after ablation, and at 3-month intervals thereafter.

Currently, various imaging modalities are being used for guidance of minimally invasive or surgical procedures. However, only MRI combines characteristics such as high soft tissue contrast as well as spatial resolution, precise vascular conspicuity, multiplanar imaging capabilities, and lack of radiation exposure. Furthermore, visualization by means of MRI offers options for temperature mapping, and therefore MRI is able to define treatment end points by providing immediate feedback regarding the extent of coagulative necrosis during the ablation (39) (Fig. 13.2). With those attributes, MRI has won increasing acceptance as an interventional procedure guidance for aspirations, biopsies, and drainages as well as for monitoring ablation. To date, a continuous effort to further develop MRI guidance techniques has concentrated mainly on local treatment of cancer and cancer metastases using percutaneous MRI-guided thermal tumor ablation procedures (Fig. 13.1E,F).

Interventional MRI Suite

The early years of MRI were characterized by relatively long imaging times in closed-bore superconducting cylindrical systems. Those initial configurations made MRI an unlikely guidance and monitoring modality for radiologic procedures. Increasingly, many of these disadvantages have been overcome through system hardware and pulse sequence improvements that have allowed the development of rapid imaging techniques. Therefore, early experiences with thermal ablation procedures during which access to the patient was not necessarily required for the monitoring process, were gathered in various institutions employing conventional cylindrical superconducting systems (40–42).

The use of MRI for more complex interventional procedure guidance includes the manipulation of thermal ablation electrodes by radiologists. This form of more active intervention requires a departure from conventional diagnostic concepts and traditional imaging systems. The development of an open magnet configuration has facilitated the patient access necessary to perform more extensive manipulative maneuvers during interventional procedures (43–46). Many open MRI system designs have been used to guide percutaneous procedures; each system has emphasized the constant trade-off between field strength and its homogeneity, as well as the stability of the static and gradient magnetic fields that result in direct effects on the signal-to-noise ratio, access to the patient, usable field of view, and expense (47).

Modern MRI magnets now provide sufficient image quality for the interventional guidance phase of minimally invasive procedures. Image acquisition times of 1 to 3 seconds or less per image provide the necessary temporal resolution (48,49). Furthermore, through the development of in-room, high-resolution,

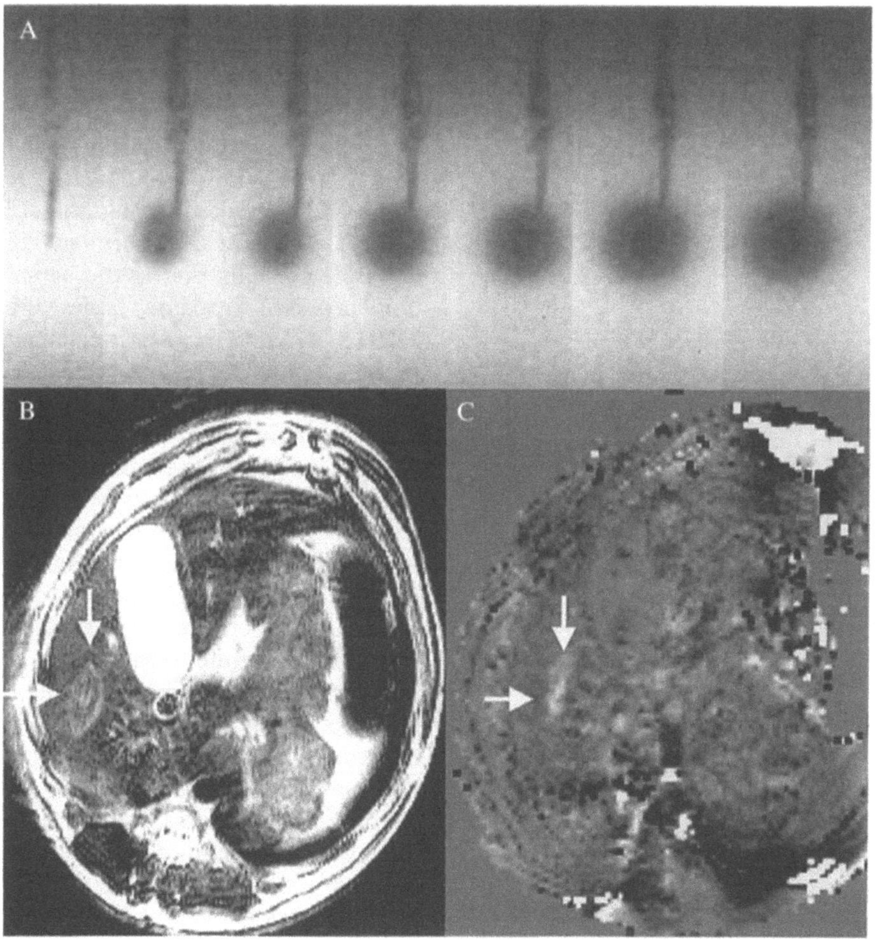

FIGURE 13.2. Magnetic resonance thermometry based on changing T1 relaxation times, diffusion weighting, and chemical shift phenomenon allows precise monitoring of thermal lesion growth, as shown in image series (A). Furthermore, strong direct correlation is observed between morphologic changes as visualized on T2-weighted magnitude MRI (B), and the tissue damage predicted by direct temperature measurement, using the chemical shift phenomenon as imaged on MR phase images (C) in a canine liver model.

RF-shielded monitors, the interventional radiologist has the ability to operate the scanner and view images at the scanner side within the magnetic fringe field throughout the entire procedure. In combination with direct patient access allowed by open imaging systems, this capability permits the entire procedure to be performed with the operator sitting next to the patient throughout the procedure (Fig. 13.3).

In addition, thermal ablation electrodes have been developed that are undeflected by the magnetic field and that create little or no external field distortions or image degradation (50,51). Their appearance on the image is due mainly to the displacement of proton-containing tissue that produces the actual MR signal and to the metal intrinsic to the instrument or paramagnetic markers that is incorporated into the instrument. These factors lead to the formation of areas of increased susceptibility, and therefore contribute to areas of signal void in the images (52).

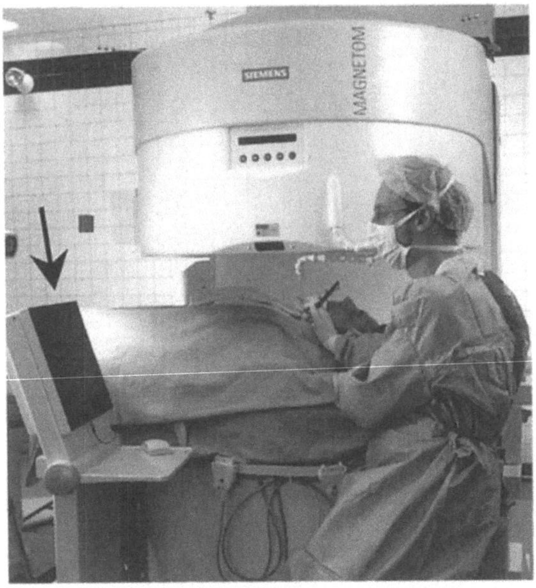

FIGURE 13.3. C-arm system for percutaneous intervention. For immediate monitoring of thermal ablation electrode placement and subsequent RF thermal ablation acquired breath-hold images are presented to the interventionalist on a shielded liquid crystal display (LCD) monitor (arrow) adjacent to the scanner. A computer mouse on the LCD console and foot pedals (not shown) allow the scanner to be operated by the radiologist throughout the procedure.

The modification and development of rapid gradient-echo pulse sequences that facilitate a wide range of tissue contrast in a time frame sufficient for device tracking even at low field strength and with the suboptimal coil position sometimes required to access a puncture site, have proven their capability and usefulness in interactive guidance procedures during device placement. Furthermore, the inherent inability of MRI to monitor actively a thermal lesion as it is created, due to imaging interference caused by the RF source, has been overcome. New software and hardware modifications have been developed that allow RF energy to be deposited during imaging with short interruptions during the sampling periods, thereby maintaining tissue temperature, while making interference-free real-time monitoring possible (53,54).

Safety Issues for Interventional MRI During Radiofrequency Energy Deposition

In contrast to widespread imaging modalities used for interventional guidance, such as ultrasound and computed tomography (CT), which interact with human tissue and the interventional device only during the actual visualization process, a major basic difference of MRI is its continuous strong magnetic field. Although risks are less prominent with the low and medium magnetic field strengths of 0.2 to 0.5T typically used for MRI-guided procedures, hazardous consequences can result when ferromagnetic instruments become attracted to and are accelerated in the fringe field of the MRI unit. Serious or even fatal injuries can occur. Therefore, the generally accepted rule is that no ferromagnetic materials should be brought within the 5-gauss line of any MR scanner. Electric burns can result from direct electromagnetic induction in a conductive loop, induction in a resonant conducting loop, or electric field resonant coupled with a wire (55,56). Acoustic noise during interventions on open low- and medium-field scanners normally does not reach the occupational exposure limit of 15 minutes per day at 115dB.

Adequate visualization of the target pathology and surrounding anatomy is crucial, especially in interventional MRI. Because of the need for high temporal resolution during the advancement and final placement of the thermal ablation electrode, the resultant images do not have the quality expected from a purely diagnostic sequence. Different, nearly real-time pulse sequences are available, thus allowing multiple tissue contrasts to be obtained, depending on the sequence design as well as the implemented parameters (57).

The most commonly used sequences for the guidance phase for MRI of RF thermal ablations are fast imaging with steady-state precession (FISP) techniques, with a temporal resolution of 1 to 3 seconds per image, FISP sequences with balanced gradients in all spatial directions (true FISP), characterized by an acquisition speed of 1 second per image, and finally a time-reversed version of the FISP sequence (known as PSIF) with a temporal resolution of 4 to 5 seconds per image. However, those gradient echo sequences are associated with more prominent susceptibility artifacts from thermal ablation electrodes than with the relatively slower spin echo or turbo spin echo sequences. Therefore, to reduce artifactual needle widening, the use of turbo spin echo imaging for position confirmation should be strongly considered when electrode placement within 5 mm of a major neurovascular structure is contemplated (58).

After successful placement of the thermal ablation electrode, MRI provides incomparable techniques for monitoring lesion formation and morphology. The development of temperature-sensitive MR sequences enables accurate online monitoring of heat deposition (59). The relationship of MR signal intensity change to tissue temperature is a complex phenomenon, and precise MR temperature measurement is difficult. However, the phase transition from viable to necrotic tissue can be imaged directly using changes in the tissue relaxation parameters, T1 and T2, that occur in the process of necrosis formation (60,61).

When applying the relatively high currents necessary to perform RF ablation procedures successfully, system grounding through an adequate surface area is crucial. This is due to the fact that when RF current passes through a patient's body and closes its complete electric circuit, an equal amount of current is deposited at the return electrodes, such as the grounding pad, compared to the source electrode (62). The optimal outcome of an RF ablation session is the generation of a thermal lesion that covers the whole targeted tumor plus a safety margin comparable to the 0.5- to 1-cm rim generally targeted during surgery. While undertreatment is obviously an unacceptable outcome, overablation also is not free from risks. Injury of vital structures adjacent to the target tumor can complicate the treatment. In addition to the concern about collateral damage, it is also important when planning extensive ablations to consider whether sufficient organ function can be preserved and to be aware that large-volume tissue necrosis is associated with a higher incidence of infection and the postablation syndrome.

Economic Considerations

The cost-effectiveness of interventional MRI has been debated primarily because conventional, less expensive, and widely available imaging modalities seemed adequate in the past. Compared to current ultrasound and CT-guided procedures, MRI guidance is still slightly more expensive. However, when thermal therapy guidance, monitoring, and evaluation are the issues, the unparalleled ability of MRI to detect residual untreated tumor foci during the ablation session outweighs the extra cost associated with the use of this technology. In fact, in many institutions in which thermal therapy is performed under ultrasound or CT guidance, the patient is ultimately transferred to the MR scanner following ablation to confirm the extent of necrosis.

Compared to the surgical approach, the use of MRI guidance for RF thermal ablations is associated with tremendous cost reduction, from a decrease in the cost of the procedure itself relative to surgery, to the equal or greater savings realized by avoiding the intensive care unit as well as routine hospitalization. This is in addition to the patient benefits that result from the reduction in morbidity, mortality, postprocedure discomfort, and recovery time when open surgical procedures can be avoided (63).

Applications

MRI-Guided Radiofrequency Thermal Ablation of the Liver

Over the past decade, hepatic malignancies, such as primary hepatocellular carcinomas (17) and hepatic metastasis (64), have evolved as prime abdominal therapeutic sites amenable to treatment with RF-induced thermal ablation. The anatomic structure of the liver capsule and the liver parenchyma accounts for the relatively low incidence of complications, such as bleeding following insertion of interventional devices of various calibers, and therefore substantiate the rationale to use hepatic RF thermal ablation in the liver (65).

Prior to the clinical application of this technique, however, a representative *small animal model* focusing on implantation, harvesting, and subsequent MRI-guided RF thermal ablation treatment in the rabbit liver was developed at our institution (21) (Fig. 13.4). It demonstrated that the absence of major interventional complications, the mean treatment duration of 44 minutes including all evaluation by MRI, and the ability to monitor tissue damage during and immediately after the procedure confirmed the feasibility of this approach. Important information concerning the correlation of image appearance of the induced coagulative necrosis and gross pathologic evaluation revealed a difference of less than 2mm. T2-weighted imaging continuously overestimated the lesion size, consistent with other studies (66). Remaining tumor within the liver was best identified on T2-weighted turbo spin echo sequences; these results followed those of animal studies performed at other anatomic locations (67,68). Follow-up examinations consisting of T2-weighted turbo spin echo sequences and intravenous gadopentetate dimeglumine–enhanced T1-weighted imaging were able to demonstrate an accuracy of estimating RF thermal lesion size within 2 to 3mm.

Experience gathered during the development phase of the hepatic RF thermal ablation technique in the animal model is of paramount importance for establishing this form of treatment within the clinical routine environment (Fig. 13.5). The efficacy and success of percutaneous RF thermal ablation can be diminished by a tumor mass of more than 30% of the complete liver volume, extrahepatic tumor extension, or severe dilatation of the intrahepatic biliary system.

The probability of a successful outcome with MRI-guided RF ablation increases with smaller tumor size, less than 3 to 4cm. Studies performed in our institution showed that T2-weighted turbo spin echo and short-tau inversion recovery (STIR) sequences utilized after the RF thermal ablation demonstrate the zone of tissue damage with similar precise conspicuity compared to contrast-enhanced T1-weighted spin echo sequences. Especially the contrasts within the thermally induced lesion, the edematous surrounding hyperintense rim, and the physiologic surrounding liver tissue imaged with T2-weighted turbo spin echo and STIR sequences are comparable to con-

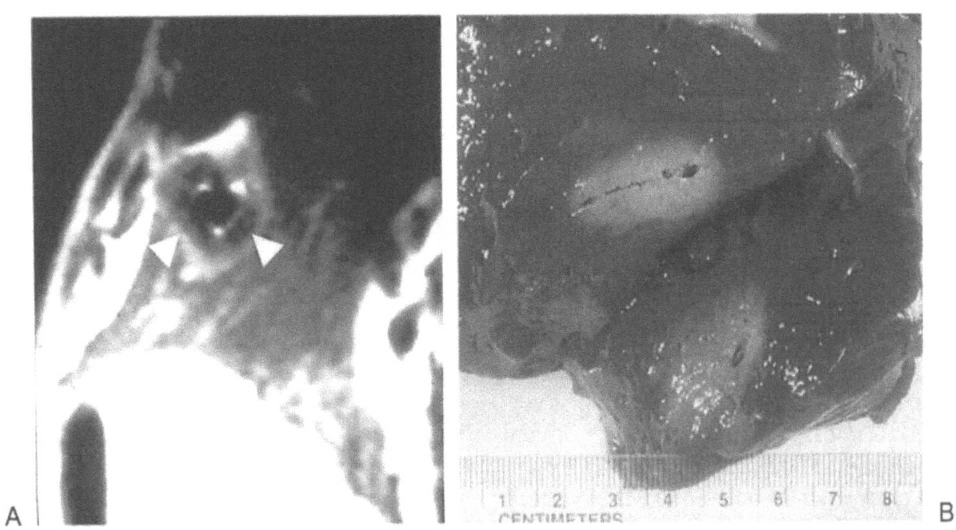

FIGURE 13.4. Small animal model demonstrating the feasibility of MRI-guided liver ablation in a rabbit specimen. Area of low signal intensity (A) (arrowheads) on T2-weighted image developing around electrode during RF ablation correlates closely with measurements on gross pathology (B) and histology (see ref. 66). Animal experiments in multiple organ systems were used to document the ability of this method of imaging tissue damage to be used to tailor the treatment phase of MRI-guided thermal ablation.

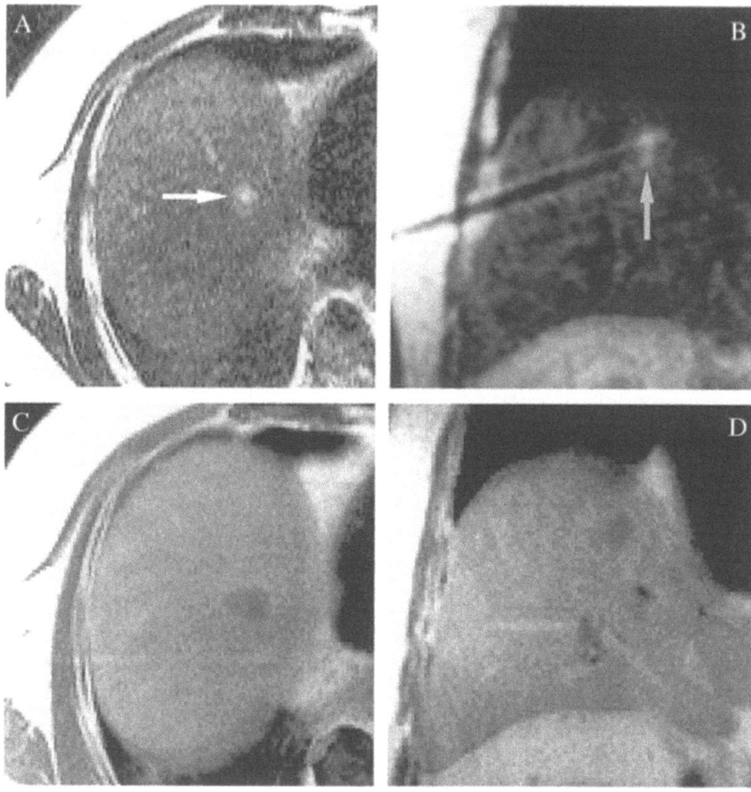

FIGURE 13.5. Images of a 74-year-old patient with three known metastases from a previously resected leiomyosarcoma of the stomach. T2-weighted axial image (A) through the right lobe of the liver demonstrates a 1-cm bright tumor nodule (arrow). T2-weighted coronal image (B) demonstrates the titanium electrode identified as a dark band with its tip through the center of the tumor nodule (arrow). Transverse (C) and coronal (D) T1-weighted contrast-enhanced images obtained after ablation and removal of the electrode demonstrate a central low- signal necrotic core replacing the bright tumor nodule, with a thin, bright rim of surrounding edema. By tailoring this region of tumor necrosis as depicted on MRI, lesions of variable size and shape can be effectively ablated along with a margin of surrounding tissue.

trast media–enhanced sequences. Thus repeat images are obtained during the thermal RF ablation, because of the contrast media independence of these sequences (69).

MRI-Guided Radiofrequency Thermal Ablation of Kidney Tissue and Tumors

The proliferation of cross-sectional imaging techniques has led to an increase in the incidental visualization and therefore early detection of renal malignancies (70). Furthermore, high-risk patients who underwent cross-sectional imaging for suspected cancer have benefited from the earlier detection of smaller masses (71,72). With the increasing ability to detect renal malignancies, nephron-sparing therapies have been developed that are aimed at the preservation of renal function. This preservation is of paramount importance in an anatomically or functionally solitary kidney or in conditions such as Von Hippel–Lindau disease linked to the occurrence of recurrent renal cell carcinomas. Studies have demonstrated that minimally invasive and nephron-sparing treatments of small renal malignancies have the same efficacy as radical nephrectomy (73–75). Minimally invasive, image-guided

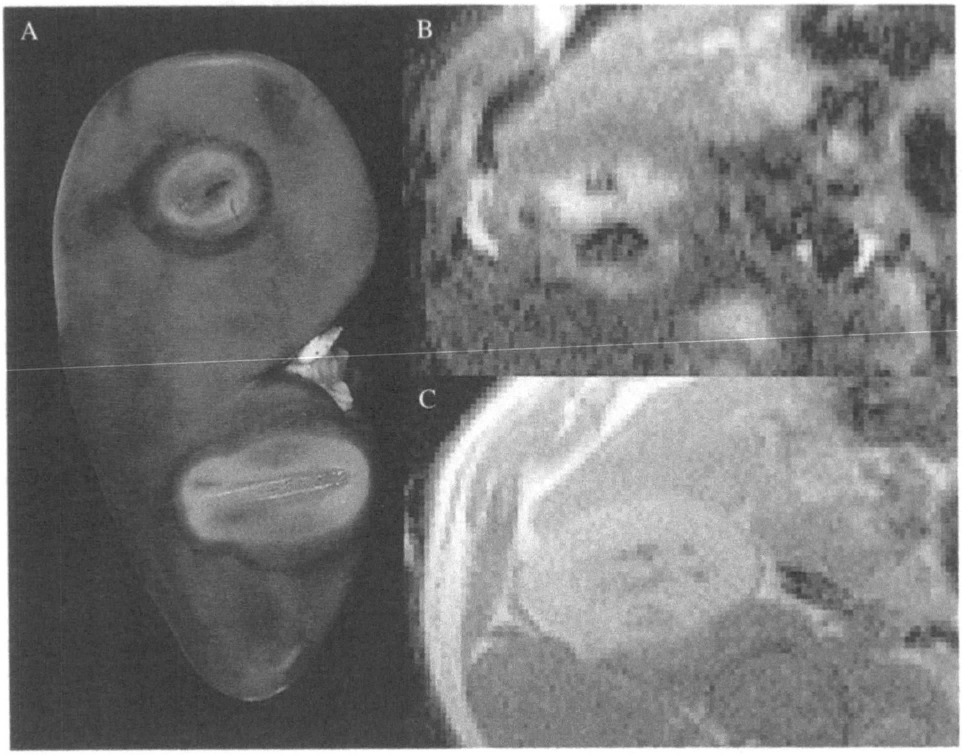

FIGURE 13.6. Animal model presenting the feasibility of MRI-guided kidney ablation and the correlation with porcine gross pathology specimen (A) and short-tau inversion recovery (STIR) (B), as well as contrast-enhanced T1-weighted MRI (C).

renal tissue ablation has been described using techniques such as cryotherapy, focused ultrasound, and microwave application (76–79).

Radiofrequency thermal energy to treat malignant lesions within the kidneys was not described prior to the development of an animal model to prove the feasibility and safety of this approach (24) (Fig. 13.6). Under MRI guidance, the desired insertion site in the retroperitoneal kidneys was accessed without difficulty with the RF ablation probe. The excellent vessel conspicuity of MRI facilitates the avoidance of large vessels during the placement of the ablation electrode. However, due to the high vascularity of the targeted site, the development of small puncture-related hematomas was observed in 30% of porcine kidney RF ablations. However, small hemorrhages immediately visualized by MRI are not an uncommon complication of interstitial thermotherapy in the kidney, with an occurrence rate up to 100% of cases during cryoablation (80). The procedure time required to perform interventional thermal ablation in the kidney was measured at a mean of 11 minutes. By employing MRI during the procedure, the growth and morphology of the coagulative necrosis were monitored successfully, allowing repositioning of the ablation electrode immediately. It was proven that MRI succeeded in predicting the size and morphology of an induced thermal lesion within porcine kidneys.

At our institution, a phase II clinical trial focusing on interactive MRI-guided interstitial RF thermal ablations of primary kidney tumors was initiated with the purpose of evaluating long-term follow-up examinations of a cohort of patients (Fig. 13.7). The trial specifically was designed to demonstrate efficacy of this treatment modality and to analyze patient discomfort or any complications associated with this procedure. Complete ablation of renal masses was achieved in 93% of all patients treated and in 100% of patients with tumors of 4 cm diameter or less, based on postprocedure and follow-up examinations on T2-weighted and STIR images. Due to the proximity of the developing thermal lesion to the renal pelvis, further RF application could not be performed in one larger tumor in which a small rim of hyperintense material was still visible on T2-weighted and STIR images. In 40% of all treated patients, oral analgesia was administered on the evening after the procedure; however, none of these patients required pain medication on discharge.

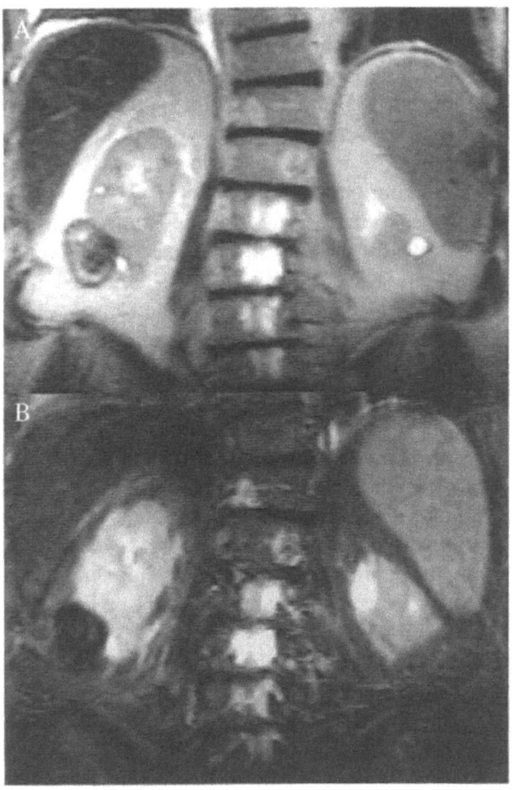

FIGURE 13.7. Follow-up examination 20 months after RF thermal ablation of the right kidney in a patient with renal cell carcinoma. T2-weighted (A) and STIR (B) coronal images demonstrate typical encasing scar of a prior successfully ablated exophytic renal cell carcinoma. On turbo spin echo (TSE) T2-weighted images (A), the fat surrounding the shrinking low-signal tumor scar remains bright, but is suppressed on STIR images (B).

Patients with complete coagulative necrosis of their renal malignancy showed no clinical or imaging evidence of tumor recurrence with a mean follow-up of 366 ± 129 days. On volumetric analysis, it was demonstrated that the thermal lesion increased in size by approximately 2 mL on the 2-week follow-up examination, compared to the images obtained at the conclusion of the ablation session. Subsequently, the lesion volume slowly decreased during the follow-up period. Signal intensity remained low on T2-weighted and STIR images throughout the follow-up period for all successful ablation procedures. The ability to detect inadequately treated portions of the renal malignancy and interactively reposition the electrode during therapy was critical in this investigation. Despite the relatively small sizes of the masses, manipulation of the electrode into untreated tumor was necessary in 80% of the treated patients to achieve complete tumor ablation. This relatively high proportion is undoubtedly related to the high vascularity of both the tumor and the adjacent renal parenchyma.

With mean follow-up examinations of greater than 1 year, this clinical study suggests that interactive MRI-guided RF renal ablation for treatment of primary renal tumors has a high success rate to achieve complete ablation and a low level of tumor recurrence; it is also extremely well tolerated by patients (81).

Research and Future Directions

The feasibility and safety of RF thermal ablations performed under MRI guidance for other body organs have been investigated in animal models. Multiple reports have proven the applicability of this technique to more than the current clinically recognized applications. Positive results from pancreatic (27), long bone (82), and vertebral (83) ablation sites (Fig. 13.8) promise to expand the future of cancer treatment by taking advantage of the minimally invasive nature of RF ablation along with the superb value of MRI for guiding and monitoring RF thermal treatment.

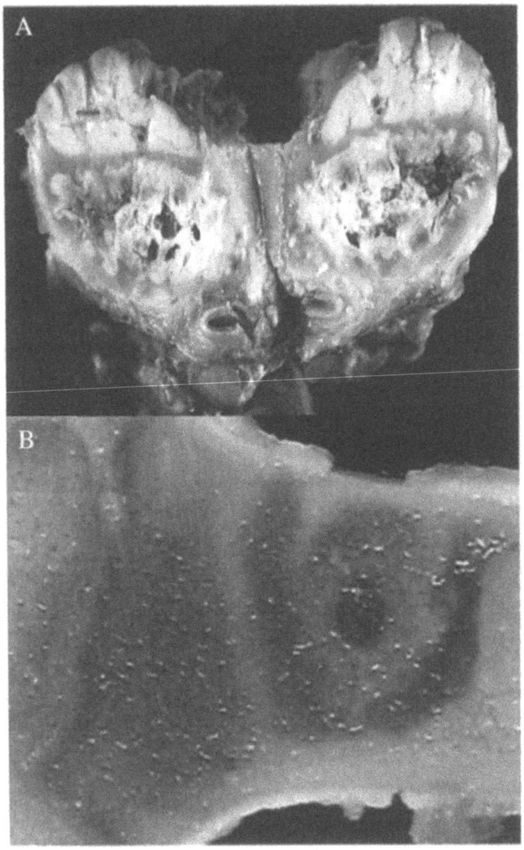

FIGURE 13.8. The feasibility and safety of RF thermal ablation performed under MRI guidance also have been investigated and successfully performed in animal models in other body organs such as the pancreas (A) and long bone (B).

Further development of the RF technology will be necessary to create larger thermal lesions with the least number of RF electrode insertions. This is of paramount importance for reducing such risks as tumor seeding, bleeding, and infection, and is also important to reduce the procedure time and thus improve patient compliance, particularly when managing large tumors. Techniques already investigated include the use of multiple-probe RF electrode arrays that allow a higher maximum energy to be deposited into the tissue (36,84).

Ongoing extensive interventional MR physics research is primarily focused on MR pulse sequence development (57) and device tracking optimization. Interactive MRI scan plane definition for rigid interventional devices, such as RF thermal electrodes, without the need for stereotactic cameras, is now possible using wireless, tuned fiducial markers mounted to the device (85).

References

1. Allport JR, Weissleder R. In vivo imaging of gene and cell therapies. Exp Hematol 2001; 29(11):1237–1246.
2. Yang X, Atalar E, Li D, et al. Magnetic resonance imaging permits in vivo monitoring of catheter-based vascular gene delivery. Circulation 2001; 104(14):1588–1590.
3. Guerquin-Kern JL, Volk A, Chenu E, et al. Direct in vivo observation of 5-fluorouracil release from a prodrug in human tumors heterotransplanted in nude mice: a magnetic resonance study. NMR Biomed 2000;13(5):306–310.
4. Calvo BF, Semelka RC. Beyond anatomy: MR imaging as a molecular diagnostic tool. Surg Oncol Clin North Am 1999;8(1):171–183.
5. Fuss M, Wenz F, Essig M, et al. Tumor angiogenesis of low-grade astrocytomas measured by dynamic susceptibility contrast-enhanced MRI (DSC-MRI) is predictive of local tumor control after radiation therapy. Int J Radiat Oncol Biol Phys 2001;51(2):478–482.
6. Mack MG, Straub R, Eichler K, et al. [Needle holder for reducing radiation burden of examiners in CT-assisted puncture. Technical contribution]. Radiologe 2001;41(10):927–929.
7. Huber PE, Jenne JW, Rastert R, et al. A new noninvasive approach in breast cancer therapy using magnetic resonance imaging-guided focused ultrasound surgery. Cancer Res 2001; 61(23):8441–8447.
8. Chen JC, Moriarty JA, Derbyshire JA, et al. Prostate cancer: MR imaging and thermometry during microwave thermal ablation-initial experience. Radiology 2000;214(1):290–297.
9. Mala T, Samset E, Aurdal L, Gladhaug I, Edwin B, Soreide O. Magnetic resonance imaging-estimated three-dimensional temperature distribution in liver cryolesions: a study of cryolesion characteristics assumed necessary for tumor ablation. Cryobiology 2001;43(3):268–275.
10. Brodkey JS, Miyazaki Y, Ervin FR, Mark VH. Reversible heat lesions with radiofrequency current: a method of stereotactic localization. J Neurosurg 1964;21:49–53.

11. Tew JM Jr, Keller JT. The treatment of trigeminal neuralgia by percutaneous radiofrequency technique. Clin Neurosurg 1977;24:557–578.
12. Hitchcock ER, Teixeira MJ. A comparison of results from center-median and basal thalamotomies for pain. Surg Neurol 1981;15(5):341–351.
13. Laitinen LV, Bergenheim AT, Hariz MI. Leksell's posteroventral pallidotomy in the treatment of Parkinson's disease. J Neurosurg 1992;76(1): 53–61.
14. Rosomoff HL, Brown CJ, Sheptak P. Percutaneous radiofrequency cervical cordotomy: technique. J Neurosurg 1965;23(6):639–644.
15. Zervas NT, Kuwayama A. Pathological characteristics of experimental thermal lesions. Comparison of induction heating and radiofrequency electrocoagulation. J Neurosurg 1972;37(4):418–422.
16. Farahani K, Mischel PS, Black KL, De Salles AA, Anzai Y, Lufkin RB. Hyperacute thermal lesions: MR imaging evaluation of development in the brain. Radiology 1995;196(2):517–520.
17. Rossi S, Di Stasi M, Buscarini E, et al. Percutaneous RF interstitial thermal ablation in the treatment of hepatic cancer. AJR 1996;167(3): 759–768.
18. Lewin JS, Connell CF, Duerk JL, et al. Interactive MRI-guided radiofrequency interstitial thermal ablation of abdominal tumors: clinical trial for evaluation of safety and feasibility. J Magn Reson Imaging 1998;8(1):40–47.
19. Zervas NT. Eccentric radio-frequency lesions. Confin Neurol 1965;26(3):143–145.
20. Chung YC, Duerk JL, Lewin JS. Generation and observation of radiofrequency thermal lesion ablation for interventional magnetic resonance imaging. Invest Radiol 1997;32(8):466–474.
21. Merkle EM, Boll DT, Boaz T, et al. MRI-guided radiofrequency thermal ablation of implanted VX2 liver tumors in a rabbit model: demonstration of feasibility at 0.2T. Magn Reson Med 1999;42(1):141–149.
22. Nicoli N, Casaril A, Marchiori L, Mangiante G, Hasheminia AR. Treatment of recurrent hepatocellular carcinoma by radiofrequency thermal ablation. J Hepatobiliary Pancreat Surg 2001; 8(5):417–421.
23. Buscarini L, Buscarini E, Di Stasi M, Vallisa D, Quaretti P, Rocca A. Percutaneous radiofrequency ablation of small hepatocellular carcinoma: long-term results. Eur Radiol 2001;11(6): 914–921.
24. Merkle EM, Shonk JR, Duerk JL, Jacobs GH, Lewin JS. MR-guided RF thermal ablation of the kidney in a porcine model. AJR 1999;173(3): 645–651.
25. Pavlovich CP, Walther MM, Choyke PL, et al. Percutaneous radiofrequency ablation of small renal tumors: initial results. J Urol 2002;167(1): 10–15.
26. Lewin JS, Connell CD, Duerk JL, Nour SG, Resnick MI, Haaga JR. A phase II clinical trial of interactive MR-guided interstitial radiofrequency thermal ablation of primary kidney tumors: preliminary results. Proceedings of the Radiological Society of North America 87th Meeting, 2001:261.
27. Merkle EM, Haaga JR, Duerk JL, Jacobs GH, Brambs HJ, Lewin JS. MR imaging-guided radiofrequency thermal ablation in the pancreas in a porcine model with a modified clinical C-arm system. Radiology 1999;213(2):461–467.
28. Syed AH, Stewart LH, Hargreave TB. Day-case local anaesthetic radiofrequency thermal ablation of benign prostatic hyperplasia: a four-year follow-up. Scand J Urol Nephrol 2000;34(5): 309–312.
29. Zlotta AR, Djavan B, Matos C, et al. Percutaneous transperineal radiofrequency ablation of prostate tumour: safety, feasibility and pathological effects on human prostate cancer. Br J Urol 1998;81(2):265–275.
30. Izzo F, Thomas R, Delrio P, et al. Radiofrequency ablation in patients with primary breast carcinoma: a pilot study in 26 patients. Cancer 2001;92(8):2036–2044.
31. Wood BJ, Bates S. Radiofrequency thermal ablation of a splenic metastasis. J Vasc Intervent Radiol 2001;12(2):261–263.
32. Dupuy DE, Zagoria RJ, Akerley W, Mayo-Smith WW, Kavanagh PV, Safran H. Percutaneous radiofrequency ablation of malignancies in the lung. AJR 2000;174(1):57–59.
33. McGahan JP, Gu WZ, Brock JM, Tesluk H, Jones CD. Hepatic ablation using bipolar radiofrequency electrocautery. Acad Radiol 1996;3(5): 418–422.
34. Rossi S, Buscarini E, Garbagnati F, et al. Percutaneous treatment of small hepatic tumors by an expandable RF needle electrode. AJR 1998; 170(4):1015–1022.
35. Goldberg SN, Gazelle GS, Solbiati L, Rittman WJ, Mueller PR. Radiofrequency tissue ablation: increased lesion diameter with a perfusion electrode. Acad Radiol 1996;3(8):636–644.
36. Lorentzen T. A cooled needle electrode for radiofrequency tissue ablation: thermodynamic aspects of improved performance compared

with conventional needle design. Acad Radiol 1996;3(7):556–563.
37. Solbiati L, Goldberg SN, Ierace T, et al. Hepatic metastases: percutaneous radio-frequency ablation with cooled-tip electrodes. Radiology 1997; 205(2):367–373.
38. Solbiati L, Ierace T, Goldberg SN, et al. Percutaneous US-guided radio-frequency tissue ablation of liver metastases: treatment and follow-up in 16 patients. Radiology 1997;202(1):195–203.
39. Chung YC, Duerk JL, Shankaranarayanan A, Hampke M, Merkle EM, Lewin JS. Temperature measurement using echo-shifted FLASH at low field for interventional MRI. J Magn Reson Imaging 1999;9:138–145.
40. Kahn T, Harth T, Bettag M, et al. Preliminary experience with the application of gadolinium-DTPA before MR imaging-guided laser-induced interstitial thermotherapy of brain tumors. J Magn Reson Imaging 1997;7(1):226–229.
41. Vogl TJ, Mack MG, Straub R, Roggan A, Felix R. Magnetic resonance imaging–guided abdominal interventional radiology: laser-induced thermotherapy of liver metastases. Endoscopy 1997; 29(6):577–583.
42. Liu H, Martin AJ, Truwit CL. Interventional MRI at high-field (1.5T): needle artifacts. J Magn Reson Imaging 1998;8(1):214–219.
43. Lewin JS, Nour SG, Duerk JL. Magnetic resonance image-guided biopsy and aspiration. Top Magn Reson Imaging 2000;11(3):173–183.
44. Lufkin R, Teresi L, Hanafee W. New needle for MR-guided aspiration cytology of the head and neck. AJR 1987;149(2):380–382.
45. Gronemeyer DH, Kaufman L, Rothschild P, Seibel RM. [New possibilities and aspects of low-field magnetic resonance tomography]. Radiol Diagn (Berl) 1989;30(4):519–527.
46. Lewin JS. Interventional MR imaging: concepts, systems, and applications in neuroradiology. AJNR 1999;20(5):735–748.
47. Hinks RS, Bronskill MJ, Kucharczyk W, Bernstein M, Collick BD, Henkelman RM. MR systems for image-guided therapy. J Magn Reson Imaging 1998;8(1):19–25.
48. Duerk JL, Lewin JS, Wendt M, Petersilge C. Remember true FISP? A high SNR, near 1-second imaging method for T2-like contrast in interventional MRI at .2T. J Magn Reson Imaging 1998;8(1):203–208.
49. Chung YC, Merkle EM, Lewin JS, Shonk JR, Duerk JL. Fast T(2)-weighted imaging by PSIF at 0.2T for interventional MRI. Magn Reson Med 1999;42(2):335–344.
50. Ladd ME, Erhart P, Debatin JF, Romanowski BJ, Boesiger P, McKinnon GC. Biopsy needle susceptibility artifacts. Magn Reson Med 1996; 36(4):646–651.
51. Lewin JS, Duerk JL, Jain VR, Petersilge CA, Chao CP, Haaga JR. Needle localization in MR-guided biopsy and aspiration: effects of field strength, sequence design, and magnetic field orientation. AJR 1996;166(6):1337–1345.
52. Bakker CJ, Smits HF, Bos C, et al. MR-guided balloon angioplasty: in vitro demonstration of the potential of MRI for guiding, monitoring, and evaluating endovascular interventions. J Magn Reson Imaging 1998;8(1):245–250.
53. Zhang Q, Chung YC, Lewin JS, Duerk JL. A method for simultaneous RF ablation and MRI. J Magn Reson Imaging 1998;8(1):110–114.
54. Patel KC, Duerk JL, Zhang Q, et al. Methods for providing probe position and temperature information on MR images during interventional procedures. IEEE Trans Med Imaging 1998; 17(5):794–802.
55. Dempsey MF, Condon B, Hadley DM. Investigation of the factors responsible for burns during MRI. J Magn Reson Imaging 2001;13(4):627–631.
56. Nitz WR, Oppelt A, Renz W, Manke C, Lenhart M, Link J. On the heating of linear conductive structures as guide wires and catheters in interventional MRI. J Magn Reson Imaging 2001; 13(1):105–114.
57. Duerk JL, Butts K, Hwang KP, Lewin JS. Pulse sequences for interventional magnetic resonance imaging. Top Magn Reson Imaging 2000;11(3): 147–162.
58. Lewin JS, Petersilge CA, Hatem SF, et al. Interactive MR imaging-guided biopsy and aspiration with a modified clinical C-arm system. AJR 1998; 170(6):1593–1601.
59. Botnar RM, Steiner P, Dubno B, Erhart P, von Schulthess GK, Debatin JF. Temperature quantification using the proton frequency shift technique: in vitro and in vivo validation in an open 0.5 tesla interventional MR scanner during RF ablation. J Magn Reson Imaging 2001;13(3): 437–444.
60. Matsumoto R, Oshio K, Jolesz FA. Monitoring of laser and freezing-induced ablation in the liver with T1-weighted MR imaging. J Magn Reson Imaging 1992;2(5):555–562.
61. Bleier AR, Jolesz FA, Cohen MS, et al. Real-time magnetic resonance imaging of laser heat deposition in tissue. Magn Reson Med 1991;21(1): 132–137.

62. Goldberg SN, Solbiati L, Halpern EF, Gazelle GS. Variables affecting proper system grounding for radiofrequency ablation in an animal model. J Vasc Intervent Radiol 2000;11(8):1069–1075.
63. Lewin JS. MR guides intervention and keeps costs down. Diagn Imaging (San Franc) 1998; Suppl Open MRI:MR22–MR24.
64. Livraghi T, Goldberg SN, Monti F, et al. Saline-enhanced radio-frequency tissue ablation in the treatment of liver metastases. Radiology 1997; 202(1):205–210.
65. Wildhirt E, Moller E. [Experience with nearly 20,000 blind liver punctures]. Med Klin 1981; 76(9):254–255,279.
66. Boaz TL, Lewin JS, Chung YC, Duerk JL, Clampitt ME, Haaga JR. MR monitoring of MR-guided radiofrequency thermal ablation of normal liver in an animal model. J Magn Reson Imaging 1998;8(1):64–69.
67. Anzai Y, Lufkin R, DeSalles A, Hamilton DR, Farahani K, Black KL. Preliminary experience with MR-guided thermal ablation of brain tumors. AJNR 1995;16(1):39–48.
68. Anzai Y, Brunberg JA, Lufkin RB. Imaging of nodal metastases in the head and neck. J Magn Reson Imaging 1997;7(5):774–783.
69. Aschoff AJ, Rafie N, Jesberger JA, Duerk JL, Lewin JS. Thermal lesion conspicuity following interstitial radiofrequency thermal tumor ablation in humans: a comparison of STIR, turbo spin-echo T2-weighted, and contrast-enhanced T1-weighted MR images at 0.2T. J Magn Reson Imaging 2000;12(4):584–589.
70. Smith SJ, Bosniak MA, Megibow AJ, Hulnick DH, Horii SC, Raghavendra BN. Renal cell carcinoma: earlier discovery and increased detection. Radiology 1989;170(3 pt 1):699–703.
71. Bosniak MA, Rofsky NM. Problems in the detection and characterization of small renal masses. Radiology 1996;198(3):638–641.
72. Rofsky NM, Bosniak MA. MR imaging in the evaluation of small (< or =3.0cm) renal masses. Magn Reson Imaging Clin North Am 1997;5(1): 67–81.
73. Motzer RJ, Bander NH, Nanus DM. Renal-cell carcinoma. N Engl J Med 1996;335(12):865–875.
74. Lerner SE, Hawkins CA, Blute ML, et al. Disease outcome in patients with low stage renal cell carcinoma treated with nephron sparing or radical surgery. 1996. J Urol 2002;167(2 pt 2):884–889.
75. Licht MR, Novick AC, Goormastic M. Nephron sparing surgery in incidental versus suspected renal cell carcinoma. J Urol 1994;152(1):39–42.
76. Kigure T, Harada T, Yuri Y, Satoh Y, Yoshida K. Laparoscopic microwave thermotherapy on small renal tumors: experimental studies using implanted VX-2 tumors in rabbits. Eur Urol 1996;30(3):377–382.
77. Lotfi MA, McCue P, Gomella LG. Laparoscopic interstitial contact laser ablation of renal lesions: an experimental model. J Endourol 1994;8(2): 153–156.
78. Watkin NA, Morris SB, Rivens IH, ter Haar GR. High-intensity focused ultrasound ablation of the kidney in a large animal model. J Endourol 1997;11(3):191–196.
79. Uchida M, Imaide Y, Sugimoto K, Uehara H, Watanabe H. Percutaneous cryosurgery for renal tumours. Br J Urol 1995;75(2):132–136.
80. Chosy SG, Nakada SY, Lee FT Jr, Warner TF. Monitoring renal cryosurgery: predictors of tissue necrosis in swine. J Urol 1998;159(4): 1370–1374.
81. Lewin J, Nour S, Connell C, Sulman A, Duerk J, Resnick MI. Followup Findings of a Phase II Clinical Trial of Interactive MR-Guided Interstitial Radiofrequency Thermal Ablation of Primary Kidney Tumors. Proceedings of the International Society of Magnetic Resonance in Medicine 2002;1:740.
82. Aschoff AJ, Merkle EM, Emancipator SN, Petersilge CA, Duerk JL, Lewin JS. Femur: MR imaging-guided radio-frequency ablation in a porcine model-feasibility study. Radiology 2002;225(2):471–478.
83. Nour SG, Aschoff AJ, Mitchell IC, Emancipator SN, Duerk JL, Lewin JS. MR imaging-guided radio-frequency thermal ablation of the lumbar vertebrae in porcine models. Radiology 2002; 224(2):452–462.
84. Goldberg SN, Gazelle GS, Dawson SL, Rittman WJ, Mueller PR, Rosenthal DI. Tissue ablation with radiofrequency using multiprobe arrays. Acad Radiol 1995;2(8):670–674.
85. Flask C, Elgort D, Wong E, Shankaranarayanan A, Lewin J, Wendt M. A method for fast 3D tracking using tuned fiducial markers and a limited projection reconstruction FISP (LPR-FISP) sequence. J Magn Reson Imaging 2001; 14(5):617–627.

14
Image Guidance and Control of Thermal Ablation

Ferenc A. Jolesz

The physical and biologic principles of localized high-temperature thermal therapy are well understood. If the targeted tissue volume is heated beyond 57° to 60°C, the threshold for protein denaturation, then coagulation necrosis occurs. This type of thermal treatment results in irreversible cell damage in both normal and neoplastic tissues. Since heat energy deposited above this critical level is not selective, thermal ablation is more comparable to surgery than to the more selective hyperthermia. In the case of cryoablation, the underlying physical and biologic principles are less well understood; nevertheless multiple freezings at a relatively low temperature also result in cell death.

Despite the straightforwardness of the thermal ablation approach, the clinical implementation of various ablative techniques has been challenging. There are multiple reasons for the slow and gradual translation of promising experimental results into clinical practice. Initially, these were mostly technical difficulties because of the lack of small, percutaneously introducible energy-delivery probes that fulfill the requirements of a minimally invasive intervention.

The use of optical fibers for interstitial laser therapy (ILT) and the medical application of radiofrequency (RF) and microwave devices significantly advanced the ablation field by allowing percutaneous treatment (1–4). Similarly, by substituting the larger liquid nitrogen–based probe that uses gas with much smaller devices, percutaneous cryoablation became a viable alternative to cryosurgery (5,6). Even a noninvasive, targeted heat deposition method, high-intensity focused ultrasound (HIFU), has reached technical maturity (7,8). This improvement and refinement of heat delivery devices are the primary reasons for the current emergence of minimally invasive ablation therapies. There are, however, additional obstacles that hinder a broader acceptance and further evolution of ablation methods. Among those the most important is the lack of appropriate "closed-loop" control of efficient and safe energy deposition.

Heat or cold transfer into deep-seated organs requires the introduction of the heat-conducting probes into the target volume without significant collateral tissue damage. Although most of the ablation methods use a relatively small-diameter probe, and therefore they are, in general, minimally invasive, these probes impose major limitations on the size and shape of thermally induced tissue injury. The thermal diffusion originating from these probes is influenced by the physical properties of the tissue, and the resulting geometry may not exactly correspond to the shape of the treated tumor. This mismatch can be corrected only if the size of the treated tissue volume increases to the extent that the irregular tumor outline fits into the larger geometrically fixed object boundary. This may result in the destruction of a substantial normal tissue margin, which sometimes is preferred in treating malignancies. The lesion size, however, in most cases cannot be increased indefinitely because of the developing balance or steady state between the rate of energy deposition and absorption. In most cases, tissue perfusion and the presence of blood flow profoundly influence and limit the size of the ablation.

The original intents of thermal ablative therapies are to confine the thermal coagulation to the target volume, and to prevent injury to the surrounding normal tissues. This goal cannot be achieved unless the exact three-dimensional (3D) extent of the target, and the spread (diffusion and convection) of the heat within and outside the targeted tissue volume are measured and monitored. To satisfy these fundamental requirements, image-guidance and image-guided therapy delivery control are necessary. Although thermal ablation of tumors is a well-known alternative to surgical excision, the control of destructive energy deposition has hitherto been an unresolved issue. The necessity for spatial and temporal temperature control is most obvious for the brain, where thermal damage must be limited to the target. It is less obvious in the liver that has plenty of tissue to "waste," unless the targeted volume is close to critical structures. It is imperative to establish the basic principles of image-guidance and image-based control for thermal ablative therapies.

The Principles of Image Guidance

In therapeutic procedures that require image guidance, imaging methods are used for localization, targeting, monitoring, and control (9). To develop and clinically implement image-guided ablations, it is essential to use all these components to achieve complete treatment of the targeted tissue volume, while minimizing the associated collateral damage to surrounding normal tissue.

Localization

The localization of tumor margins and the 3D definition of the targeted tumor volume are essential requirements for image-guided thermal therapy. The localization process is part of the preprocedural diagnostic workup and planning; this information must be updated by intraprocedural imaging as well The purpose of this localization is to identify and confine the exact spatial extent of the diseased tissue to be ablated, as well as to delineate the adjacent anatomic structures around that target volume. The full understanding of anatomic relationship within the entire operational volume is essential to define the potential access trajectories through which the thermal probes can be introduced with minimal tissue impairment (Fig. 14.1).

Localization not only provides a diagnostically relevant description of the target, but also is a target definition process used to plan and execute the therapy. The 3D model of the target and the operational volume within which the intervention will be carried out can be generated from localization that comes from multimodality imaging. For correct localization, not only tumor margins are defined, but also intratumoral features are important, for example, to differentiate the solid from the cystic part of a tumor and to distinguish necrotic tumor from viable neoplastic tissue. Contrast agents play a major role in characterizing tumor vascularity and/or tumor boundaries. Dynamic contrast enhancement can characterize tumor perfusion, which is essential information for thermal ablation.

Localization of tumors is required to define the ultimate target volume. The target volume is not necessarily identical to the tumor volume. In thermal therapies, as in surgery, when possible the target should be larger than the targeted tumor to assure a substantial "surgical" margin. This is the case with liver and breast tumors during which the parenchyma beyond the detected tumor boundary can be ablated. In the case of prostate ablation, the treatment should be confined to an anatomically defined target, irrespective of tumor margins. Therapy planning for brain tumor ablation should consider the presence of essential functional areas that may overlap with the tumor, and in that case, the target may be smaller than the tumor volume. In the case of benign tumor ablation, such as uterine fibroids, we may elect partial tumor ablation so the target may represent only a fraction of the overall tumor volume.

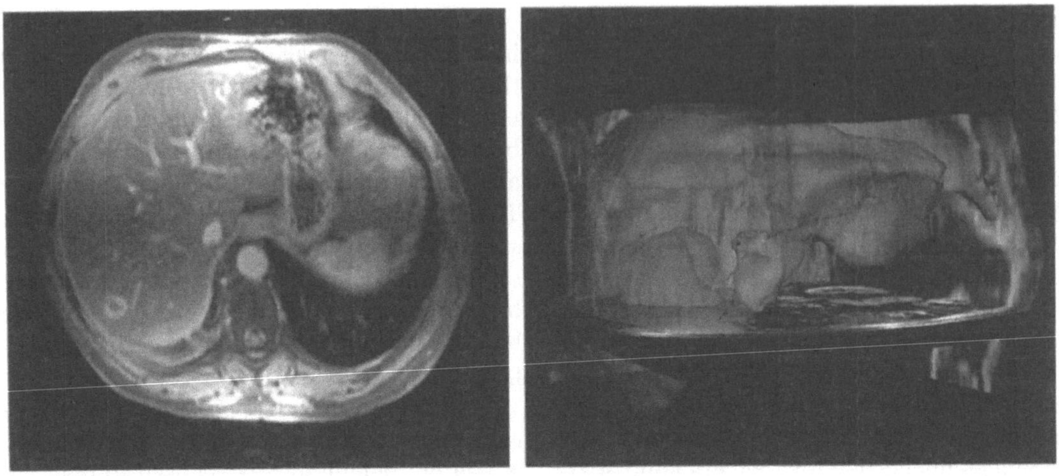

FIGURE 14.1. Localization of the tumor is the initial step in an image-guided thermal ablation procedure. This takes place during the diagnosis and planning stages of a patient's care. The purpose is to identify the location and spatial extent of the diseased tissue. (A) The axial contrast-enhanced MRI reveals a solitary 2×2 cm metastasis in segment 7 of the liver in a 62-year-old man. (B) Three-dimensional (3D) visualization of the patient's image data provides anatomic context for the tumor. Superimposed in this 3D space are the original axial MRI images (seen just below the gallbladder, perpendicular to the plane of the Figure). (Images provided by Stuart G. Silverman.)

Complete tumor destruction of most malignant tumors is unachievable because of ill-defined tumor margins and the limited sensitivity of imaging. The frequent failure of thermal therapy methods is the direct consequence of this inaccurate target definition. Cure is easier if the tumor is well defined. Conversely, in cases of ill-defined, diffuse, infiltrative malignant tumor, cure is an extremely difficult task and likely impossible. Tumor-seeking contrast agents and biomarkers can improve not only the detection of tumors, but also the effectiveness of thermal therapies. Improving image quality and spatial resolution by applying multimodality imaging is essential to define the full extent of more invasive malignancies, such as cerebral glioma and breast cancer.

Targeting

Target definition is followed by the selection of potential access routes. This targeting process is essentially therapy planning that involves choosing a single trajectory from multiple possible trajectories. This targeting allows the insertion of thermal probes and matching of the predefined thermal volume with the target volume.

Conceptually, the single-trajectory biopsy is a key element of several therapeutic procedures in which the insertion of needles or other therapy-delivery probes becomes necessary. For accurate targeting, a more or less correct anatomic model has to be generated from preprocedural or intraprocedural images. In the case of preoperatively obtained image data, this model should be registered to the actual patient. If there are shifts and/or deformations of soft tissues, the preoperative image-based 3D models should be updated or corrected using elastic warping algorithms or other more elaborate computer-based methods.

Single trajectory procedures like biopsy or thermal probe insertion require intraprocedural imaging for targeting, especially in the case of mobile, deformable, or unstable soft tissue organs. The combined or integrated localization and targeting process can be achieved either with real-time or close to real-time imaging methods like x-ray fluoroscopy, computed tomography (CT) fluoroscopy, ultrasound (US), or intraoperative magnetic resonance imaging (MRI). Projectional or two-dimensional imaging methods, especially when integrated with navigational techniques, are suitable for interactive targeting; this involves real-time planning by the interventionalist. Using nearly real-time cross-sectional methods, such as US, CT, or MRI fluoroscopy, interactive localization and targeting are possible if the probe position can be tracked continuously during the procedure by various optical and nonoptical sensors. Interventional MRI systems (IMRI) with multiplanar imaging capability and with navigational tools can operate like US by using interactive scanning of the entire operational volume (Fig. 14.2) (10).

This selection of optimal trajectories for thermal probes is the only image-guidance method in most currently practiced thermal ablations. Only a limited number of application sites create a 3D model of the operational volume, target volume, and predicted thermal treatment volume. These 3D models should be distinctly separated from each other and should be individually highlighted to facilitate the simulation and planning process.

Planning for thermal ablation and radiation therapy has substantial similarities. Both require the creation of a 3D volumetric model, target definition, optimization of access routes, and the avoidance of important normal anatomic structures. Radiation plans are based entirely on predictions for delayed biologic effects. Plans for thermal ablation also should include thermal dosimetry, as well as the estimation of acute and late effects.

Monitoring

Real-time or nearly real-time monitoring of temperature and thermally induced changes and other functional or physical parameters that may be altered or modified during ablation procedures is possible. Direct measurement or mapping of temperature distribution is possible only with multiple invasive probes. The number of temperature-sensitive probes usually is insufficient to monitor properly the 3D distribution of energy. Besides, these measurements do not signal the irreversible cellular impairment that is the desired end point of these thermal ablations.

The various physical probes that are used with the imaging system reflect the interaction between the thermal energy and the tissue. A wide variety of imaging parameters can be used to monitor temperature. There are considerable differences between imaging systems and how they detect the spread of thermal energy. Each imaging modality has its own limitations that are defined by their physical characteristics. The monitoring capabilities of imaging systems can be compared, using certain specific attributes such as temperature-sensitivity, temporal resolution, adequacy for volumetric imaging, and ease of use during procedures. Real-time monitoring devices, x-ray fluoroscopy and US are inexpensive methods to monitor the location and position of thermal probes, but they are insensitive to thermal changes. Similarly, CT has no substantial sensitivity to detect temperature changes. Temperature-sensitive MRI techniques are fundamental for MRI-guided interventional procedures or for MRI-guided ablations. The ability of MRI to detect temperature changes initiated and motivated the evolution of IMRI from a relatively simple image-guidance method used for biopsies to a complex tool to monitor and control thermal ablations, other minimally invasive percutaneous procedures, and eventually endoscopies and open surgery (Fig. 14.3).

The 3D extent of the thermal injury cannot be verified without volumetric imaging. To kill tissue with heat, the critical dose of thermal energy has to be delivered, and at least a 60°C isotherm should envelop the entire mass. This requires not only accurate target definition in 3D, but also temperature-sensitive imaging methods that can limit the deposition of destructive energy within the lesion and detect potential thermal energy spread to the surrounding normal tissue. This monitoring permits the thermal ablative treatment to be highly effective and, at the same time, relatively safe. During monitoring of thermal ablations, tissue characterization still is essential. It is needed to provide

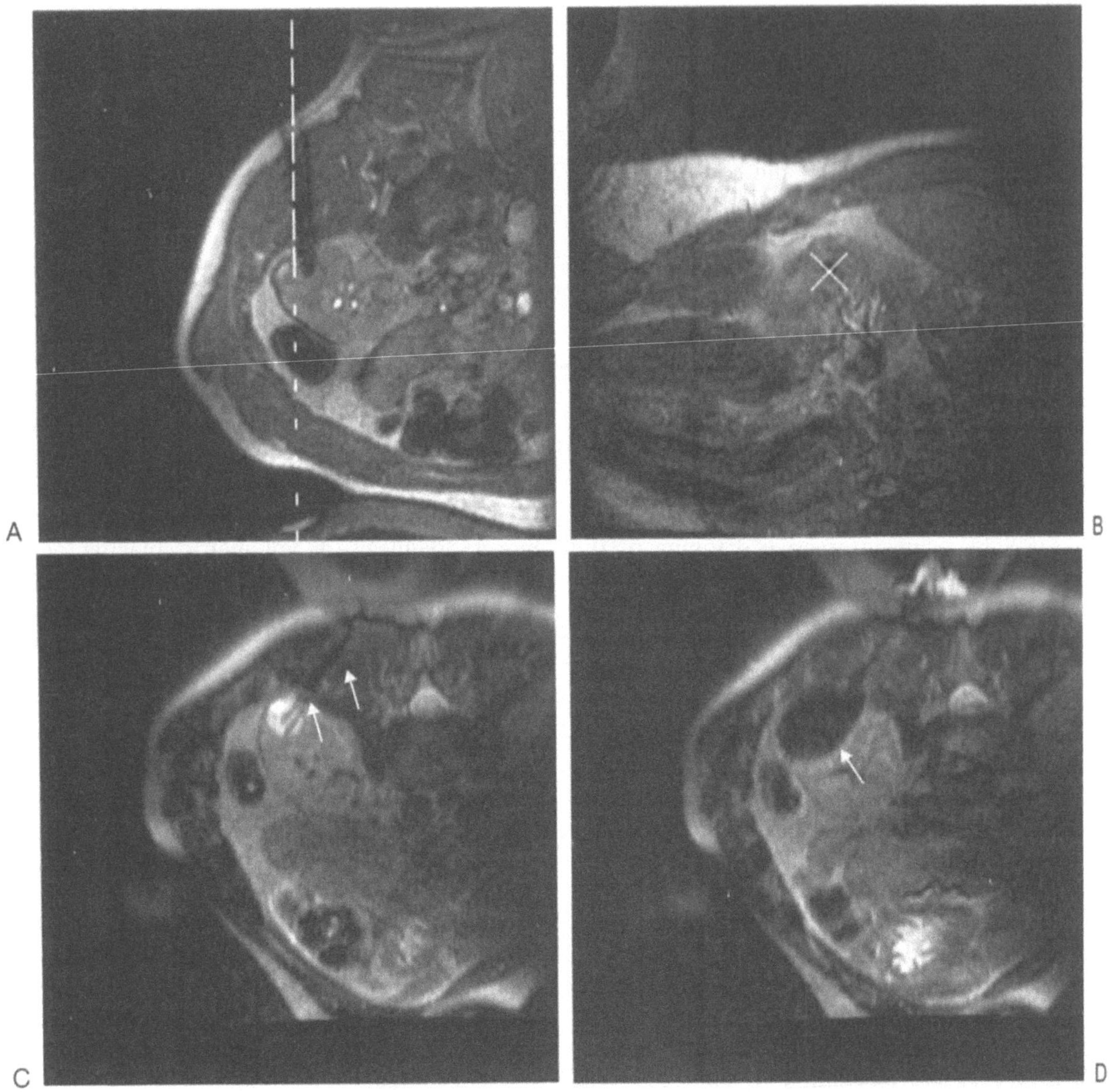

FIGURE 14.2. Targeting is performed intraprocedurally. It relies on localization and planning efforts, as well as intraprocedural imaging. This targeting process implements the treatment planning and involves choosing a single trajectory from multiple possible trajectories for the insertion of each thermal probe, and matching the predefined thermal volume with the target volume. Here, a kidney tumor is targeted for percutaneous cryoablation under prone MRI guidance. (A) An oblique axial image is acquired in plane with a needle during the procedure. The image data are supplemented by an icon (central, vertical dashed line) that is registered to the handle of the needle and assists in the targeting. The oblique sagittal image (B) is orthogonal to A, and is perpendicular to the needle; the icon (crosshair) provides added trajectory information. (C) Targeting is complete with the placement of two probes (arrows) for effective coverage of the hyperintense tumor by the iceball (signal void in D) (arrows). (Images provided by Stuart G. Silverman.)

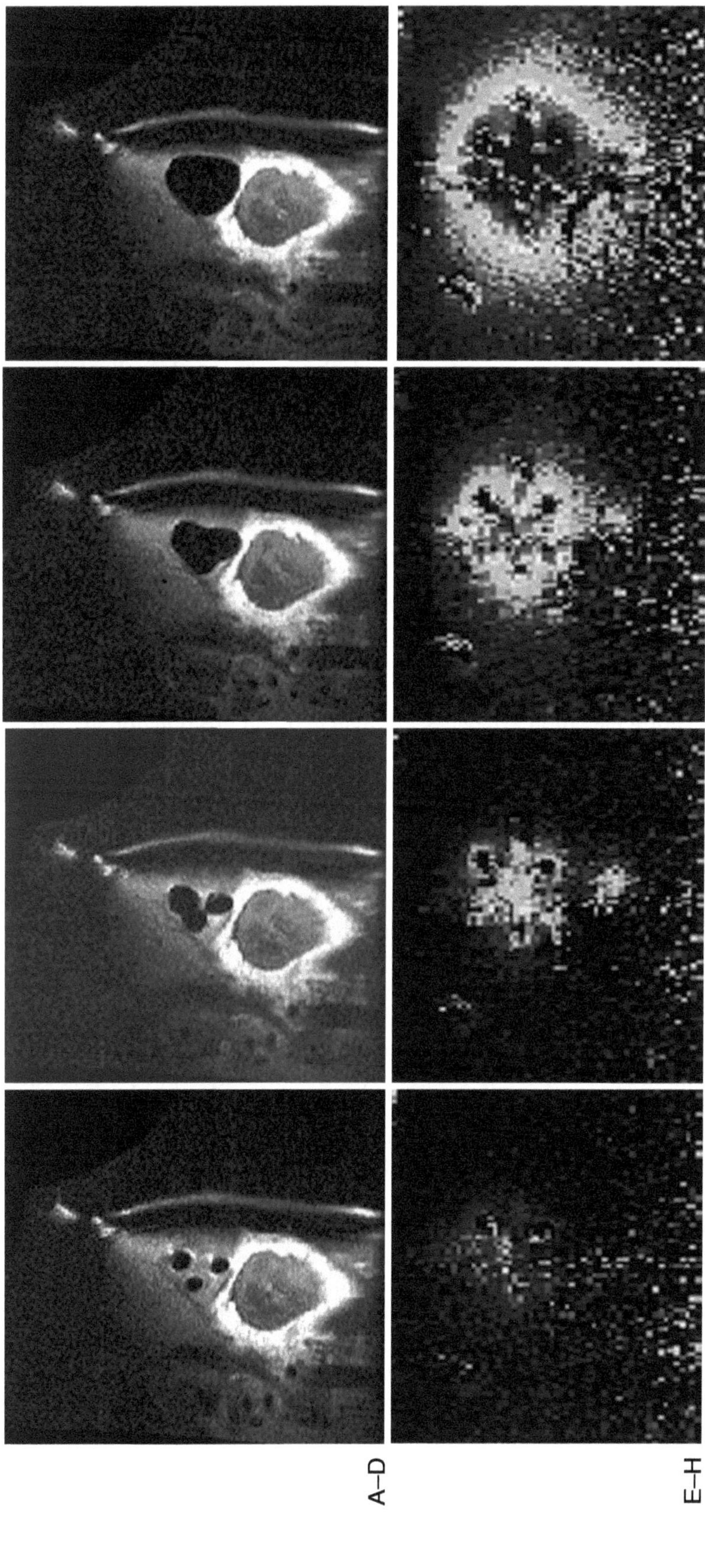

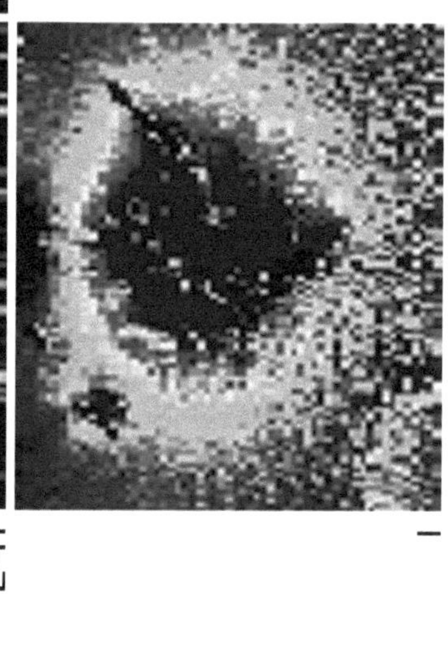

FIGURE 14.3. (A–I) Monitoring must provide suitable spatial and temporal resolution for visualization of the thermal event in tissue. "Real-time" imaging of a more slowly developing iceball during cryotherapy does not require the frequency of image updates that a more rapid radiofrequency (RF) ablation does. In the top row, three-probe cryotherapy in the liver is monitored by MRI; the ice is seen clearly as the developing region of signal void. In the bottom row, heating with an array-type RF probe is monitored by fast thermal MRI. (Cryotherapy images provided by Stuart G. Silverman; RF images provided by Osamu Kainuma.)

information as the procedure progresses and the original tissue undergoes phase transitions. The detection of these coagulative processes provides a relatively simple way to follow the progress of thermal ablations by detecting the changes in tissue integrity. In a limited way, both CT and US can be used for this "thumb-printing" method when the ablated tissue is somewhat distinguishable from the intact one. Sequential imaging steps can follow the progressive tissue coagulation.

Thermally induced phase transitions are best revealed on MR images; therefore, short of thermal monitoring, this thumb-printing method is applicable for MRI-guided thermal interventions. The temperature-sensitivity of various MR parameters [primarily inversion time (TI), diffusion, and chemical shift] can be exploited to detect temperature changes within a critical temperature range (11–14). Also, appropriate MR sequences can distinguish phase transitions within the thermally treated tissue volume, and can verify normal margins that encompass the thermal lesions. Beyond these edges, the temperature elevation still is visible with MR, but is low enough to rule out cell necrosis.

The role of MRI in thermal ablative therapy is twofold. First, real-time MRI with temperature-sensitive pulse sequences can detect the transient temperature elevations. Using this intraoperative information, the operator can confine the thermal treatment to the target tissue and can prevent the unwanted heating of surrounding normal tissue by discontinuing the energy delivery. The second role of MRI is to delineate irreversible tissue necrosis. MR images taken intraprocedurally, but immediately after the actual treatment (i.e., delivery of a thermal dose), can verify the permanent changes within the treated tissue volume and present important information about the spatial extent of thermal ablation. For the safe and efficient delivery of destructive energy, however, images should be taken not only after, but also during the energy transfer.

Monitoring of temperature changes and/or thermally induced tissue changes is essential within the targeted volume to achieve complete tissue kill. Heterogeneous thermal maps are useful, and cold spots within RF and laser ablations have been shown. Similarly, hot spots can be present within on iceball during cryotherapy. Outside the target volume, these changes also should be monitored to assure safety and prevent damage of normal tissue.

Control

Originally the role of image guidance during thermal ablations was limited to the introduction of various probes through which the treatment was accomplished. Although correct positioning of the probes within the lesions is extremely important, imaging should continue during the energy delivery as well. The increased role of monitoring should result in the implementation of quantitative imaging, based on control techniques with heat sensitive advanced image-guidance methods.

Imaging is important for optimal energy delivery during thermal ablations. This image-based control can be accomplished only if the temperature-sensitivity of the imaging systems and the technical capabilities of the therapy devices are matched and are functionally integrated. To monitor the progressive enlargement and reduction of the "iceball" or the expansion of heat-treated tissue volumes, the time constant of the freezing process or thermal diffusion should be matched with the temporal resolution of the particular imaging modality. Within this time limit, multiplanar, multislice, or volumetric imaging should be applied to provide a correct 3D description of the process (Fig. 14.4).

Both the temporal and spatial resolution of imaging has to satisfy the requirements for the closed loop control of a thermal ablation. The magnitude and time constants of thermal diffusion should be seriously considered before an image-guided therapy procedure is conceived, developed, and implemented. For feasibility, the limitations of the imaging systems, compatibility between the imaging and therapy devices, and the safety features of both, should be taken into account before the initiation of the full integration process.

The immediate visibility of a physiologic effect of a thermal intervention (such as perfusion or metabolic response to elevated temperature) is potentially achievable for sophisticated control of the procedure. Such control assures that

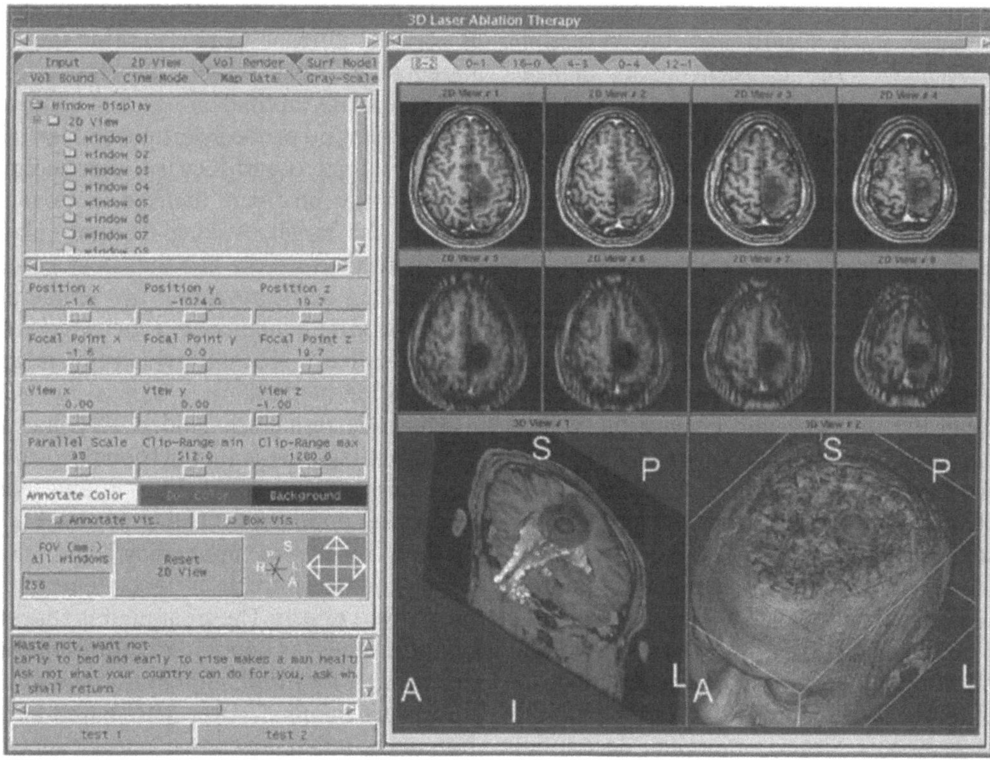

FIGURE 14.4. Control of ablation is an extension of monitoring. It is achieved by the interpretation of the visualized effects. This requires an understanding of the relationship between the reversible thermal effects and irreversible sequelae. Further, this must be done in the context of the relevant anatomy—both the targeted tissues and those adjacent structures to be spared. The figure shows the user interface of thermal therapy control software that provides a multiplanar presentation of intraprocedural data. In the upper half of the display screen, a set of eight contiguous axial images through the head is displayed. In the lower half of the display screen are 3D views of the tumor with a superimposed colorization of the temperature (left) and thermal dose (right). (Image provided by Pairash Saiviroonporn.)

the temperature-induced physiologic effect never reaches a critical threshold of irreversible thermal damage. During thermal treatment, there are significant changes in the state of blood vessels. Both vasoconstriction and vasodilatation can occur, depending on the actual temperature levels. These functional data can be used to control energy deposition and adjust the level of temperature within the treated volume.

Discussion

Interstitial laser thermotherapy (ILT), RF heating, and cryoablation all have important constraints in delivering the required energy dose through a probe placed within tumors. The probe's size and position, the physical properties of the tissue, and the form and duty cycle of the energy delivery ultimately will limit the spatial distribution of the effects. The size and shape of the thermal coagulation has to conform to the 3D configuration of the tumor. Preoperative 3D treatment planning and dosimetry are essential to optimize energy delivery (2). However, in some cases this solution is impractical because it requires successive repositioning of the probes or the insertion of multiple probes, all of which increase the likelihood of complications.

The limitation of heat-induced, probe-delivered thermal ablations is the presence of a large thermal gradient that results in the ambiguity of the demarcation zone between the irreversible tissue death and the reversible tissue damage. The transient tissue damage results in tissue survival and subsequent tumor recurrence. The unpredictable separation of treated and untreated volumes remains an unresolved problem. The only solution is to use only the central, high-temperature zone of the large thermal gradient for tumor treatment, and to disregard the rest of the heat deposition as most likely ineffective. This requires temperature sensitive imaging with MRI techniques. This real-time MRI monitoring is useful in recognizing the diffusion and convection of heat within the inhomogeneous tissue environment, where both the presence of variable microvasculature and the occurrence of larger blood vessels can modify the treatment plans. Flow and tissue perfusion both can influence the rate and extent of energy delivery and the resulting size of the treated tissue volumes. Constant monitoring of the procedure provides input for potential control methods that optimize treatment protocols. Since the original description of MRI monitoring and control of laser-tissue interactions (15), MRI-guided tissue ablation has become a clinically tested and an accepted minimally invasive treatment option. It is a relatively simple, straightforward method that can be well adapted to the interventional MRI environment.

Although RF treatment is basically the same as ILT (both based on thermal coagulation), there are differences in the resulting lesion size. The optical laser fiber has a relatively small heating surface, while the RF probe can cook a larger tissue volume. The tip of the optical fiber can be extremely hot, resulting in charring, which prevents the spread of the optical energy. The RF probe never reaches that high temperature (by internal cooling or stepwise power increases), and thus the thermal diffusion effect can be enhanced. Most RF treatments have been accomplished without temperature-sensitive imaging, and MRI has been used only to detect the resulting coagulative lesion. The incompatibility of RF energy deposition and MRI has been resolved, and MRI-guided RF ablations have become a reality (16–18).

The most appealing thermal ablation method is focused ultrasound (FUS). This method is based on primary acoustic energy deposition and secondary thermal effects. It is noninvasive and requires no probe insertion, and the appropriately targeted and focused high-energy US beam causes no tissue damage in front of or beyond the target. Among thermal ablations, the noninvasive FUS has the most potential. Introducing and integrating the temperature-sensitive MRI guidance into the targeting and energy delivery process revived this relatively old ablation method.

Magnetic resonance–guided FUS has some key advantages: It is nonincisional, so there is no entry tract of destruction. Spatial control is precise, predictable, and reproducible. The method results in nonhemorrhagic, sharply demarcated lesions. It is instantaneous, with no delayed effects. The treatment is repeatable multiple times (as opposed to radiosurgery). Its effects are localized and nonsystemic; aftereffects are minimal. After MRI-based localization of the target, low power energy deposition is used to target—a nondestructive "test" pulse. The MRI-detectable small temperature elevation within the few-millimeter diameter focal spot causes no permanent tissue damage, but can be located. When targeting is accomplished, the power level can be increased to achieve irreversible tissue damage. This method is now under clinical testing for the treatment of benign and malignant breast lesions, uterine fibroids, and brain tumors (7,8).

The most serious shortcoming of thermal ablative treatment of malignant tumors is the lack of precise target definition by MRI. The surgical concept of well-defined tumor masses is incorrect. Instead, there are spatially disseminated tumor cells that may spread beyond the reach of the thermal treatment. This is a serious handicap for both conventional and minimally invasive approaches. Nevertheless, if cure is not anticipated, a less invasive procedure is more justifiable for palliation.

Image-guided thermal ablation requires the integration of therapeutic devices with imaging systems. This integration is a prerequisite of image-guided therapy: both location and feedback control of the energy disposition call for a fully integrated system. We are entering a new area of combined diagnostic and therapeutic applications that involve high technology. There are still unresolved problems, and most important is the lack of sufficient data to establish the clinical efficacy of the minimally invasive techniques under trial. The few MRI-guided thermal ablations already performed contribute to the evaluation of the feasibility of these techniques.

Image-guided thermal therapy is an interdisciplinary effort. Not only radiologists but also other medical disciplines, computer scientists, engineers, and physicists are contributing to the development of this exciting new application. The goal is to take advantage of advanced imaging technologies—MRI, therapy systems, and computers—to make this exciting technology clinically more applicable, safe, and efficient.

References

1. Bleier AR, Jolesz FA, Cohen MS, et al. Real time magnetic resonance imaging of laser heat deposition in tissue. Magn Reson Med 1991;21:132–137.
2. Puccini S, Bar, N-K, Bublat M, Kahn T, Busse H. Simulations of thermal tissue coagulation and their value for the planning and monitoring of laser-induced interstitial theremotherapy (LITT). Magn Reson Med 2003;49:351–362.
3. Livraghi L, Goldberg SN, Lazzaroni S, Meloni F, Solbiati L, Gazelle GS. Small hepatocellular carcinoma: treatment with radio-frequency ablation versus ethanol injection. Radiology 1999;210:655–661.
4. Goldberg SN, Stein MC, Gazelle GS, Sheiman RG, Kruskal JB, Clouse ME. Percutaneous radiofrequency tissue ablation: optimization of pulsed-radiofrequency technique to increase coagulation necrosis. J Vasc Intervent Radiol 1999;10:907–916.
5. Silverman SG, Tuncali K, Adams DF, et al. MR imaging-guided percutaneous cryotherapy of liver tumors: initial experience. Radiology 2000;217:657–664.
6. Matsumoto R, Mulkern RV, Hushek SG, Jolesz FA. Tissue temperature monitoring for thermal interventional therapy: comparison of TI-weighted MR sequences. J Magn Reson Imaging 1994;4:65–70.
7. Jolesz FA, Hynynen K. Magnetic resonance image-guided focused ultrasound surgery. Cancer J 2002;8(suppl 1):S100–12.
8. Hynynen K, Pomeroy O, Smith DN, et al. MR imaging-guided focused ultrasound surgery of fibroadenomas in the breast: a feasibility study. Radiology 2001;219:176–185.
9. Jolesz FA. Image-guided procedures and the operating room of the future. Radiology 1997;204:601–612.
10. Jolesz FA, Nabavi A, Kikinis R. Integration of interventional MRI with computer-assisted surgery. J Magn Reson Imaging 2001;13:69–77.
11. Kuroda K, Chung AH, Hynynen K, Jolesz FA. Calibration of water proton chemical shift with temperature for noninvasive temperature imaging during focused ultrasound surgery. J Magn Reson Imaging 1998;8:175–181.
12. Stollberger R, Ascher PW, Huber D, Renhart W, Radner H, Ebner F. Temperature monitoring of interstitial thermal tissue coagulation using MR phase images. J Magn Reson Imaging 1997;8:188–196.
13. Chung AH, Hynynen K, Colucci V, Oshio K, Cline HE, Jolesz FA. Optimization of spoiled gradient-echo phase imaging for in vivo localization of a focused ultrasound beam. Magn Reson Med 1996;36:745–752.
14. Kuroda K, Abe K, Tsutsumi S, Ishihara Y, Suzuki Y, Sato K. Water proton magnetic resonance spectroscopic imaging. Biomed Thermol 1994;13:43–62.
15. Jolesz FA, Bleier AR, Jakab P, Ruenzel PW, Huttl K, Jako GJ. MR imaging of laser-tissue interactions. Radiology 1988;168:249–253.
16. Lewin JS, Connell CF, Duerk JL, et al. Interactive MRI-guided radiofrequency interstitial thermal ablation of abdominal tumors: clinical trial for evaluation of safety and feasibility. J Magn Reson Imaging 1998;8:40–45.
17. Steiner P, Botnar R, Dubno B, Zimmermann GG, Gazelle GS, Debatin JF. Radio-frequency-induced thermoablation: monitoring with T1-weighted and proton-frequency-shift MR imaging in an interventional 0.5T environment. Radiology 1998;206:803–810.
18. Zhang Q, Chung YC, Lewin JS, Duerk JL. A method for simultaneous RF ablation and MRI. J Magn Reson Imaging 1998;8:110–114.

Section IV
Methods of Ablation

15 Percutaneous Ethanol Injection Therapy

Tito Livraghi and Maria Franca Meloni

Percutaneous ethanol injection therapy (PEIT) is one of the most widely used local procedures to treat hepatocellular carcinoma (HCC). Local-regional therapies are specific ablation modalities that introduce a damaging agent directly into the neoplastic tissue percutaneously. These techniques are capable of destroying the tissue chemically, such as with sterile ethanol acetic acid, ,or thermally by laser, microwave, or radiofrequency (1–3). Percutaneous ethanol injection therapy was the first method to be proposed (4). It was conceived independently at the University of Chiba in Japan and at the Vimercate Hospital in Milan, Italy.

Initially PEIT was targeted as a palliative treatment for nonsurgical patients who had primary or metastatic liver lesions (4). At the Barcelona Conference in 2000, percutaneous techniques were classified as a curative treatment for HCC (5), based on complete response obtained in selected patients (6,7). Hepatocellular carcinoma is a multicentric disease; indeed, the first nodule is only a prelude to others. Local-regional therapies can be used alone or in combination with other treatment modalities for long-range therapy.

Principles and Procedure

Alcohol acts by diffusion into cells and causes immediate dehydration of cytoplasmic proteins with consequent coagulation necrosis. This is followed by fibrosis. By entering into the circulation, alcohol induces necrosis of endothelial cells and platelet aggregation; consequent thrombosis of small vessels is followed by ischemia of the neoplastic tissue. Two characteristics of HCC favor the toxic action of ethanol: hypervascularization and the different consistency of neoplastic versus cirrhotic tissue. Since the neoplastic tissue of HCC is softer than the surrounding cirrhotic tissue, ethanol diffuses within it easily and selectively. Similarly, hypervascularization facilitates the uniform distribution of alcohol within the rich network of neoplastic vessels.

Percutaneous ethanol injection therapy is performed in multiple sessions in an ambulatory regimen (conventional technique), or, when the tumor is more advanced, in a single session under general anesthesia with hospitalization. The former technique is generally used for a single HCC that is less than 4 to 5 cm in diameter or for multiple HCCs with two to three nodules, <3 cm in diameter. The latter technique is adopted for intermediate HCCs, single or multiple, that do not occupy more than 30% of the hepatic volume, and with no tumor thrombus in the main portal vein branches or in the hepatic veins.

Equipment

Percutaneous ethanol injection therapy usually is performed under ultrasound (US) guidance because real-time control allows faster execution, precise centering of the needle in the target, continuous monitoring of ethanol distribution, and determination of the appropriate amount of ethanol to be injected. In some centers computed tomography (CT) guidance is used (8,9). The advantage of CT is greatest in treating large tumors, in which multiple needle placements may be necessary to ablate the lesion completely. In these cases, CT enables direct visualization of areas of tumor necrosis, and identifies potentially untreated areas within the tumor. However, CT guidance does not permit real-time visualization of the diffusion of ethanol.

We use a commercially available US scanner with a 3.5-MHz convex probe that has an incorporated, lateral needle guide. The needle is fine-caliber (21 gauge) with a closed conical tip and three terminal side holes (PEIT, Hakko, Tokyo, Japan). The alcohol is sterile 95%.

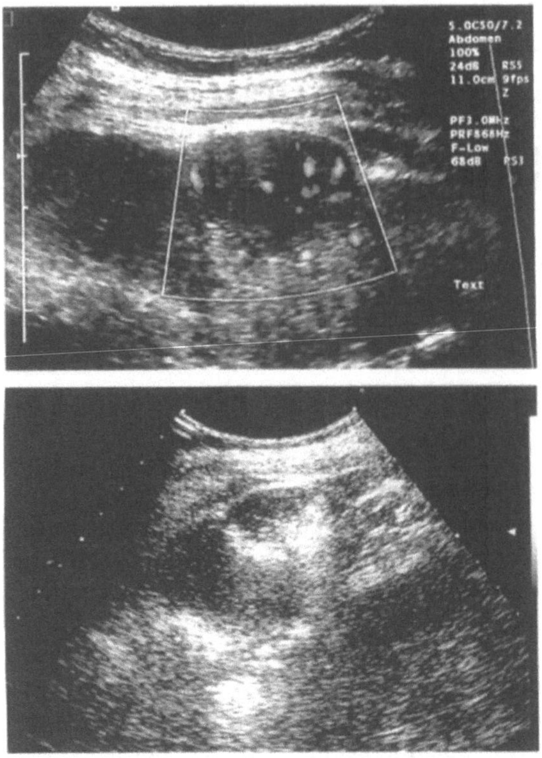

A
B

FIGURE 15.1. (A) Encapsulated hepatocellular carcinoma, 2.5 cm in size, located in segment 6 and vascularized on the power-doppler. (B) Treatment with PEI in multiple sessions: the ethanol echogenic diffuses within the neoplastic vessels shown by power-doppler.

Conventional Technique

The treatment usually is performed without sedation or local anesthesia. Patients must fast because nausea may occur, although it is rare. After local disinfection of skin with iodized alcohol, which also is used as a contact medium, the best approach is chosen. For lesions situated in the right lobe of the liver, an intercostal approach with the patient lying on the left side often is preferable. During insertion and retraction of the needle, the patient is asked to stop breathing, and during the injection to breathe slowly. In the same session, 1 to 8 mL of ethanol are injected, with one or more injections, in different areas depending on the distribution of ethanol, the tolerance of the patient, the size of the tumor, the degree of vascularizaton, and the presence or absence of septations. The area perfused by ethanol clearly is visible as hyperechoic. The ethanol is injected slowly and the diffusion is controlled by real-time US monitoring (Fig. 15.1). The alcohol usually diffuses for a radius of 2 to 3 cm around the needle tip toward the periphery of the tumor.

The injection is stopped if there is a significant leakage of ethanol outside the lesion, or if diffusion is not clearly visible. The infusion can be repeated after a few minutes. Significant leakage of ethanol is unusual because the surrounding cirrhotic tissue, of greater consistency, forms a barrier. Good diffusion of ethanol is not seen in the focal multinodular confluent variant of HCC because the fibrotic component alternates with neoplastic tissue.

Durig the initial session of PEIT, when the tumor is still largely viable, ethanol is easily eliminated by the rich neoplastic circulation. Injection is continued intermittently in small boluses until the ethanol is seen to remain within the lesion. Since alcohol reflux can cause pain, the needle is left within the tumor for 30 to 40 seconds after the injection, particularly in the case of superficial lesions, and then is removed slowly.

The site of the injection is chosen before each session to ensure perfusion of the areas previously considered untreated. Color-Doppler examination, particularly with echo enhancers, indicates the areas of viable tissue in which signs of vascularization persist. Each session generally requires 10 to 20 minutes, and the patient remains in the waiting room for 1 to 2 hours after the procedure. The treatment usually is performed twice weekly. Therapy is finished when perfusion of the tumor is considered complete, and when no vascular signs are detectable after US-contrast enhancement (Fig. 15.2).

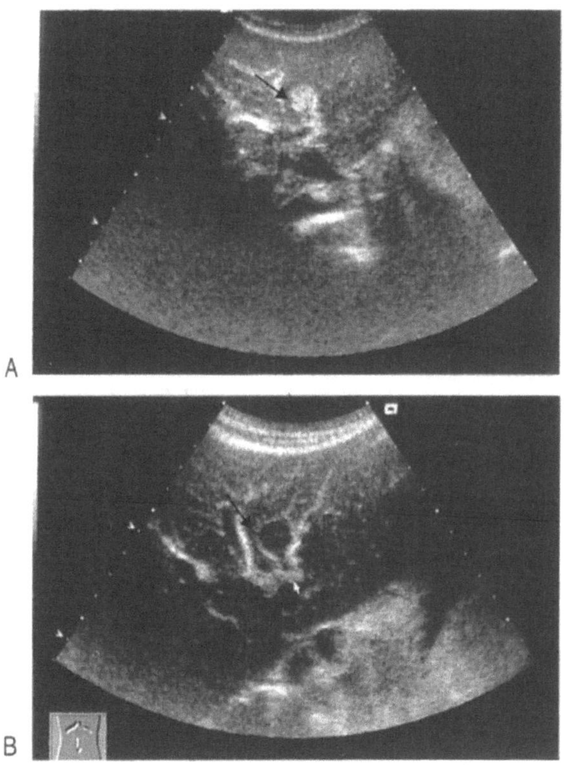

FIGURE 15.2. (A) Small hepatocellularcarcinoma 1.2 cm in size located in the left lobe vascularized at the USCA examination. (B) No enhancement immediately after PEI multisession treatment at contrast-enhanced examination.

We treat lesions <2 cm in size in three to four sessions, those of 2 to 3 cm in four to six sessions, and lesions of 3.5 to 5 cm in six to ten sessions. The number of sessions is thus approximately twice the diameter of the lesion, although it is difficult to establish a priori the number of sessions or the exact quantity of ethanol to be administered. This therapy also can be used to treat tumor thrombus with portal vein (10) when the thrombus is segmental or subsegmental or to arrest progression toward the main branches. In this case, the tip of the needle is positioned precisely within the thrombus, so the ethanol can diffuse selectively.

Single-Session Technique

Treatment in a single session is performed with the patient under general anesthesia, with tracheal intubation, and mechanical ventilation, to administer an *ad libitum* quantity of ethanol. The technique adapts well to operative requirements, for example, to obtain a period of controlled apnea in the respiratory phase judged most appropriate. The deepest portions of the lesion are treated first, followed by the central portion, and last, the most superficial portions of the lesions. This sequence prevents an initial superficial diffusion of ethanol, which, owing to its hyperechogenicity, would impede the guidance of successive injections. Direct injection of ethanol into hepatic veins must be avoided, because sudden, high concentrations of alcohol in the bloodstream may lead to prolonged hypoxemia, followed by cardiopulmonary collapse.

The treatment is concluded when the tumor appears completely hyperechoic (Fig. 15.3). The total time required for the procedure ranges from 20 to 60 minutes, depending on the number and size of the lesions to be treated. In any case, the total amount of ethanol always is less than the volume of the tumor. In the days immediately following the treatment, formation of gas within the lesion occurs, particularly when more than 50 mL of ethanol have been administered.

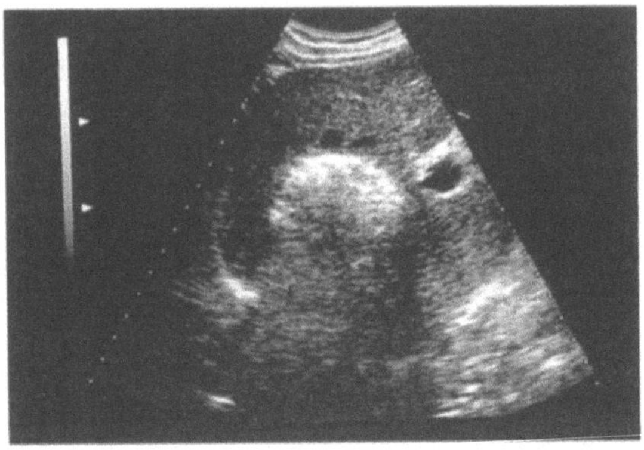

FIGURE 15.3. Single encapsulated hepatocellular carcinoma 6 cm in size, shown by US, located in the right lobe, at the end of the treatment with single-session PEI is quite echogenic.

Adverse Effects and Complications

Conventional Treatment

Most patients complain of mild pain during or immediately after the injection, but it is usually well tolerated and does not prevent normal daily activities. The pain usually is restricted to the injection site, but patients sometimes complain of pain in the right shoulder or epigastric region. Patients who complain of severe pain after the first session are given an analgesic before each subsequent session.

No death occurred in 1623 patients treated with conventional PEIT, collected from various series (6). In a multicenter study that included 1066 patients, one death (0.09%) was reported due to hemoperitoneum and subsequent hepatic coma (11). Two other anecdotal cases of death have been reported: one due to a massive area of hepatic necrosis distant from the site of injection of ethanol, and one to myocardial infarction. In the latter case, there was no direct correlation between the two events (12); in the former case, the massive hepatic necrosis was caused by an intratumoral arterioportal shunt that allowed ethanol to spread through the blood vessels (13). Major complications are rare, and occur in 1.3% to 3.2% of cases; they generally are treated conservatively (6,11).

Cases of neoplastic seeding along the needle tract have been reported, particularly in moderately differentiated tumors (6,11,14).

Single-Session Treatment

Greater volumes of ethanol per session correlate with a higher complication rate (15). Some cases of alcohol intoxication have been observed, but they do not require therapy. High levels of alcoholemia normalize within 24 hours. Abdominal pain may last 2 to 3 days, and is controlled with analgesic treatment. Hyperpyrexia for a few days is observed routinely in patients administered more than 50 mL of alcohol. During the first day of treatment, there is an increase in transaminases, bilirubin, d-dimer, and white blood cells, and a reduction in fibrinogen, haptoglobin, hemoglobin, platelets, and red blood cells. These effects usually normalize within 2 weeks. The changes are due to necrosis of neoplastic tissue, and diffuse intra- and peritumoral microthrombosis and hemolysis. In our initial 111 treatments, when contraindications were not yet well known, there was one death due to bleeding from esophageal varices; this occurred on the third postprocedural day in a Child's class C patient who had a single encapsulated HCC.

Major complications included intraperitoneal hemorrhage that required transfusion, hepatic decompensation in a Child's B patient, transient renal insufficiency, and two cases of infarction of a segment adjacent to the tumor. Minor complications included slight bleeding and transitory hepatic decompensation. The mortality rate was 0.7%, and major complications 4.6% (16,17). In another series, the mortality rate was 6% (five patients): three patients died from rupture of esophageal varices, one patient from rupture of a subcapsular HCC, and one patient from hepatic failure (18).

Contraindications

Contraindications depend on the general condition of the patient (advanced cirrhosis or severe coagulation disorders). We do not perform PEIT in Child's C patients or when prothrombin time is significantly prolonged and platelets <40,000/mm^3. Contraindications depend on the tumor stage, extrahepatic metastases, the presence of thrombosis in main portal branches, tumor volume >30% of the hepatic volume, or a diffuse form of HCC. Single-session therapy is contraindicated in the following situations-marked portal and/or pulmonary hypertension, esophageal varices at risk for bleeding, increased fibrinolysis, cardiac ischemia, major disorders of myocardial conduction, large subcapsular lesions, severe coagulation disorders, and chronic renal insufficiency.

Evaluation of Therapeutic Efficacy

To evaluate therapeutic response, that is, to determine whether the tumor has become completely necrotic or whether areas of neoplastic tissue are still present, a combination of investigations and serum assays for tumor markers is used. The follow-up tests are the same exams as for initial staging. Although many studies are virtually comparable, we prefer to use contrast-enhanced US, currently with second-generation echo enhancers (e.g., Sono Vue, Bracco, Milan, Italy) and spiral CT with biphasic technique (4–5 mL/sec, 20 and 60 seconds after the injection of contrast medium) (Fig. 15.4).

Other examinations or biopsy are performed only in unusual problem cases of partial versus complete response. If areas of tissue are still viable but are very small beyond the present degree of resolution, they obviously will not be detectable. However, they will be identified at successive examinations as they become apparent as zones of enhancement on CT or as they increase in volume.

Response is considered complete when CT shows total disappearance of enhancement within the neoplastic tissue, and is confirmed on successive examinations (Fig. 15.5). The absence of enhancement implies absence of blood flow due to necrotic and fibrotic effects. Even with complete necrosis, the dead tissue occupies space and remains visible in place of the tumor, but reduced in size (Fig. 15.6). Contrast-enhanced US can be useful, but it should not be used as the only test to establish follow-up, because it is less sensitive than CT in demonstrating vascularity of small viable areas.

For tumor markers, we use α-fetoprotein (AFP) and des-γ-carboxy-prothrombin (DCP), which are often complementary. Nevertheless, their effect is useful only if they are initially high. When the imaging shows complete response, but AFP or DCP levels remain high, it means that neoplastic tissue is not detected or is growing elsewhere. An increase always suggests local recurrence or the appearance of new lesions. Contrast-enhanced US, CT, and serum assay of tumor markers are carried out a month after treatment and then every 4 to 6 months thereafter.

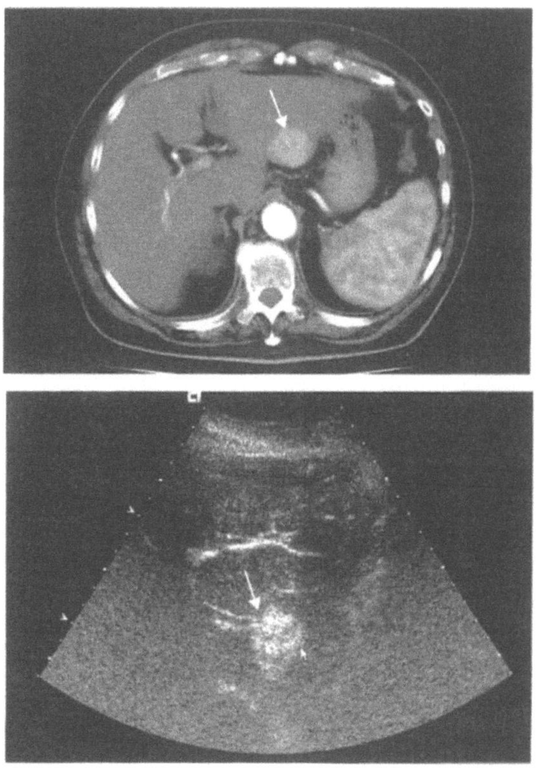

A

B

FIGURE 15.4. Hepatocellular carcinoma located in the left lobe: contrast-enhanced computed tomography (CT) (A), and enhanced US (B) demonstrate hypervascular lesion (arrows).

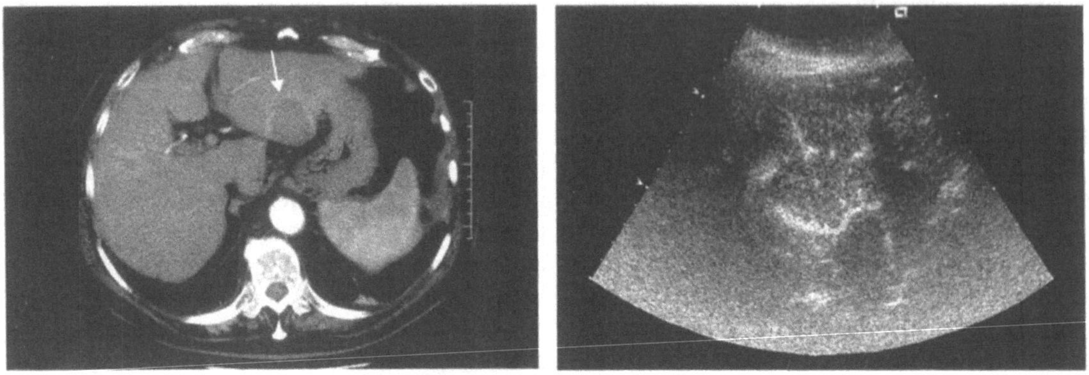

A B

FIGURE 15.5. Hepatocellular carcinoma the day after radiofrequency: contrast-enhanced CT (A), and USCA (B), demonstrate the absence of enhancement within the lesion and a hypervascular inflammatory ring (arrow).

Results

Many long-term survival curves have been published. A total of 112 patients have been treated at the University of Chiba—93 patients with one, 16 with two, and three with three lesions, all ≤3 cm in diameter. Survival at 1, 3, and 5 years, respectively, was 96%, 72%, and 51% for 60 patients with Child's A; 90%, 62%, and 48% for 33 Child's B patients; and 94%, 25%, and 0% for 19 patients with Child's C disease (19). Shiina et al (20) treated 50 patients with single or multiple lesions of diameters varying from 1.2 to 6 cm. Overall survival at 1, 3, and 5 years was 87%, 62%, and 43%, respectively. Comparison of Child's A versus Child's C disease ($p < .0001$), diameter ≤3 cm versus ≥4 cm ($p < .0002$), and number ≤3 versus ≥4 lesions ($p < .02$) showed significant differences.

Lencioni et al (21) treated 184 patients. A select group of 70 patients with well-compensated cirrhosis and a single HCC 3 cm or less in diameter had 3- and 5-year survival of 89% and 63%, respectively. A multicenter Italian study enrolled 746 patients (6). In Child's A patients ($n = 293$), B ($n = 149$), or C ($n = 20$) with a single HCC <5 cm in diameter, survival at 1, 3, and 5 years, respectively, was 98%, 79%, and 47% for Child's A; 93%, 63%, and 29% for Child's B; and 64%, 12%, and 0% for Child's C. In Child's

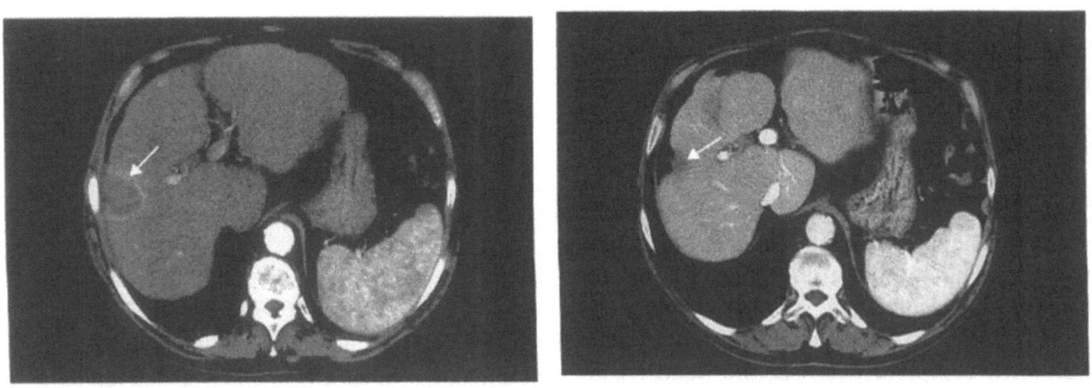

A B

FIGURE 15.6. Hepatocellular carcinoma (arrows) treated with radiofrequency: the day after therapy (A), and 2 years later (B).

A patients with multiple HCCs (n = 121), survival was 94%, 68%, and 36% at 1, 3, and 5 years, respectively. A multicenter Japanese study enrolled 110 Child's A patients with HCC 3cm or less and 3 lesions or less: their 3- and 5-year survival was 83% and 53%, respectively (22). As regards HCC >5cm in diameter, a study of 108 patients reported a 3-year survival of 57% in patients with encapsulated HCC measuring 5 to 8.5cm in diameter and 42% in patients with infiltrating HCC measuring 5 to 10cm or multiple lesions (16).

In all the aforementioned patients, the main cause of death in Child's A patients was progression of the neoplastic disease due mainly to the appearance of new lesion; in Child's C patients it was hepatic insufficiency. The incidence of appearance of new lesion at 5 years in the group of patients from the University of Chiba was 87%, in the Shiina group 64%, and in the Lencioni group 78%. In our study, the overall incidence was 87%. In patients with a single HCC, new lesions occurred in 74%, and in patients with multiple HCCs the incidence was 98%.

The incidence of local recurrences (i.e., due to an increase in size or the appearance of viable areas within the lesion treated with PEIT) was 4% in the series of Ebara et al (19) (in lesions <3cm in diameter), 7% in the series of Shiina et al (20) (in lesions <4–5cm in diameter), and 17% in our series (in lesions <5cm in diameter). Many of the recurrences were treated with additional cycles of PEIT.

Discussion

The rationale to utilize to PEIT is based on the following points:

1. The expansive type of HCC initially shows regional growth, so a local therapy like PEIT can be used.
2. Ultrasound screening of cirrhotic populations identifies HCC at an early stage, when the tumor is still small, generally less than 5cm.
3. Ethanol shows a selective diffusion in HCC owing to the tumor's soft consistency with respect to the surrounding cirrhotic tissue and its hypervascularity.
4. Alcohol therapy does not have the disadvantage of loss or damage of nonneoplastic parenchyma. In contrast, it is likely that the loss of healthy tissue due to multisegmental resection or parenchymal damage following a massive transarterial chemoembolization may result in deterioration of hepatic function and potentially terminal insufficiency (23, 24).
5. Percutaneous ethanol injection therapy is a low-risk method. In series published thus far, the mortality rate has been minimal, and the highest complication rate is 3.2%, with most complications treated in a conservative manner. The absence of mortality with conventional PEIT is in marked ontrast with the perioperative mortality due to surgery, which even though much lower than in the past, is a factor to take into consideration, especially in centers with little experience. Centers with extensive surgical experience report a mortality rate of 1.4% to 11% and a complication rate as high as 58% (6). In this regard, it should be remembered that patients selected by ultrasound screening are asymptomatic and that, even if untreated, they have a life expectancy of more than 1 year (25).
6. Percutaneous ethanol injection therapy can be repeated easily when new lesions appear, as happens in most patients within 5 years. The incidence of appearance of new lesions in surgical series varies from 67% to 100% (6). In our series treated with PEIT, it was 65% to 98%. This factor of multicentricity in patients with HCC and chronic hepatitis always should be taken into consideration whenever a choice of treatment is necessary. This means that the first lesion seen at ultrasound is usually the prelude to others, and that surgery, even if radical for resected lesions, is generally only palliative because of the natural history of the disease. Patients should be followed frequently to treat lesions as soon as possible when they are still small. An advantage of PEIT is that the patient is followed by the same physician in the diagnostic as well as in the therapeutic phase. Moreover, it is now possible with single-session PEIT to intervene further in the course of the disease in select patients who would not have benefited from conventional PEIT.

7. The low cost of the material and easy execution of the procedure make it possible to perform PEIT readily. Patients generally are treated on an outpatient basis. The cost of material is not expensive: in Italy, one PEIT cycle is about $1000, the cost of an orthotopic liver transplantation is about $125,000, and that of a partial hepatectomy is about $30,000. The number of patients who will develop the disease is about 20,000 to 25,000 in Japan and about 12,000 in Italy. Thus the problem of cost is quite important (6).

8. The local therapeutic efficacy of PEIT is rather high. Histopathologic studies of resected lesions carried out, particularly in the initial period of this procedure demonstrated the effectiveness of PEIT. Shiina et al (13) demonstrated complete necrosis in 16 of 23 lesions (69.6%), 90% necrosis in six lesions, and 70% necrosis in one lesion. Their study showed that viable tissue was present in small satellite nodules around the main lesions, along the lesion margins, or in septations.

9. Long-term results with PEIT are satisfactory. No controlled studies have reported PEIT compared to no treatment, but the same is true for surgery. It was evident from the beginning that PEIT was an efficacious treatment with few risks.

Comparisons with no treatment are based only on historical data. Two studies of untreated patients with comparable disease showed a 5-year survival of 0% in 27 patients, and in a second study of 73 patients, a rate of 11% (19,25). A controlled study of Child's class A patients with HCC less than 4 cm in diameter confirmed the validity of PEIT compared to no treatment, as survival at 3 years was 71% and 21%, respectively (27).

In a comparative study based on historical data, the mean overall survival at 5 years for 628 patients with lesions less than or equal to 5 cm in diameter and compensated cirrhosis treated with PEIT was 48%, whereas that of 1272 patients undergoing surgical resection with a similar presentation was 49% (6). This comparability was confirmed in a cohort study (28), and, more recently, by a multicenter Japanese study, in which survival of 445 patients undergoing resection at 5 years was 54%, versus 110 patients treated with PEIT, in which it was 53% (22). The substantial comparability can probably be attributed to a balance between the advantages and disadvantages of the two therapies: the greater percentage of complete ablation with resection favors surgery, while for PEIT it is the absence of perioperative mortality, the absence of normal tissue loss, the insufficient evaluation of prognostic factors in resected patients, and the upstaging of imaging examinations.

The large number of patients enrolled in US-screening programs has created a demand for an effective, safe, repeatable, and economic treatment that can be made available in many centers; PEIT satisfies all such requisites. In the absence of randomized studies and on the basis of reported results, PEIT is indicated as the treatment of choice for most patients found positive by US screening, excluding those who are candidates for liver transplantation or for surgical resection; unfortunately, the former is available only for few patients. Regarding the indication for surgery, the Liver Cancer Study Group of Japan has reported factors predictive for a long-term prognosis (29). By multivariate analysis, the most important predictive factors, in decreasing order, were AFP level, tumor size, number of lesions, age of the patient, stage of cirrhosis, margins of resection, and portal thrombosis. Univariate analysis showed capsular infiltration, tumor extent, and Edmondson-Steiner classification to be the most important predictive factors. In our opinion, PEIT is therefore indicated in patients who are (a) not candidates for liver transplantation; (b) not resectable; (c) resectable, but presenting with one of the negative prognostic factors of the aforementioned multivariate analysis (high AFP, age over 70 years, multinodularity, Child's class B disease, vascular infiltration); or (d) resectable with only enucleation, since such surgery does not remove eventual peritumoral satellites (which is also a limitation of PEIT). Patients undergoing enucleation, in addition to having a significantly shorter survival than those who undergo segmentectomy or subsegmentectomy, also have a shorter survival than that obtained with PEIT (30).

References

1. Seki T, Wakabayashi M, Nakagawa T, et al. Percutaneous microwave coagulation therapy for solitary metastatic liver tumors from colorectal cancer: a pilot clinical study. Am J Gastroenterol 1999;94:322–327.
2. Amin Z, Donald JJ, Masters A, Kant R, Bown SG, Lees WR. Hepatic metastases: interstitial laser photocoagulation with real-time US monitoring and dynamic CT evaluation of treatment. Radiology 1993;187:339–347.
3. Rossi S, Buscarini E, Garbagnati F, et al. Percutaneous treatment of small hepatic tumors by an expandable RF needle electrode. AJR 1998;170: 1015–1022.
4. Livraghi T, Festi D, Monti F, Salmi A, Vettori C. US-guided percutaneous alcohol injection of small hepatic and abdominal tumors. Radiology 1986;161:309–312.
5. Bruix J, Sherman M, Llovet JM, et al. Clinical management of hepatocellular carcinoma. Conclusions of the Barcelona-2000 EASL Conference. J Hepatol 2000.
6. Livraghi T, Giorgio A, Marin G, et al. Hepatocellular carcinoma and cirrhosis in 746 patients: long-term results of percutaneous ethanol injection. Radiology 1995;197:101–108.
7. Livraghi T, Benedini V, Lazzaroni S, Meloni F, Torzilli G, Vettori C. Long-term results of single session PEI in patients with large hepatocellular carcinoma. Cancer 1998;83:48–57.
8. Redvanly RD, Chezmar JL. Percutaneous ethanol ablation therapy of malignant hepatic tumors using CT guidance. Semin Intervent Radiol 1993;10:82–87.
9. Lee MJ, Mueller PR, Dawson SL, et al. Percutaneous ethanol injection for the treatment of hepatic tumors: indications, mechanism of action, technique, and efficacy. AJR 1995;164: 215–220.
10. Livraghi T, Grigioni W, Mazziotti A, Sangalli G, Vettori C. Percutaneous ethanol injection of portal thrombosis in hepatocellular carcinoma: a new possible treatment. Tumori 1990;76:394–397.
11. Di Stasi M, Buscarini L, Livraghi T, et al. Percutaneous ethanol injection in the treatment of hepatocellular carcinoma: a multicentric survey of evaluation practices and complication rates. Scand J Gastroenterol 1997;32:1168–1173.
12. Taavitsainen M, Vehmas T, Kauppila R. Fatal liver necrosis following percutaneous ethanol injection for hepatocellular carcinoma. Abdom Imaging 1993;18:357–359.
13. Boucher E, Carsin A, Raoul JL, Marchetti C, Joram F, Kerbrat P. Massive hepatic necrosis secondary to treatment of hepatocellular carcinoma by percutaneous ethanol injection. Gastroenterol Clin Biol 1998;22:559–561.
14. Ishii H, Okada S, Okusaka T, et al. Needle tract implantation of hepatocellular carcinoma after percutaneous ethanol injection. Cancer 1998;82: 1638–1642.
15. Giorgio A, Tarantino L, Francica G, et al. One-shot percutaneous ethanol injection of liver tumors under general anesthesia: preliminary data on efficacy and complications. Cardiovasc Intervent Radiol 1996;19:27–31.
16. Giorgio A, Tarantino L, Francica G, et al. One-shot percutaneous ethanol injection of liver tumors under general anesthesia. CVIR 1996;19:27–31.
17. Meloni F, Lazzaroni S, Livraghi T. Percutaneous ethanol injection: single session treatment. Eur J Ultrasound 2001;13:107–115.
18. Giorgio A, Tarantino L, Mariniello N, et al. Percutaneous ethanol injection under general anesthesia for hepatocellular carcinoma: 3 year survival in 112 patients. Eur J Ultrasound 1998; 8:201–208.
19. Ebara M, Otho M, Sugiura N, Okuda K, Kondo K. Percutaneous ethanol injection for the treatment of small hepatocellular carcinoma: study of 95 patients. J Gastroenterol Hepatol 1990;5: 616–626.
20. Shiina S, Tagawa K, Niwa Y, et al. Percutaneous ethanol injection therapy for hepatocellular carcinoma: results in 146 patients. AJR 1993;160: 1023–1028.
21. Lencioni R, Pinto F, Armillotta N, et al. Long-term results of percutaneous ethanol injection for hepatocellular carcinoma in cirrhosis: a European experience. Eur Radiol 1997;7:514–519.
22. Ryu M, Shimamura Y, Kinoshita T, et al. Therapeutic results of resection, TAE and PEI in 3225 patients with hepatocellular carcinoma: a retrospective multicenter study. Jpn J Clin Oncol 1997;27:251–257.
23. Yamashita Y, Torashima M, Ognuni T, et al. Liver parenchymal changes after transcatheter arterial embolization therapy for hepatoma. CT evaluation. Abdom Imaging 1993;18:352–356.
24. Groupe d'Etude et de Traitment du Carcinome Hepatocellulare. A comparison of lipiodol chemoembolization and conservative treatment for unresectable hepatocellular carcinoma. N Engl J Med 1995;332:1256–1261.

25. Livraghi T, Bolondi L, Buscarini L, et al. No treatment, resection and ethanol injection in hepatocellular carcinoma: a retrospective analysis of survival in 391 patients with cirrhosis. J Hepatol 1995;22:522–526.
26. Shiina S, Tagawa K, Unuma T. Percutaneous ethanol injection therapy for hepatocellular carcinoma: a histopathologic study. Cancer 1991;68: 1524–1530.
27. Orlando A, Cottone M, Virdone R, et al. Treatment of small hepatocellular carcinoma associated with cirrhosis by percutaneous ethanol injection. Scand J Gastroenterol 1997;32:598–603.
28. Castells, A, Bruix J, Bru C. Treatment of small hepatocellular carcinoma in cirrhotic patients: a cohort study comparing surgical resection and percutaneous ethanol injection. Hepatology 1993;18:1121–1126.
29. The Liver Cancer Study Group of Japan. Predictive factors for long-term prognosis after partial hepatectomy for patients with hepatocellular carcinoma. Cancer 1994;74:2772–2780.
30. Takayama T, Makuuchi M. Surgical resection. In: Livraghi T, Makuuchi M, Buscarini L, eds. Diagnosis and Treatment of Hepatocellular Carcinoma. London: Greenwich Medical Media, 1997:279–286.

16
Radiofrequency Ablation

Riccardo Lencioni and Laura Crocetti

The goal of radiofrequency (RF) ablation is to induce thermal injury to the tissue through electromagnetic energy deposition. The term *radiofrequency* refers to the alternating electric current that oscillates in the range of high frequency (200–1200kHz). In RF ablation, the patient is part of a closed-loop circuit that includes an RF generator, an electrode needle, and a large dispersive electrode (ground pads). An alternating electric field is created within the tissue of the patient. Because of the relatively high electrical resistance of tissue in comparison with the metal electrodes, there is marked agitation of the ions present in the target tissue that surrounds the electrode, since the tissue ions attempt to follow the changes in direction of alternating electric current. The agitation results in frictional heat around the electrode. The discrepancy between the small surface area of the needle electrode and the large area of the ground pads causes the generated heat to be focused and concentrated around the needle electrode (1).

The thermal damage caused by RF heating is dependent on both the tissue temperature that is achieved and the duration of heating. Heating of tissue at 50° to 55°C for 4 to 6 minutes produces irreversible cellular damage. At temperatures between 60° and 100°C nearly immediate coagulation of tissue is induced, with irreversible damage to mitochondrial and cytosolic enzymes of the cells. At more than 100° to 110°C, tissue vaporizes and carbonizes. For adequate destruction of tumor tissue, the entire target volume must be subjected to cytotoxic temperatures. Thus, an essential objective of ablative therapy is achievement and maintenance of a 50° to 100°C temperature throughout the entire target volume for at least 4 to 6 minutes. However, the relatively slow thermal conduction from the electrode surface through the tissues increases the duration of application to 10 to 30 minutes. On the other hand, the tissue temperature should not be increased over these values to avoid carbonization around the tip of the electrode from excessive heating (1,2).

Another important factor that affects the success of RF thermal ablation is the ability to ablate all viable tumor tissue and an adequate tumor-free margin. The most important difference between surgical resection and RF ablation of hepatic tumors is the surgeon's insistence on a 1-cm-wide tumor-free zone along the resection margin. To achieve rates of local tumor recurrence with RF ablation that are comparable to those obtained with hepatic resection, physicians should produce a 360-degree, 1-cm-thick tumor-free margin around each tumor (3) (Fig. 16.1). This cuff is necessary to assure that all microscopic invasion around the periphery of a tumor has been eradicated. Thus, the target diameter of an ablation must be ideally 2cm larger than the diameter of the tumor that undergoes treatment (4,5). Eradication of a tumor, therefore, can be achieved with a single ablation if the diameter of the tumor is 2cm less than the diameter of tissue ablated. For example, a 5-cm ablation device can be used to treat a 3-cm-diameter tumor. Other-

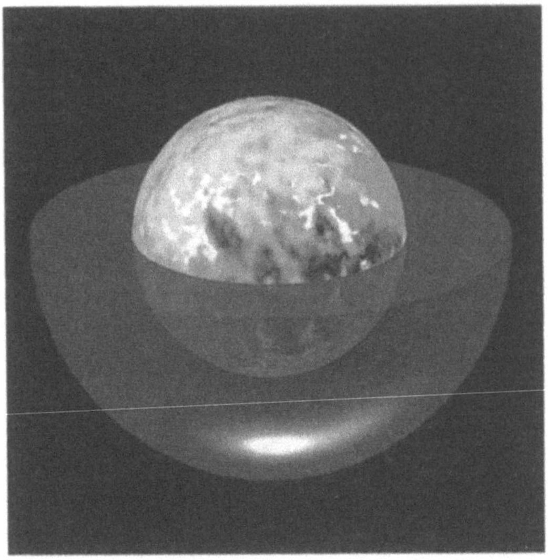

FIGURE 16.1. Computer art demonstrating concept of 360-degree, 1-cm margin around a tumor.

wise, multiple overlapping ablations can be performed (1,4).

Heat efficacy is defined as the difference between the amount of heat produced and the amount of heat lost. Therefore, effective ablation can be achieved by optimizing heat production and minimizing heat loss within the area to be ablated. The relationship between these factors has been characterized as the "bioheat equation". The bioheat equation governing RF-induced heat transfer through tissue has been previously described by Pennes (6). The equation has been simplified to a first approximation by Goldberg and colleagues (7):

$$\text{Coagulation} = \text{Energy Deposited} \times \text{Local Tissue Interactions} - \text{Heat Lost}$$

Heat production is correlated with the intensity and duration of the RF energy that is deposited. Tissues cannot be heated to greater than 100° to 110°C without vaporizing, and this process produces significant gas that both serves as an insulator and retards the ability to effectively establish an RF field. On the other hand, heat conduction or diffusion usually is explained as a factor of heat loss in regard to the electrode tip. Heat is lost mainly through convection by means of blood circulation (5). These processes, together with the rapid decrease in heating at a distance from the electrode, limit the extent of induced coagulation from a single, unmodified monopolar electrode to no greater than 1.6cm in diameter (7,8).

Therefore, most investigators have devoted their attention to strategies that increase the energy deposited into the tissues. Several corporations have manufactured new RF-ablation devices based on technologic advances that increase heating efficacy. To accomplish this increase, the RF output of all commercially available generators has been increased to 150 to 200W, which potentially may increase the intensity of the RF current deposited in the tissues. Expandable, multineedle electrodes permit the deposition of this energy over a larger volume. In addition, this design decreases the distance between the tissue and the electrode, thereby ensuring more uniform heating that relies less on heat conduction over a large distance (9).

The commercially available devices also were developed strategically to monitor the ablation process so that high-temperature coagulation can occur without exceeding a 110°C maximum temperature threshold. One device (RITA Medical Systems) relies on direct temperature measurement throughout the tissue to prevent any electrode in a multi-tined configuration from exceeding 110°C. The two other commercially available devices (Radionics and Radiotherapeutics) rely on an electrical measurement of tissue impedance to determine that tissue boiling is taking place. These impedance rises can be detected by the generator, which then can reduce the current output to a preset level.

One of the manufacturers markets a system with retractable needle electrodes (Starburst XL and Starburst XLi; RITA Medical Systems). The needle electrodes consist of a 14-gauge insulated outer needle that houses nine retractable curved electrodes of various lengths. When the electrodes are extended, the device assumes the approximate configuration of a Christmas tree, with the length and diameter of the electrode clusters measuring a maximum of 5cm. Five of the electrodes are hollow and contain thermocouples in their tips that are used to measure the temperature of the adjacent tissue. The alternating electric current generator is available in a 150- or 200-W model. To perform a typical ablation, two grounding pads are placed on the patient's thighs. The tip of the needle (with retracted electrodes) is advanced to the proximal edge of the lesion, and the electrodes are deployed approximately step by step from 2 cm to the desired expansion. The generator is turned on, and can run manually or by an automated program. The temperature at the tips of the electrodes are controlled, and the peak power is maintained until the temperature exceeds the preselected target temperature (typically between 90° and 100°C). After the target temperature is achieved, the curved electrodes can be advanced as previously described to full deployment, while maintaining the target temperature. When the electrodes are fully deployed, the program maintains the target temperature by regulating the wattage. As the tissue begins to desiccate, the amount of power needed to maintain the target temperature decreases. At the end of the procedure, when the generator runs off, a "cool-down cycle" is automatically performed. After retracting the hooks, coagulation of the needle tract can be done (tract ablation) maintaining temperature above 70°C.

Another RF-ablation device (LeVeen Needle Electrode; Radiotherapeutics) has retractable curved electrodes and an insulated 14-gauge outer needle that houses 10 solid retractable curved electrodes that, when deployed, assume the configuration of an umbrella (10). The electrodes are manufactured in different lengths. Two ground pads are used with the device; both are placed on the patient's thighs. For use, the tip of the needle is advanced to the target tissue and the curved electrodes are deployed to full extension. The generator is switched on, and energy is administered until a rapid rise in impedance occurs. The ablation algorithm is based on tissue impedance, rather than tissue temperature. The impedance of the tissue increases as the tissue desiccates. It is believed that an ablation is successful if the device impedes out.

Alternate strategies to increase the energy deposited from a single RF electrode also have been developed. A third manufacturer (Radionics) uses an internally cooled electrode designed to minimize carbonization and gas formation around the needle tip by eliminating excess heat near the electrode. The needle has an exposed tip of variable length. The tip of the needle is closed and contains a thermocouple to record the temperature of the adjacent tissue. The shaft of the needle has two internal channels to allow the needle to be perfused with chilled water. Conceptually, the cooling is believed to prevent desiccation and charring around the needle tip. To increase the size of the ablation, the company placed three of the cooled needles in a parallel triangular cluster with a common hub. This device produces a significantly larger ablation than does a single cooled needle (11–13). Pulsing of RF energy (i.e., alternation of very high RF current for several seconds, followed by minimal RF deposition for a defined period) also has been described as a method to increase current deposition.

Despite technologic advances and electrode modifications that have effectively increased RF energy deposition and tissue heating, inadequate coagulation is a clinical problem in some circumstances, due not only to the large size of lesions. Key culprits implicated in inadequate coagulation include the other two elements of the bioheat equation: (a) heterogeneity of tissue composition, by which differences in tumor tissue density, including fibrosis and calcification, alter electrical and thermal conductance; and (b) blood flow, by which perfusion-mediated tissue cooling (vascular flow) reduces the extent of thermally induced coagulation (Fig. 16.2). These limitations have led investigators to study adjuvant therapies that modify the underlying tumor physiologic characteristics in an attempt to improve RF thermal ablation, either in conjunction with, or as an alternative to, multiple ablations of a given tumor. These adjuvant therapies can be classified, on the basis of the bioheat equation, as: (a) strategies that permit an increase in the overall deposition of energy through an alteration in tissue electrical conductivity;

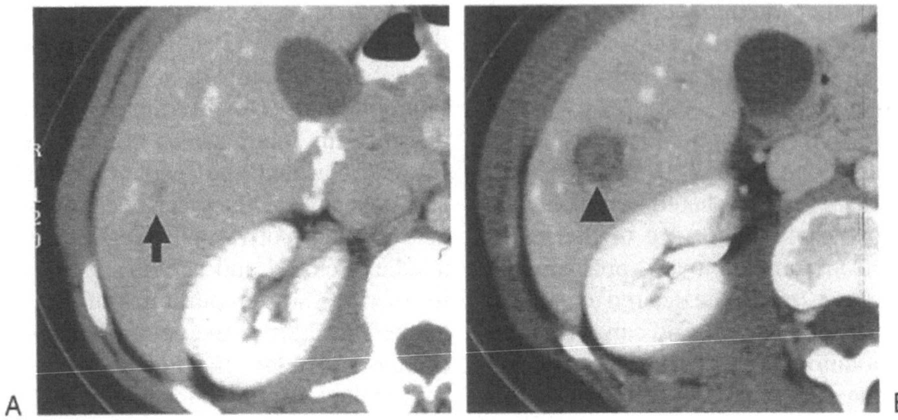

FIGURE 16.2. A 14-year-old girl with gastrointestinal stromal tumor metastatic to the liver. (A) Contrast-enhanced computed tomography (CT) scan through the caudal aspect of the right lobe of the liver shows a 1-cm tumor (arrow) in segment 6. (B) Contrast-enhanced CT scan of the liver performed immediately after percutaneous radiofrequency ablation demonstrates an 18-mm ablation (arrowhead) of the tumor. The ablation was performed with the Radionics cluster electrode and a 12-minute automated ablation cycle. Note the relatively small ablation, which was limited in size due to hyperdynamic blood flow through the liver.

(b) strategies that improve heat retention within the tissue; and (c) strategies that decrease the tolerance of tumor tissue to heat (7).

For a given RF current, power deposition is strongly dependent on local electrical conductivity. Intratumoral injection of saline solution prior to, or during the application of, RF current alters tissue conductivity, thereby allowing greater deposition of RF current and increased tissue heating and coagulation. Experimental findings demonstrate that ablative temperatures can be generated farther from an RF electrode by increasing tissue electrical conductivity with NaCl solution injection. This method permits greater energy deposition without inducing tissue boiling, which, in effect, flattens the heat distribution curve (14). However, because both volume and concentration of saline solutions influence tissue heating and the coagulation diameter in a nonlinear fashion, optimal parameters for injection of saline solution must be determined for each type of RF apparatus and for the different types of tumor and tissue to be treated. A major concern for the feasibility of adjuvant percutaneous injection strategies is the possibility of nonuniform alteration of tissue electrical conductivity, because of the difficulty of achieving uniform fluid diffusion and distribution. Irregularly shaped areas of coagulation have been observed previously with RF during simultaneous saline injection, and are attributed to nonuniform saline distribution (15). Saline-enhanced ablation may lead to distortion of the lesion shape at coagulation owing to the spread of hot fluid along the path of least resistance and thus causing thermal damage off-target, as has been demonstrated in cow udder tissue in vitro (16,17). Goldberg et al (14) have observed this phenomenon in tissue samples in which large volumes of saline were injected (25 mL). The administration of only relatively small volumes of fluid may potentially minimize the issue of NaCl solution diffusion over larger volumes by obtaining maximal tissue heating and coagulation.

Perfusion-mediated tissue cooling reduces the extent of coagulation produced by thermal ablation (14,18,19). Modeling of the bioheat equation shows that for a given tissue and power deposition, the effects of tissue blood flow predominate. RF-induced coagulation is also more limited and variable in vivo, particularly in clinical practice than ex vivo. Coagulation in vivo often is shaped by vasculature in the vicinity of the ablation. Experiments in which hepatic perfusion is altered by mechanical or pharmacologic means during RF ablation of normal liver tissue and tumors show that blood flow is largely responsible for this reduction in observed coagulation (20,21). Several strategies to reduce blood flow during ablation therapy have been proposed. Total portal inflow occlusion (Pringle maneuver) has been used at open laparotomy and at laparoscopy. Angiographic balloon occlusion of the hepatic artery can be used, but has proven helpful only for hypervascular tumors (21). Embolization prior to ablation with particles that occlude sinusoids such as absorbable gelatin sponge or iodized oil may overcome this limitation. Pharmacologic modulation of blood flow and antiangiogenesis therapy are theoretically possible, but currently should be considered experimental (20).

As far as decreasing tissue resistance to heat, combining thermal ablation with other therapies such as chemotherapy or chemoembolization are considerations. The findings of preliminary experiments suggest that adjuvant chemotherapy may increase the ablation volume compared with RF-ablation therapy alone (22). Further research to determine optimal methods of combining chemotherapeutic regimens (both agent and route of administration) with RF ablation is ongoing.

Targeting of the lesion can be performed with ultrasonography (US), computed tomography (CT), or magnetic resonance imaging (MRI), and ablation may be delivered by means of open surgery, percutaneous access, or, in case of abdominal procedures, laparoscopy (23). The guidance system is chosen largely on the basis of operator preference and local experience. Although acoustic shadowing due to nitrogen bubbles and obscuration of the US image by the RF current are major disadvantages, US is still accepted as a viable modality for guidance or monitoring during RF ablation (Fig. 16.3). The recent development of CT fluoroscopic systems may result in a larger role for CT in the future. Similarly, the developments of open-architecture MRI systems and MRI-compatible interventional equipment have resulted in increased interest in the use of this modality to help guide interventional procedures (24).

In the clinical arena, RF ablation has been used for the treatment of a variety of neoplasms, including osteoid osteoma, hepatocellular carcinoma, renal cell carcinoma, non–small-cell lung cancer (NSCLC), and hepatic, lung, cerebral, osseous, and retroperitoneal metastases from a variety of primary tumors.

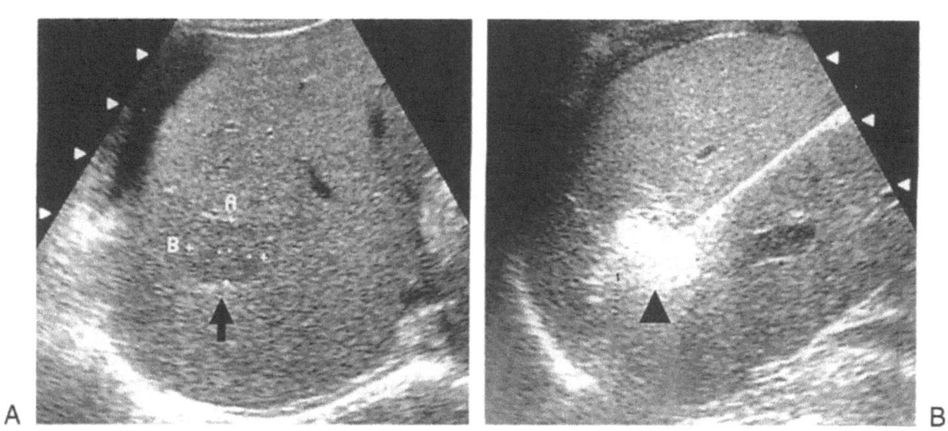

FIGURE 16.3. A 48-year-old man with hepatitis B–induced cirrhosis. (A) Axial sonogram demonstrates a 2-cm hepatocellular carcinoma (arrow) in segment 8 of the liver. (B) Oblique sonogram through the right lobe of the liver during radiofrequency ablation shows the hyperechoic reaction caused by microbubble formation produced by the high temperatures induced during the ablation process.

Liver Tumor Ablation

Hepatocellular carcinoma (HCC) and metastases from colorectal carcinoma are the two most common malignant tumors to affect the liver. It has been estimated that only 5% to 15% of patients with HCC or hepatic metastases are eligible for resection (25–27). For those patients who undergo hepatic resection, there is considerable postoperative morbidity, a small but real risk of death related to the operation, significant monetary expense, and only a modest improvement in long-term prognosis. The 5-year survival rate for patients undergoing resection of HCC or hepatic metastases is only 20% to 40% (25–27). Most patients die from recurrent hepatic tumors. Although in some instances surgery may be repeated to resect recurrent tumor, at most institutions hepatic resection is a "one-shot" therapy. In light of these shortcomings, an effective, minimally invasive technique is needed to treat these tumors, and one that can be repeated as necessary to treat recurrent tumor.

Preoperative CT or MRI is the fundamental imaging examination on which the candidacy of a patient for RF ablation is based. These imaging studies are used to determine the number and size of tumors and their relationship to surrounding structures such as blood vessels, bile ducts, gallbladder, diaphragm, and bowel. To be considered eligible for treatment by RF thermal ablation, patients must meet some general requirements. First, as RF ablation is a local treatment, disease ideally should be confined to the liver, without evidence of vascular invasion or extrahepatic metastases (28). In addition, the tumor must be a focal, nodular-type lesion. The presence of a clear and easy-to-detect target for needle placement is crucial for the outcome of treatment. The tumor must be either uninodular or, when multinodular, preferentially with a maximum of four to five lesions. Tumor size ideally should be smaller than 4 to 5cm in the greatest dimension. Nevertheless, larger lesions, especially HCCs, also can be treated by using newer RF generators and RF needles, as well as by performing RF ablation after occlusion of tumor blood supply (21).

Treatment of lesions adjacent to the gallbladder or to the hepatic hilum entails the risk of thermal injury of the biliary tract. In contrast, treatment of lesions located in the vicinity of hepatic vessels is possible, since flowing blood usually "refrigerates" the vascular wall, protecting it from thermal injury. In these cases, however, the risk of incomplete ablation of the area of neoplastic tissue adjacent to the vessel may increase because of the heat loss caused by the vessel itself. Lesions located along the surface of the liver can be considered for RF ablation, although their treatment requires experienced hands and may be associated with a higher risk of complications (Fig. 16.4). Finally, the treatment of subcapsular tumors abutting other abdominal viscera poses the risk of damage to those organs. Of greatest concern in this regard is the possibility of inducing thermal necrosis in an adjacent loop of bowel (23).

It has to be noticed that in HCC tumors, RF treatment tends to produce a volume of thermal necrosis that matches that of the original lesion (Fig. 16.5). This is mainly due to the differences in tissue impedance between tumor interior and surrounding cirrhotic tissue. Radiofrequency waves do not progress easily outside the lesion because of the reduced conductivity of cirrhotic tissue. This phenomenon has the advantages of sparing the surrounding nonneoplastic tissue and of enhancing the heat deposition within the tumor, thus increasing the effectiveness of the procedure. However, it entails the disadvantage of lacking control over extracapsular daughter nodules (29–32).

Metastases do not have a clear lesion-to-liver interface like nodular-type HCCs, but tend to strand into the surrounding liver parenchyma. Hence, if the necrosis volume produced by RF treatment is nearly equivalent to that of the visible native lesion, tumor recurrence caused by microscopic tests of tumor along the boundary is likely to occur. Therefore, to successfully ablate liver metastases, it is necessary to produce a thermal necrosis volume that exceeds that of the original lesion, with ideally a 1-cm safety margin of coagulation necrosis in the liver parenchyma all around the lesion

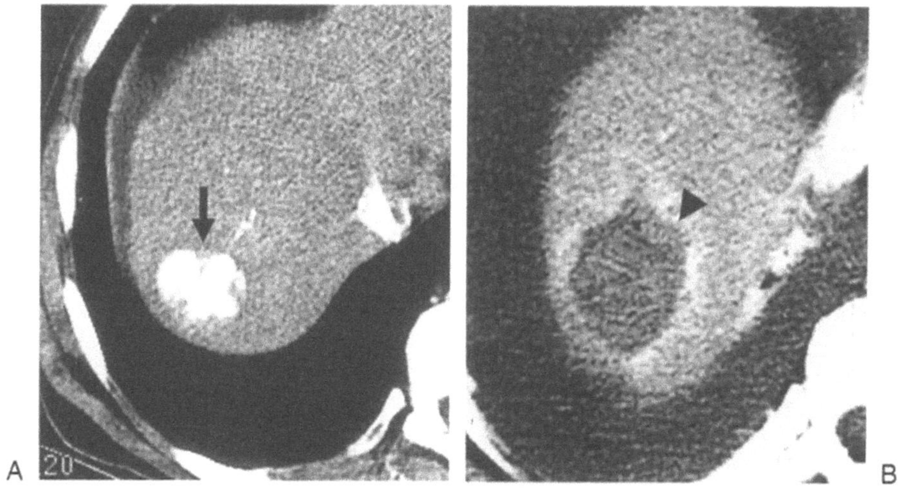

FIGURE 16.4. A 52-year-old man with subcapsular hypervascular hepatocellular carcinoma in segment 7. (A) Preablation contrast-enhanced CT scan through the dome of the liver shows a 2 × 3 cm hypervascular hepatocellular carcinoma (arrow). (B) Contrast-enhanced CT scan performed immediately following ablation demonstrates the hypovascular-induced state of the ablated tumor (arrowhead). Note the subcapsular and subdiaphragmatic location of the ablation, performed without complication.

(Fig. 16.6). This safety margin can be achieved in the case of metastatic lesions, because the progression of RF waves outside the lesion is not impaired by the poor conductivity of cirrhotic tissue as in HCC, provided that the lesion is not located in the vicinity of major vascular structures. Flowing blood within the vessels acts as a heat sink and may limit the necrotizing effect of RF treatment in the adjacent tissue (29,33–35).

Whenever possible RF ablation is performed percutaneously. Percutaneous treatment has several advantages over other approaches. The percutaneous approach is the least invasive, produces minimal morbidity, requires only conscious sedation, is relatively inexpensive,

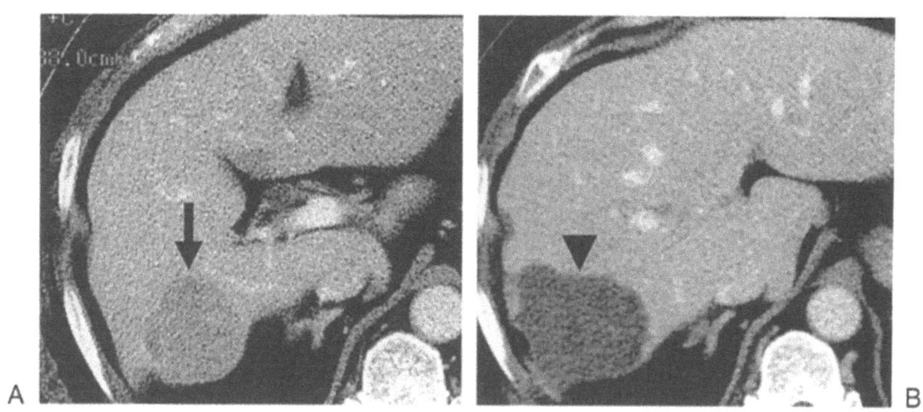

FIGURE 16.5. A 53-year-old man with hepatitis B–induced cirrhosis with a hepatocellular carcinoma in segment 6. (A) Contrast-enhanced CT scan demonstrates an approximately 4-cm hepatocellular carcinoma (arrow). (B) Contrast-enhanced CT scan performed immediately following ablation demonstrates an avascular region of coagulative necrosis (arrowhead) that closely matches the configuration of the tumor except in the region of the watershed zone where the ablation was potentiated.

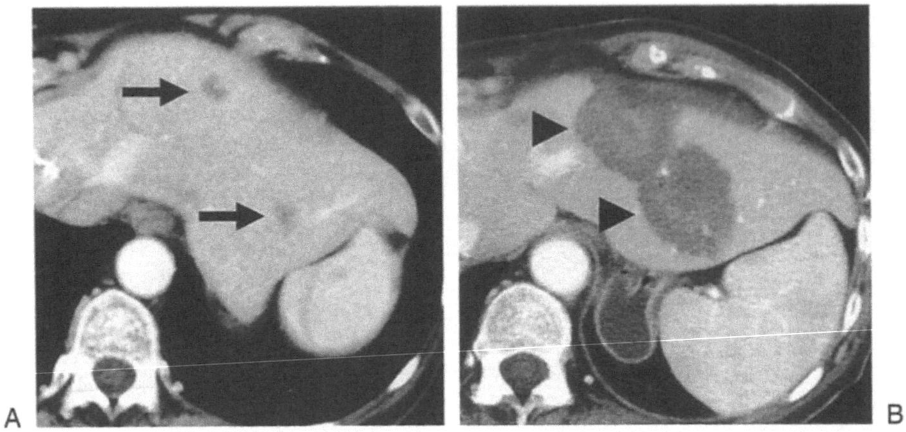

FIGURE 16.6. A 65-year-old woman with breast carcinoma metastatic to the liver. (A) Contrast-enhanced CT scan through the left lobe of the liver shows two 1-cm tumors (arrows). (B) Contrast-enhanced CT scan performed immediately after ablation demonstrates two large zones of coagulative necrosis (arrowheads) at the site of the treated 1-cm tumors. Note that the ablations substantially exceed the size of the treated tumors and clearly create a greater than 1-cm tumor-free margin around each tumor.

and can be repeated as necessary to treat recurrent tumor. However, advocates of laparoscopic thermal ablation of hepatic tumors claim that the laparoscopic approach provides some distinct advantages over the percutaneous approach (36). With the laparoscopic technique, the entire liver can be imaged with a high-frequency transducer placed directly on the surface of the liver. This technique allows the visualization (and treatment) of small tumors that cannot be detected using any other imaging technique. Furthermore, with laparoscopy the extent of a tumor can be staged more accurately. The identification of previously undetected surface lesions or peritoneal implants may lead to the appropriate cancellation of the planned RF ablation. This is important if the goal of the procedure is potential cure. Additionally, advocates of a laparoscopic approach argue that they can perform a Pringle maneuver (temporary occlusion of the hepatic artery and portal vein) and thus enhance the size of a thermal ablation (36). The disadvantages of a laparoscopic approach include the added invasiveness of the procedure, with the associated complications and added costs, and the technical difficulties of the procedure. In particular, the placement of the needle electrode can be problematic. Unlike the percutaneous technique in which the US probe and RF needle can be moved to any position over the right upper quadrant to achieve the best angle of approach to treat a tumor, the laparoscopic technique is hampered by limited access through the existing laparoscopic ports. Furthermore, no needle guides currently are available that can be attached to the laparoscopic US transducers, and the RF needles cannot be placed parallel to the transducers. Most commonly, the needles are placed either perpendicular or oblique to the US transducers. The manipulation of the needle from these angles is technically challenging and is not easily mastered (36).

Other investigators have published their experiences with RF ablation performed via open surgical treatment (28). Disadvantages of this technique include the associated morbidity and mortality of an open procedure and general anesthetic, the added expense of the procedure and associated recovery time, and that the technique typically is a one-shot therapy. Some of the advantages of the technique are the same as for the laparoscopic approach—namely, the ability to scan the whole liver with high-frequency transducers and to accurately stage the extent of the tumor. Additionally, the open approach allows a great deal of freedom in placing the US transducer and RF needle. Difficult lesions adjacent to the diaphragm, bowel, or gallbladder may be treated better with the open technique. These organs can be removed or isolated from the mobilized liver to prevent damage during the ablation of a tumor. Finally, the blood supply to the liver may be temporarily stopped during RF ablation. A Pringle maneuver, which causes temporary occlusion of the portal vein and hepatic artery, decreases blood supply to both the targeted tumor and the adjacent hepatic parenchyma. The result is a larger thermal injury than is possible with normal blood flow (28).

Extrahepatic Tumor Ablation

Tumors in several other organ sites have been treated with RF (2). Rosenthal et al (37,38) treated over 100 osteoid osteomas by using percutaneously placed conventional monopolar electrodes. Pain, the primary clinical manifestation of this lesion, was eradicated in more than 95% of cases; 12 recurrent lesions were successfully re-treated with percutaneous techniques. In addition, the length of hospital stay compared with that after surgical excision, previously the therapy of choice, decreased from 6.8 to 2.6 days.

Percutaneous image-guided thermal ablation of metastatic neoplasms involving bone may offer an alternative to conventional therapies for pain management in terminally ill patients. Dupuy et al (39) reported treating 10 patients with painful metastatic bone lesions by using CT guidance and 18-gauge internally cooled electrodes. Subjective pain relief was reported in 90% and lasted a minimum of 4 months without further treatment. Callstrom et al (40) treated 12 patients with severe pain from metastatic lesions involving bone that were refractory to radiation therapy, chemotherapy, surgery, or analgesic medicines or, alternatively, who had refused to undergo these standard therapies. Patients included in the study had pain resulting from no more than two sites of metastatic disease. Patients with lesions within 1 cm of the spinal cord, brain, aorta, inferior vena cava, bowel, or bladder and patients with impending fracture at the potential ablation site were not eligible for this study. All patients experienced a decrease in pain over the course of the follow-up period. Patients derived benefit from the RF-ablation treatment within 1 week. The patients showed greater benefit from RF ablation with time, reporting mean decreases for pain 4 weeks after treatment. In addition to providing pain relief, RF ablation resulted in improved quality of life with decreased interference from pain in the activities of daily living. The mechanism of action responsible for decreased pain at the metastatic site after RF ablation is unclear. Radiofrequency ablation might provide an alternative treatment for palliation of painful metastatic lesions that are resistant to radiation and in cases in which further radiation therapy is not possible because of limitations of dose to normal structures. It is also possible that RF ablation will play an adjunctive role to the use of radiation therapy for palliation of painful metastatic lesions (40). Prospective comparison studies of RF ablation and radiation therapy may be useful to help distinguish the relative benefits of these therapies for palliation of painful metastatic lesions.

Additional reports have begun to appear describing the use of RF ablation in other sites and organs. Polascik et al (41) reported their experience with saline-enhanced RF-ablation treatment of VX2 tumors that had been implanted beneath the renal capsule in rabbits. Zlotta et al (42) reported the treatment of three focal renal tumors in two patients by using hooked electrodes. Extensive coagulation necrosis was found throughout these tumors at subsequent nephrectomy. McGovern et al (43) reported the successful treatment of a single 3-cm renal cell carcinoma (RCC) by using an 18-gauge internally cooled RF electrode placed percutaneously with US guidance.

In a recent series, by Gervais et al (44), 42 RCCs were ablated with a total of 140 overlapping ablations with acceptable morbidity and no procedure-related mortality. The number of ablated tumors allowed statistical analysis of the effect of tumor location on results of RF ablation of large tumors, and the authors were able to achieve complete ablation of all exophytic tumors up to 5.0cm in size. Although the mean follow-up period in this study was short (13.2 months) with respect to the natural history of RCC, the results observed during the longest follow-up period (3.5 years) were encouraging in terms of the continued long-term evaluation of this technique. The absence of tumor recurrences over the time course was also very encouraging. Still, because many small RCC tumors can be expected to grow at a rate of 1 to 3mm per year, longer-term follow-up of surviving patients to assess rates of local recurrence and occurrence of possible metastatic disease is needed. Small exophytic RCC tumors (as large as 5.0cm) are the ideal tumors for treatment with RF ablation. For patients with an actual or functionally solitary kidney who undergo complete ablation of RCC, RF ablation provides a treatment option that does not subject them to the inconvenience and morbidities of dialysis. Even in the absence of complete ablation, RF ablation may play a role in palliation of disease in patients who find dialysis unacceptable. This palliative role of RF ablation in the treatment of RCC is an interesting area for further study, especially for large tumors with a central component (44).

Dupuy et al (45) reported their experience in treating lung malignancies. Three patients with unresectable lung tumors were treated with RF ablation. Zagoria et al (46) published a case report in which two lung metastatic nodules in a patient with RCC were ablated without major complications. Steinke et al (47) described a case of a pulmonary metastasis resected after RF ablation, in which histologic proof of complete necrosis was obtained. VanSonnenberg et al (48) reported their initial clinical experience in six patients with either primary or secondary unresectable lung tumors, who had exhausted radiation and chemotherapy alternatives.

In all cases, extensive necrosis, manifested as no enhancement on the postprocedure contrast-enhanced MRI, was seen. One intraprocedural pneumothorax was encountered, and treated intraprocedurally with a small-bore (7-Fr) percutaneous cathether that allowed the procedure to continue. Wallace et al (49) also treated patients with either primary or secondary unresectable lung malignancies. In their series of 12 patients with 16 lesions, follow-up CT contrast densitometry demonstrated a significant drop in mean enhancement of treated tumors 1 to 2 months after the ablation. Complications included pneumothoraces requiring catheter drainage ($n = 4$), pleural effusion ($n = 3$), and pain ($n = 2$). Dupuy et al (50) treated 27 patients, 14 with primary lung cancer and 13 with metastases from various primary tumors. Radiofrequency ablation was tolerated in all patients, and the pneumothorax rate was 14%.

In this series, residual tumor or tumor recurrence at the treated site was identified in nine patients after a mean follow-up of 4.4 months. Lencioni et al (51) reported a series of 10 patients with unresectable, biopsy-proven NSCLC of 3cm or less in greatest dimension (range, 1.1–3cm; mean, 2.1 ± 0.6cm) undergoing RF ablation. In this study, correct placement of the electrode needle within the lesion was achieved in all cases, and single-session ablation was successfully performed. Pneumothorax was observed in four of 10 patients, two of whom required drainage. No other complication occurred. Pulmonary function tests did not show any significant worsening with respect to baseline. CT studies obtained 1 month after treatment showed areas of thermal injury encompassing the native tumor in all cases. At 3-month CT studies, treated areas showed reduction in size with no signs of recurrence in any case. Complete tumor response was confirmed in six of six patients who also were assessed 6 months after the procedure. Glenn et al (52) treated 10 nonsurgical patients with colorectal lung metastases. Radiofrequency ablation was technically successful in 14 of 15 pulmonary tumors. Baseline tumor size was 2.6 ± 1.9cm (range 0.8–8.0). Computed tomography lesion size after ablation decreased from 1 month to 3 months in all lesions with 3-month follow-up. Complications requiring intervention occurred in three patients and included pneumothorax (three) and pleural effusion (one).

References

1. Rhim H, Goldberg SN, Dodd GD III, et al. Essential techniques for successful radiofrequency thermal ablation of malignant hepatic tumors. Radiographics 2001;21:S17–S35.
2. Gazelle GS, Goldberg SN, Solbiati L, Livraghi T. Tumor ablation with radiofrequency energy. Radiology 2000;217:633–646.
3. Cady B, Jenkins RL, Steele GD Jr, et al. Surgical margin in hepatic resection for colorectal metastasis: a critical and improvable determinant of outcome. Ann Surg 1998;227:566–571.
4. Dodd GD III, Soulen M, Kane R, et al. Minimally invasive treatment of malignant hepatic tumors: at the threshold of major breakthrough. RadioGraphics 2000;20:9–27.
5. Patterson EJ, Scudamore CH, Owen DA, Nagy AG, Buczkowski AK. Radiofrequency ablation of porcine liver in vivo: effects of blood flow and treatment time on lesion size. Ann Surg 1998; 227:559–565.
6. Pennes HH. Analysis of tissue and arterial blood temperatures in the resting human forearm. J Appl Physiol 1948;1:93–122.
7. Goldberg SN, Gazelle GS, Mueller PR. Thermal ablation therapy for focal malignancy: a unified approach to underlying principles, techniques, and diagnostic imaging guidance. AJR 2000;174: 323–331.
8. Goldberg SN, Gazelle GS, Halpern EF, Rittman WJ, Mueller PR, Rosenthal DI. Radiofrequency tissue ablation: importance of local temperature along the electrode tip exposure in determining lesion size and shape. Acad Radiol 1996;3:212–218.
9. Rossi S, Buscarini E, Garbagnati F, et al. Percutaneous treatment of small hepatic tumors by an expandable RF electrode needle. AJR 1998;170: 1015–1022.
10. LeVeen RF. Laser hyperthermia and radiofrequency ablation of hepatic lesions. Semin Intervent Radiol 1997;14:313–324.
11. Goldberg SN, Gazelle GS, Solbiati L, Rittman WJ, Mueller PR. Radiofrequency tissue ablation: increased lesion diameter with a perfusion electrode. Acad Radiol 1996;3:636–644.
12. Goldberg SN, Gazelle GS. Radiofrequency tissue ablation and techniques for increasing coagulation necrosis. Hepatogastroenterology 2001;48: 359–367.
13. Goldberg SN, Solbiati L, Hahn PF, et al. Large-volume tissue ablation with radiofrequency by using a clustered, internally cooled electrode technique: laboratory and clinical experience in liver metastases. Radiology 1998;209:371–379.
14. Goldberg S, Ahmed M, Gazelle GS, et al. Radiofrequency thermal ablation with NaCl solution injection: effect of electrical conductivity on tissue heating and coagulation—phantom and porcine liver study. Radiology 2001;219:157–165.
15. Livraghi T, Goldberg SN, Lazzaroni S, et al. Saline-enhanced radio-frequency tissue ablation in the treatment of liver metastases. Radiology 1997;202:205–210.
16. Böhm T, Hilger I, Mueller W, Reichenbach JR, Fleck M, Kaiser WA. Saline enhanced radiofrequency ablation of breast tissue: an in-vitro feasibility study. Invest Radiol 2000;35:149–157.
17. Boehm T, Malich A, Goldberg SN, et al. Radiofrequency tumor ablation: internally cooled electrode versus saline-enhanced technique in an aggressive rabbit tumor model. Radiology 2002;222:805–813.
18. Goldberg SN, Solbiati L, Halpern EF, Gazelle GS. Variables affecting proper system grounding for radiofrequency ablation in an animal model. J Vasc Intervent Radiol 2000;11:1069–1075.
19. Goldberg SN, Hahn PF, Tanabe KK, et al. Percutaneous radiofrequency tissue ablation: does perfusion-mediated tissue cooling limit coagulation necrosis? J Vasc Intervent Radiol 1998;9: 101–115.
20. Goldberg SN, Hahn PF, Halpern E, Fogle R, Gazelle GS. Radio-frequency tissue ablation: effect of pharmacologic modulation of blood flow on coagulation diameter. Radiology 1998; 209:761–767.
21. Rossi S, Garbagnati F, Lencioni R, et al. Percutaneous radio-frequency thermal ablation of nonresectable hepatocellular carcinoma after occlusion of tumor blood supply. Radiology 2000;217: 119–126.
22. Goldberg SN, Saldinger PF, Gazelle GS, et al. Percutaneous tumor ablation: increased necrosis with combined radio-frequency ablation and intratumoral doxorubicin injection in a rat breast tumor model. Radiology 2001;220:420–427.
23. McGahan JP, Dodd GD III. Radiofrequency ablation of the liver: current status. AJR 2001; 176:3–16.
24. Lewin JS, Connell CF, Duerk JL, et al. Interactive MR-guided radiofrequency interstitial thermal ablation of abdominal tumors: clinical trial for evaluation of safety and feasibility. J Magn Reson Imaging 1998;8:40–47.

25. Franco D, Capussotti L, Smadja C, et al. Resection of hepatocellular carcinoma: results in 72 European patients with cirrhosis. Gastroenterology 1990;98:733–738.
26. Hughes KS, Rosenstein RB, Songhorabodi S, et al. Resection of the liver for colorectal carcinoma metastases: a multi-institutional study of long-term survivors. Dis Colon Rectum 1988; 31:1–4.
27. Castells A, Bruix J, Bru C, et al. Treatment of small hepatocellular carcinoma in cirrhotic patients: a cohort study comparing surgical resection and percutaneous ethanol injection. Hepatology 1993;18:1121–1126.
28. Curley SA, Izzo F, Delrio P, et al. Radiofrequency ablation of unresectable primary and metastatic hepatic malignancies: results in 123 patients. Ann Surg 1999;230:1–8.
29. Lencioni R, Cioni D, Bartolozzi C. Percutaneous radiofrequency thermal ablation of liver malignancies: techniques, indications, imaging findings, and clinical results. Abdom Imaging 2000; 26:345–360.
30. Rossi S, Di Stasi M, Buscarini E, et al. Percutaneous radiofrequency interstitial thermal ablation in the treatment of small hepatocellular carcinoma. Cancer J Sci Am 1995;1:73–77.
31. Livraghi T, Goldberg SN, Lazzaroni S, et al. Small hepatocellular carcinoma: treatment with radiofrequency ablation versus ethanol injection. Radiology 1999;210:655–661.
32. Lencioni R, Allgaier HP, Cioni D, et al. A randomized comparison of radiofrequency thermal ablation and percutaneous ethanol injection for the treatment of small hepatocellular carcinoma in cirrhosis. Radiology 2003;228:235–240.
33. Lencioni R, Goletti O, Armillotta N, et al. Radiofrequency thermal ablation of liver metastases with a cooled-tip electrode needle: results of a pilot clinical trial. Eur Radiol 1998;8:1205–1211.
34. Solbiati L, Goldberg SN, Ierace T, et al. Hepatic metastases: percutaneous radiofrequency ablation with cooled-tip electrodes. Radiology 1997; 205:367–373.
35. Gillams AR, Lees WR. Survival after percutaneous, image-guided, thermal ablation of hepatic metastases from colorectal cancer. Dis Colon Rectum 2000;43:656–661.
36. Siperstein AE, Rogers SJ, Hansen PD, Gitomirsky A. Laparoscopic thermal ablation of hepatic neuroendocrine tumor metastases. Surgery 1997;122:1147–1155.
37. Rosenthal DI, Alexander A, Rosenberg AE, Winfield D. Ablation of osteoid osteomas with a percutaneously placed electrode: a new procedure. Radiology 1992;183:29–33.
38. Rosenthal DI, Springfield DS, Gebhart MC, Rosenberg AE, Mankin HJ. Osteoid osteoma: percutaneous radio-frequency ablation. Radiology 1995;197:451–454.
39. Dupuy DE, Safran H, Mayo-Smith WW, Goldberg SN. Radiofrequency ablation of painful osseous metastases. Radiology 1998;209(P):389.
40. Callstrom MR, Charboneau JW, Goetz MP, et al. Painful metastases involving bone: feasibility of percutaneous CT- and US-guided radiofrequency ablation. Radiology 2002;224:87–97.
41. Polascik TJ, Hamper U, Lee BR, et al. Ablation of renal tumors in a rabbit model with interstitial saline-augmented radiofrequency energy: preliminary report of a new technology. Urology 1999;53:465–472.
42. Zlotta AR, Wildschutz T, Raviv G, et al. Radiofrequency interstitial tumor ablation (RITA) is a possible new modality for treatment of renal cancer: ex vivo and in vivo experience. J Endourol 1997;11:251–258.
43. McGovern FJ, Wood BJ, Goldberg SN, Mueller PR. Radiofrequency ablation of renal cell carcinoma via image guided needle electrodes. J Urol 1999;161:599–600.
44. Gervais DA, McGovern FJ, Arellano RS, McDougal WS, Mueller PR. Renal cell carcinoma: clinical experience and technical success with radio-frequency ablation of 42 tumors. Radiology 2003;226:417–424.
45. Dupuy DE, Zagoria RJ, Akerley W, Mayo-Smith WW, Kavanaugh PV, Safran H. Percutaneous RF ablation of malignancies in the lung. AJR 2000;174:57–60.
46. Zagoria RJ, Chen MY, Kavanagh PV, Torti FM. Radio-frequency ablation of lung metastases from renal cell carcinoma. J Urol 2001;166: 1827–1828.
47. Steinke K, Habicht J, Thomsen S, Soler M, Jacob LA. CT-guided radiofrequency ablation of a pulmonary metastasis followed by surgical resection. Cardiovasc Intervent Radiol 2002;25:543–546.
48. VanSonnenberg E, Shankar S, Tuncali KT, Silverman SG, Morrison PR, Jaklitsch M. Initial clinical experience with RF ablation of lung tumors. Radiology 2002;225(P):291.
49. Wallace AB, Suh RD, Sheehan RE, Heinze SB, Goldin JG. Contrast nodule densitometry to assess the efficacy of radiofrequency ablation of pulmonary malignancies. Radiology 2002; 225(P):292.

50. Dupuy DE, Mayo-Smith WW, Di Petrillo T, Ridlen MS, Murphy BL, Cronan JJ. Clinical experience of pulmonary radiofrequency ablation in 27 patients. Radiology 2001;221(P): 389.
51. Lencioni R, Crocetti L, Cioni R, Mussi A, Angeletti CA, Bartolozzi C. Percutaneous radiofrequency thermal ablation of small unresectable non-small cell lung cancer. Radiology 2003; 226:38A.
52. Glenn DW, Clark W, Morris DL, King J, Zhao J. Percutaneous radiofrequency ablation of colorectal pulmonary metastases. Radiology 2001; 221(P):315.

17a
Microwave Coagulation Therapy for Liver Tumors

Toshihito Seki

As treatment for hepatocellular carcinoma (HCC), surgical resection, transcatheter arterial embolization (TAE), and ultrasound (US)-guided local treatment have been performed alone or in combination. Surgical resection is not a viable option for all patients due to poor liver function induced by hepatic cirrhosis, and TAE sometimes is ineffective because of angioneogenesis in small HCCs. For these reasons, US-guided percutaneous local treatment has been adopted independently or in combination with TAE.

Percutaneous ethanol injection therapy (PEIT) was widely performed for patients with small HCCs as a local treatment in Japan when surgery was not indicated. Because PEIT was tolerated by most patients, it could be carried out easily in those with hepatic cirrhosis. However, PEIT was evaluated histopathologically and clinically, and the injected ethanol did not always cause complete necrosis of the tumor.

It is common to see HCCs surrounded by a fibrous capsule. However, formation of a fibrous capsule around the tumor often is incomplete in small HCCs. In such instances, injected ethanol may spread to the noncancerous peripheral tissue or may flow into large vessels around the tumor instead of remaining within the tumor, causing failure of tumor necrosis. Even when a fibrous capsule exists, but the encapsulated area or its periphery has been infiltrated by tumor cells, the injected ethanol may be blocked by the capsule and fail to reach tumor cells that have spread outside the capsule. Often viable cancer cells persist in the extra- or intracapsular area in surgically resected or autopsy specimens after PEIT. These viable cells have the potential to cause local recurrence, as well as intrahepatic or distant metastases.

To address these problems, we developed US-guided percutaneous microwave coagulation therapy (PMCT) as a local percutaneous treatment to induce complete tumor necrosis (1,2). Regardless of the presence of a capsule, microwave irradiation is most reliable to induce tissue coagulation if the tip of the electrode is located in the target lesion.

Initially, treating HCC, microwave coagulation was used in hepatic resection during open surgery for tissue coagulation and hemostasis (3). Several studies have reported excellent results (4,5). For percutaneous treatment, we could not use the electrode designed for hepatic resection because the shaft of the electrode for surgical use is too thick (1 cm in diameter). For percutaneous use of microwave coagulation, it was necessary to develop a thin electrode. Furthermore, it had to be designed so that this electrode caused tissue coagulation at the tip of the electrode, but did not burn the skin. We designed a thin electrode with decreased heat conduction through the shaft of the electrode.

In this chapter, both the mechanisms of microwave coagulation and the technique of PMCT for HCCs are elucidated. Clinical data using PMCT for HCCs including complications of PMCT are discussed as well.

Microwave Tissue Coagulation

In tissue, microwave irradiation from a monopolar antenna causes water molecules in the dielectric substance to vibrate dramatically at a frequency of 2450 MHz. This generates frictional heat in the water molecules and leads to thermal coagulation of tissue (5). Microwaves with a frequency of 2450 ± 50 MHz and a wavelength of 12-cm are recognized internationally as an industrial, scientific, and medical (ISM) band.

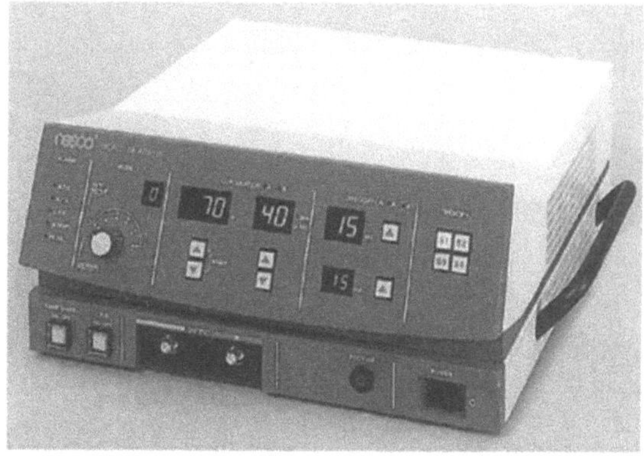

FIGURE 17a.1. Microwave generator: Microtaze: AZM-520, AZWELL, Osaka, Japan.

Microwave Coagulation System

The extent of the coagulation achieved by microwave irradiation is related to the amount of electric power and the irradiation time. To achieve tissue coagulation of not only the tumor but also neighboring noncancerous tissue, it is necessary to apply high energy efficiently to heat the tissue. For this purpose, the microwave irradiation power (in watts) must be sufficiently high and the electrodes must be able to withstand the conditions. As for irradiation time, long irradiation can induce extensive tissue coagulation, but is stressful for patients. Therefore, irradiation time should be shortened as much as possible.

Microwave Generator

The microwave is generated by a magnetron in a microwave generator (Microtaze: AZM-520, AZWELL, Osaka, Japan) (Fig. 17a.1). The electric energy of the microwave is supplied to a high-frequency coaxial cable with an impedance of 50 ohms via an isolated sympathizer cavity in the generator, and then conducted to an electrode attached to the other end of the cable for irradiation from the tip to the tissue. For easy manipulation, we use a coaxial cable, 2.5 m long with a diameter of 5.7 mm. To avoid unintended and unexpected irradiation, the generator is equipped with a fail-safe system so that the microwave cannot be irradiated unless both the inner and outer electrodes completely contact the tissue.

Microwave Electrode

The structure of the electrode (AZWELL) from the tip to the other end consists of an antenna 10 mm long made of stainless steel, an insulator 2 mm long made of polytetrafluorethylene (PTFE), and then a coaxial system 238 mm long, of which the inner conductive rod is made of silver-plated tool steel and is electrically connected to the antenna. The outer conductor of the coaxial construction is made of nickel-plated brass and this is the electrode. The electrode measures 2.0 mm in diameter and 25 cm in length. To prevent adhesion of the coagulated tissue to the electrode, the surfaces of the center and outer conductors are coated with PTFE (Fig. 17a.2).

It is known from the specific absorption rate (SAR) distribution that heating is limited to the area adjacent to the antenna. The electrode generates an electromagnetic field that surrounds the insulator, and the heated area of the tissue is limited to and focused on the area adjacent to the tip of the electrode.

Power Output Assessment

In vitro evaluation of coagulation capability was performed using resected pig liver. With irradiation at 80 W for 5 minutes, the coagulated area was elliptical, with maximal and minimal diameters of 3.5 cm and 2.5 cm, respectively (Fig. 17a.3). At this power and duration,

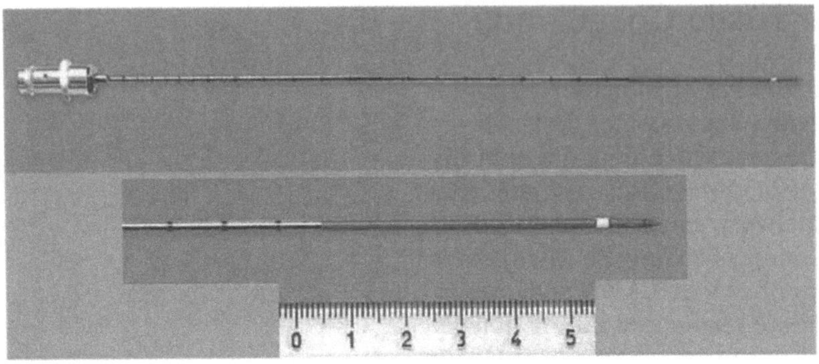

FIGURE 17a.2. Microwave electrode.

the temperature of the shaft of the electrode did not exceed 46°C. If the power and duration of irradiation exceeded 80W and 5 minutes, respectively, the temperature of the shaft was over 50°C. At this temperature, the skin may burn where the electrode has been inserted.

Percutaneous Microwave Coagulation Therapy (PMCT)

Methods (Fig. 17a.4)

1. After the location of the tumor is confirmed, the puncture line from the point of insertion of the electrode to the mass lesion is determined. Local anesthesia is induced along the puncture line by introducing 0.5% lidocaine from the insertion point at the skin to the peritoneum.
2. The insertion point of the skin is incised.
3. Under ultrasonic guidance, a 13-gauge guide needle is inserted in the vicinity of the tumor.
4. The inner needle of the guide is removed.
5. The microwave electrode is inserted through the outer needle of the guide into the tumor.
6. The tumor is irradiated with microwaves at 80W for 5 minutes. The microwave electrode is rotated axially during microwave irradiation to prevent the coagulated tissue from adhering to the tip of the electrode.
7. During microwave irradiation, the shaft of the electrode and the guide needle are heated. Therefore, to prevent the heat injury, the shaft of the electrode and the guide needle are cooled by cold saline using a cooling device.
8. The electrode and the outer needle of the guide are removed. The puncture line is irradiated with microwaves to prevent both bleeding from the hepatic surface and cancer cells from seeding along the puncture line when the electrode is removed.

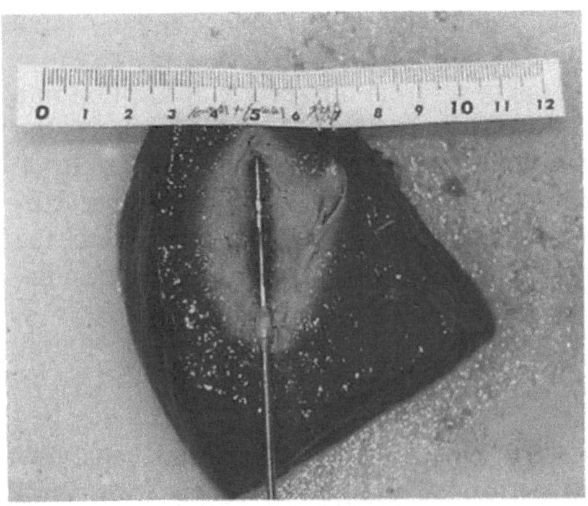

FIGURE 17a.3. Experimental study using resected liver. With irradiation at 80W for 5 minutes, the coagulated area is elliptical, with maximal and minimal diameters of 3.5cm and 2.5cm, respectively.

At each session, one to three electrode insertions at different sites are performed for the tumor. Microwave irradiation at 80W for 5 minutes is performed for each electrode insertion. The end point is the hyperechoic changes that cover the tumor and the neighboring noncancerous tissue to obtain a treated margin of

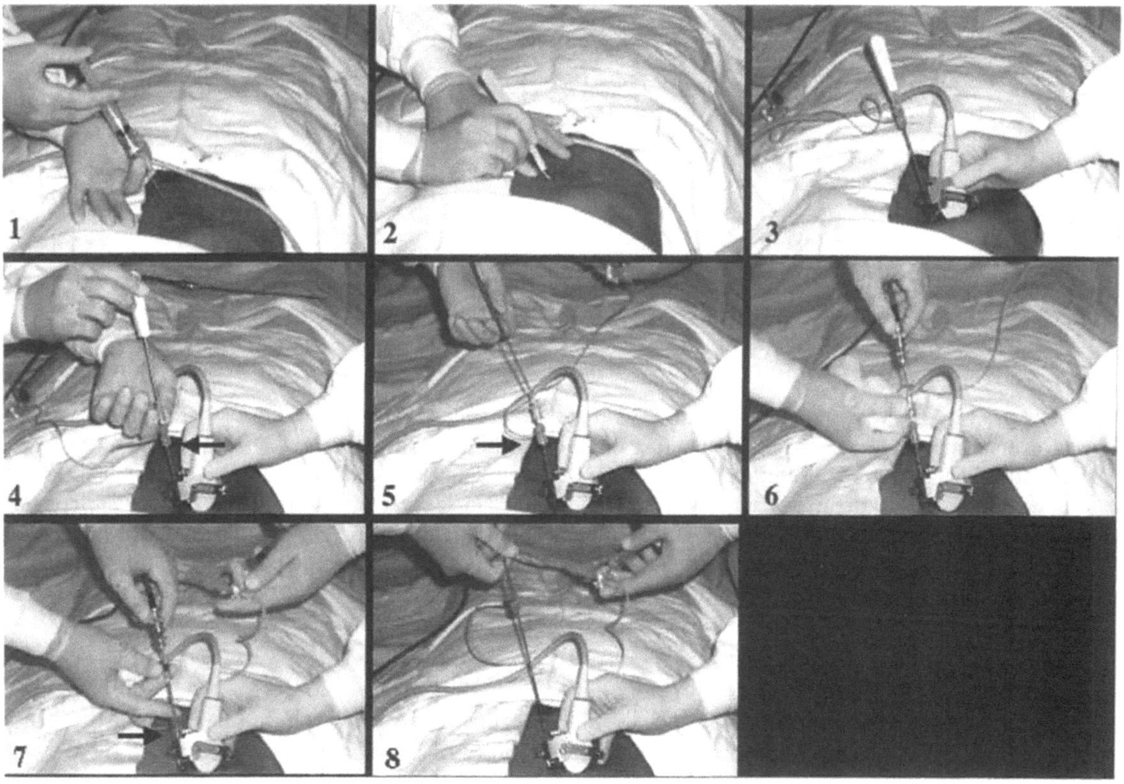

FIGURE 17a.4. Method of percutaneous microwave coagulation therapy (PMCT). Black arrows show a cooling device.

≥5 mm (Fig. 17a.5). When this change in the echo texture is achieved, the initial session is completed. It is important that the approach to the tumor should be multidirectional, for example, subcostal and intercostal, to produce extensive necrosis (Fig. 17a.6).

Microwave irradiation changes the low echo image of a tumor to hyperechoic. However, it is difficult to assess the therapeutic effect of PMCT using US, because the echogenic change indicates not only tissue necrosis, but also water vapor that is generated by the microwave irra-

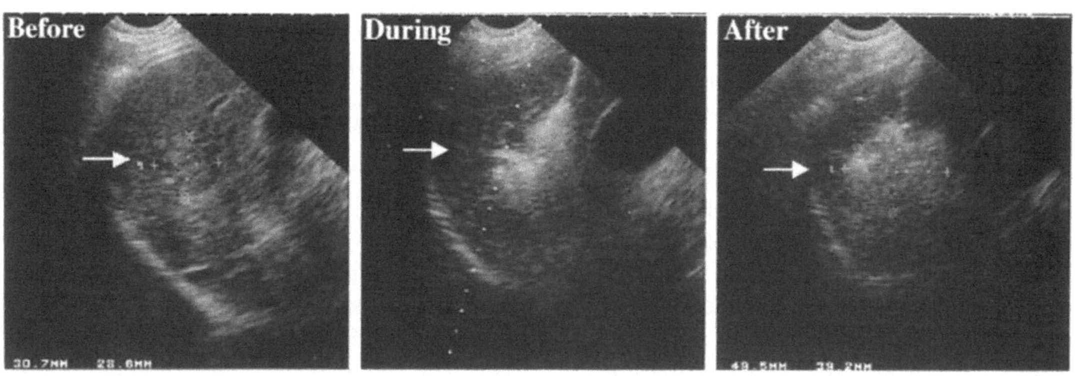

FIGURE 17a.5. Sonographic changes before, during, and after PMCT. The hepatocellular carcinoma (HCC) measuring 3.0 cm in diameter (white arrow) was treated with two punctures and microwave irradiation. Note hyperechogenicity obscuring the treated tumor.

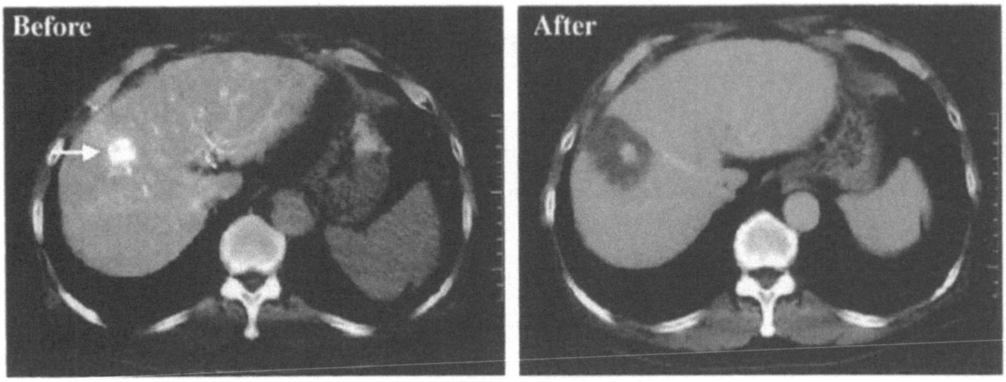

FIGURE 17a.6. A 56-year-old man with an HCC that was located in segment 8. CT obtained before and 1 week after PMCT treatment. Before treatment (CT-A), the tumor site (white arrow, tumor size 1.8 cm in greatest dimension) appears as an enhanced area. The tumor was treated with two subcostal and intercostal probe insertions. One week after treatment (dynamic CT, portal phase). PMCT induced a sufficient treatment margin. The tumor and the surrounding area did not enhance. Accumulation of iodized oil was observed in the tumor. The coagulated area was 3.7 cm in maximal diameter and 3.3 cm in minimal diameter.

diation. Therefore, the therapeutic effect should be confirmed by dynamic computed tomography (CT), dynamic magnetic resonance imaging (MRI), or enhanced US.

To assess the necrotic area, dynamic CT is performed 2 to 3 days after each treatment in our hospital. When the initial session fails to obtain a desired treated margin, the next session is performed under US guidance with reference to postdynamic CT images taken after the initial session. Thus, the total number of sessions is determined by dynamic CT findings. In our experience, PMCT can be completed with a single electrode insertion for most HCCs measuring 2 cm or less in diameter (Fig. 17a.7). Likewise, three electrode insertions suffice for HCCs measuring more than 2 cm, but not more than 3.0 cm in diameter.

Percutaneous microwave coagulation therapy is performed twice weekly in our hospital when indicated. In some patients, an iodized oil (4–6 mL, Lipiodol, Andre Guerbet, Aulnay-sous-Bois, France) is injected in the hepatic artery to evaluate the grade of cancer.

Tumors showing extrahepatic extension are excluded from PMCT because of difficulty in maintaining the puncture line. Similarly, tumors located near the gallbladder or gastrointestinal organs also were excluded because of the possibility of bile leakage or gastric or bowel perforation by heat injury.

Results of Percutaneous Microwave Coagulation Therapy

One hundred thirty-one patients with hepatic cirrhosis and a solitary nodular HCC measuring 3 cm or less in diameter (tumor size ≤2 cm, 81 patients; >2 to ≤3 cm, 50 patients) who were admitted to Kansai Medical University and its affiliated hospital between September 1994 and March 2002 underwent PMCT alone.

In patients with recurrence, we performed transcatheter arterial chemoembolization (TACE) and PMCT, or TACE alone.

Survival

The 5- and 7-year survival rates of patients with HCC measuring 2 cm or less in diameter treated with PMCT were 71% and 56%, respectively. The 5-year survival rate of patients with HCCs measuring more than 2 cm, but no more than 3.0 cm in diameter, treated with PMCT was 52%. At present, the 7-year survival rate of

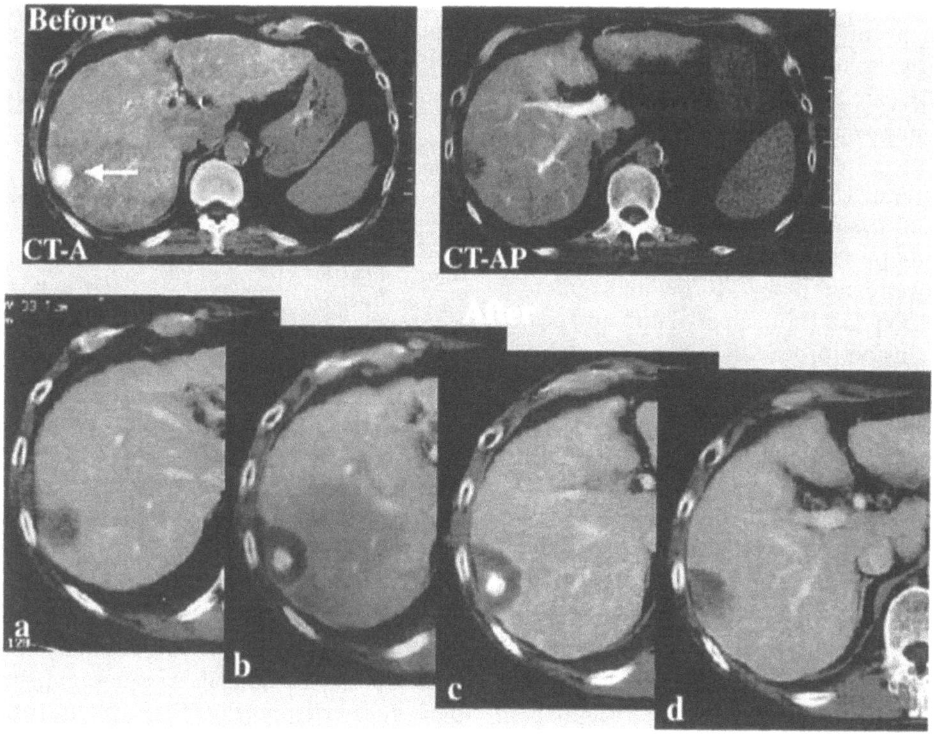

FIGURE 17a.7. A 72-year-old woman with HCC that was located in segment 6 with underlying hepatic cirrhosis (HCV). Before treatment (CT-A and CT-AP), the tumor (white arrow, tumor size 2.0cm in greatest dimension) enhanced with contrast material. The tumor was treated with one needle pass. Sequence of enhanced CT (portal phase) scans (slice width: 1 cm, A–D) one week after PMCT. The CT images show an extensive avascular area surrounding the tumor.

patients with HCCs measuring more than 2cm but no more than 3cm in diameter with PMCT is unknown.

Cancer-Free Survival and Local Recurrences

The 3- and 5-year cancer-free survival rates of patients with HCC measuring 2cm or less in diameter treated with PMCT were 40% and 15%, respectively, while 3- and 5-year survival rates of patients with HCCs measuring more than 2.0cm but no more than 3.0cm in diameter with PMCT were 40% and 20%, respectively.

The incidence of definite local recurrence of HCC measuring 2.0cm or less in diameter after PMCT within 2 years was 6%. On the other hand, among patients with HCC measuring more than 2.0cm, but no more than 3.0cm in diameter after treatment with PMCT, the local recurrence rate was 16%.

Combination Therapy (PMCT After TACE)

Transcatheter arterial chemoembolization can reduce the cooling effect for microwave thermal coagulation by decreasing hepatic arterial flow, and thus play a primary role in inducing tumor destruction. Furthermore, TACE with a combination of iodized oil and gelatin sponge particles can reduce the portal flow around the tumor transiently by filling the peripheral portal veins around the tumor with injected iodized oil that passes through multiple arterioportal communications (6,7). This decrease of portal flow also may reduce the cooling effect. Moreover, edematous changes (water retention) in the tumor that include the surrounding area induced by ischemia and inflammation after TACE (8) can enlarge the coagulation area, because microwaves act mainly on the watery component (water molecules) and produce dielectric heat (5). With an increasing watery component, tissue necrosis induced by microwave irradiation is enlarged (9). Furthermore, it has been reported that PMCT with segmental hepatic blood flow (both arterial flow and portal flow) occlusion produced extensive necrosis with a single needle insertion and subsequent microwave irradiation (10,11).

TABLE 17a.1. Complications associated with percutaneous microwave coagulation therapy.

Complication	No. of cases
Bleeding	
Intraabdominal	2
Hemothorax	1
Subcapsular	1
Bile duct stricture	3
Hepatic infarction	0
Pleural effusion	4
Ascites	1
Tract seeding	0
	12/356 cases

Adverse Effects and Complications (Table 17a.1)

At present, PMCT alone or in combination with TACE was performed in 356 patients having primary or recurrent nodules in our hospital. All patients complained of a slight heat sensation in the upper abdominal region during PMCT. Half of the patients felt some pain during treatment, but it was not serious enough to warrant treatment.

Local dissemination of the cancer cells along the tract was not encountered. However, complications such as intraabdominal bleeding, hemothorax, subcapsular hematoma, intrahepatic duct stricture (Fig. 17a.8), pleural effusion, and ascites did occur.

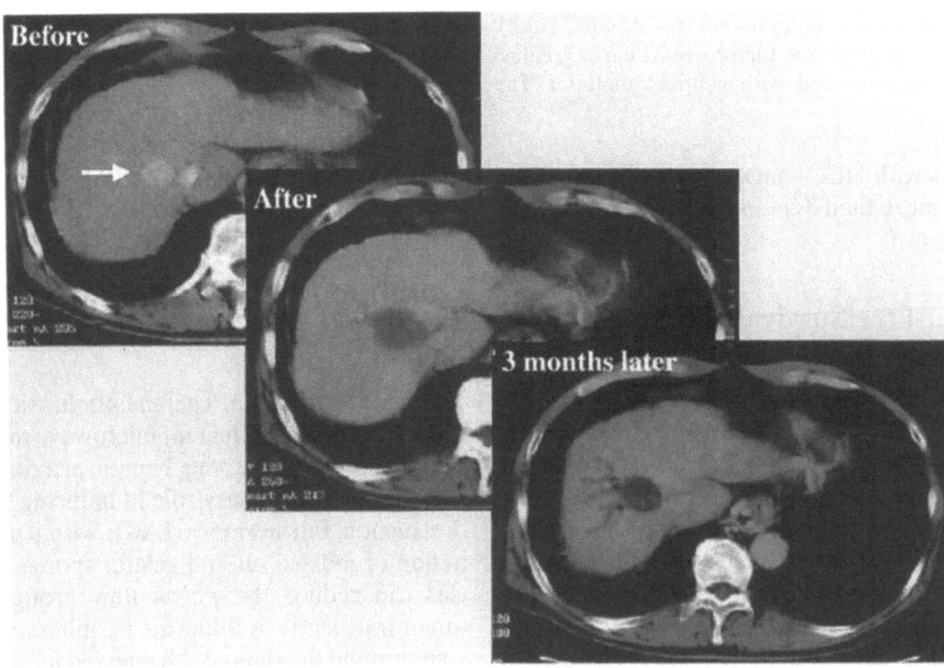

FIGURE 17a.8. Intrahepatic bile duct stricture after PMCT. A 65-year-old man with an HCC that was located in segment 8. Single microwave irradiation with 80 W for 5 minutes was performed for the HCC (white arrow). About 3 months later, the stricture was detected by the presence of dilated intrahepatic bile ducts. The patient is being observed without treatment.

There is a possibility that PMCT may induce complications from direct heat injury by the microwave irradiation. Accordingly, close observation is required posttherapy.

The Choice Between PMCT and Percutaneous Radiofrequency Ablation (PRFA) Therapy for HCC

It is reported that lesions created by PRFA for HCC with one needle insertion for 10 to 20 minutes ranged in diameter from 3 to 4 cm (12–15). RFA requires a longer ablation time than microwave, but a larger area can be ablated per session. Recently, it has been reported that PRFA and PMCT have equivalent therapeutic effects, but that PRFA could be achieved with fewer sessions. Thus, PRFA is recommended for small HCCs (16). Currently PMCT is in early stages of development, and despite good coagulation capability, treated areas induced by PMCT with one microwave electrode insertion are small (1). However, PMCT can produce extensive necrosis with one needle insertion and 5 minutes microwave irradiation using the newer microwave coagulation systems.

Prolonged RF ablation may be stressful for patients and may result in tumor tract seeding. It can be hypothesized that internal pressure within the HCC that is encased by a capsule is elevated by the heat from RF ablation or microwave coagulation. If this rise in the internal pressure is prolonged, the risk of tumor cells escaping into the peritoneal cavity along the tract and/or hepatic vessels may be increased during ablation (17). Llovet et al (18) reported that RF ablation with a cooled-tip probe for poorly differentiated HCCs located along the liver surface is associated with a high risk of tract seeding. On the other hand, we have not experienced tumor tract seeding associated with PMCT. However, we believe that the short ablation time of PMCT may decrease the risk of tract seeding. Thus, PMCT using the newest microwave coagulation system may be advantageous for small HCCs, although further clinical studies are required.

Laparoscopic Microwave Coagulation Therapy (LMCT)

When tumors have extrahepatic extension, we utilize laparoscopic microwave coagulation therapy (LMCT). Recently, various microwave electrodes and instruments for LMCT have been developed (Fig. 17a.9). LMCT is performed for HCCs that extend from the liver edge (Fig. 17a.10). Thirty-six patients have been treated with LMCT in our hospital; five died of

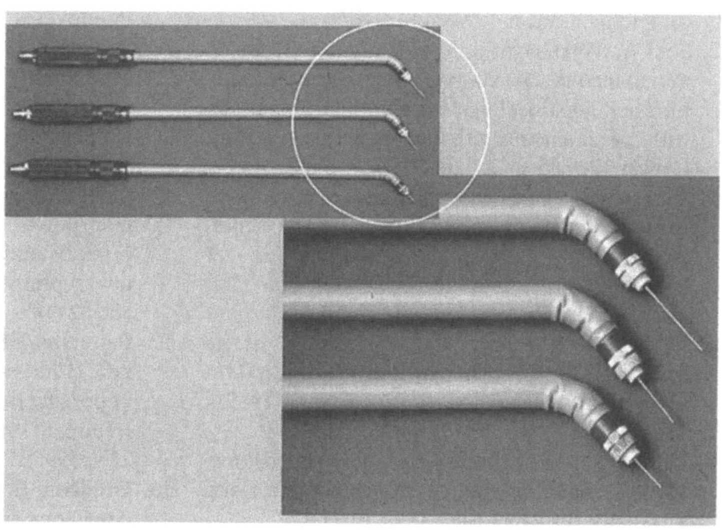

FIGURE 17a.9. Microwave electrodes (End-Angle electrode: AZWELL, Osaka, Japan) for laparoscopic microwave coagulation therapy (LMCT). This electrode has a flexible head for easy needle insertion.

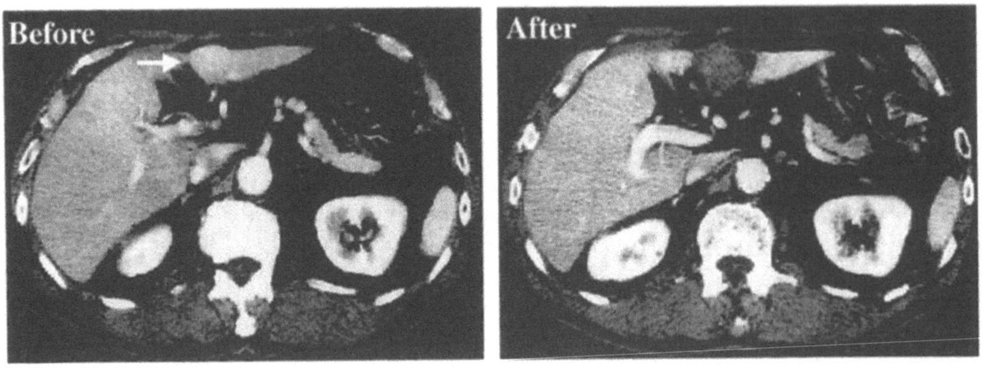

FIGURE 17a.10. A 66-year-old man with an HCC that was located in segment 3. Dynamic CT images before (arterial phase) and after (portal phase) LMCT. White arrow indicates the pretreatment lesion. There were six needle insertions and microwave irradiation (80W for 60 seconds) was performed. After LMCT, the tumor and surrounding area did not enhance.

the advanced HCC. However, at present, there are only two patients with definite local recurrence. Using laparoscopic ultrasonography (Laparo-US) can be quite difficult, and skill and training are required (19). In cases of HCCs that exist under the diaphragm and cannot be visualized under laparoscopy and Laparo-US, thoracoscopy is used (20).

References

1. Seki T, Wakabayashi M, Nakagawa T, et al. Ultrasonically guided percutaneous microwave coagulation therapy for small hepatocellular carcinoma. Cancer 1994;74:814–825.
2. Seki T, Wakabayashi M, Nakagawa T, et al. Percutaneous microwave coagulation therapy for small hepatocellular carcinoma: Comparison with percutaneous ethanol injection therapy. Cancer 1999;85:1694–1702.
3. Tabuse K, Katsumi M. Application of microwave tissue coagulator to hepatic surgery. The hemostatic effects of spontaneous rupture of hepatoma and tumor necrosis. Arch Jpn Chir 1981;50:571–579.
4. Tabuse K, Katsumi M, Kobayashi Y, et al. Microwave surgery: hepatectomy using microwave tissue coagulator. World J Surg 1985;9: 136–143.
5. Tabuse K. Basic knowledge of a microwave tissue coagulator and its clinical applications. J Hepatol Bil Pancr Surg 1998;5:165–172.
6. Kan Z, Sato M, Ivancev K, et al. Distribution and effect of iodized poppyseed oil in the liver after hepatic artery embolization: experimental study in several animal species. Radiology 1993;186: 861–866.
7. Chung JW. Transcatheter arterial chemoembolization of hepatocellular carcinoma. Hepato-Gastroenterology 1998;45(suppl 3):1236–1241.
8. Yoshioka H, Nakagawa K, Shindou H, et al. MR imaging of the liver before and after transcatheter hepatic chemo-embolization for hepatocellular carcinoma. Acta Radiol 1990;31:63–67.
9. Seki T, Tamai T, Nakagawa T, et al. Combination therapy with transcatheter arterial chemoembolization and percutaneous microwave coagulation therapy for hepatocellular carcinoma. Cancer 2000;89:1245–1251.
10. Murakami T, Shibata T, Ishida T, et al. Percutaneous microwave hepatic tumor coagulation with segmental hepatic blood flow occlusion in seven patients. AJR 1999;172:637–640.
11. Shibata T, Murakami T, Ogata N. Percutaneous microwave coagulation therapy for patients with primary and metastatic hepatic tumors during interruption of hepatic blood flow. Cancer 2000; 88:302–311.
12. Patterson EJ, Scudamore CH, Owen DA, Nagy AG, Buczkowski AK. Radiofrequency ablation of porcine liver in vivo. Effects of blood flow and treatment time on lesion size. Ann Surg 1998; 227:559–565.
13. Goldberg SN, Hahn PF, Tanabe KK, et al. Percutaneous radiofrequency tissue ablation: Does

perfusion-mediated tissue cooling limit coagulation necrosis? J Vasc Intervent Radiol 1998;9: 101–111.
14. de Baere T, Denys A, Wood BJ, et al. Radiofrequency liver ablation: experimental comparative study of water-cooled versus expandable systems. AJR 2001;176:187–192.
15. Goldberg SN, Gazelle GS. Radiofrequency tissue ablation: physical principles and techniques for increasing coagulation necrosis. Hepato-Gastroenterology 2001;48:359–367.
16. Shibata T, Iimuro Y, Yamamoto Y, et al. Small hepatocellular carcinoma: comparison of radiofrequency ablation and percutaneous microwave coagulation therapy. Radiology 2002;223:331–337.
17. Seki T, Tamai T, Ikeda K, et al. Rapid progression of hepatocellular carcinoma after transcatheter arterial chemoembolization and percutaneous radiofrequency ablation in the primary tumor region. Eur J Gastroenterol Hepatol 2001;13: 291–294.
18. Llovet JM, Vilana R, Bru C, et al. Increased risk of tumor seeding after percutaneous radiofrequency ablation for single hepatocellular carcinoma. Hepatology 2001;33:1124–1129.
19. Ido K, Isoda N, Kawamoto C, et al. Laparoscopic microwave coagulation therapy for solitary hepatocellular carcinoma performed under laparoscopic ultrasonography. Gastrointest Endosc 1997;45:415–420.
20. Yamashita Y, Sakai T, Maekawa T, Watanabe K, Iwasaki A, Shirakusa T. Thoracoscopic transdiaphragmatic microwave coagulation therapy for a liver tumor. Surg Endosc 1998;12:1254–1258.

17b
Microwave Ablation: Surgical Perspective

Andrew D. Strickland, Fateh Ahmed, and David M. Lloyd

The Field Effect of Microwave Heating

Thermal destruction by microwaves has been used effectively for many years for ablation of both small liver metastases and primary lesions. Microwaves produce effective ablation without islands of viable cells in a rapid and reproducible fashion. The microwave region of the electromagnetic spectrum is well suited to such a role due to the efficient conversion of electromagnetic energy to heat. This translation of energy is a result of the strong interaction between polar molecules and microwaves that causes oscillation of molecules, which is expressed as heat.

Water is a highly polar molecule, abundant in both normal liver tissue and hepatic neoplasms; it is the interaction between the microwaves and water that is principally responsible for the rise in temperature. The interaction between water and the entire range of frequencies in the microwave bandwidth is particularly strong. It is no coincidence that the fastest form of heating foodstuffs in the domestic kitchen is the microwave oven, principally due to the interaction between water molecules and microwaves.

Another advantage of microwave ablation is the manner in which the heating occurs. Unlike the alternative ablative devices such as radiofrequency or cryotherapy, the passage of heat is not solely reliant on conduction. The fundamental reason why microwave energy is unique and efficient is that it is transmitted from a suitable applicator or probe as a "field" around its tip. Direct heating of water molecules occurs within the whole microwave field, not simply by conduction of heat from the surface of a hot probe. A whole spherical area, perhaps the size of a tennis ball, is heated simultaneously and uniformly within minutes. Heating is not reliant on conduction through the tissues. Cytotoxic increases in temperature are reached rapidly. Beyond the microwave field, however, heating of the adjacent tissue does occur by thermal conduction.

The distinction between conductive heating and direct field heating is important, as conduction through water-laden tissue is slow and inefficient, particularly when the effects of local blood flow act as a heat sink. The interaction between the microwave field and water molecules of the target tissue within that field occurs very rapidly; consequently, the temperature climbs quickly. Theoretically, microwave coagulation should be the most efficient method for the destruction of large liver tumors.

Until recently the production of large, predictable ablations with microwave devices has not been possible unless multiple insertions of a probe or needle were used, similar to radiofrequency ablation (RFA). This constraint has limited its use among liver surgeons and interventional radiologists for ablation of colorectal metastases and small primary hepatocellular carcinomas in cirrhotic patients. Currently, the treatment of larger tumors has been possible only by multiple placements of a microwave probe that produce overlapping volumes of ablation. This is undesirable, as the technique requires highly skilled, accurate placements of the probe to avoid leaving islands of viable islands of cells in the target tumor. It also means that many patients will undergo multiple treatment sessions.

The Development of a New Microwave Applicator for Large Liver Tumor Ablation

Over the last decade a new form of microwave treatment applicator, the microwave endometrial ablation (MEA) applicator, has been developed by Microsulis Medical Ltd., UK in conjunction with scientists at the University of Bath, UK. The initial focus was in the field of gynecology. A microwave applicator was designed specifically to treat women with menorrhagia using an 8.5-mm-diameter antenna that was able to produce a heated microwave field from a generator delivering a frequency of 9.2GHz. Microwave endometrial ablation now is an established method to destroy the endometrium. It has been successfully used to treat more than 30,000 patients worldwide and the safety and efficacy of this treatment has been extensively validated in randomized controlled trials (Fig. 17b.1) (1). The uniqueness of the applicator is its ability to transmit microwave energy via a coaxial cable with extremely efficient heating of tissue within its microwave field.

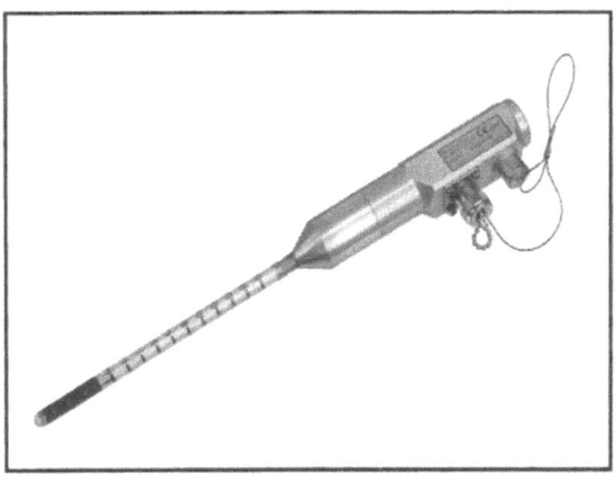

FIGURE 17b.1. The microwave endometrial ablation (MEA) applicator designed by Microsulis Medical Ltd., UK.

The data gained from the experiments into the microwave properties of tumor tissue and normal liver parenchyma have given physicists more knowledge of the electromagnetic properties of target tissues and how they change during treatment. Using this information, accurate computer models have been constructed to test the efficacy of novel applicator designs, thereby avoiding the need to "bench-test" every new probe. The models assess radiation of the microwave into the tissues and the degree of reflection that will occur.

Animal Experiments on Production of Large Ablation Volumes by Microwave Energy

Female pigs (body weight 45–50kg) were anesthetized and underwent a laparotomy to allow good exposure of the liver. Once adequately exposed, the novel microwave applicators were inserted into the hepatic parenchyma and ablations were carried out at varying times (1 to 3 minutes) and power settings (45 to 250W). The most remarkable finding was that the microwave equipment was able to produce large volume ablations (5 to 8cm in diameter) quickly, and were spherical in nature. The results were reproducible, and there was a linear relationship between the size of burn and the power output for any given time (2,3). Thus, accurate treatment volumes could be calculated for any given tumor size. The animals tolerated the production of multiple liver ablations extremely well. A large, 7-cm liver ablation with a single insertion is seen in Figure 17b.2, produced by using the 6.4-mm probe, powered at 150W, at a frequency of 2.45GHz.

Clinical Studies with Large Ablations

Although microwave liver ablation has been used extensively in the Far East over the past 20 years to treat primary liver tumors in cir-

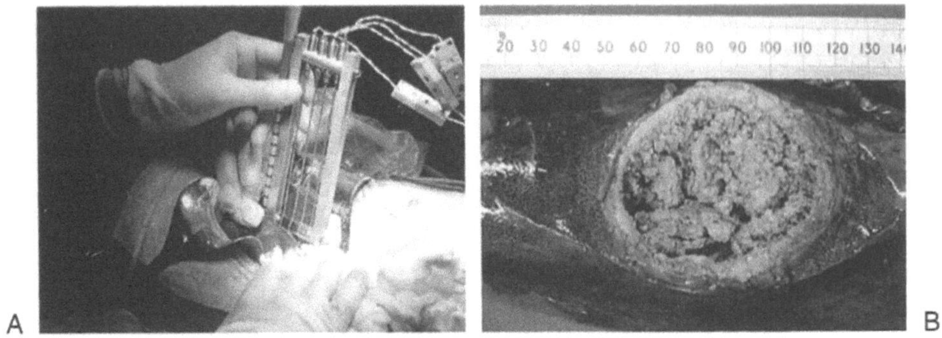

FIGURE 17b.2. Experimental liver ablation in a large animal model. The applicator is seen (with centimeter markings) (A) adjacent to thermocouples in a holder (left) with the production of a 7-cm-diameter ablation within 3 minutes (B).

rhotic patients, the results have been mixed, and limited by the size of the needle applicator that can treat only small lesions (<2 cm) unless multiple punctures are utilized. Developments in radiofrequency (RF) probes are encouraging, but RF also is limited because large tumor ablation (>5 cm) is associated with high recurrence rates.

We have used the large microwave applicator clinically with encouraging early results. There is no need for a conduction plate to be placed on the body, thereby eliminating the potential for skin complications that can occur with RFA. It also reduces the chance of bile duct damage caused by RF electric currents that can potentiate the "heat-sink" effect, as the high energy has to travel through tissues (bile ducts and vessels) to complete the electric circuit.

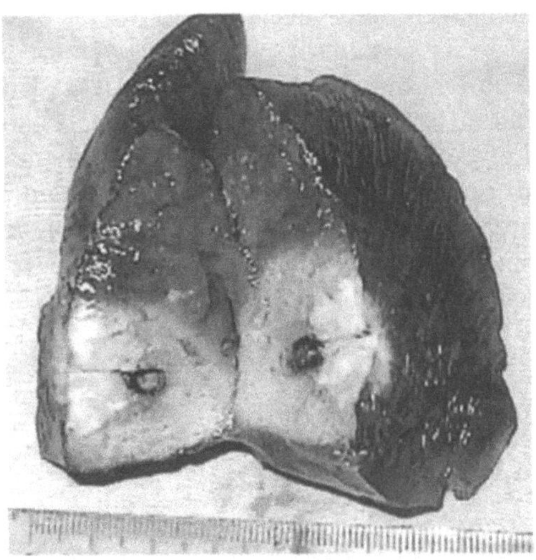

FIGURE 17b.3. Microwave ablation of a liver tumor using the novel microwave applicator. A 2-cm tumor is seen surrounded by a large area of ablation.

To date, our experience has included 22 patients with inoperable liver cancer who were entered into a clinical study. The study was approved by our institution's ethical committee. Six patients had inoperable primary liver cancer, 15 had inoperable colorectal metastases, and one had multiple neuroendocrine tumors. The age range was 38 to 79 years with a median age of 72 years. Four patients underwent simultaneous resection of the colorectal primary, and 12 underwent liver resection as well as microwave ablation.

Patients with tumors greater than 5 cm in diameter were treated for 3 or 4 minutes using the lower frequency of 2.45 GHz with the 6.4-mm-diameter probe at 150 W. Those with smaller tumors were treated for between 1 and 3 minutes at 9.2 GHz frequency at 45 W (Fig. 17b.3). Over 60 total ablations were performed, with the mean number of treatments being four per patient (range 1–9).

No complications were seen, and no early recurrences have occurred at the ablation sites with a mean follow-up of 12 months. There were two deaths in the colorectal group and one in the primary hepatocellular carcinoma (HCC) group, which occurred within 30 days. One patient treated for a large, 5.5-cm HCC was readmitted to the hospital with liver decompensation 5 weeks posttreatment. None of these deaths was directly attributable to the microwave ablation. The two patients who died in the colorectal group were elderly and frail and were awaiting triple coronary bypass grafting for severe ischemic heart disease. Both of these patients were rejected for cardiac surgery because of the presence of inoperable liver tumors. The microwave ablations in both of these patients were minimal, as only a few 2-cm metastatic lesions were treated, and did not contribute to the deaths of these patients.

The mean survival for the 22 patients in this initial study group was 12 months, with most patients dying of causes unrelated to their liver treatment. Several patients died of sepsis secondary to urinary tract infection or pneumonia 8 or 9 months after discharge from hospital, and other patients developed thoracic metastases. There was no evidence that any of these patients developed local recurrence at the site of a microwave ablation, although some patients developed liver tumors in other parts of the liver.

An example of the microwave procedure is demonstrated in a 74-year-old retired general practitioner with known liver cirrhosis who developed a 6.5-cm primary liver tumor in the right lobe of the liver (Fig. 17b.4).

Although a trial dissection was attempted, it was abandoned because of bleeding secondary to portal hypertension. During the procedure, it was elected to treat the tumor with the 6.4-mm probe with a frequency of 2.45 GHz for 3 minutes. No bleeding occurred at the time of ablation. The patient has remained well for 2½ years. His α-fetoprotein levels fell from 6000 units preoperatively to 40 units within a few months after the ablation. He had a slow-growing pleural metastasis that probably accounted for the slightly raised α-fetoprotein. Follow-up computed tomography (CT) scans confirmed he had complete regression of his liver primary.

A second patient was deemed to have inoperable hepatic metastases from a colorectal carcinoma. This 59-year-old woman failed to respond to chemotherapy. There were five large tumor deposits in the right liver and one large one (6 cm diameter) within the left lateral segment (Fig. 17b.5).

The patient underwent resection of four segments (segments 2, 3, 5, and 6) with four metastases. Microwave ablation of the two lesions in segments 7 and 8 was performed. She did well following the surgery, and remained in the hospital for 14 days. The follow-up scans taken at 2 months postablation showed no viable recurrence in the ablation areas or the remaining liver (Fig. 17b.6).

The new applicator can be used for both laparotomy and laparoscopy. Large ablations can be treated. For example, a 37-year-old woman presented with pain in her right upper quadrant, and was found to have a 6.4-cm benign adenoma in the middle of the right lobe. Rather than subject her to a formal right hemihepatectomy, she was treated laparoscopically using a 5.5-mm microwave probe. She under-

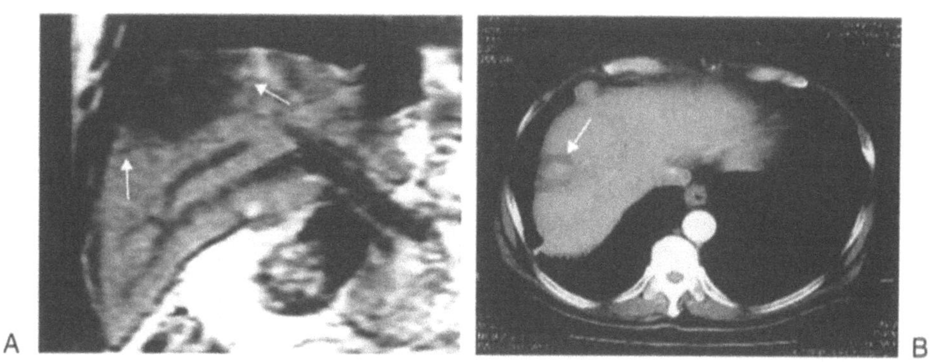

FIGURE 17b.4. (A) Coronal magnetic resonance imaging (MRI) scan of a patient with a 6.5-cm primary liver tumor (HCC) in the dome of the right hepatic lobe is seen as the lower-intensity mass (arrows). (B) Two years after microwave ablation treatment, the lesion (arrow) remains small and inactive on the contrast-enhanced computed tomography (CT) scan.

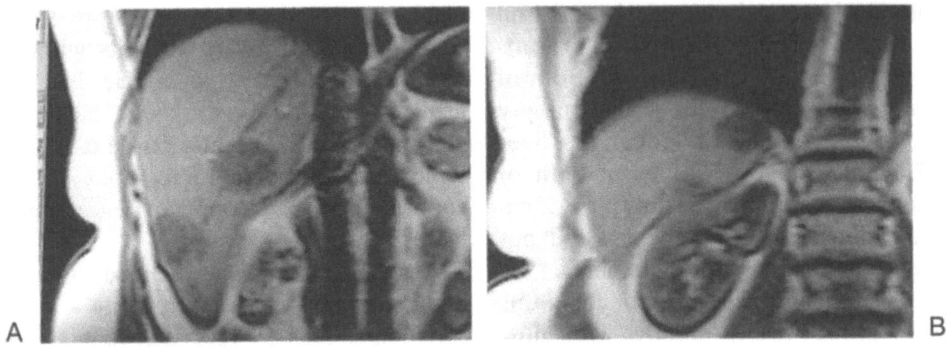

FIGURE 17b.5. (A,B) MRI scan of a patient with six large colorectal metastases in the liver. Three tumors in segments 5, 6, and 8 are shown. The 6-cm tumor in segments 2 and 3 is not shown.

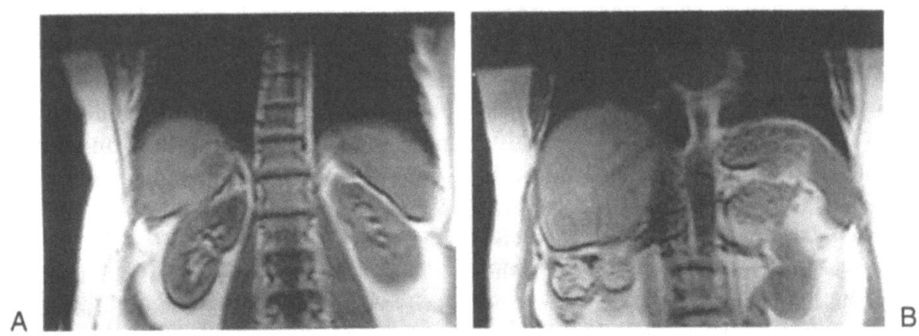

FIGURE 17b.6. (A,B) Follow-up MRI scans show two areas of ablated lesions (segments 7 and 8) in the hypertrophied liver.

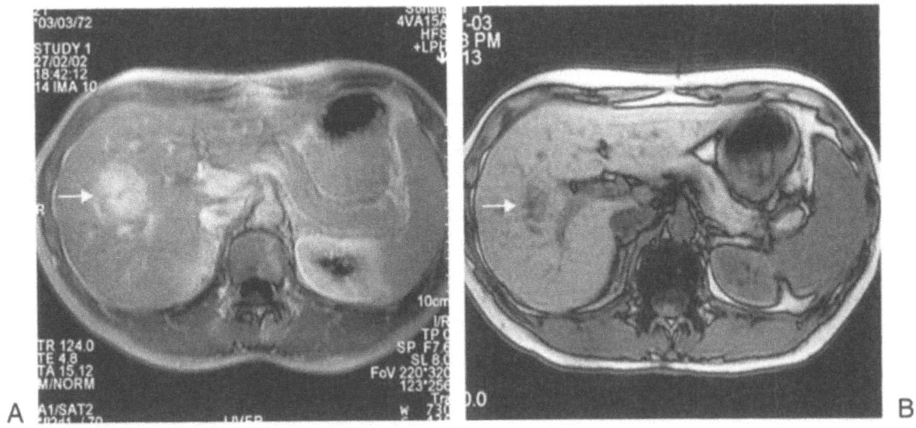

FIGURE 17b.7. (A,B) The preablation MRI scan of a 5.5-cm adenoma is seen on the left as a high-intensity mass (arrow). Six months following microwave ablation, a scar (arrow) remains.

went ablation using 150 W at 2.45 GHz for only 2 minutes. The preoperative and 6-month follow-up MRI scans of her liver are shown in Figure 17b.7.

Conclusion

These early data confirm that microwave ablation is safe, very quick, and efficient to destroy liver tumors within minutes. Large ablations can be achieved quickly and safely. We have not experienced any specific microwave-related complications during or after surgery. Large-volume ablations greater than 5 cm in diameter are achieved, and ablations of 8 cm in diameter may be accomplished. While large ablations have been achieved at open surgery, they are also feasible laparoscopically. Thinner probes for percutaneous treatments are being developed as well.

References

1. Cooper KC, Bain C, Parkin DE. Comparison of microwave endometrial ablation and transcervical resection of the endometrium for treatment of heavy menstrual loss: a randomised trial. Lancet 1999;354:(9193):1859–1863.
2. Swift B, Strickland A, West K, Clegg P, Cronin N, Lloyd DM. The histological features of microwave coagulation therapy: an assessment of a new applicator design. Int J Exp Pathol 2003;84(1): 17–30.
3. Strickland AD, Clegg PJ, Cronin NJ, et al. Experimental study of large volume microwave ablation in the liver. Br J Surg 2002;89(8):1003–1007.

18
Percutaneous Laser Therapy of Primary and Secondary Liver Tumors and Soft Tissue Lesions: Technical Concepts, Limitations, Results, and Indications

Thomas J. Vogl, Ralf Straub, Katrin Eichler, Stefan Zangos, and Martin Mack

Percutaneous laser therapy is one of the general percutaneous ablation therapy strategies. In principle, laser therapy is possible using fibers or by laser-induced thermotherapy (LITT). The LITT procedure currently is performed at laparotomy, by laparoscopic control intraoperatively, or percutaneously. Monitoring is essential for percutaneous interventions; magnetic resonance imaging (MRI) has proven to be the most reliable thermal measure, while ultrasound has been unable to show an adequate estimation of the thermal changes induced by the applied energy. Laser-induced thermotherapy makes available a photothermal tumor destruction technique that allows solid tumors within parenchymal organs to be destroyed. The laser energy is transmitted via thin optic fibers and causes a well-defined area of coagulative necrosis. This effect results in destruction of tissue by direct heating, while limiting damage to surrounding structures. Magnetic resonance imaging has proven to be an ideal clinical instrument to define the exact position of the optical fibers in the target area, provides real-time monitoring of the thermal effects, and the subsequent evaluation of the extent of coagulative necrosis.

Several clinical indications for the use of minimally invasive laser applications currently are under investigation. By far the most frequent use is in the liver, followed by soft tissue tumor ablation, ablation and of lung, breast, head and neck, and renal tumors. From the oncologic point of view, therapeutic decisions have to be made according to curative, palliative, and symptomatic indications.

This chapter presents the technical requirements, the methodology, and the results of MRI-guided LITT in the field of liver and head and neck tumors, and general oncologic issues.

The liver as a large solid organ is very suitable for interventional radiology procedures, due to the short transcostal access and its excellent functional capacity. It is the most common site of metastatic tumor deposits, especially for colorectal cancer, which is the third leading cause of death in Western communities, outnumbered only by lung and breast cancer. At the time of death, approximately two thirds of patients with colorectal cancer present with liver metastases.

As metastatic disease is so prevalent in the liver, new treatment protocols currently are under investigation. Laser-induced thermotherapy recently has been applied as a minimally invasive technique to treat liver metastases. The percutaneous approach avoids laparotomy and uses local anesthesia with outpatient management, which are the main advantages of this new therapy.

After cure of the primary tumor, hepatic metastases have a decisive influence on survival. Therapeutic strategies for malignant liver lesions are based on a number of factors, such as the underlying primary tumor, location, stage of the tumor, and general factors, such as age and any existing concomitant illness. For example, when hepatocellular carcinoma (HCC) is curable, liver resection, hemihepatic resection, or liver transplant is the treatment of choice. If there are contraindications, transarterial chemoembolization combined with local alcohol injection is used as a palliative therapeutic strategy. Interstitial procedures such as LITT show a high rate of controlling the tumor, and are being evaluated clinically.

Strategies for liver metastases are considerably more complex. Up to now, surgical resection of solitary lesions has been the only potential curative treatment. However, the high rate of intrahepatic relapse, and the possible potentiation of intrahepatic growth of metastases because of tumor stimulation caused by release of growth-stimulating substances, are considered problematic. For these reasons, over the past few years there has been great interest in development of interstitial procedures such as laser coagulation or radiofrequency ablation.

Laser Application Techniques

For the theoretical and clinical use of LITT, the tissue-destroying effect is dependent on the choice of both radiation capacity and time. This means that parameters must be preselected in such as way that all tumor cells, if possible, are exposed to the coagulative effect. There also must be a safety margin of at least 10 mm in width around the tumor. Adjacent sensitive structures must not be damaged. Selecting the right laser is based on an optimal depth effect in tissue that is determined by the absorption properties of water and hemoglobin. This can be achieved with a wavelength between 1060 and 1200 nm. The neodymium: yttrium-aluminum-garnet (Nd:YAG) and semiconductor lasers with wavelengths of 1060 nm or 900 nm fulfill these requirements. The Nd:YAG laser is the solid-state laser used most often, and it comes with a wavelength of 1064 nm. The laser can be both pulsed and operated continuously, and supplies output power of up to 100 W. The tissue-dependent penetration depth of the photons is an essential parameter of the absorption in various depths of tissue layers. The range of the resulting temperature rise is not restricted to the optical penetration depth, but is substantially extended by thermal conduction. Normal cells are less sensitive to thermal exposure, while malignant cells are more sensitive. The altered metabolic state of malignant cells with pronounced hypoxia causes this high sensitivity.

To do justice to the coagulation of three-dimensional tumor geometry, it must be possible to heat an approximately spherical volume of tissue throughout. For this reason, application systems of defined space radiation have been developed, the distal ends of which are designed such that the result is an even circumference of radiation. With conventional applicators, almost spherical coagulation zones with a diameter of 20 to 25 mm are achieved. Apart from the applicator geometry, the radiation capacity and time are crucial parameters for the dimensions of the coagulation zone, as are specific tissue properties such as optical parameters and perfusion rate.

The temperature-dependent effects of the laser light on the tissue include enzyme induction, edema formation, and membrane relaxation in a temperature range of 40° to 45°C. At 60°C protein denaturation takes place, at 80°C collagen denaturation, and over 150°C carbonization.

Applicators and Application Techniques

Tissue carbonization must be avoided to achieve large-volume coagulation zones and to be able to guarantee safe application. The critical value is a power density of approximately 5 W/cm^2. Depending on the applicator, this means laser power of 3 to 10 W. At this point, migration of the photons deep into the tissue through absorption into the resulting "carbon layer" is impeded, and only "a hot spot" is produced. The heat diffusion that is still active limits the LITT zone to a small volume (diameter of 1 cm).

To avoid the carbonization effect that greatly reduces the volume, a dome-shaped applicator (scattering dome) has been developed. The

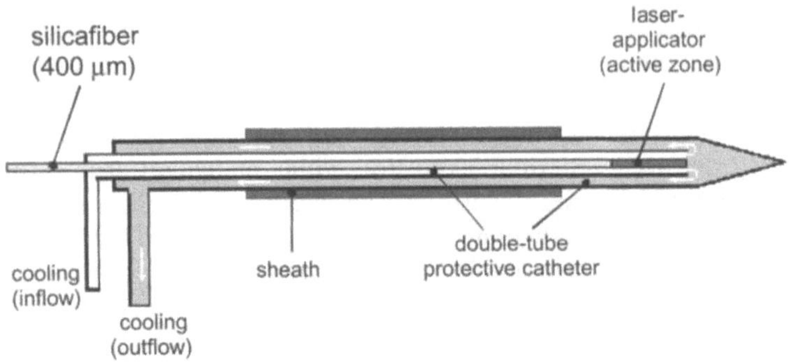

FIGURE 18.1. Illustration of the internally cooled power laser system.

scattering dome applicator can achieve the maximum penetration depth of the photons into the tissue. Because of absorption and convection, additional heat propagation results in deeper heating and hence "expansion" of the applicator, through which the diffusion processes of the heat propagation becomes dominant. It is technically easy and effective to adapt the scatter applicator to the therapeutic situation (Fig. 18.1). Radiation times over 30 minutes do not lead to any substantial additional expansion of the damaged tissue (diffusion equilibrium).

An essential step in clinical LITT is the development of application systems that can be applied percutaneously, laparoscopically, or operatively. First, a conventional system was available that consisted of a scattering dome applicator, a sluicing system, and a thermostable sheathed catheter, via which the LITT applicator was positioned (Fig. 18.2A).

Development of an irrigation system further expanded laser-induced necrosis, and optimized the treatment. This system has been developed from a 9-French sluicing system with centimeter markings, and a 7-French sheathed catheter with double lumina for irrigation. A sterile salt solution at room temperature is a proven irrigation medium. With a pump system integrated into the laser, irrigation rates of 30 to 60 mL per minute can be reached, thus providing reliable cooling of the applicator zone.

The following application techniques permit further treatment optimization; for the monoapplication, an application system is placed in the lesion percutaneously and is removed after application of heat.

A method of modifying the size and morphology of necrosis is a multiapplication with unifocal access ("pull-back" technique). After the end of the first heat application, the laser fibers are withdrawn by 1 and 2 cm through the percutaneous access point in the puncture pathway, while further heat application is applied.

As well as monoapplicators, multiapplicators can be utilized (multiapplications with multifocal access). Here, two or even up to four applicators are laid parallel and operated simultaneously. Prerequisites are the corresponding number of laser devices or beam splitters that help treat larger malignant lesions more rapidly. The disadvantage is the higher number of punctures that are required.

Treatment Monitoring

Magnetic resonance tomography (MRT) and MR thermometry (MRTE) are the optimum imaging methods to monitor treatment. Multiplanar representation and the high soft tissue contrast of MRT highlight the value of these techniques (Fig. 18.2).

Magnetic resonance sequences that emphasize perfusion and diffusion are temperature dependent and thus can be used for noninvasive temperature measuring. These parameters include the diffusion coefficient of water, the photon resonance frequency or chemical shift, and the T1 relaxation time. Due to the relatively low sensitivity with regard to motion artifacts, their wide availability, and the speed of data acquisition, thermosensitive T1-weighted

A–C

D–G

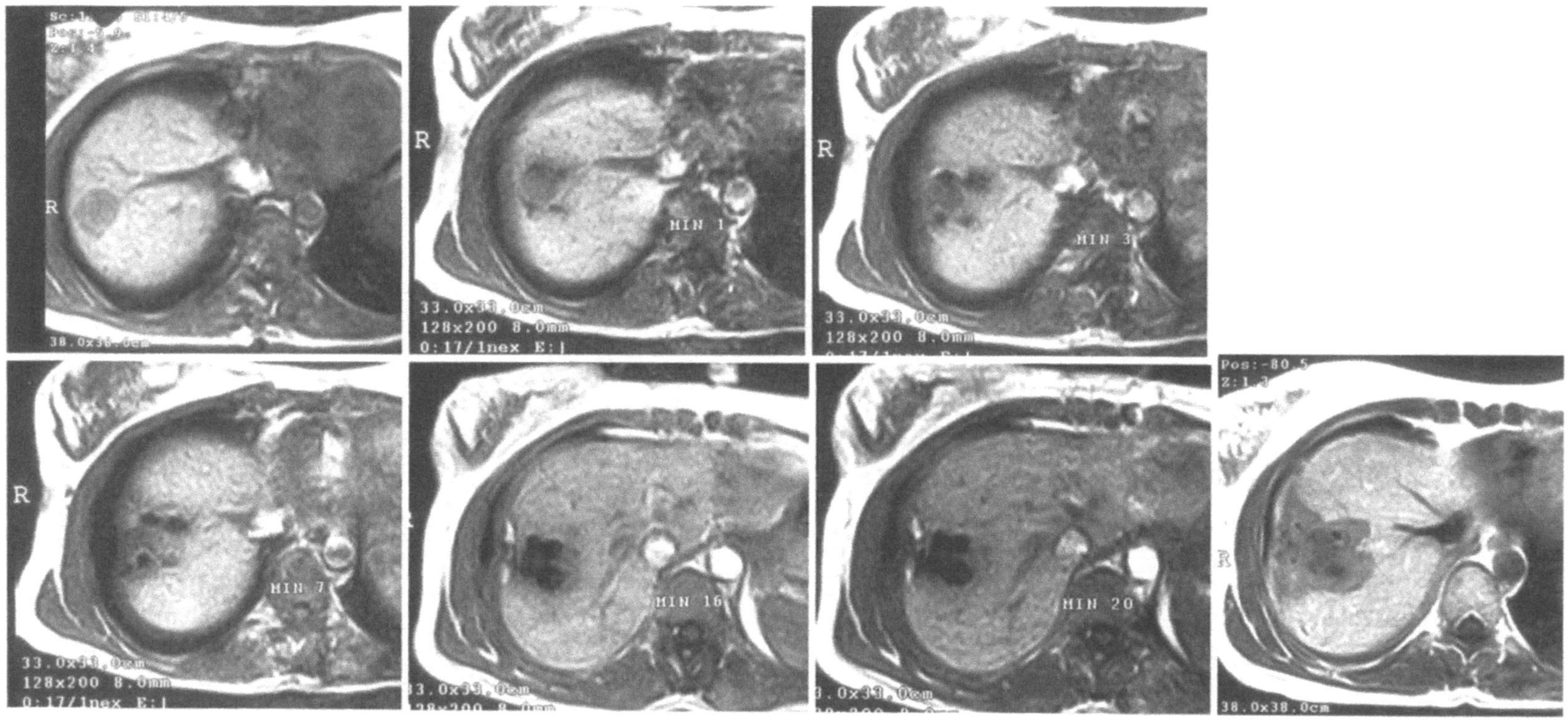

FIGURE 18.2. (A) A 35-year-old woman with liver metastasis from a colorectal carcinoma (initial tumor stage pT3, N1, M1). The T1-weighted thermosensitive gradient echo sequence in axial tomographic orientation shows the metastasis in liver segment 8 before starting the laser. (B) T1-weighted thermosensitive gradient echo sequence in axial tomographic orientation in the 1st minute. Clear drop in the signal intensity in the heated area. (C) T1-weighted thermosensitive gradient echo sequence in sagittal tomographic orientation in the 3rd minute. Further drop in signal intensity in the heated area. (D) T1-weighted thermosensitive gradient echo sequence in sagittal tomographic orientation in the 7th minute. Drop in signal intensity in the heated area. (E) T1-weighted thermosensitive gradient echo sequence in sagittal tomographic orientation in the 16th minute. Wider reduction in signal intensity in the heated area. (F) T1-weighted thermosensitive gradient echo sequence in sagittal tomographic orientation in the 20th minute. Low signal intensity in the heated area. (G) T1-weighted spin echo sequence in axial tomographic orientation after the administration of gadolinium–diethylenetriamine pentaacetic acid (DTPA) (0.1 mL per kg body weight). Sharp demarcation of the laser-induced thermotherapy (LITT)-induced necrosis with a safety margin surrounding the lesion.

MRTE sequences are used for clinical implementation of hepatic LITT. The longitudinal or spin-lattice relaxation time of a tissue is temperature dependent, and a local rise in temperature results in a signal drop in the MRT image. In vivo examinations and the findings of ours and other teams have shown a virtually linear correlation between the drop in signal in the image and the temperature. Appropriately weighted gradient echo sequences [fast low-angle shot (FLASH) and turbo-FLASH] with measuring times between 6 and 15 seconds in breath-hold technique have proved suitable for depicting the laser-induced temperature changes ranging from 60° to 110°C.

Before and after LITT a test of T1- and T2-weighted spin echo and gradient echo sequences is used for treatment planning and control. In addition, contrast agents [0.1 mmol gadolinium–diethylenetriamine pentaacetic acid (Gd-DTPA) per kilogram of body weight] optimize T1-weighted sequences (Figs. 18.3 and 18.4).

Computer-aided treatment planning that has been developed through in vivo comparative tests is available to further aid therapy. This makes it possible to calculate the optimum parameters for radiation capacity and time for each individual fiber before carrying out the laser treatment. The progress of the current temperature and the irreversible damage distribution can be monitored simultaneously as progress of treatment with real-time simulation, so that magnetic resonance tomography with indirect monitoring is available as an extension of virtual on-line monitoring.

Implementing and evaluating computer-aided thermoplanning for LITT applications is costly. The expected irreversible damage zone depends on various complex parameters. Influencing factors are laser capacity, radiation time, applicator characteristics, and optical

FIGURE 18.3. LITT of pleomorphic adenoma. (A) Thermo-turbo FLASH image (TR/TE/TI/flip angle = 7/3/400/8°) demonstrates the tumor recurrence (arrows) of the pleomorphic adenoma in the pre-styloid compartment of the right parapharyngeal space nearly isointense to muscle tissue. A subzygomatic approach was used for positioning of the laser applicator. Note the signal loss of the laser applicator due to the magnetite marker. The active zone (length 2 cm) of the laser applicator starts 1 cm before the end of the magnetite marker. (B) Thermo-turbo FLASH image obtained 12 minutes after starting the laser shows a signal loss around the active zone of the laser applicator (arrow) after an increase of tissue temperature due to an increase in T1 relaxation time. (C) Left image before LITT, middle image 2 days after LITT, right image 1 week after LITT. *Left image:* The contrast-enhanced (0.1 mmol/kg b.w. Gd-DTPA) T1-weighted spin echo (SE) image (TR/TE = 700/15) demonstrates the recurrent pleomorphic adenoma in the pre-styloid compartment of the left parapharyngeal space with a strong contrast enhancement, displacing the internal carotid artery on the left side posteriorly (arrows). *Middle image:* Contrast-enhanced image 2 days after LITT with 5.8 W over 20 minutes demonstrates the induced coagulative necrosis (N) with strong enhancement in the border of the lesion most likely representing postinterventional reactive changes. *Right image:* The contrast-enhanced image 1 week after LITT shows decreasing postablation reactive changes and an increase in size of zone of coagulative necrosis (N). (D) Left image 4 weeks after LITT, middle image 3 months after LITT, right image 2 years after LITT. *Left image:* Contrast-enhanced (0.1 mmol/kg b.w. Gd-DTPA) T1-weighted SE image (TR/TE = 700/15) demonstrates a further decrease of the reactive changes in the border of the treated recurrent tumor (arrows). However, in the anterior portion of the tumor pathologic contrast enhancement still could be visualized. Therefore, a second LITT treatment was performed to treat this part of the recurrent tumor. *Middle image:* The contrast-enhanced image 3 months after LITT demonstrates the induced coagulative necrosis (N) with some residual reactive changes in the border of the lesion. *Right image:* The contrast-enhanced image 2 years after LITT shows decreasing postablation reactive changes (arrows). (E) The plain T1-weighted SE image (TR/TE = 700/15) obtained 4 years after laser treatment demonstrates mainly residual scar tissue in the pre-styloid compartment of the left parapharyngeal space. (F) The contrast-enhanced (0.1 mmol/kg b.w. Gd-DTPA) T1-weighted SE image (TR/TE = 700/15) demonstrates no pathologic contrast enhancement in the pre-styloid compartment of the left parapharyngeal space, indicating lack of viable tumor.

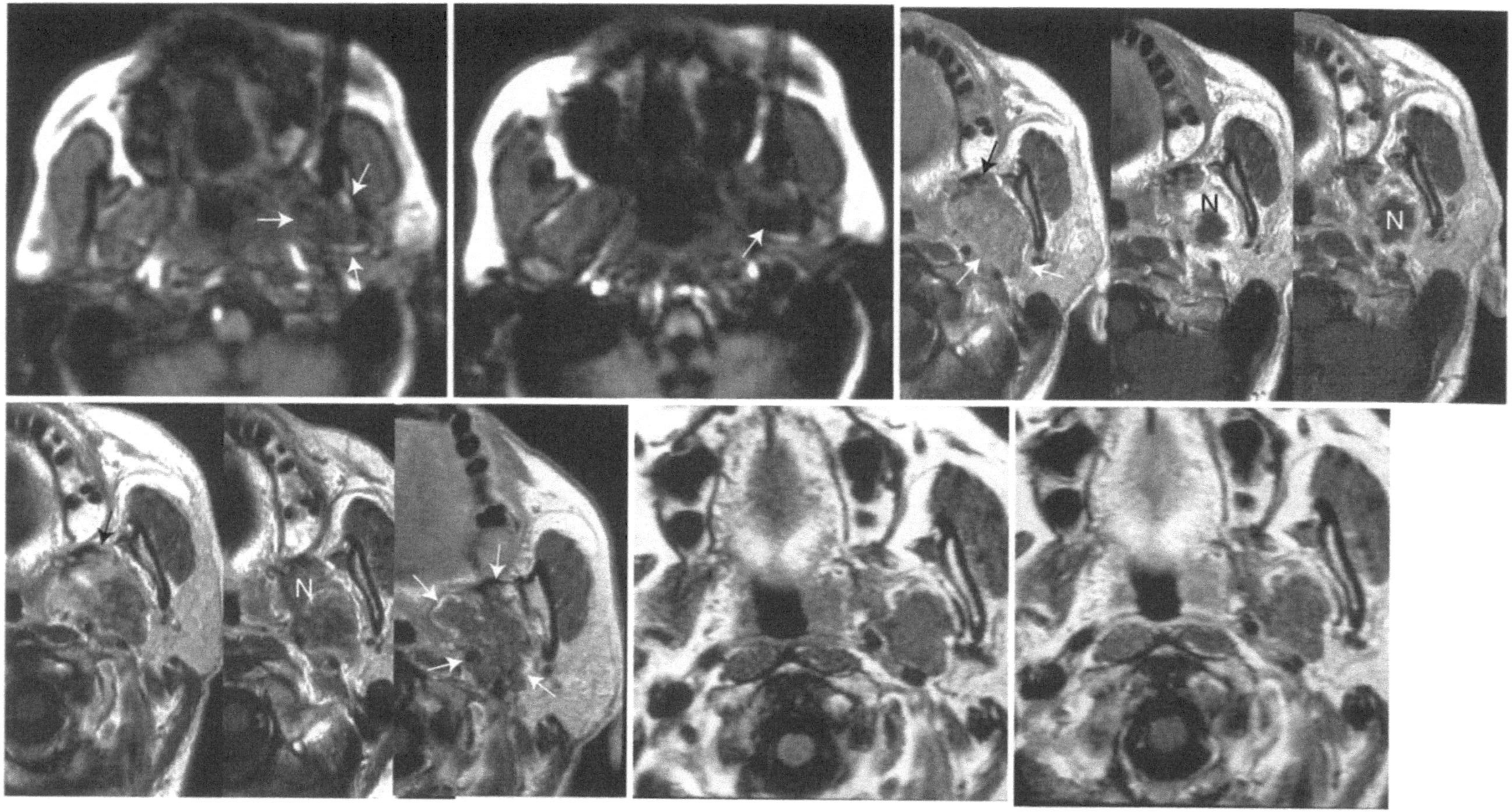

A–C

D–F

and thermal tissue parameters such as tissue perfusion and blood flow. Initial applications of this type of system lead us to expect further improvements in precision during treatments.

Standard Laser-Induced Thermotherapy Procedure to Treat Malignant Liver Tumors

Laser coagulation uses an Nd:YAG laser light with a wavelength of 1064 nm (MediLas 5060, MediLas 5100, Dornier Germering, Germany). It is delivered through optic fibers whose tips end in a specially developed diffusor. Originally, a diffusor tip with a glass dome of 0.9-mm diameter that was mounted at the end of a 10-m-long silica fiber (diameter 400 μm) was used. Since 2000, a flexible diffuser tip has been used with a diameter of 1.0 mm; this facilitates laser applications since the risk of damage to the diffuser tip has decreased to almost zero. The active length of the diffuser tip ranges from 20 to 40 mm in length. The laser power is adjusted to 12 W per centimeter active length of the laser applicator.

The laser application kit (SOMATEX, Berlin, Germany) consists of a cannulation needle, a sheath system, and a protective catheter that prevents direct contact of the laser applicator with the treated tissues and allows cooling of the tip of the laser applicator. The closed end of the protective catheter enables complete removal of the applicator even in the unlikely event of damage to the fiber during treatment. This simplifies the procedure and makes it safer for the patient.

The laser itself is installed outside the MR examination room, and the light is transmitted through a 10-m-long optic fiber. All patients are examined using an MRI protocol including gradient-echo (GE) T1-weighted plain and contrast-enhanced scans (Gd-DTPA 0.1 mmol/kg body weight). T1- and T2-weighted sequences are obtained to localize the target lesion and plan the interventional procedure. The scanners are a conventional 1.5-T magnet system (Siemens, Erlangen, Germany) and a 0.5-T system (Elscint Privileg).

Imaging During Therapy

After informing the patient about the advantages, disadvantages, and potential complications of LITT, consent is obtained. The metastasis is localized on computed tomographic scans and the injection site is infiltrated with 20 mL of 1% lidocaine. The laser application system is inserted under computed tomography (CT) guidance using the Seldinger technique. The patient then is transferred to MRI. After the patient is positioned on the MRI table, the laser catheter is inserted into the protective catheter. The MR sequences are performed in three perpendicular orientations before and during LITT; MRI is obtained every 30 seconds to assess the progress in heating of the lesion and the surrounding tissue. Heating is manifested as signal loss on the T1-weighted gradient-echo images as a result of the heat-induced increase of the T1 relaxation time.

Depending on the geometry and intensity of the signal loss and the speed of heat distribution, readjustment can be made in the position of the laser fibers, the laser power, and the cooling rate. The treatment is stopped after total coagulation of the lesion, and a safety margin from 5 to 15 mm surrounding the lesion is visualized on MR images. After switching off the laser, T1-weighted contrast-enhanced FLASH–two-dimensional (2D) images are obtained to verify the necrosis. After the procedure, the puncture channel is sealed with fibrin glue. Follow-up examinations using plain and contrast-enhanced MRI sequences are performed at 24 to 48 hours, and every 3 months following the LITT procedure. Quantitative and qualitative parameters, including size, morphology, signal behavior, and contrast enhancement are evaluated to decide whether treatment can be considered successful or whether subsequent treatment sessions are required.

Qualitative and Quantitative Evaluation

Laser-induced effects are evaluated by comparing images of lesions and surrounding liver parenchyma obtained before and after treat-

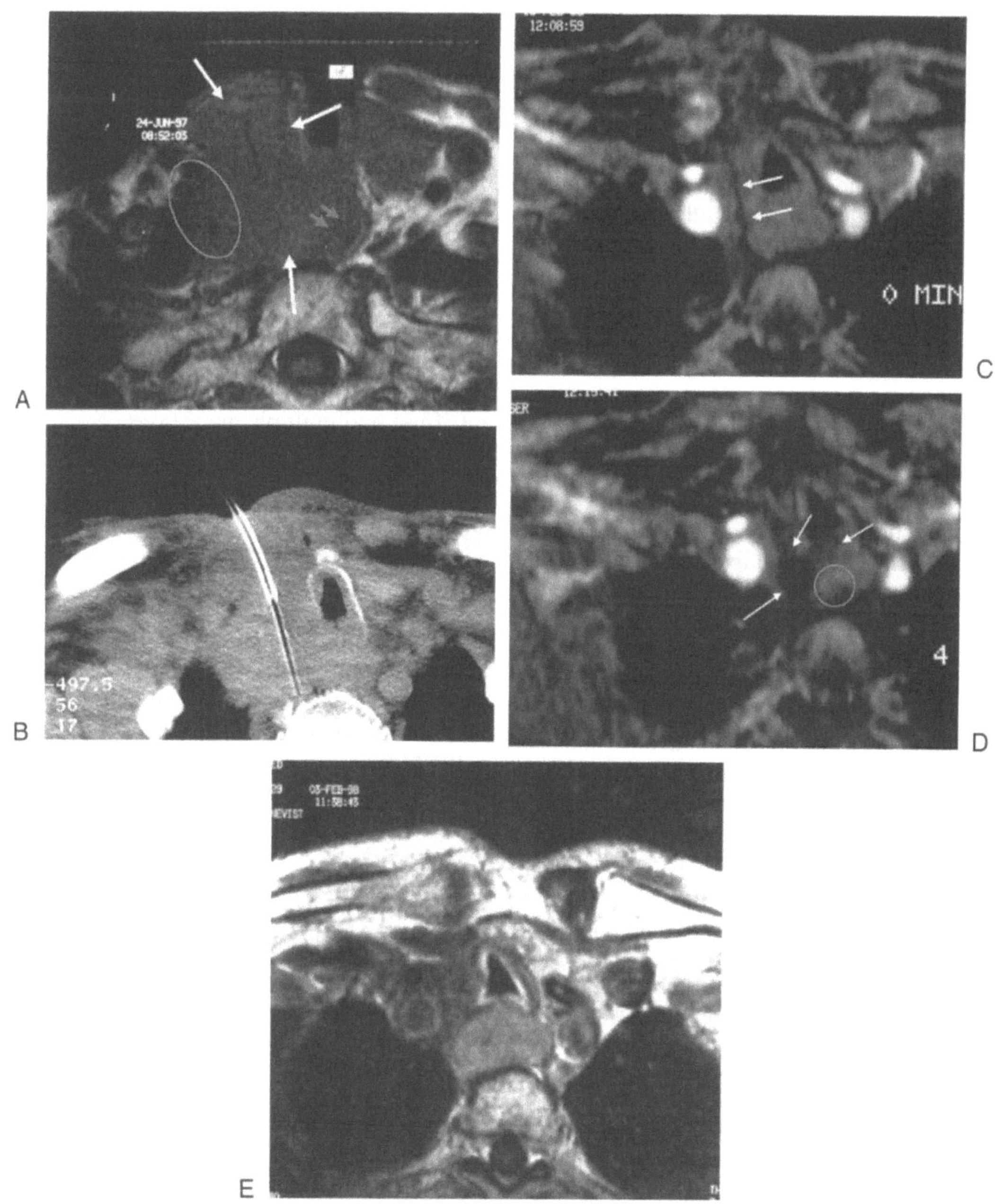

FIGURE 18.4. Laser treatment of a parastomal recurrent squamous cell carcinoma after laryngectomy. (A) Contrast-enhanced T1-weighted SE image demonstrates recurrent tumor on the right side with an infiltration of more than 180 degrees of the circumference of adjacent vascular structures with strong contrast enhancement (arrows). (B) The CT image demonstrates the positioning of the laser application set with the sheath system (arrows) and the protective catheter. A power application set was used. (C) The FLASH-2D MR image in axial slice orientation verifies the position of the application set. A specially designed magnetite marker is already inserted into the application set (arrows). (D) Thermo-FLASH-2D image 4 minutes after starting the laser demonstrates the close relationship of the induced necrosis to the vascular structures and the esophagus (circle). (E) Contrast-enhanced T1-weighted SE image obtained 6 months after LITT treatment shows an excellent result of this combined treatment protocol.

ment, and at follow-up examinations. Tumor volume and volume of coagulative necrosis are calculated using three-dimensional MR images and measurements of the maximum diameter in three planes (A, B, and C). The volume is calculated using the formula $(A \times B \times C) \times 0.5$. The results are tested for significance using the analysis of variance (ANOVA) test. Survival rates are calculated using the Kaplan-Meier method.

Indications

The primary therapeutic goal is defined as local tumor control in patients with limited hepatic malignant tumor. The majority of patients in our experience have had liver metastases from colorectal cancer. However, solitary hepatic metastases from other primary tumors, like breast cancer, carcinoid, and other malignancies also are treatable. According to our inclusion criteria, patients who are eligible for this treatment have fewer than five lesions, a maximum diameter of 50mm, are unfit for surgical resection, do have unresectable tumors in both hepatic lobes, or refuse surgical resection.

Those patients who have had partial resection of one hepatic lobe and develop a new lesion in the remaining liver also are suitable for this laser therapy. Requirements in the latter group are complete resection of the primary tumor and absence of extrahepatic metastases.

Indications and Inclusion Criteria for LITT of Hepatic Tumors

- Maximum of five lesions
- Maximum diameter of 50mm
- Patients with tumor recurrence after surgery, radiation, or chemotherapy
- New metastases after hepatic resection
- No response to chemotherapy
- Metastases in both lobes of the liver
- Lesions in high-risk locations, for example, near the bile duct
- LITT as a replacement for chemotherapy if patient refusal

LITT for Soft Tissue Tumors

- Recurrent head and neck tumors
- Tumor recurrence in the pelvis
- Lymph node metastases in the abdomen, the head and neck region, and the retroperitoneum

Exclusion Criteria for LITT

- Extensive extrahepatic tumor spread
- Contraindications for MRI (pacemaker)
- Ascites, apparent infection, coagulation disorder
- Diffuse and multiple metastases

Comparison with Alternative Methods

Surgery

Surgical resection of liver metastases still is considered one of the best options for radical treatment of malignant tumors, but only 20% of patients are candidates. Clinical conditions such as the presence of lesions in both hepatic lobes or poor overall status of the patient excludes surgical treatment. Additional liver surgery is associated with a mortality rate of approximately 3 to 8%. A major problem after surgical resection is tumor recurrence in up to 70% of cases. Only in selected cases is re-resection possible, so that further surgery is untenable for most patients.

Magnetic resonance imaging–guided LITT offers the option of multiple retreatment sessions. For new hepatic lesions the same inclusion criteria are applied as for the initial LITT.

In the literature Stangl followed up 1099 consecutive patients with colorectal liver metastases; 566 of them (51.5%) received no treatment for their hepatic metastases; 340 (31%) underwent hepatic resection; 123 (11.2%) received regional chemotherapy; and 70 (6.4%) received systemic chemotherapy. Thirty-four patients died within 30 days, as a result either of postoperative complications or advanced disease; 48 were excluded, because they developed a second primary cancer. After hepatic resection, 60% of these patients survived 5 years (median survival 30 months). In patients who underwent regional or systemic chemotherapy, the median survival was 12.7 and 11.1 months, respectively. In the untreated group, 31.3% of the patients were alive after 1 year, 7.9% after 2 years, 2.6% after 3 years, and 0.9% after 4 years. Considering these data, our results are comparable to those of surgery. The lack of perioperative mortality and low rate of side effects combined with an outpatient management are responsible for high patient tolerance. Patients with unresectable liver tumors need multimodality therapy for palliation, while preserving a good quality of life. But LITT alone, or combined with systemic or locoregional chemotherapy, transarterial chemoembolization, or surgical resection improves local tumor control and tumor-free survival in patients with metastatic discase.

Percutaneous Ethanol Injection

Magnetic resonance imaging–guided ethanol ablation is used to reduce tumor bulk and cancer pain, but mostly in low-risk regions, and it has been used particularly to treat HCC. Among the limitations of this agent is the lack of an instrument to monitor the effects in both normal and pathologic tissue. Comparisons between interstitial laser coagulation and percutaneous alcohol injection to treat colorectal hepatic metastases have shown that there were no major complications after either method, but that pain during alcohol injection was more severe and tumor control was less. In summary, alcohol injection is an accepted therapy method for small HCC nodules, but it is not a treatment option for metastases.

Cryotherapy

At present, cryotherapy is carried out using laparotomy and ultrasound guidance. Single and multiprobe arrays are possible. Tumor tissue is frozen at temperatures approaching −190 degrees, and then thawed. The double-freezing technique results in reliable destruction of tumor cells. Inclusion criteria are similar to LITT as to size and number of lesions. Cryotherapy under MRI guidance has been investigated in clinical studies, and MRI is promising for real-time monitoring of the progress of freezing and thawing. Hospitalization of about 7 to 10 days is typical with surgical cryotherapy.

Radiofrequency Ablation

Radiofrequency (RF) ablation is another modality for thermal coagulation of tumors. Heating is caused by high tissue impedance between two applicator tips. Solbiati demonstrated the feasibilty of tumor destruction with conventional and cooled-tip monopolar RF electrodes in patients with metastatic gastrointestinal carcinomas. The same inclusion criteria for LITT are used, but problems exist with monitoring of the procedure. Interference between RF systems and MRI devices prevents simultaneous imaging, monitoring, and treatment.

Focused Ultrasound

Noninvasive therapy using focused, high-intensity ultrasound beams was first proposed as a therapeutic modality for destruction of central nervous system tissue. Recently, a novel approach has been used for real-time monitoring of focused ultrasound using only MRI to demonstrate temperature elevation during sonication and to delineate tissue necrosis. This promising modality is under evaluation for soft tissue tumors in the brain and the breast. Problems are the rapid increase of temperature and reaching larger volumes with a small focus. So far, focused ultrasound is not used to treat liver metastases due to breathing artifacts.

Transarterial Chemoembolization

Transarterial chemoembolization (TACE) is defined as a local infusion of chemotherapy into tumor vessels to treat HCC nodules and neuroendocrine hepatic metastases. The goal is palliative, to reduce tumor bulk and to decelerate tumor progression.

Systemic and Regional Chemotherapy

All the above-mentioned techniques are restricted regionally to the liver, so the adjunctive use of systemic chemotherapy is essential in most cases. Protocols, doses, and intervals depend on the primary tumor and data from staging.

Results

In Vitro Studies

In vitro studies using porcine liver demonstrated a reproducible loss of signal intensity in MRI in accordance with increasing tissue temperature. Using an energy of 5W and an application time of 12 minutes, the maximum diameter of signal loss was 25mm. This effect was best monitored using the thermo-turbo-FLASH sequence at TI values of 300 to 400ms; this provided a nearly linear, inverse correlation between signal intensity and temperature, as well as with thermo-FLASH-2D sequences.

A mean size of necrosis of 2 cm^3 with an ellipsoid morphology may be achieved by an application time of approximately 20 minutes and a power of 5 to 6W using one applicator system. There are several possibilities to enlarge the necrosis volume: first is the pullback technique, that allows a longitudinal enlargement of necrosis. Second is the multiapplicator technique. The placement of two or three applicator systems results in a volume of necrosis of up to 17 cm^3. The use of an internally cooled laser applicator at power settings between 25 and 30W for 10 to 20 minutes also produces significant enlargement of the coagulative necrosis volume.

Patients

From 1993 to July 2002, we treated 1159 patients with a total of 2505 liver metastases from colorectal carcinoma, esophageal, gastric, pharyngeal, testicular, and pancreatic tumors. A total of 9470 laser applications were performed. The laser-induced necrosis was quantified by comparing the pre- and posttherapeutic unenhanced and contrast-enhanced MRI. Parameters such as size, morphology, and contrast enhancement were compared to pretherapeutic MRI. Successful therapy has been defined by a geometrically shaped necrotic area without enhancement along with a reliable safety margin.

Local tumor control rates for data from 1997 to 2000 are 98.1% after 3 months, and 97.3% after 6 months in liver lesions smaller than 50 mm. Mean survival time for all patients is 45 months using the Kaplan-Meier method (95% confidence interval: 40.9 to 49.2 months, median 39.8 months, maximum survival 74.6 months) (Fig. 18.5).

The most homogeneous group of patients are those with hepatic metastases from primary

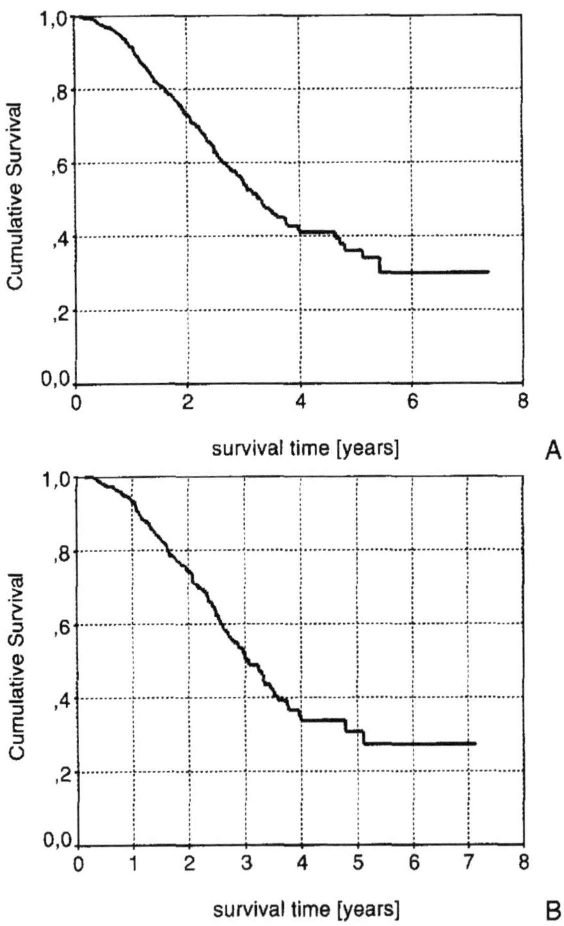

FIGURE 18.5. (A) The mean survival time in the total population of patients with liver metastases is 48.0 months (95% confidence interval: 44.4–52.8 months). (B) For patients with liver metastases from colorectal carcinoma the mean survival time is 41.8 months (95% confidence interval, 37.3–46.4 months).

colorectal carcinoma. The mean survial rate is 42.6 months (95% confidence interval: 37.7 to 47.5 months, median 36.7 months).

Survival did not differ significantly ($p > .05$) between men and women, or between patients with colorectal metastases and those with metastases from other primary tumors.

Complications

All patients tolerated the procedure well under local anesthesia. The following side effects were documented by clinical examination or imaging studies: pleural effusion in 7.28%, subcapsular hematoma in 2.46%, intrahepatic abscess in 0.8%, intraabdominal bleeding in 0.11%, and local infection at the site of the puncture in 0.2%.

All complications except the following did not require therapy—in 0.8% of cases pleural effusion had to be treated by percutaneous drainage. All abscesses were treated by percutaneous drainage. Three patients died of LITT within 4 weeks. One patient with a suspected colonic perforation had surgical repair.

Head and Neck and Extrahepatic Tumors

Twenty-six patients (eight women and 18 men, mean age 64 years, range 57–77 years) with recurrent tumors of the head and neck were treated with LITT. In all these patients the primary tumor was located in the head and neck region. Recurrent squamous cell carcinoma occurred in the majority of patients. Two patients with pleomorphic adenoma in the parapharyngeal space were treated for tumor recurrence after primary surgery (Figs. 18.3 and 18.4). All patients tolerated the procedure well under local anesthesia. No side effects were observed.

The procedure was judged successful if postinterventional MRI revealed a sharply delineated necrosis that exceeded the diameter of the pretherapeutic tumor. Reduction of clinical symptoms, such as pain, was observed in 11 patients. Amelioration of swallowing problems and symptoms of nerve compression occurred in six patients.

Fourteen patients with abdominal lymph node tumors or recurrent primary pelvic tumors were treated successfully using MRI-guided LITT. Reduction of clinical symptoms was seen in 68% these patients.

Magnetic resonance imaging–guided LITT allows accurate online thermometry during these interventional procedures. Dynamic gadolinium-enhanced MRI is suitable for early and late follow-up studies for lesions treated with LITT. Follow-up studies indicate that these laser-induced effects lead to reliable palliation in recurrent head and neck tumors.

Conclusions

Percutaneous MRI-guided interstitial laser-induced thermotherapy (LITT) of malignant liver tumors is a reliable treatment method to destroy tumors palliatively, and it is also potentially curative. The treatment concept should be differentiated according to the underlying histology: for hepatocellular carcinoma a local ablative procedure instead of, or in combination with, local alcohol instillation or transarterial chemoembolization (TACE) can be used.

In the case of liver metastases, the therapeutic situation must be discussed within the context of the primary tumor. Today, using MRI-guided LITT for hepatic metastases restricted to a local area without extrahepatic tumor can be justified clinically. Magnetic resonance tomography is a valuable tool to monitor and control percutaneous LITT. Magnetic resonance imaging also is used for follow-up. It is proven to be the optimal imaging examination to detect very small tumor recurrences.

The ultimate goal of MRI-guided LITT is 100% eradication of local tumor, as MRI online thermometry allows precise guidance of the interventional procedure. Magnetic resonance imaging provides unparalleled topographic accuracy due to its excellent soft tissue contrast and high spatial resolution. Therefore, early detection of local complications such as bleeding, as well as the desired effect of coagulative necrosis are all possible. Dynamic contrast-enhanced MRI represents the optical method to evaluate the treated lesions, short- and long-term.

Bibliography

Adson MA, Heerden van J, Adson MH, Wagner JS, Ilstrup DM. Resection of hepatic metastases from colorectal cancer. Arch Surg 1984;119:647–651.

Amin Z, Bown SG, Lees WR. Local treatment of colorectal liver metastases: a comparison of interstitial laser photocoagulation (ILP) and percutaneous alcohol injection (PAI). Clin Radiol 1993; 48(3):166–171.

Anzai Y, Desalles AA, Black KL, et al. Interventional MR imaging. Radiographics 1993;13(4): 897–904.

Bozzetti F, Doci R, Bignami P, Morabito A, Gennari L. Patterns of failure following surgical resection of colorectal cancer liver metastases. Ann Surg 1987;205(3):264–269.

Brewer WH, Austin RS, Capps GW, Neifeld JP. Intraoperative monitoring and postoperative imaging of hepatic cryosurgery. Semin Surg Oncol 1998;14: 129–155.

Butler J, Attiyeh FF, Daly JM. Hepatic resection for metastases of the colon and rectum. Surg Gynecol Obstet 1986;162(2):109–113.

Cady B, Stone MD, McDermott WV, et al. Technical and biological factors in disease-free survival after hepatic resection for colorectal cancer metastases. Arch Surg 1992;127:561–569.

Charnley RM, Doran J, Morris DL. Cryotherapy for liver metastases: a new approach (comment in Br J Surg 1990;77:354). Br J Surg 1989;76: 1040.

Cline HE, Hynynen K, Hardy CJ, Watkins RD, Schenck JF, Jolesz FA. MR temperature mapping of focused ultrasound surgery. Magn Reson Med 1994;31(6):628–636.

Cline HE, Hynynen K, Watkins RD, et al. Focused US system for MR imaging-guided tumor ablation. Radiology 1995;194(3):731–737.

Cline HE, Schenck JF, Hynynen K, Watkins RD, Souza SP, Jolesz FA. MR-guided focused ultrasound surgery. J Comput Assist Tomogr 1992; 16(6):956–965.

Cline HE, Schenck JF, Watkins RD, Hynynen K, Jolesz FA. Magnetic resonance-guided thermal surgery. Magn Reson Med 1993;30(1):98–106.

Doci R, Gennari L, Bignami P, Montalto F, Bozzetti F. One hundred patients with hepatic metastases from colorectal cancer treated by resection: analysis of prognostic determinants. Br J Surg 1991; 78:797–801.

Ekberg H, Tranberg KG, Andersson R, Hägerstrand I, Ranstam J, Bengmark S. Determinants of survival in liver resection for colorectal secondaries. Br J Surg 1986;73:727–731.

Feifel G, Schüdder G, Pistorius G. Kryochirurgie—Renaissance oder echter Fortschritt? Der Chirurg 1999;70:154–159.

Fortner JG, Silva JS, Golbey RG, Cox EB, Maclean BJ. Multivariate analysis of a personal series of 247 consecutive patients with liver metastases from colorectal cancer. Ann Surg 1984;199:306–315.

Fried MP, Morrison PR, Hushek SG, Kernahan GA, Jolesz FA. Dynamic T1-weighted magnetic resonance imaging of interstitial laser photocoagulation in the liver: observations on in vivo temperature sensitivity. Lasers Surg Med 1996; 18(4):410–419.

Gayowski TJ, Iwatsuki S, Madariaga JR. Experience in hepatic resection for metastatic colorectal cancer: analysis of clinical and pathological risk factors. Surgery 1994;116:703–710.

Gewiese B, Beuthan J, Fobbe F, et al. Magnetic resonance imaging-controlled laser-induced interstitial thermotherapy. Invest Radiol 1994;29(3):345–351.

Goldberg SN, Gazelle GS, Solbiati L, et al. Ablation of liver tumors using percutaneous RF therapy. AJR 1998;170:1023–1029.

Griffith KD, Sugarbaker PH, Chang AE. Repeat hepatic resections for colorectal metastases. Surgery 1990;107:101–104.

Harned RK, Chezmar JL, Nelson RC. Recurrent tumor after resection of hepatic metastases from colorectal carcinoma: location and time of discovery as determined by CT. AJR 1994;163(1):93–97.

Herfarth C, Heuschen UA, Lamade W, Lehnert T, Otto G. Rezidiv-Resektionen an der Leber bei primären und sekundären Lebermalignomen. Chirurg 1995;66:949–958.

Hill CR. Optimum acoustic frequency for focused ultrasound surgery. Ultrasound Med Biol 1994; 20(3):271–277.

Hohenberger P, Schlag P, Schwarz V, Herfarth C. Leberresektion bei Patienten mit Metastasen colorektaler Carcinome. Ergebnisse und prognostische Faktoren. Chirurg 1988;59:410–417.

Holm A, Bradley E, Aldrete JS. Hepatic resection of metastases from colorectal carcinoma. Morbidity, mortality and pattern of recurrence. Ann Surg 1989;209(4):428–434.

Hughes KS, Simon R, Songhorabodi S, et al. Resection of the liver for colorectal carcinoma metastases: a multi-institutional study of indications for resections. Surgery 1988;103(3):278–288.

Hughes KS, Simon R, Songhorabodi S, et al. Resection of the liver for colorectal carcinoma metastases: a multi-institutional study of pattern of recurrence. Surgery 1986;100(2):278–284.

Iwatsuki S, Shaw BW, Starzl TE. Experience with 150 liver resections. Ann Surg 1983;197(3):247–253.

Jolesz FA, Bleier AR, Jakab P, Ruenzel PW, Huttl K, Jako GJ. MR imaging of laser-tissue interactions. Radiology 1988;168(1):249–253.

Jolesz FA, Blumenfeld SM. Interventional use of magnetic resonance imaging. Magn Reson Q 1994; 10(2):85–96.

Kahn T, Bettag M, Ulrich F, et al. MRI-guided laser-induced interstitial thermotherapy of cerebral neoplasms. J Comput Assist Tomogr 1994;18(4): 519–532.

Lee FT, Mahavi DM, Chosy SG, et al. Hepatic cryosurgery with intraoperative US guidance. Radiology 1997;202:624–632.

Lee TH, Anzai Y, Lufkin RB. Magnetic resonance imaging-guided needle biopsy of head and neck lesions. West J Med 1993;159(1):69.

Lencioni R, Goletti O, Armillotta N, et al. Radiofrequency thermal ablation of liver metastases with a cooled-tip electrode needle: results of a pilot clinical trial. Eur Radiol 1998;8:1205–1211.

Lewin JS, Connell CF, Duerk JL, et al. Interactive MRI-guided radiofrequency interstitial thermal ablation of abdominal tumors: clinical trial for evaluation of safety and feasibility. J Magn Reson Imaging 1998;8:40–47.

Livraghi T, Giorgio A, Marin G, et al. Hepatocellular carcinoma and cirrhosis in 746 patients: long-term results of percutaneous ethanol injection. Radiology 1995;197(1):101–108.

Livraghi T, Goldberg N, Lazzaroni S, Meloni B, Solbiati L, Gazelle GS. Small hepatocellular carcinoma: treatment with radiofrequency ablation versus ethanol injection. Radiology 1999;210: 655–661.

Livraghi T, Goldberg S, Monti F, et al. Saline-enhanced radiofrequency tissue ablation in the treatment of liver metastases. Radiology 1997; 202:205–210.

Livraghi T, Lazzaroni S, Meloni F, Torzilli G, Vettori C. Intralesional ethanol in the treatment of unresectable liver cancer. World J Surg 1995;19(6): 801–806.

Lopez RL, Pan SH, Lois JF, et al. Transarterial chemoembolization is a safe treatment for unresectable hepatic malignancies. Am Surg 1997;63: 923–926.

Lorentzen T. A cooled needle electrode for radiofrequency tissue ablation: thermodynamic aspects of improved performance compared with conventional needle design. Acad Radiol 1996;3(7):556–563.

Lorenz M, Rossion I. Adjuvante und palliative regionale Therapie von Lebermetastasen kolorektaler Tumoren. Dtsch Med Wochenschr 1995;120: 690–697.

Lorenz M, Staib-Sebler E, Rossion I, Koch B, Gog C, Encke A. Ergebnisse der Resektion und adjuvanten Therapie von Lebermetastasen kolorektaler Primärtumoren—eine Literaturübersicht. Zentralbl Chir 1995;120:769–779.

Lufkin RB, Robinson JD, Castro DJ, et al. Interventional magnetic resonance imaging in the head and neck. Top Magn Reson Imaging 1990;2(4): 76–80.

Martin M, Tarara D, Wu YM, et al. Intrahepatic arterial chemoembolization for hepatocellular carcinoma and metastatic neuroendocrine tumors in the era of liver transplantation. Am Surg 1996; 62:724–732.

Masters A. Cryotherapy for liver metastases [letter; comment]. Br J Surg 1990;77(3):354.

Masters A, Steger AC, Lees WR, Walmsley KM, Bown SG. Interstitial laser hyperthermia: a new approach for treating liver metastases. Br J Cancer 1992;66(3):518–522.

Matsumoto R, Oshio K, Jolesz FA. Monitoring of laser and freezing-induced ablation in the liver with T1-weighted MR imaging. J Magn Reson Imaging 1992;2(5):555–562.

McDannold N, Hynynen K, Wolf D, Wolf G, Jolesz F. MRI evaluation of thermal ablation of tumors with focused ultrasound. J Magn Reson Imaging 1998;8:91–100.

Nordlinger B, Guiguet M, Vaillant JC, et al. Surgical resection of colorectal carcinoma metastases to the liver. A prognostic scoring system to improve case selection, based on 1568 patients. Assoc Franc Chirurg Cancer 1996;77(7):1254–1262.

Nordlinger B, Vaillant J-C. In *Hepatobiliary Cancer*, Sugarbaker, P, editor. Repeat Resections for Recurrent Colorectal Liver Metastases. Boston: Kluwer Academic, 1994:57–61.

Ohlsson B, Stenraum U, Tranberg KG. Resection of colorectal liver metastases: 25-year experience. World J Surg 1998;22:268–276.

Onik GM, Atkinson D, Zemel R, Weaver ML. Cryosurgery of liver cancer. Semin Surg Oncol 1993;9:309–317.

Ravikumar TS, Kane R, Cady B, Jenkins R, Clouse M, Steele G. A 5-year study of cryosurgery in the treatment of liver tumors. Arch Surg 1991;126: 1520–1524.

Ringe B, Bechstein WO, Raab R, Meyer H-J, Pichlmayr R. Leberresektion bei 175 Patienten mit colorektalen Metastasen. Chirurg 1990;61: 272–279.

Roberts HRS, Paley M, Sams VR, et al. Magnetic resonance imaging control of laser destruction of hepatic metastases: correlation with post-operative helical CT. Min Invas Ther Allied Technol 1997;6:53–64.

Rossi S, Di Stasi M, Buscarini E, et al. Percutaneous RF interstitial thermal ablation in the treatment of hepatic cancer. AJR 1996;167:759–768.

Sanz-Altamira PM, Spence LD, Hubermann LS, et al. Selective chemoembolization in the management of hepatic metastases in refractory colorectal carcinoma: a phase II trial. Dis Colon Rectum 1997;40:770–775.

Sarantou T, Bilchik A, Ramming KP. Complications of hepatic cryosurgery. Semin Surg Oncol 1998;14: 156–162.

Scheele J, Altendorf-Hofmann A, Stangl R, Schmidt K. Surgical resection of colorectal liver metastases: gold standard for solitary and completely resectable lesions. Swiss Surg Suppl 1996;4:4–17.

Scheele J, Stangl R, Altendorf Hofmann A, Gall FP. Indicators of prognosis after hepatic resection for colorectal secondaries. Surgery 1991;110(1):13–29.

Schlag P, Hohenberger P, Herfarth C. Resection of liver metastases in colorectal cancer—competitive analysis of treatment results in synchronous versus metachronous metastases. Eur J Surg Oncol 1990; 16:360–365.

Schwarzmaier HJ, Kahn T. Magnetic resonance imaging of microwave induced tissue heating. Magn Reson Med 1995;33(5):729–731.

Shiina S, Tagawa K, Unama T, et al. Percutaneous ethanol injection therapy of hepatocellular carcinoma: analysis of 77 patients. AJR 1990;155: 1221–1226.

Sironi S, De Cobelli F, Livraghi T, et al. Small hepatocellular carcinoma treated with percutaneous ethanol injection: unenhanced and gadolinium-enhanced MR imaging follow-up. Radiology 1994; 192(2):407–412.

Solbiati L, Goldberg SN, Ierace T, et al. Hepatic metastases: percutaneous radio-frequency ablation with cooled-tip electrodes. Radiology 1997; 205(2):367–373.

Stangl R, Altendorf Hofmann A, Charnley RM, Scheele J. Factors influencing the natural history of colorectal liver metastases. Lancet 1994;343(8910): 1405–1410.

Steele G Jr. Cryoablation in hepatic surgery. Semin Liver Dis 1994;14(2):120–125.

Steele G, Osteen RT, Wilson RE, et al. Patterns of failure after surgical cure of large liver tumors. Am J Surg 1984;147:554–559.

Sugihara K, Hojo K, Moriya Y, Yamasaki S, Kosuge T, Takayama T. Pattern of recurrence after hepatic resection for colorectal metastases. Br J Surg 1993;80(8):1032–1035.

van Hillegersberg R. Fundamentals of laser surgery. Eur J Surg 1997;163:3–12.

Viadana E, Bross IDJ, Pickren JW. The metastatic spread of cancers of the digestive system in man. Oncology 1978;35:114–126.

Vogl TJ, Eichler K, Straub R, et al. Laser-induced thermotherapy of malignant liver tumors: general principles, equipment, procedure, side-effects, complications, and results. Eur J Ultrasound 2001;13(2):117–127.

Vogl TJ, Mack M, Straub R, Engelmann K, Eichler K, Zangos S. Interventional MRI: interstitial therapy. Eur Radiol 1999;9:1479–1487.

Vogl TJ, Mack MG, Straub R, Roggan A, Felix R. Magnetic resonance imaging-guided abdominal interventional radiology: laser-induced thermotherapy of liver metastases. Endoscopy 1997; 29:577–583.

Vogl TJ, Mack M, Straub R, Roggan A, Felix R. Percutaneous MRI-guided laser-induced thermotherapy for hepatic metastases for colorectal cancer. Lancet 1997;350:29.

Vogl TJ, Mack MG, Straub R, et al. MR-guided laser-induced thermotherapy of malignant liver lesions: technique and results. Onkologie 1998;21:412–419.

Vogl TJ, Muller PK, Hammerstingl R, et al. Malignant liver tumors treated with MR imaging-guided laser-induced thermotherapy: technique and prospective results. Radiology 1995;196(1):257–265.

Vykhodtseva NI, Hynynen K, Damianou C. Pulse duration and peak intensity during focused ultrasound surgery: theroretical and experimental effects in rabbit brain in vivo. Ultrasound Med Biol 1994;20(9):987–1000.

Weaver ML, Ashton JG, Zemel R. Treatment of colorectal liver metastases by cryotherapy. Semin Surg Oncol 1998;14:163–170.

Weiss L, Grundmann E, Torhorst J, et al. Haematogenous metastatic patterns in colonic carcinoma: an analysis of 1541 necropsies. J Pathol 1986;150(3): 195–203.

Wingo PA, Tong T, Bolden S. Cancer statistics, 1995. CA Cancer J Clin 1995;45(1):8–30.

Yeh KA, Fortunato L, Hoffmann JP, Eisenberg BL. Cryosurgical ablation of hepatic metastases from colorectal carcinomas. Am Surg 1997;63(1): 63–67.

Zhou X-D, Tang Z-Y, Yu Y-Q, et al. The role of cryosurgery in the treatment of hepatic cancer: a report of 113 cases. J Cancer Res Clin Oncol 1993; 120:100–102.

19
Cryoablation: History, Mechanism of Action, and Guidance Modalities

Sharon M. Weber and Fred T. Lee, Jr.

History of Cryoablation

Cold temperatures have been used to decrease inflammation and relieve pain since the time of the ancient Egyptians. James Arnott (1797–1883), an English physician, is credited with being the first to use cold to destroy tissue, using a combination of ice and salt to produce tissue necrosis (1). Because this cryogen needed to be applied topically to tumors, he was able to treat only tumors of the cervix and breast; he reported decreases in tumor size and palliation of pain in patients treated by cryoablation (1).

The utility of liquid air and carbon dioxide (CO_2) as cryogens was popularized in the late 1890s. The use of these substances was based on a principle that has since been used for air conditioning and refrigeration—atmospheric gases warm when compressed and cool during expansion. The first clinical application of liquid air was reported by White, who used it to treat various skin conditions. He also described its potential curative action for carcinoma. Liquid CO_2 was first used in the early 1900s by a number of investigators, including Pusey, Cranston-Low, Whitehouse, and Hall-Edwards. These investigators described liquid CO_2 to treat skin conditions with minimal resultant scarring. Part of the appeal of liquid CO_2 was that it was both easier to obtain and simpler to maintain in liquid form than liquid air. Both Pusey and Whitehouse made initial observations regarding the relationship between pressure on the skin and increasing depth of penetration (1). These techniques became fairly widespread, and are currently still used for a variety of skin conditions. During this time, the clinical sequelae of freezing skin were well described in many medical journals. The clinical manifestations included bulla formation, followed by superficial crusting, then eschar formation, and finally healing to form a superficial scar.

In the 1950s, Allington became one of the first to recognize the importance of liquid nitrogen for surgical applications. He described a technique of dipping cotton swabs into liquid nitrogen followed by direct application to benign skin lesions. In the late 1960s, the clinical indications for low-temperature therapy expanded to treat other organ sites including oral cancers, ophthalmologic, and gynecologic conditions. Also in the 1960s, the invention of other devices, including a liquid nitrogen spray in a hand-held form, helped popularize the use of cryoablation for skin lesions. These devices improved the depth of penetration of the cryolesion, and thus improved the efficacy for treatment of many skin lesions (2).

In 1963 Cooper (3), a New York neurosurgeon, reported on a liquid nitrogen probe capable of achieving a temperature of –196°C. The Cooper device was an automated system that utilized the continuous flow of liquid nitrogen through a closed, self-contained cryoprobe. This unit was one of the first to use pressurized liquid nitrogen pumped through a cryoprobe, and was capable of temperature-controlled regulation of the freezing process. This device made possible the ability to rapidly create a continuous large-volume freeze in deep-seated tissue. The probes initially were used to treat inoperable brain tumors and Parkinson's disease by focally ablating affected areas in the brain.

The novel idea of using liquid nitrogen to cool a probe for placement into less accessible body spaces was instrumental in ushering in the modern era of cryoablation and increasing the number and variety of applications. Up to this point, freezing of tissue had been limited to easily accessible organs and small volumes of tissue. Development of liquid nitrogen cryoprobes dramatically augmented the volume of tissue that could be frozen by low probe temperatures, and increased the types of tissues that could be ablated. The continued development of systems based on this technology has helped to broaden the clinical applications of cryoablation. In the 1970s and 1980s, several other indications for cryoablation using liquid nitrogen systems were investigated, including ablation of prostate, kidney, and liver cancers.

Despite the increased interest and investigation into tumor ablation by low temperatures, cryoablation of deep-seated thoracoabdominal and pelvic tumors did not become a clinically important tool until the 1980s. The main reason for this was simple—physicians could not adequately control the extent of freezing and tissue death caused by powerful cryoprobes that used liquid nitrogen. Several clinical series demonstrated the ability to kill targeted tissue effectively, but the methods for monitoring the freeze were crude at best. In most cases, the freeze was controlled by inspection and palpation of the iceball. In other words, the physician had to rely primarily on physical examination to determine whether the targeted tissue had been adequately treated without inadvertently freezing nontargeted tissue. The results of cryoablation monitored by physical examination were predictably mixed. Most reports during this period showed some efficacy in terms of tumor kill, but severe complications also were common. Tissue vulnerable to cryoablation (bile ducts, urethra, bowel, etc.) often was irreparably damaged (1). For instance, in prostate cryotherapy, these complications often resulted in prolonged catheter drainage due to damage to the urethra (1). The complication rate for cryoablation monitored by physical examination was high enough that the technique rapidly lost favor, and was only revived in the mid-1980s.

The key development that sparked renewed interest in cryoablation was the fusing of cryoablation with real-time imaging guidance in the form of intraoperative ultrasound (4,5). Liver tumors were the first cancer to be approached with this method. During the early to mid-1980s, surgeons had become increasingly aware of the segmental anatomy of the liver, and the importance of the blood supply to individual hepatic segments (6). Knowledge of this anatomy allowed hepatic surgeons to resect liver tumors more safely and aggressively. As a result, the morbidity and mortality from hepatic surgery have greatly decreased during the past two decades, accompanied by a concomitant increase in overall and disease-free survival (7). During this period of increased interest in hepatic surgery, intraoperative ultrasound was discovered to be an excellent tool to define liver anatomy for resection and to evaluate the liver for the presence of occult metastatic disease. Intraoperative ultrasound is now widely considered to be the gold standard for imaging the liver (8–10).

It was Onik et al's (4,5) discovery of the highly echogenic nature of the iceball that forms during hepatic cryoablation that sparked renewed interest in hepatic cryoablation and ultimately led to the development of other thermal ablation devices and techniques. Subsequent animal studies showed a close correlation between the sonographically visible iceball and the zone of cell death (11,12). The ability to monitor the formation of the iceball precisely helped overcome the primary limitation of cryoablation to that time—the uncontrolled and poorly monitored freezing process. With intraoperative ultrasound monitoring, cryoprobes could now be placed precisely with real-time guidance into the tumor, thus decreasing injury to hepatic vessels and bile ducts by the probes. The cryolesion also could be controlled well enough to allow for freezing of the targeted tumor and a margin of normal liver, while decreasing the frequency of injuries to the bile ducts and extrahepatic structures. This process has become more precise over the ensuing decades, and many reports of low complication rates coupled with complete tumor kill in a high percentage of cases are now common in the scientific literature (13–16). While initially developed to monitor hepatic cryoablation, Onik et al (4,17) and others (18,19) have since used intraoperative ultrasound in combination with cryoablation to treat prostate, renal, and various other benign and malignant conditions.

The next technical breakthrough that prompted further development of cryoablation techniques was the introduction of argon gas systems based on the Joule-Thompson principle (20). These systems increased the convenience of freezing, decreased the procedure time, and allowed for smaller (some as small as 17-gauge), yet highly effective cryoprobes. Most recently, the small probes used with argon systems have led to the development of minimally invasive cryoablation techniques that can be performed through small incisions, laparoscopic ports, or percutaneously under cross-sectional image guidance (4,18,21).

Mechanism of Cell Destruction by Cold Temperature

In the past 50 years, the biologic effects of freezing have been studied, primarily using liquid nitrogen–based systems. During freezing, ice crystals form within the intra- and extracellular spaces. Intracellular ice crystal formation leads to cell death by injury to either the cellular membrane or structures within the cell, or both (22). However, intracellular ice forms only with freezing that occurs rapidly or freezing to extremely low temperatures (22). Extracellular ice forms when freezing is slower, and causes cell death by creating an osmotic gradient that results in intracellular fluid moving into the extracellular space; this results in dehydration and subsequent cell death (22–24). It also has been hypothesized that extracellular ice crystals cause deformation and rupture of the cell membrane itself (25). Another important mechanism of cell death after cryoablation is local tissue ischemia due to small-vessel thrombosis (26,27).

To destroy tumor cells, it has become clear that temperatures must reach a certain critical threshold that is unique to the cell type and thermal environment of the targeted tissue. Estimates of the critical temperature for complete tissue destruction range between –20 and –50°C, depending on the tissue. In addition, studies on isolated cell suspensions have shown that multiple freeze cycles, an increased rate of freezing, and colder temperatures all contribute to a decrease in viable cells after cryoablation (28–30).

There is experimental evidence that suggests that a single freeze–thaw cycle results in complete cell death in large animal models; however, these models tested cryoablation in normal tissue, not tumor (27,31). When cryoablation has been tested in small animal tumor models, it appears that multiple freeze–thaw cycles result in a greater likelihood of complete cell death. It is likely that because tumors are more fibrotic than normal tissue, they are more resistant to freezing. This has been shown in small animal tumor models in which viable cells survived after a single freeze cycle (29,30). In these subcutaneously implanted tumors, repetitive freeze–thaw cycles resulted in improved rates of local tumor control (30). Clinically, the standard treatment for patients consists of two freeze–thaw cycles.

Different cell types are relatively more or less sensitive to cold than others. Melanocytes are one of the most sensitive, which accounts for the depigmentation of skin after freezing (32). On the other hand, collagen and elastin fibers are some of the most resilient (33). A study by Gage and colleagues (34), in which large arteries in dogs were isolated and liquid nitrogen was passed through them for 10 minutes, first reported this observation. The authors showed that after cryoablation, followed by normal blood flow through the arteries, there were no episodes of wall rupture. Although there were some minor histologic changes in the vessel wall 2 to 4 weeks after freezing, there was no change in function, either in the early or late postoperative period. Modern studies have redemonstrated the ability of vessel walls to withstand freezing, although tissue up to the vessel wall is ablated if the temperature is cold enough (27). Computed tomography (CT) scans following cryoablation of liver tissue routinely demonstrate patent vessels coursing through the area of tissue necrosis, even in the presence of complete ablation of the tumor. Unfortunately, the bile ducts, urethra, bowel, and ureter are not as immune to the effects of cryoablation. Freezing of these structures can result in necrosis and infarction after freezing, often leading to stricture, sloughing, and perforation (1,34,35). This clearly limits the use of cryoablation in certain anatomic areas, unless warming of the vulnerable structure can be accomplished. Urethral, ureteral, and bile duct warming during cryoablation all have been described as techniques to decrease the damage to these structures during cryoablation (1,26).

Cryoablation Equipment

Between the 1960s and early 1990s, liquid nitrogen–based systems were the only commercially available cryoablation devices in the United States. The most recent manufacturers of these devices were Cryomedical Sciences (Accuprobe, Rockville, MD) and Candela Corporation (Cryotech, Wayland, MA). These devices were based on the circulation of liquid nitrogen through probes of varying sizes [3–8 mm outer diameter (OD)]. Up to five probes could be employed during a single freeze. While highly effective in freezing tissue, these devices were quite large, and required large stainless steel dewars to store the liquid nitrogen, as well as large insulated probe cables. The dewars and fill tanks were prone to leakage, and therefore liquid nitrogen could not be stored for more than a few days at a time. Consequently, it was difficult to perform cryoablation on short notice, a major disadvantage when unexpected tumors were encountered during liver surgery. Other disadvantages of liquid nitrogen–based systems included the relatively slow formation of the iceball, as well as slow switching between the freeze and thaw modes. As a result, repositioning of a frozen cryoprobe could take several minutes, during which the probe needed to be thawed, repositioned, and refrozen. In addition, the relatively large probe sizes were generally placed using a multistep Seldinger technique that could be complicated and time-consuming. During the late 1980s and early 1990s, liver and prostate tumors were the two main indications for cryoablation. However, the length and complexity of the procedures and the awkward, difficult-to-use equipment as well as the requirement for high-quality intraoperative ultrasound discouraged widespread use. Several studies were published in which experienced liver and prostate surgeons were unable to successfully perform these procedures without serious complications or failure to ablate tumors completely (36,37).

The development of argon gas–based systems based on the Joule-Thompson principle in the early 1990s represented a major advance in cryoablation. Argon systems have largely replaced liquid nitrogen units. The Joule-Thompson principle states that low temperatures are created by the rapid expansion of high pressure inert gas. The probe tips in argon gas–based systems reach a temperature of approximately −150°C. Temperatures at the probe tips of argon systems may appear warmer than those achieved by liquid nitrogen devices (−196°C), but much of this temperature discrepancy can be explained by the difference in location at which the temperatures are measured. For example, in one argon-based system, temperatures are measured at the probe tip. This is in contrast to the most popular liquid nitrogen system in which temperatures are measured as the nitrogen enters the probe and is not yet susceptible to the warming effects of tissue. When tip temperatures are measured and compared directly, they are similar, regardless of the type of system (20,38). Therefore, this difference is likely not clinically significant.

There are two manufacturers of argon-based cryoablation systems in the United States (CRYOcare™, EndoCare Inc., Irvine, CA, and CryoHit®™, Seed Net™, Galil Medical, Wallingford, CT). The advantages of these systems over liquid nitrogen units primarily are related to the use of high-pressure argon gas as a cryogen. Because of the relatively low viscosity of argon gas compared to nitrogen, it can be circulated very rapidly and at high pressure through small probes (currently down to 17-gauge). As a result, iceball formation commences very rapidly after the initiation of the freezing process. Thawing can also be started and stopped rapidly which allows for much more rapid repositioning of cryoprobes. Low temperatures are reached more quickly than nitrogen-based systems, which is important since in vivo studies suggest that rapid cooling may improve tissue destruction (28). In both systems, multiple probes can be used simultaneously to ablate larger lesions or lesions in different locations (CRYOcare™: eight probes from 2.4–4.9mm OD, Seed Net™: up to fifteen 17-gauge probes, or eight 3.0mm probes). Both manufacturers make sharp-tipped cryoprobes that can be directly placed into tumors. A modified Seldinger-like device (Fast-Trak™, Endo-Care, Irvine, CA) has also become available recently that speeds probe placement compared to first-generation Seldinger systems. The Galil system is the only cryoablation unit that has MRI compatible cryoprobes.

An important aspect of both cryoablation systems available in the United States is the ability to use multiple cryoprobes and to adjust the argon flow rate to "sculpt" the iceball to a precise shape. This is particularly important in prostate cryoablation in which it is often necessary to create a conglomerate iceball using six to eight 3.0mm cryoprobes (or up to fifteen 17-gauge probes) to adequately ablate a prostate gland of asymmetric shape. Prostate cryoablation often is monitored by both transrectal biplane ultrasound and thermosensors placed in critical areas (Denonvillier's fascia, neurovascular bundles) (39). Depending on the location of the tumor, it may be important to assure a hard freeze of at least –40°C in certain locations as determined by thermosensors. An important advantage of cryoablation over single probe thermal ablation devices (specifically radiofrequency ablation) is the ability to incrementally adjust the amount of flow to specific probes (or place an additional probe in an area that is not reaching critical temperatures). This results in a high degree of control over the eventual shape of the zone of necrosis that is not possible with other thermal ablation techniques.

Imaging Guidance for Cryoablation

There are three main cross-sectional imaging techniques that are used to guide cryoablation: ultrasound (percutaneous or intraoperative), CT (percutaneous), and MRI (percutaneous). These will each be considered separately.

Ultrasound Guidance for Cryoablation

Intraoperative ultrasound to guide cryoablation was first described by Onik in 1984 (5). This seminal observation is largely responsible for the entire field of focal tumor ablation that began with intraoperative cryoablation, and has since expanded to include many percutaneous thermal ablation techniques. Since the original use of ultrasound, this method has become the dominant modality to guide cryoablation of the liver and prostate. The main advantages of ultrasound for cryoablation are the real-time capabilities to safely guide probe placement, the high spatial resolution of intraoperative ultrasound, the highly visible nature of the iceball, and the excellent correlation between the location of the iceball and the zone of cell death (11,12).

The ability to place cryoprobes under real-time ultrasound guidance helps to assure that the probe does not cross major vessels, bile ducts, or other vulnerable structures. In addition, the ability to correct the path of the probe rapidly helps minimize procedure time and the number of passes through the tumor. This may help to decrease the risk of tumor seeding. For liver cryoablation, many different ultrasound probes can be used to guide probe placement and to monitor the iceball. The initial description of intraoperative ultrasound guidance for cryoablation used T-shaped side-fire transducers that display the liver parenchyma from the liver surface (Fig. 19.1). This side-fire configuration minimizes interference by probe cords during scanning of the liver. This is particularly important because of the small space between the diaphragm and liver surface into which intraoperative probes must fit.

These high-frequency (5–12MHz) transducers come in linear and curvilinear probe faces,

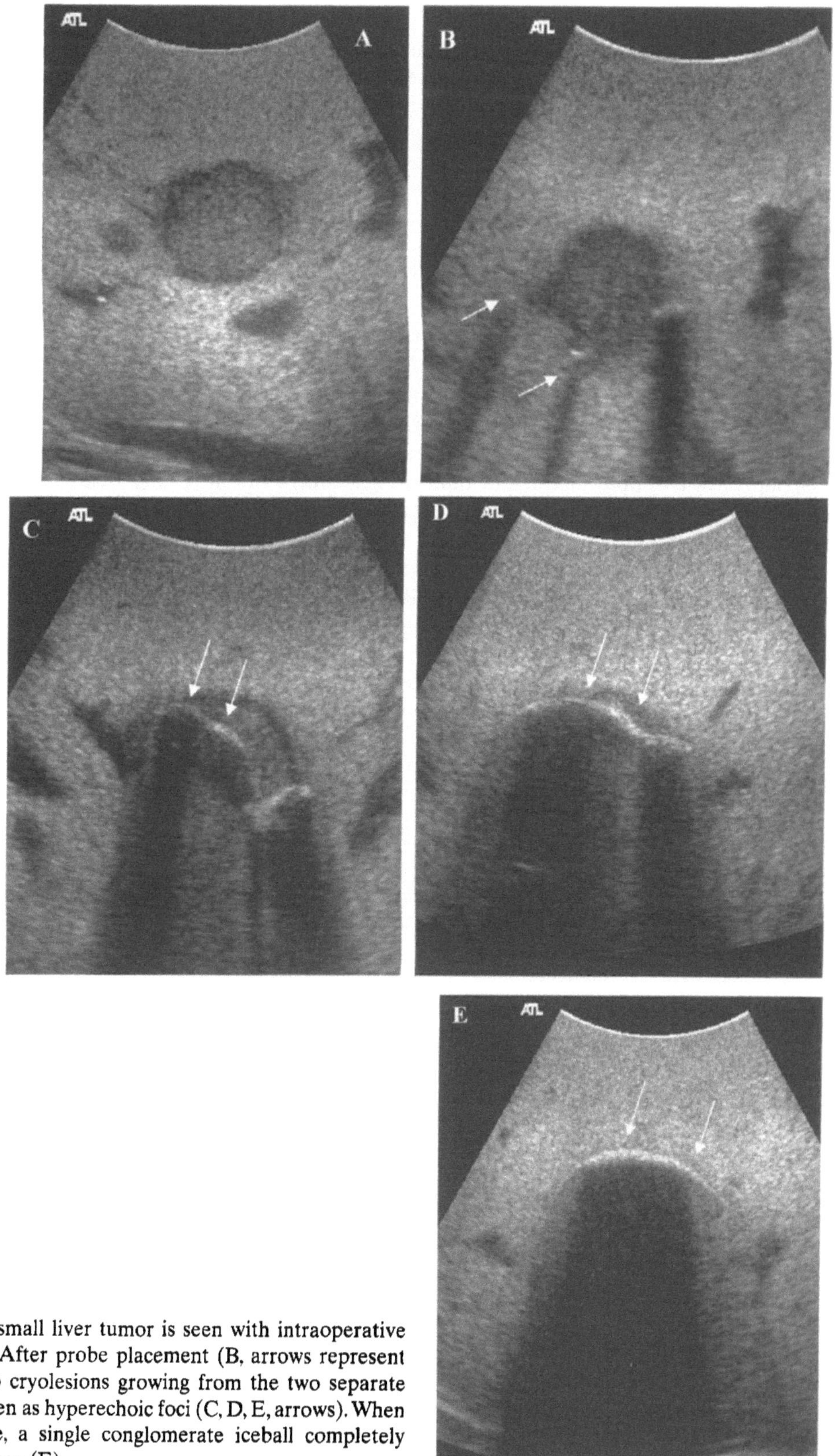

FIGURE 19.1. A small liver tumor is seen with intraoperative ultrasound (A). After probe placement (B, arrows represent probes), the two cryolesions growing from the two separate probes can be seen as hyperechoic foci (C, D, E, arrows). When the iceballs fuse, a single conglomerate iceball completely obscures the tumor (E).

and remain the most widely used transducers for hepatic cryoablation. Other transducers frequently used for liver cryoablation include an I-shaped side-fire transducer in a sagittal configuration for longitudinal imaging, laparoscopic ultrasound transducers, and transvaginal/endorectal end-fire probes that can be used for open or cryoablation performed via a minilaparotomy. For the latter, a small incision can be made in the anterior abdominal wall through which a transvaginal or endorectal transducer can be introduced, with the cryoprobe directly mounted on the ultrasound transducer (21). Punctures of left lobe or anterior right lobe tumors can then be performed precisely using an electronic puncture guide. This approach is simpler and faster than using a laparoscopic ultrasound transducer to guide laparoscopic cryoablation (Fig. 19.2).

For prostate cryoablation, a transrectal, biplane ultrasound transducer is mandatory. Due to the need for true orthogonal imaging, an end-fire transducer is not adequate.

Under ultrasound visualization, the cryolesion is a highly echogenic structure that prevents the transmission of sound (Fig. 19.1). As a result, no information can be obtained from structures that are engulfed by the iceball, and acoustic shadowing limits visualization posterior to the cryolesion. This can be a serious problem during prostate cryotherapy when the iceball is monitored strictly from a transrectal approach posterior to the iceball. Once freezing of the posterior probes have commenced, a lack of ultrasound information concerning the anterior probes results. The use of thermosensors in areas not well visualized by ultrasound has become an important method to assure proper size of the zone of necrosis, particularly in prostate cryoablation when it is often not possible to create a large ablative margin. Temperatures of –40°C and below at a thermosensor can substantially increase confidence that tissue at that specific location has been ablated (28). For liver cryoablation performed at open surgery, unlike prostate cryoablation, it is often possible to monitor the iceball from more than one surface. When this is not feasible because of adhesions or other anatomic limitations, it is important to place the cryoprobes in such a

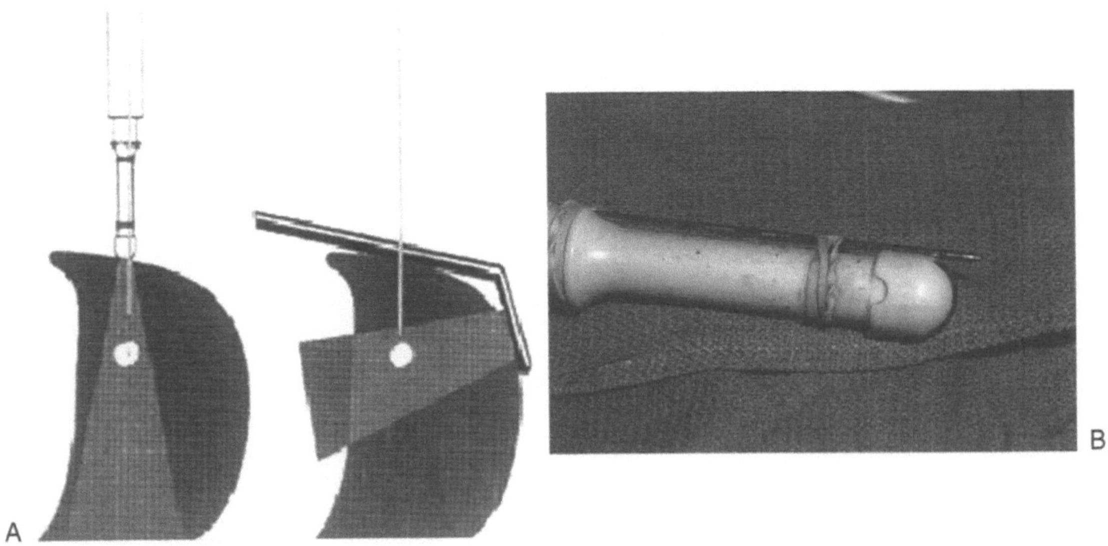

FIGURE 19.2. (A) Minilaparotomy using a direct puncture technique. The cryoprobe is directly placed on a transvaginal or transrectal ultrasound transducer (B). This allows a direct puncture of an anterior liver lesion using an electronic biopsy guide (A, left panel). This is in contrast to the more difficult technique of conventional laparoscopic guidance of cryoablation (A, right panel). For laparoscopic ultrasound-guided cryoablation, the cryoprobe and laparoscopic ultrasound transducer are not in a fixed plane, thus making it difficult to simultaneously image the target, cryoprobe, and probe path.

manner as to ensure that the deep margin is adequately frozen because this margin will not be monitored easily from the anterior liver surface. In our practice, because of this problem, we place more probes closer to the deep margin to ensure an adequate enlation in this area.

Several troublesome ultrasound artifacts can be encountered during ultrasound-monitored cryoablation. Depending on the type of ultrasound transducer used, a "critical angle effect" can be present at the edge of the iceball that can increase the apparent size of the iceball (35). This is due to the speed of sound differences between soft tissue and ice that causes refraction of the sound beam. This artifact is exacerbated when using vector transducers, and is lessened with linear transducers that minimize the amount of sound that strikes the iceball at oblique angles. It is important for the physician to understand this artifact and adjust when necessary. An additional artifact that often is encountered during ultrasound-monitored cryoablation is a reverberation artifact from the highly echogenic surface of the iceball (Fig. 19.3). This can lead to the spurious assignment of echoes within the iceball.

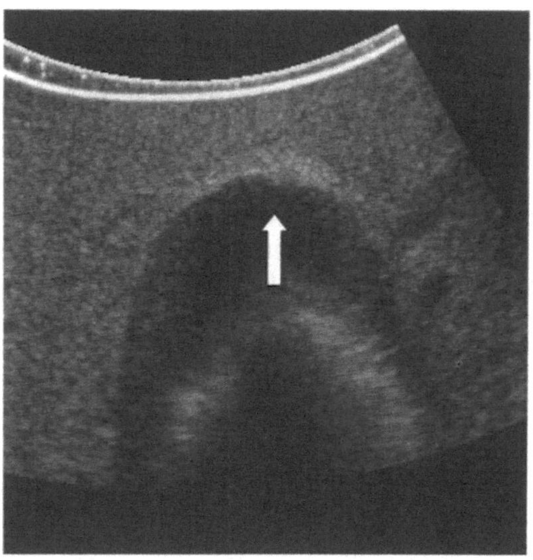

FIGURE 19.3. Reverberation artifact during liver cryoablation. Note the spurious assignment of echoes within the iceball caused by reverberation between the transducer face and the highly reflective iceball (arrow). (Case courtesy of Michael Ledwidge, BS, RDMS, RVT, Madison, WI.)

Mirror image artifacts also can be encountered when imaging the iceball, similar to the artifact encountered when imaging the diaphragm or other highly echogenic structures.

When the freezing process is complete and the cryolesion has been thawed, it is often possible to visualize the extent of the zone of necrosis. The area where the iceball was located becomes less echogenic than the surrounding tissue, and thus ablative margins can be determined (Fig. 19.4). This effect is particularly pronounced in the liver where adjacent unablated tissue allows for comparison.

Computed Tomography Guidance of Cryoablation

The development of cryoprobes suitable for percutaneous use has spurred the development of CT-guided cryoablation. To date, CT has been used to guide percutaneous cryoablation of liver, kidney, lung, and body wall masses (18,19,39–42). Prostate cryoablation has not yet been performed with CT guidance due to the requirement for the patient to be in the lithotomy position for the transperineal placement of cryoprobes.

Computed tomography has several features that make it a feasible, and in some ways a nearly ideal, method to guide and monitor percutaneous cryoablation of accessible tumors. The first important feature of CT guidance for cryoablation is that it is often the imaging modality that was used initially to detect the tumor. Thus, the physician performing the procedure can have confidence that the targeted area is indeed what was seen on the initial CT scan. In many cases, CT is used to follow the patient postablation (43), and correlation of the intraprocedural images with follow-up scans can be extremely helpful. Computed tomography also can image most structures (or the anatomic region where the structure is located) that might be injured by the freezing process, namely, bowel, central bile ducts, and nerves. Computed tomography scanners are also available in virtually every radiology practice in the

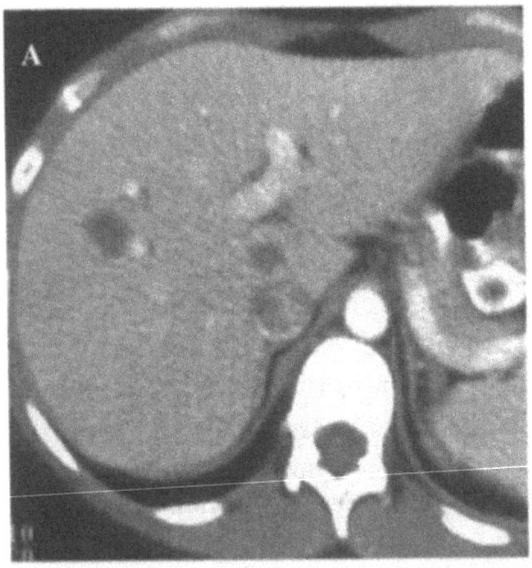

FIGURE 19.4. Metastatic neuroendocrine metastases in segments 1, 5, and 8 (A). The tumor in segment 1 (calipers) is visualized anterior to the inferior vena cava (B), and a cryoprobe (arrows) has been placed in it using intraoperative ultrasound guidance (C). After freezing, a hypoechoic zone is seen (D, arrows) surrounding the tumor. This zone corresponds to the region of tissue death.

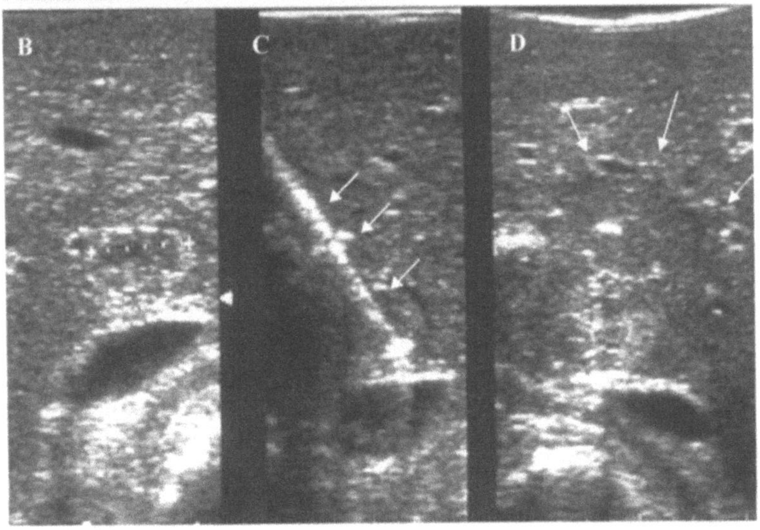

United States, and radiologists are comfortable with CT-guided punctures for biopsy or fluid drainage. Thus, the expertise needed to perform CT-guided cryoablation is widespread. For these reasons, combined with a growing understanding of the nearly painless nature of the procedure (44), the number of cryoablation cases performed under CT guidance is expected to grow dramatically in the coming years.

Until recently, CT-guided procedures were handicapped by the lack of true real-time guidance capability. Probes or needles were placed, and intermittent scans helped determine the *post facto* location of the device. This could result in the unfortunate placement of needles in undesirable locations, potentially increasing the complication rate. Because of the large probe sizes associated with cryoablation, either a large number of intermediate monitoring scans were needed, or the procedure needed to be done in several steps using the Seldinger technique. Both of these techniques could potentially increase the accuracy of probe placement, but came at the cost of lengthening the procedure time and increasing radiation exposure. Some CT-guided procedures could take several hours with this method.

The development of CT fluoroscopy has helped increase the acceptance of CT-guided cryoablation (45). Intermittent scanning can substantially decrease the time needed for checking probe position. In addition, it is even possible to perform nearly real-time imaging of probe placement. However, this requires continuous fluoroscopy, and the radiation dose to the patient and operator can be quite high. With CT fluoroscopy, it is possible to directly and rapidly place sharp cryoprobes by the trocar rather than Seldinger technique. The operator simply makes several quick checks to confirm proper probe trajectory during placement. The use of CT fluoroscopy, therefore, can substantially decrease procedure time.

Perhaps the most important reason that CT is becoming an increasingly important modality to guide and monitor cryoablation is that the iceball is seen very well when compared to soft tissue, and the visible iceball has a good correlation in relation to the eventual zone of cell death (43,46,47). In most cases, the iceball in liver, kidney, or muscle measures approximately 0 Hounsfield units (HU). As a result, an approximately 50 to 70 HU difference between the iceball and soft tissue makes it simple to determine the extent of the freezing process using CT. In many cases, the tumor and iceball margin both are well seen (Fig. 19.5), even with noncontrast CT, so an exact ablative margin can be determined. If necessary, the patient can receive a small bolus of contrast material to help visualize tumors seen only by contrast-enhanced scans. When cryoprobes of 3.0 mm OD or larger are used, streak artifact can degrade image quality. However, in most cases this artifact does not substantially interfere with the monitoring of freezing because of the highly visible iceball. This streak artifact is much less severe when using 2.0-mm probes. Artifact can also be minimized by pulling back the cryoprobes just prior to CT scanning.

After the freezing process has finished and the iceball has melted, it is still possible to see the frozen zone due to its decreased attenuation compared to unfrozen tissue. This is analogous to the zone of decreased echogenicity of thawed tissue seen by ultrasound. After the administration of contrast material, this zone does not enhance, and therefore post-contrast scans can be an excellent method to determine the exact area of tissue destruction postcryoablation.

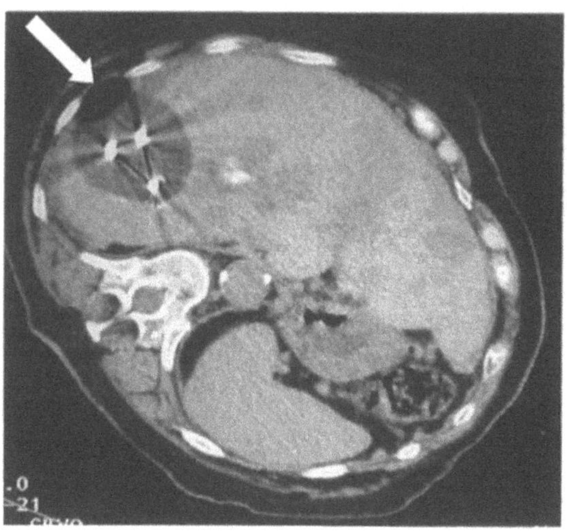

FIGURE 19.5. Computed tomography (CT)-guided cryoablation of the liver: Three cryoprobes have been percutaneously placed in a peripheral liver lesion under CT fluoroscopic guidance. Note the highly visible nature of the iceball compared to background liver. The arrow denotes a balloon inflated peripheral to the iceball to protect the chest wall from freezing damage. (Case courtesy of Peter Littrup, MD, Detroit, MI.)

Magnetic Resonance Imaging (MRI) Guidance of Cryoablation

Like CT-guided cryoablation, the development of MRI-guided cryoablation was spurred by the development of small-diameter cryoprobes suitable for percutaneous use. To date, only one manufacturer of cryoablation equipment (Galil Medical, Wallingford, CT) produces MRI-compatible cryoprobes.

Percutaneous MRI-guided cryoablation cannot be performed routinely with many clinical MRI scanners (Fig. 19.6). Dedicated midfield interventional MRI systems with a vertical magnet orientation are the best systems for percutaneous cryoablation (48,49). These have the advantage of letting the operator stand immediately adjacent to the patient during the procedure. However, cryoablation also can be performed with somewhat more difficulty in magnets with "open" horizontal architecture.

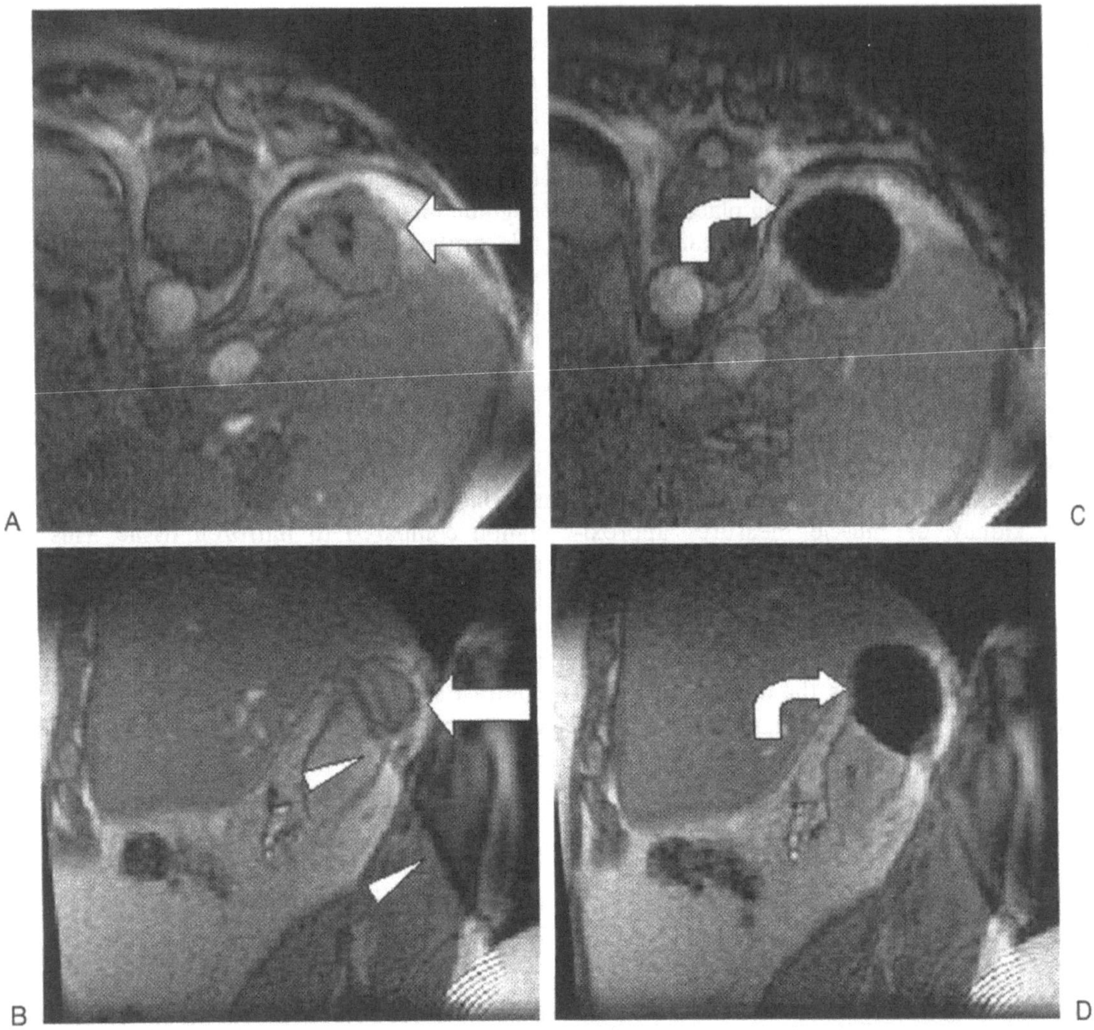

FIGURE 19.6. Percutaneous magnetic resonance imaging (MRI)-guided ablation of a renal cell carcinoma. (A) An oblique axial projection demonstrates a renal mass originating in the upper pole of the right kidney (arrow). (B) Sagittal image. Under real-time MRI guidance, a cryoprobe (arrowheads) is placed into the tumor (arrow). (C) During the freezing process, the iceball (curved arrows) is low signal intensity, and is seen to engulf the tumor in both the axial and sagittal (D) projections. (Case courtesy of Stuart Silverman, MD, Boston, MA.)

The rationale to use MRI for guidance and monitoring of cryoablation stems from the fact that MRI has a very high sensitivity for the detection of most tumors amenable to cryoablation. Compared to CT scanning without intravenous contrast, it is likely that most tumors will be more visible on noncontrast MRI due to the high inherent contrast resolution of MRI (50). This is a substantial advantage compared to CT, in which many tumors are detectable only with intravenous contrast administration. Because of the rapid circulation time of iodinated contrast materials for CT, the tumor may be detectable only transiently, limiting the ability to guide a probe into a liver tumor under real-time guidance.

In addition to tumor visualization, ice is highly visible by MRI. In general, ice is of low signal intensity on T1-weighted images, with a temperature dependence to the signal intensity

(51). As a result, MRI can be used to determine temperature in tissue during the freezing process (52).

Several other advantages of MRI guidance for cryoablation have become evident with increasing clinical experience. The nearly real-time ability to guide cryoprobes into virtually any space of the abdomen is similar to that of CT fluoroscopy (48). However, the multiplanar capability of MRI represents a substantial advantage over CT for both placing probes and monitoring the freezing process.

Comparison with Other Focal Ablative Techniques

Thermal ablation techniques cause tissue destruction by creating ionic agitation [in the case of radiofrequency (RF) and microwave ablation] and heat, which results in tissue boiling and the creation of water vapor. If lethal temperatures are reached, protein denaturation and vascular thrombosis result. A zone of partial tissue destruction up to 8 mm in diameter is seen surrounding the thermal lesion. The mechanism of tissue destruction by heat is different from that created by cryoablation. In cryoablation, the freezing and thawing process destroys cell membranes and organelles due to the mechanical stresses associated with the phase change from ice formation. At gross pathology, this results in a well-defined zone of tissue destruction (Fig. 19.7).

Secondary vascular thrombosis can result, adding to the eventual tissue death, but it is not as prominent a feature as with the heat-based ablation modalities. Because the cell death due to cryoablation is primarily mechanical, cell destruction can be readily appreciated immediately postfreeze at the light microscopic level. Cell membranes are destroyed and cells are clearly seen as nonviable. This differs from the immediate postablation appearance of the heat-based modalities in which the cells appear nearly normal, with some subtle changes in the nucleus and organelles (Fig. 19.8). Some authors feel that the rapid destruction of cell membranes and the relative lack of protein denaturation associated with freezing is responsible for a more severe form of systemic response ("cryoshock") than is present with tissue destruction by heat. The hypothesis is that intact cellular elements are more readily delivered into the bloodstream by freezing than with heat ablation, and this can result in thrombocytopenia and hepatic and renal failure in severe cases (42). The actual incidence

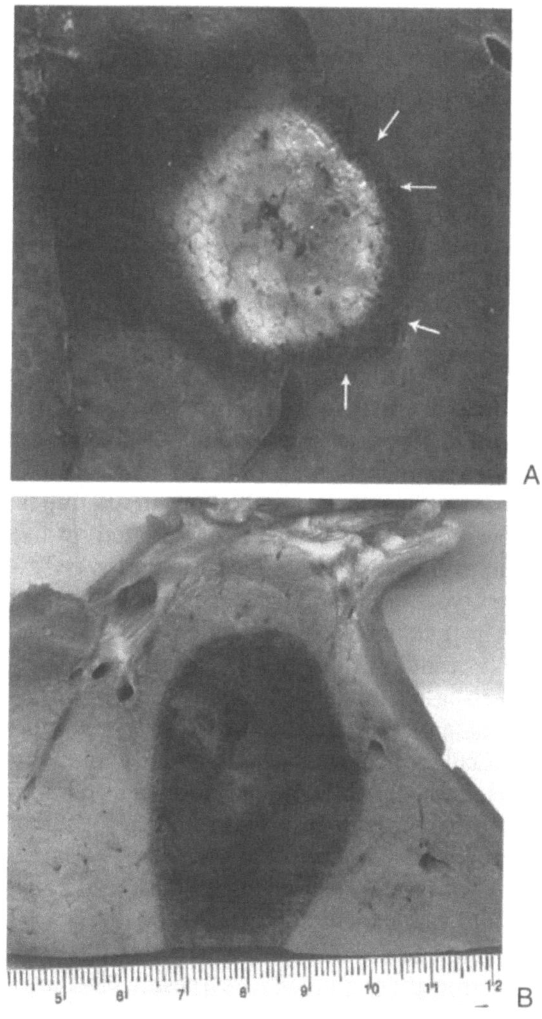

FIGURE 19.7. Pathology of radiofrequency (RF) vs. cryoablation. (A) Radiofrequency ablation lesion in normal pig liver demonstrates a central pale zone corresponding to the area of coagulation necrosis. The surrounding red zone (arrows) represents an area of liver injury with some remaining viable tissue. (B) Cryoablation lesion in normal pig liver. Note the abrupt transition between normal and necrotic liver, and the lack of a zone of partial necrosis.

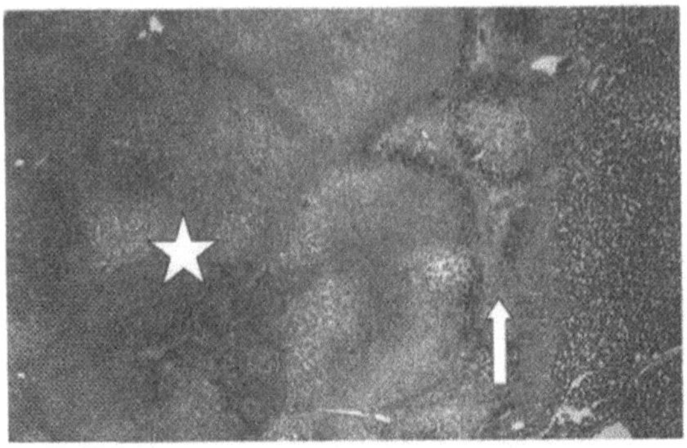

FIGURE 19.8. Cryoablation, histology. Cryolesion 24 hours after ablation reveals marked disruption of cellular integrity with absence of cell membranes. No viable cells are present within the area of the freeze. An abrupt transition between nonviable (left, star) and viable tissue (right) is present, bordered by a thin zone of inflammation (arrow).

of cryoshock has probably been overestimated in many reports, as a review of the world literature of cryoablation found a 3% incidence of major complications (53).

Over time, postcryoablation tissue breaks down more rapidly than tissue ablated by heat due to the existence of patent blood vessels in the cryoablation site. This exposes the necrotic tissue to inflammatory mediators and scavenger cells of the reticuloendothelial cell system (42). Heat-based modalities cause vascular thrombosis, and thus the zone of necrosis is more avascular than with cryoablation. Tissue subjected to heat ablation therefore takes a longer time to undergo resorption and fibrosis than cryoablated tissue.

Heat-based ablation modalities cause profound vascular thrombosis. In fact, the first RF ablation device was a modification of the Bovie electrocautery unit (54). As a result, bleeding is an unusual complication of RF ablation. In contrast, cryoablation has minimal intrinsic hemostatic properties, and has been associated with substantial hemorrhage during large-volume freezes performed at open laparotomy (53). In general, this is a result of cracking of the iceball during thawing. However, percutaneous cryoablation does not appear to have a high bleeding rate, perhaps because in contrast to laparotomy, percutaneous ablation does not have the iceball–air interface, is not performed in a low-pressure environment, and has the benefit of surrounding tissues for tamponade (37,47,49).

The phase change seen with cryoablation proceeds along a smoother and more predictable front than the tissue heating associated with RF and microwave ablation. This leads to smooth, regular-appearing, reproducible zones of freezing during cryoablation (Fig. 19.7). Cryoablation lesions are almost always round or oval in appearance. There is little deviation of the iceball by various tissue types, with the exception of vascular structures. Similar to heat-based ablation, patent blood vessels limit the ability to cause tissue necrosis because of the constant inflow of relatively warm blood. Thus viable tumor cells may be preserved next to blood vessels (Fig. 19.9), unless additional attempts to achieve complete freezing are utilized, such as using multiple probes. However, because of the ability to freeze several probes simultaneously, vascular warming often can be overcome, and tissue can be ablated up to large blood vessels (portal vein, inferior vena cava) if the probes are clustered and placed close enough to the heat source (Fig. 19.10).

Comparing the relative effectiveness of tissue destruction between RF and cryoabla-

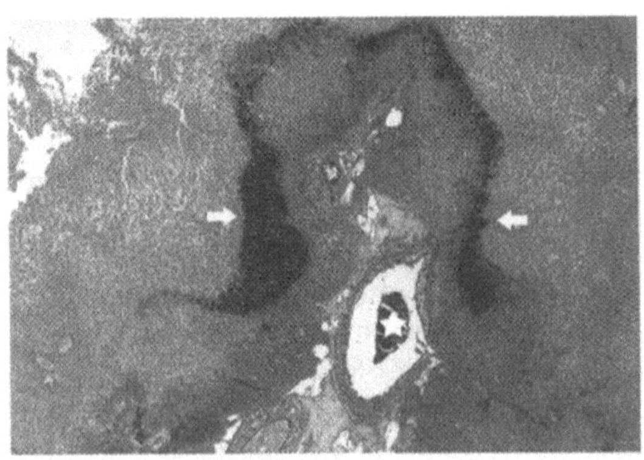

FIGURE 19.9. Postcryoablation viable tumor (arrows) surrounding a large patent blood vessel (star) in this rabbit VX2 animal model. Tumor in proximity to patent blood vessels often is preserved due to the inflow of warm blood. Ablating tumor near large blood vessels is a problem for all thermal-based ablation modalities.

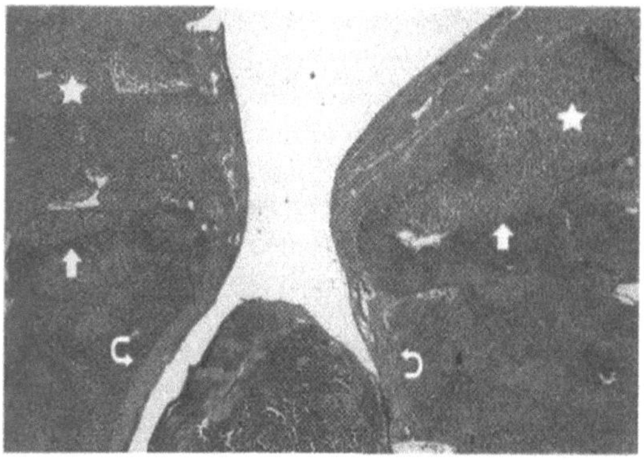

FIGURE 19.10. Cryoablation up to a vessel wall. Cryoablation in normal porcine liver demonstrates the ability to ablate tissue immediately adjacent to a vessel wall when the probes are placed in proximity. In this case, there is an abrupt transition (arrows) between normal liver (stars) and completely necrotic liver. Note the complete ablation of tissue up to the vessel wall (curved arrow) with preservation of the patent portal vein.

tion is problematic, due to the lack of well-controlled studies. Most authors conclude that cryoablation has a slight advantage in the ability to cause cell death when tissue has been appropriately targeted in the laboratory (55), but appropriately controlled clinical studies have not been performed. In clinical trials of hepatic tumor ablation, local recurrence rates generally are lower with cryoablation; these studies typically were performed during open laparotomy, and most RF ablation studies were performed percutaneously, or a mix of intraoperative and percutaneous cases. The RF trial with the lowest local recurrence rates included a large proportion of patients with lesions that were ablated intraoperatively, and many with a concurrent Pringle maneuver (56).

Monitoring of tissue undergoing freezing currently is more reliable than monitoring of tissue undergoing heating, regardless of the imaging modality (CT, ultrasound, MRI), as discussed above. This is an important advantage of cryoablation, as the success of any ablation technique is dependent on the likelihood to visualize the complete destruction of the targeted tumor.

Summary

Modern cryoablation techniques have been widely used for the focal destruction of various different types of tissue for more than 20 years. Cryoablation was the modality that ushered in the modern era of focal ablation of malignant tumors under real-time cross-sectional imaging guidance. The advantages of cryoablation over other thermal ablation techniques include the ability to use multiple cryoprobes simultaneously; the ease of monitoring the formation of ice with ultrasound, CT, and MRI; the reproducible and predictable pattern of tissue destruction; and the relatively low complication rates. Disadvantages compared with heat-based modalities include the greater systemic effects seen acutely due to the lysis of cell membranes, and the heretofore reluctance to use cryoablation in a percutaneous fashion due to the relatively large probe sizes and theoretical risk of uncontrollable bleeding. The risk of bleeding during percutaneous use appears to have been overestimated, and emerging percutaneous applications are being actively investigated.

References

1. Gage AA. History of cryosurgery. Semin Surg Oncol 1998;14:99–109.
2. Cooper SM, Dawber RP. The history of cryosurgery. J R Soc Med 2001;94:196–201.
3. Cooper IS. A new method of destruction or extirpation of benign or malignant tissues. N Engl J Med 1963;263:741–749.
4. Onik G, Gilbert J, Hoddick W, et al. Sonographic monitoring of hepatic cryosurgery in an experimental animal model. AJR 1985;144:1043–1047.
5. Onik G, Cooper C, Goldberg HI, Moss AA, Rubinsky B, Christianson M. Ultrasonic characteristics of frozen liver. Cryobiology 1984;21:321–328.
6. Fortner JG, Blumgart LH. A historic perspective of liver surgery for tumors at the end of the millennium. J Am Coll Surg 2001;193:210–222.
7. Fong Y, Fortner J, Sun RL, Brennan MF, Blumgart LH. Clinical score for predicting recurrence after hepatic resection for metastatic colorectal cancer: analysis of 1001 consecutive cases. Ann Surg 1999;230:309–318.

8. Takigawa Y, Sugawara Y, Yamamoto J, et al. New lesions detected by intraoperative ultrasound during liver resection for hepatocellular carcinoma. Ultrasound Med Biol 2001;27:151–156.
9. Bloed W, van Leeuwen MS, Borel RI. Role of intraoperative ultrasound of the liver with improved preoperative hepatic imaging. Eur J Surg 2000;166:691–695.
10. Cervone A, Sardi A, Conaway GL. Intraoperative ultrasound (IOUS) is essential in the management of metastatic colorectal liver lesions. Am Surg 2000;66:611–615.
11. Weber SM, Lee FT, Warner TF, Chosy SG, Mahvi DM. Hepatic cryoablation: US monitoring of extent of necrosis in normal pig liver. Radiology 1998;207:73–77.
12. Steed J, Saliken JC, Donnelly BJ, Ali-Ridha NH. Correlation between thermosensor temperature and transrectal ultrasonography during prostate cryoablation. Can Assoc Radiol J 1997;48:186–190.
13. Cha C, Lee FT Jr, Rikkers LF, Niederhuber JE, Nguyen BT, Mahvi DM. Rationale for the combination of cryoablation with surgical resection of hepatic tumors. J Gastrointest Surg 2001;5:206–213.
14. Ravikumar TS, Kane R, Cady B, Jenkins R. A 5-year study of cryosurgery in the treatment of liver tumors. Arch Surg 1991;126:1520–1524.
15. Zhou XD, Tang ZY, Yu YQ, et al. The role of cryosurgery in the treatment of hepatic cancer: a report of 113 cases. J Cancer Res Clin Oncol 1993;120:100–102.
16. Goering JD, Mahvi DM, Niederhuber JE, Chicks D, Rikkers LF. Cryoablation and liver resection for noncolorectal liver metastases. Am J Surg 2002;183:384–389.
17. Onik G, Cobb C, Cohen J, Zabkar J, Porterfield B. US characteristics of frozen prostate. Radiology 1988;168:629–631.
18. Lee DI, McGinnis DE, Feld R, Strup SE. Retroperitoneal laparoscopic cryoablation of small renal tumors: intermediate results. Urology 2003;61:83–88.
19. Gill IS, Novick AC, Soble JJ, et al. Laparoscopic renal cryoablation: initial clinical series. Urology 1998;52:543–551.
20. Rewcastle JC, Sandison GA, Saliken JC, Donnelly BJ, McKinnon JG. Considerations during clinical operation of two commercially available cryomachines. J Surg Oncol 1999;71:106–111.
21. Lee FT, Chosy SG, Weber SM, Littrup PJ, Warner TF, Mahvi DM. Hepatic cryosurgery via minilaparotomy in a porcine model—an alternative to open cryosurgery. Surg Endosc Ultrasound Intervent Tech 1999;13:253–259.
22. Mazur P. The role of intracellular freezing in the death of cells cooled at supraoptimal rates. Cryobiology 1977;14:251–272.
23. Gill W, Fraser J. A look at cryosurgery. Scot Med J 1968;13:268–273.
24. Whittaker DK. Mechanisms of tissue destruction following cryosurgery. Ann R Cole Surg Eng 1984;66:313–318.
25. Ishiguro H, Rubinsky B. Mechanical interactions between ice crystals and red-blood cells during directional solidification. Cryobiology 1994;31:483–500.
26. Kahlenberg MS, Volpe C, Klippenstein DL, Penetrante RB, Petrelli NJ, Rodriguez-Bigas MA. Clinicopathologic effects of cryotherapy on hepatic vessels and bile ducts in a porcine model. Ann Surg Oncol 1998;5:713–718.
27. Weber SM, Lee FT, Chinn DO, Warner T, Chosy SG, Mahvi DM. Perivascular and intralesional tissue necrosis after hepatic cryoablation: results in a porcine model. Surgery 1997;122:742–747.
28. Tatsutani K, Rubinsky B, Onik G, Dahiya R. Effect of thermal variables on frozen human primary prostatic adenocarcinoma cells. Urology 1996;48:441–447.
29. Ravikumar TS, Steele G, Kane R, King V. Experimental and clinical observations on hepatic cryosurgery for colorectal metastases. Cancer Res 1991;51:6323–6327.
30. Neel HB KA. Requisites for successful cryogenic surgery of cancer. Arch Surg 1971;102:45–48.
31. Rivoire ML, Voiglio EJ, Kaemmerlen P, et al. Hepatic cryosurgery precision: evaluation of ultrasonography, thermometry, and impedancemetry in a pig model. J Surg Oncol 1996;61:242–248.
32. Yeh CJ. Cryosurgical treatment of melanin-pigmented gingiva. Oral Surg Oral Med Oral Pathol Oral Radiol Endod 1998;86:660–663.
33. Shepherd JP, Dawber RP. Wound healing and scarring after cryosurgery. Cryobiology 1984;21:157–169.
34. Gage AA, Fazekas G, Riley EE Jr. Freezing injury to large blood vessels in dogs. With comments on the effect of experimental freezing of bile ducts. Surgery 1967;61:748–754.
35. Wong WS, Chinn DO, Chinn M, Chinn J, Tom WL. Cryosurgery as a treatment for prostate carcinoma: results and complications. Cancer 1997;79:963–974.

36. Cox RL, Crawford ED. Complications of cryosurgical ablation of the prostate to treat localized adenocarcinoma of the prostate. Urology 1995; 45:932–935.
37. Adam R, Akpinar E, Johann M, Kunstlinger F, Majno P, Bismuth H. Place of cryosurgery in the treatment of malignant liver tumors. Ann Surg 1997;225:39–48.
38. Rewcastle JC, Hahn LJ, Saliken JC, McKinnon JG. Use of a moratorium to achieve consistent liquid nitrogen cryoprobe performance. J Surg Oncol 1997;66:110–113.
39. Lee F, Bahn DK, McHugh TA, Onik GM, Lee FT Jr. US-guided percutaneous cryoablation of prostate cancer. Radiology 1994;192:769–776.
40. Adam R, Hagopian EJ, Linhares M, et al. A comparison of percutaneous cryosurgery and percutaneous radiofrequency for unresectable hepatic malignancies. Arch Surg 2002;137:1332–1339.
41. Huang A, McCall JM, Weston MD, et al. Phase I study of percutaneous cryotherapy for colorectal liver metastasis. Br J Surg 2002;89:303–310.
42. Washington K, Debelak JP, Gobbell C, et al. Hepatic cryoablation-induced acute lung injury: histopathologic findings. J Surg Res 2001;95:1–7.
43. Saliken JC, McKinnon JG, Gray R. CT for monitoring cryotherapy. AJR 1996;166:853–855.
44. Kaufman CS, Bachman B, Littrup PJ, et al. Office-based ultrasound-guided cryoablation of breast fibroadenomas. Am J Surg 2002;184:394–400.
45. Kirchner J, Kickuth R, Laufer U, Schilling EM, Adams S, Liermann D. CT fluoroscopy-assisted puncture of thoracic and abdominal masses: a randomized trial. Clin Radiol 2002;57:188–192.
46. Sandison GA, Loye MP, Rewcastle JC, et al. X-ray CT monitoring of iceball growth and thermal distribution during cryosurgery. Phys Med Biol 1998;43:3309–3324.
47. Lee FT Jr, Chosy SG, Littrup PJ, Warner TF, Kuhlman JE, Mahvi DM. CT-monitored percutaneous cryoablation in a pig liver model: pilot study. Radiology 1999;211:687–692.
48. Silverman SG, Tuncali K, Adams DF, et al. MR imaging-guided percutaneous cryotherapy of liver tumors: initial experience. Radiology 2000; 217:657–664.
49. Harada J, Dohi M, Mogami T, et al. Initial experience of percutaneous renal cryosurgery under the guidance of a horizontal open MRI system. Radiat Med 2001;19:291–296.
50. Daniel BL, Butts K, Block WF. Magnetic resonance imaging of frozen tissues: temperature-dependent MR signal characteristics and relevance for MR monitoring of cryosurgery. Magn Reson Med 1999;41:627–630.
51. Matsumoto R, Oshio K, Jolesz FA. Monitoring of laser and freezing-induced ablation in the liver with T1-weighted MR imaging. J Magn Reson Imaging 1992;2:555–562.
52. Gilbert JC, Rubinsky B, Wong ST, Brennan KM, Pease GR, Leung PP. Temperature determination in the frozen region during cryosurgery of rabbit liver using MR image analysis. Magn Reson Imaging 1997;15:657–667.
53. Seifert JK, Morris DL. World survey on the complications of hepatic and prostate cryotherapy. World J Surg 1999;23:109–113.
54. McGahan JP, Brock JM, Tesluk H, Gu WZ, Schneider P, Browning PD. Hepatic ablation with use of radio-frequency electrocautery in the animal model. J Vasc Intervent Radiol 1992;3: 291–297.
55. Collyer WC, Landman J, Olweny EO, et al. Comparison of renal ablation with cryotherapy, dry radiofrequency, and saline augmented radiofrequency in a porcine model. J Am Coll Surg 2001;193:505–513.
56. Curley SA, Izzo F, Delrio P, et al. Radiofrequency ablation of unresectable primary and metastatic hepatic malignancies: results in 123 patients. Ann Surg 1999;230:1–8.

20
Combined Regional Chemoembolization and Ablative Therapy for Hepatic Malignancies

Michael C. Soulen and Lily Y. Kernagis

Hepatic malignancies are one of the most difficult therapeutic challenges in oncology. Cure usually is not possible because of the predilection for intrahepatic recurrence, despite complete resection or ablation of the initial tumor. Nonetheless, durable local control can be achieved through vigilant monitoring and aggressive multimodality therapy coordinated by a multidisciplinary team of specialists in medical, surgical, and interventional oncology. For tumors that tend not to metastasize aggressively beyond the liver, regional control may benefit quality of life and overall survival.

Most patients with hepatic malignancies have a tumor burden in excess of what can be managed by percutaneous ablation techniques alone. While efficient in causing cell death, all methods of thermal tissue destruction inherently are limited in the volume of tumor that can be reliably ablated. Various regional liver-directed therapies exist that permit treatment of the entire liver volume; however, they lack the efficiency of thermal ablation to cause tissue necrosis. Multimodality treatment may offer synergistic advantages over individual methods alone. This chapter focuses on the results of various combinations of liver-directed regional and locally ablative therapies for treatment of primary and secondary hepatic malignancies.

Combination Therapies for Hepatocellular Carcinoma (HCC)

Neoadjuvant Therapy

Resection and transplantation are effective methods to improve survival in patients with primary liver tumors. Orthotopic liver transplant (OLT) has been shown to be the best treatment for early-stage HCC (1–3). Neoadjuvant therapies have been used to attempt to control tumor growth, prevent viability of latent hepatic foci, induce necrosis, and convert unresectable tumors to resectable ones to improve disease-free survival (DFS) and long-term overall survival (OS) (Table 20.1).

Reports of neoadjuvant therapies followed by surgical removal of the tumor are particularly instructive because they provide histopathologic assessment of response to image-guided therapy. Preoperative transarterial chemoembolization has been shown to be capable of causing partial necrosis in HCC (4). Complete necrosis occurs less commonly, but also has been demonstrated (4–6). Oldhafer et al (5) found that 29% of 21 pretransplant patients who received chemoembolization

TABLE 20.1. Neoadjuvant treatment for hepatocellular carcinoma (HCC).

Study	No. of patients	Recurrence rate (vs. control)	3-year DFS (vs. control)	3-year OS (vs. control)	Effective
Adachi (1993) (19)	46	—	52% (49%)	—	No
Uchida (1996) (20)	60	43% (52%)	—	61% (71%)	No
Harada (1996) (16)	105	—	38% (34%)	78% (68%)	No
Majno (1997) (14)	49	57% (81%*)	29% (26%)	57% (47%)	Yes (if downstaged or complete necrosis)
Paye (1998) (11)	24	58% (58%)	33% (32%)	62% (66%)	No
Oldhafer (1998) (5)	21	—	—	48% (54%)	No
Veltri (1998) (6)	38	12% (15%)	—	—	No
DiCarlo (1998) (9)	55	—	40% (20%*)	70% (38%*)	Yes (in cirrhotic)
Lu (1999) (8)	20	—	55% (22%)	53% (33%*)	Yes (in tumor >8 cm)
Wu (1995) RCT (12)	24	78% (58%)	—	—	No

RCT, randomized control trial; DFS, disease-free survival; OS, overall survival.
*Statistically significant.

developed complete necrosis, while 67% developed partial necrosis. However, no survival benefit was noted.

The addition of percutaneous ethanol injection (PEI) to chemoembolization for neoadjuvant therapy has been attempted to improve induction of necrosis. Veltri et al (6) demonstrated that 100% of patients who received preoperative chemoembolization and PEI had complete necrosis, while neoadjuvant chemoembolization alone led to complete necrosis in 24.1% of patients, and PEI alone led to complete necrosis in 80% of patients. Tumor recurrence occurred in patients who had chemoembolization only and in patients who failed to demonstrate tumor necrosis; however, patients selected to receive chemoembolization alone had more advanced disease. Despite 100% rate of complete necrosis, neoadjuvant therapy with PEI and chemoembolization did not significantly alter the recurrence rate or patient prognosis. Pre-OLT administration of chemoembolization was shown not to increase the risk of hepatic arterial complications, such as thrombosis, after patients underwent OLT (7). Therefore, the role of neoadjuvant intervention in transplant candidates is limited to prevention of tumor progression beyond the criteria for transplant eligibility.

Studies that evaluate preoperative chemoembolization for HCC prior to liver resection have conflicting results. Lu et al (8) performed a retrospective analysis of 120 cases of patients with TNM classification stage II or III HCC who underwent hepatectomy; 44 patients had chemoembolization preoperatively (20 of whom had tumor >8 cm in diameter). In patients with tumors >8 cm, the relative risk of preoperative chemoembolization for overall survival was 0.38 ($p = .017$), demonstrating that there may be some benefit to preoperative chemoembolization in patients with stage II/III tumor >8 cm who undergo hepatectomy. In another study (9), patients with tumors less than 8 cm in diameter were shown to benefit from preoperative chemoembolization. Di Carlo et al (9) found that there was a significant improvement in 3-year OS (70% vs. 38%, $p < .02$) and 3-year DFS (40% vs. 20%, $p < .05$) in pre–liver resection patients with tumors ≤5 cm in diameter who received chemoembolization for HCC. A retrospective analysis performed by Zhang et al (10) showed that in 120 patients who had received preoperative chemoembolization out of 1725 total patients who underwent hepatectomy for HCC, there was a greater DFS in patients who had received more than two chemoembolization treatments. In contrast, a comparative study by Paye et al (11) demonstrated that neoadjuvant chemoembolization produced no significant decrease in tumor size or increase in DFS. Additionally, Wu et al (12) demonstrated in a randomized controlled trial that there was an *increased* risk of extrahepatic recurrence and worse actuarial survival in patients who received chemoembolization prior to liver resection.

Preoperative chemoembolization has led to variable effects on preresection tumor size. In a study by Wu et al (12), patients who had large HCCs (maximum diameter of at least 10 cm), were demonstrated to be resectable by amount of functional liver reserve and anatomic extent of tumor. Tumor volume was decreased by a mean of 42.8% in 16 patients who received chemoembolization. Chemoembolization did not lead to complete necrosis, and there was no change in the DFS. Additional studies on the effect of neoadjuvant therapy on tumor size and conversion of unresectable tumors to resectable have led to more favorable conclusions (13–15). In a study by Majno et al (14), improvement in DFS was demonstrated in patients who were downstaged or had complete necrosis, compared to patients with no response or patients who did not receive preoperative chemoembolization. Additionally, 10% of patients became resectable after downstaging, which occurred more frequently with tumors >5 cm. A different study (16) demonstrated no significant improvement in OS and DFS; however, nearly 50% of patients who underwent neoadjuvant chemoembolization demonstrated at least 25% decrease in maximum tumor diameter (69.6% of patients with tumors less than 5 cm). While the data on chemoembolization conversion of unresectable HCC to resectable have been variable, a study using chemoradiation as neoadjuvant therapy by Sitzmann (15), showed that patients with tumors that were converted to resectable after chemoradiation survived as long as patients who were resectable initially.

Majno et al (14) showed that patients who underwent preoperative chemoembolization had an increased rate of resection of adjacent organs (58% vs. 25%, $p = .03$) compared to control patients. Other complications included adhesion of the tumor to the diaphragm, thickening of the gallbladder wall, and thickening of the hepatoduodenal ligament (17).

It appears as if preoperative chemoembolization alone may be effective in inducing at least partial necrosis and more complete necrosis when PEI is added to the neoadjuvant regimen. It has been suggested that preoperative neoadjuvant therapy should be reserved for patients with initially unresectable tumors, since preoperative chemoembolization delays surgery, can complicate further chemoembolization, and does not provide survival benefit in most studies of resectable tumors (18–20).

Treatment Combinations for HCC without Surgical Resection

Various nonsurgical treatment combinations have been attempted for patients with HCC to improve prognosis. These include liver-directed therapies such as radiofrequency ablation (RFA), microwave ablation, laser ablation, cryoablation, chemical ablation, chemoembolization, and radioembolization, as well as traditional systemic and radiation treatments.

Prospective randomized trials have demonstrated a significant improvement in response in those patients who receive chemoembolization and ethanol injection compared to patients who receive chemoembolization alone. Yamakado et al (23) demonstrated that 26 patients with unresectable HCC who received chemoembolization and transportal ethanol had 1, 3, and 5 year survivals of 87%, 72%, and 51% (18 patients received a second round of chemoembolization). Similarly, Bartolozzi et al (24) found there was significantly greater therapeutic response, lower tumor recurrences, and better rate of survival without recurrence in patients treated with chemoembolization followed by PEI, compared to patients who received repeated chemoembolization treatment for large HCCs (3.1 cm–8.0 cm diameter). Although chemoembolization-PEI patients had better survival rates (100%, 87%, 72% vs. 93%, 70%, and 43% at 1, 2, and 3 years respectively), the difference was not statistically significant. Additionally, patients who received chemoembolization and transportal ethanol injections were shown to develop more complete tumor necrosis (25).

Thermal ablative techniques are limited by the heat-sink effect from blood flow in the liver. A few investigators have attempted to combine thermal ablation with alteration in hepatic blood flow to improve local tumor control. Percutaneous microwave coagulation therapy was given to 18 patients with HCC (2–3 cm in diameter) and cirrhosis within 1–2 days of chemoembolization (26); 17/18 patients were demonstrated to have complete tumor necrosis. Although one patient developed a pleural effusion, no fatal complications presented and all patients were alive at follow-up of 12–31 months. Laser thermal ablation (LTA) was investigated in combination with chemoembolization in patients with large HCCs (3.5 cm–9.6 cm in diameter) (27). LTA preceded chemoembolization in an attempt to make the tumor more amenable to chemoembolization. Complete tumor necrosis was seen in 90% of treated cases, with cumulative survival rates of 92%, 68%, and 40% at 1, 2, and 3 years, respectively. Disease-free survival rates were 74% and 34% at 1 and 2 years, respectively, and no major complications resulted from laser therapy. Rossi et al (28) performed percutaneous RFA in 62 patients with unresectable HCC (3.5 cm–8.5 cm, mean 4.7 cm) after hepatic arterial occlusion; 90% were completely ablated by radiologic criteria after a single RFA session, and 100% after two sessions. Local recurrence was 19% at 12 months, although 45% had new intrahepatic tumors. One-year survival was 87%, with two patients subsequently undergoing surgical resection.

The encouraging early results of combining thermal and embolic therapy must be tempered by our knowledge of the limitations of imaging in measuring response. Unpublished data from our institution are sobering—90% of hepatomas treated with one or more image-guided procedures prior to liver transplantation harbor viable tumor at the time of explantation, despite "complete" radiologic responses. Furthermore, the lack of controlled studies that evaluate the impact of local treatment on the natural history of the disease is an important challenge for percutaneous therapy, particularly given the high prevalence of new tumors that appear in the liver. A nonrandomized, uncontrolled single-institution comparison of 37 patients undergoing either chemoembolization alone ($n = 24$) or chemoembolization plus RFA ($n = 13$) showed no difference in objective response, but a significant improvement in mean and 1-year survival with the combined therapy (29).

Treatment for Liver Metastases

The liver is the most common site for colorectal cancer recurrence. Patients with colorectal cancer metastasis to the liver have a poor prognosis. Liver resection is the only potentially curative option, with a 30% 5-year survival (30). Patients with unresectable colorectal liver metastasis have a median survival of 6 to 9 months without treatment (31). Multimodality treatment options with and without resection have been sought to improve outcomes in patients with liver metastasis.

Thus far, chemoembolization in combination with systemic treatment has not demonstrated promising results. In a study by Leichman et al (32), chemoembolization (doxorubicin/mitomycin C/cisplatin) and systemic 5-fluorouracil (5-FU) with leucovorin were administered to 31 patients with no improvement in survival compared to systemic treatment alone; the overall response was 29%, 1-year survival was 58%, and median time to progression was 8 months. An additional study using cisplatin and systemic 5-FU (33) yielded a median survival of 14.3 months and overall survival of 57% at 1 year and 19% at 2 years in 27 patients.

Several combination therapies have been tested as an adjunct to resection of liver metastases with more favorable results. Tono et al (34) demonstrated a beneficial effect of prophylactic hepatic arterial infusion of 5-FU after resection of colorectal metastases in nine patients (10 controls). Median DFS was 78%, 78%, and 67% at 1, 2, and 3 years, respectively, for the treated group versus 50%, 30%, and 20%. Additionally, Kemeny et al (35) studied adjuvant hepatic arterial infusion of chemotherapy (fluoxuridine/dexamethasone) through an implantable pump after resection of hepatic metastases from colorectal cancer in 74 patients. There was significant improvement in 2-year OS compared to the untreated group (86% vs. 72%) and hepatic progression-free survival at 2 years (90% vs. 60%). The benefit seemed to be confined to patients not treated previously with systemic chemotherapy.

A randomized control trial by Lorenz et al (36) demonstrated no significant improvement in 226 patients with colorectal cancer metastases to the liver who underwent hepatic artery infusion following curative resection. Patients had a median survival of 34.5 months vs. 46.8 months in the control group, and time to progression of 14.2 months vs. 13.7 months.

Rose et al (37) evaluated RFA in patients with hepatic metastases as a primary treatment or as an adjunct to resection, cryosurgical ablation, or hepatic artery infusion. They demonstrated no RFA-associated deaths, and only minimal local and systemic complications. This was confirmed in a study by Elias et al (38) in patients who underwent RFA for a central metastasis or as an adjunct to hepatectomy in patients with multiple bilateral metastases; RFA increased the rate of curative resection without complications related to the RFA. Further studies would be needed to evaluate effect on survival and recurrence.

Summary

The role of neoadjuvant and adjuvant liver-directed therapies in patients undergoing resection of liver tumors remains controversial. For the majority of patients who have unresectable disease, an impressive armamentarium of techniques is available for image-guided treatment. Combinations of these therapies may improve the efficiency of tumor cell kill and result in better immediate local control. Whether this improvement in local response alters the natural history of the disease remains to be evaluated in carefully designed and controlled trials.

References

1. Mazzaferro V, Regalia E, Doci R, et al. Liver transplantation for the treatment of small hepatocellular carcinomas in patients with cirrhosis. N Engl J Med 1996;334(11):693–699.
2. Pichlmayr R, Weimann A, Oldhafer KJ, et al. Role of liver transplantation for the treatment of unresectable liver cancer. World J Surg 1995; 19(6):807–813.
3. Selby R, Kadry Z, Carr B, Tzakis A, Madariaga JR, Iwatsuki S. Liver transplantation for hepatocellular carcinoma. World J Surg 1995;19(1): 53–58.
4. Spreafico C, Marchiano A, Regalia E, et al. Chemoembolization of hepatocellular carcinoma in patients who undergo liver transplantation. Radiology 1994;192:687–690.
5. Oldhafer KJ, Chavan A, Fruhauf NR, et al. Arterial chemoembolization before liver transplantation in patients with hepatocellular carcinoma: marked tumor necrosis, but no survival benefit? J Hepatol 1998;29:953–959.
6. Veltri A, Grosso M, Martina MC, et al. Effect of preoperative radiological treatment of hepatocellular carcinoma before liver transplantation: a retrospective study. Cardiovasc Intervent Radiol 1998;21:393–398.
7. Richard HM III, Silberzweig JE, Mitty HA, Lou WYW, Ahn J, Cooper JM. Hepatic arterial complications in liver transplant recipients treated with pretransplantation chemoembolization for hepatocellular carcinoma. Radiology 2000;214:775–779.
8. Lu C-D, Peng S-Y, Jiang X-C, Chiba Y, Tanigawa N. Preoperative transcatheter arterial chemoembolization and prognosis of patients with hepatocellular carcinomas: retrospective analysis of 120 cases. World J Surg 1999;23:293–300.
9. Di Carlo V, Ferrari G, Castoldi R, et al. Preoperative chemoembolization of hepatocellular carcinoma in cirrhotic patients. Hepato-Gastroenterology 1998;45:1950–1954.
10. Zhang Z, Liu Q, He J, Yang J, Yang G, Wu M. The effect of preoperative transcatheter hepatic arterial chemoembolization on disease-free survival after hepatectomy for hepatocellular carcinoma. Cancer 2000;89:2606–2612.
11. Paye F, Jagot P, Vilgrain V, Farges O, Borie D, Belghiti J. Preoperative chemoembolization of hepatocellular carcinoma. Arch Surg 1998;133: 767–772.
12. Wu C-C, Ho Y-Z, Ho WL, Wu T-C, Liu T-J, P'eng F-K. Preoperative transcatheter arterial chemoembolization for resectable large hepatocellular carcinoma: a reappraisal. Br J Surg 1995; 85:122–126.
13. Tang Z-Y, Yu Y-Q, Zhou X-D, et al. Cytoreduction and sequential resection for surgically verified unresectable hepatocellular carcinoma: evaluation with analysis of 72 patients. World J Surg 1995;19:784–789.

14. Majno PE, Adam R, Bismuth H, et al. Influence of preoperative transarterial lipiodol chemoembolization on resection and transplantation for hepatocellular carcinoma in patients with cirrhosis. Ann Surg 1997;226(6):688–703.
15. Sitzmann J. Conversion of unresectable liver cancer: an approach and follow-up study. World J Surg 1995;19:790–794.
16. Harada T, Matsuo K, Inoue T, Tamesue S, Inoue T, Nakamura H. Is preoperative hepatic arterial chemoembolization safe and effective for hepatocellular carcinoma? Ann Surg 1996;224(1):4–9.
17. Yu Y-Q, Xu D-B, Zhou X-D, Lu J-Z, Tang Z-Y, Mack P. Experience with liver resection after hepatic arterial chemoembolization for hepatocellular carcinoma. Cancer 1993;71:62–65.
18. Poon R, Fan S-T, Wong J. Risk factors, prevention, and management of postoperative recurrence after resection of hepatocellular carcinoma. Ann Surg 2000;232(1):10–24.
19. Adachi E, Matsumata T, Nishizaki T, Hashimoto H, Tsuneyoshi M, Sugimachi K. Effects of preoperative transcatheter arterial chemoembolization for hepatocellular carcinoma: the relationship between postoperative course and tumor necrosis. Cancer 1993;72:3593–3598.
20. Uchida M, Kohno H, Kubota H, et al. Role of preoperative transcatheter arterial oily chemoembolization for resectable hepatocellular carcinoma. World J Surg 1996;20:326–331.
21. Tanaka K, Nakamura S, Numata K, et al. Hepatocellular carcinoma: Treatment with percutaneous ethanol injection and transcatheter arterial embolization. Radiology 1992;185:457–460.
22. Matsui O, Kadoya M, Yoshikawa J, et al. Small hepatocellular carcinoma: treatment with subsegmental transcatheter arterial embolization. Radiology 1993;188:79–83.
23. Yamakado K, Nakatsuka A, Tanaka N, Matsumura K, Takase K, Takeda K. Long-term follow-up arterial chemoembolization combined with transportal ethanol injection used to treat hepatocellular carcinoma. JVIR 1999;10:641–647.
24. Bartolozzi C, Lencioni R, Caramella D, et al. Treatment of large HCC: Transcatheter arterial chemoembolization combined with percutaneous ethanol injection versus repeated transcatheter arterial chemoembolization. Radiology 1995;197:812–818.
25. Yamakado K, Hirano T, Kato N, et al. Hepatocellular carcinoma: treament with a combination of transcatheter arterial chemoembolization and transportal ethanol injection. Radiology 1994;193:75–80.
26. Seki T, Tamai T, Nakagawa T, et al. Combination therapy with transcatheter arterial chemoembolization and percutaneous microwave coagulation therapy for hepatocellular carcinoma. Cancer 2000;89(6):1245–1251.
27. Pacella C, Bizzarri G, Cecconi P, et al. Hepatocellular carcinoma: Long-term results of combined treatment with laser thermal ablation and transcatheter arterial chemoembolization. Radiology 2001;219:669–678.
28. Rossi S, Garbagnati F, Lencioni R, et al. Percutaneous radio-frequency thermal ablation of nonresectable hepatocellular carcinoma after occlusion of tumor blood supply. Radiology 2000;217:119–126.
29. Bloomston M, Binitie O, Fraiji E, et al. Transcatheter arterial chemoembolization with or without radiofrequency ablation. I: The management of patients with advanced hepatic malignancy. Am Surg 2002;68:827–831.
30. Registry of Hepatic Metastases. Resection of the liver for colorectal carcinoma metastases: a multi-institutional study of indications for resection. Surgery 1988;103(3):278–288.
31. Wagner JS, Adson MA, Van Heerden JA, Adson MH, Ilstrup DM. The natural history of hepatic metastases from colorectal cancer: a comparison with resective treatment. Ann Surg 1984;199(5):502–508.
32. Leichman CG, Jacobson JR, Modiano M, et al. Hepatic chemoembolization combined with systemic infusion of 5-fluorouracil and bolus leucovorin for patients with metastatic colorectal carcinoma. Cancer 1999;86(5):775–781.
33. Bavisotto LM, Patel NH, Althaus SJ, et al. Hepatic transcatheter arterial chemoembolization alternating with systemic protracted continuous infusion 5-fluorouracil for gastrointestinal malignancies metastatic to liver: a phase II trial of the Puget Sound Consortium (PSOC 1104). Clin Cancer Res 1999;5(1):95–109.
34. Tono T, Hasuike Y, Ohzato H, Takatsuka Y, Kikkawa N. Limited but definite efficacy of prophylactic hepatic arterial infusion chemotherapy after curative resection of colorectal liver metastases. Cancer 2000;88(7):1549–1556.
35. Kemeny N, Huang Y, Cohen AM, et al. Hepatic arterial infusion of chemotherapy after resection of hepatic metastases from colorectal cancer. N Engl J Med 1999;341(27):2039–2048.

36. Lorenz M, Muller H-H, Schramm H, et al. Randomized trial of surgery versus surgery followed by adjuvant hepatic arterial infusion with 5-fluorouracil and folinic acid for liver metastases of colorectal cancer. Ann Surg 1998;228(6):756–762.
37. Rose DM, Allegra DP, Bostick PJ, Foshag LJ, Bilchik AJ. Radiofrequency ablation: a novel primary and adjunctive ablative technique for hepatic malignancies. Am Surg 1999;65:1009–1014.
38. Elias D, Debaere T, Muttillo I, Cavalcanti A, Coyle C, Roche A. Intraoperative use of radiofrequency treatment allows an increase in the rate of curative resection. J Surg Oncol 1998;67:190–191.

21
Focused Ultrasound for Tumor Ablation

Clare Tempany, Nathan MacDonold, Elizabeth A. Stewart, and Kullervo Hynynen

This chapter reviews the basic principles of focused ultrasound therapy. The physical principles are discussed and explained. The technical requirements and instrumentation used are illustrated. The critical value of using magnetic resonance (MR) as an image guidance method for planning, delivering, and monitoring this form of ablation therapy is reviewed, and its application in uterine leiomyomas is highlighted as an example of current clinical practice.

The only known method to cause highly localized tissue destruction deep in the body noninvasively is ultrasound. The use of ultrasound for tissue destruction was demonstrated first in the 1940s. An extensive research period followed and led to clinical tests of focused ultrasound surgery in the treatment of brain disorders (1,2). These early experiments, however, did not lead to the use of ultrasound in routine practice due to the lack of image guidance and the complexity of the procedure. The recent success of minimally invasive surgeries and the ability to combine this technology with online image guidance and monitoring has led to a renewed interest in focused ultrasound ablation therapy.

The first commercial clinical devices utilized diagnostic ultrasound to aim the therapeutic beam to the target volume. These devices have been tested in the treatment of eye (3), prostate (4,5), bladder, and kidney (6) disorders with encouraging results. More detailed descriptions of the history of focused ultrasound surgery with references to the studies not covered in this chapter may be found in several review articles (4,7–10).

Propagation Through Tissue

Ultrasound is a form of vibrational energy (at a frequency above 20,000 Hz) that is propagated as a mechanical wave by the motion of molecules within tissue. The propagating pressure wave causes the tissue molecules to form compressions and rarefactions, such that the molecules oscillate around their rest position. For medical purposes, the ultrasound frequency is typically between 0.5 and 10 MHz. The speed of the propagating wave is independent of the frequency, and is about 1500 m/s in soft tissue and water. Thus, the wavelength in soft tissue at 1 MHz is about 1.5 mm, and at 2 MHz it is about 0.75 mm.

Ultrasound can be generated by piezoelectric transducers that are driven by a radiofrequency (RF) voltage at the frequency of the desired sound wave. In each piezoelectric element, the thickness changes proportionally to the amplitude of the applied voltage, so the electrical signal is converted to mechanical motion of the same frequency. The generated acoustic power is directly proportional to the driving RF power. The piezoelectric elements are most often made of a ceramic polycrystal that can be manufactured into the desired shape, such as a flat plate to generate planar waves, or a spherically curved bowl to generate focused fields.

As the ultrasound energy passes through tissue, it is attenuated according to an exponential law. At 1 MHz, the ultrasound power is attenuated approximately 50% while it propagates through 7 cm of tissue. At 2 MHz the wave is reduced to approximately 25% of its initial value by the same tissue. The attenuated energy is converted into thermal energy in the tissue.

Ultrasound is effectively transmitted from one soft tissue layer to another, with a small amount (a few percent) of the wave reflected back. At soft tissue–bone interfaces, about one third of the incident energy is reflected back at normal incidence. In addition, the amplitude attenuation coefficient of ultrasound is about 10 to 20 times higher in bone than in soft tissue. This causes the transmitted beam to be absorbed rapidly, resulting in a hot spot at the bone surface (11,12). At a soft tissue–gas interface, all of the energy is reflected back.

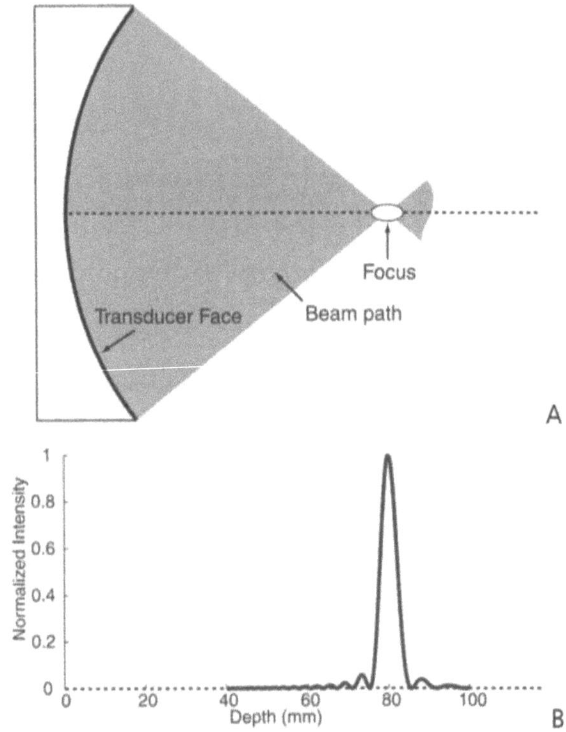

FIGURE 21.1. A focused ultrasound field can be produced by a spherically curved transducer (A). The induced temperature rise in the targeted tissue is directly proportional to the ultrasound intensity, which is highly localized in the focal region (B). This localization ensures that tissue outside of the focal zone is not damaged. Acoustic lenses, reflectors, and arrays of small transducers ("phased arrays") also can be used to create a focused ultrasound field. Phased arrays also can be utilized to move the focus and create patterns of multiple foci.

Focused Beams

Similar to optics, ultrasonic beams can be focused by radiators, lenses, or reflectors. The wavelength limits the size of the focal region (13). A focal diameter of 1 mm can be achieved in practice at 1.5 MHz with a sharply focused transducer (F number <1). The length of the focus is typically five to 20 times larger than the diameter. Since the ultrasound beam is transmitted from an applicator that is large in diameter compared to the focal spot diameter, the ultrasound intensity at the focal spot can be several hundred times higher than in the overlying tissue. Similarly, the ultrasound exposure drops off rapidly across the focus, thus limiting the high ultrasound exposure to the focus (Fig. 21.1).

Similar focusing can be achieved by using transducer arrays that are driven with signals that have the proper phase difference to obtain a common focal point (electrical focusing). Arrays with a large number of elements allow multiple focal points to be induced simultaneously. Large tissue volumes thus can be exposed with such arrays with optimized energy deposition patterns (12,14).

Tissue Effects

The ultrasound beam can interact with tissue by elevating the temperature due to energy absorption from the wave. The temperature elevation during short (a few seconds) sonications follows closely the ultrasound field distribution. At longer exposures, thermal conduction and perfusion smooth the temperature distribution and result in less sharp gradients and a more variable temperature elevation. The induced temperature elevation is directly proportional to the rate of energy absorption, but it also depends on the heat transfer by thermal conduction and blood perfusion in the tissue. In addition, tissue close to large blood vessels will be cooled by the flow (15–17). Since the ultrasound absorption coefficient and the blood perfusion are highly variable from location to location, even in the same organ, the absolute temperature elevation is difficult to predict based on the power output of the transducer. Therefore, temperature monitoring is required if predictable temperature elevations are to be induced.

Different degrees of thermal damage to the tissue depend on the temperature reached and the duration of the exposure (18–21). For exposures of a few seconds, temperatures of above approximately 60°C are needed to cause irreversible tissue damage (24). The elevated temperature can block the microvasculature and stop blood perfusion in the coagulated tissue volume. Occlusion of larger blood vessels by thermal effects of ultrasound also has been demonstrated (22–24). The temperature elevation also may be useful to localize gene therapy (25). When the temperatures reach 100°C, the tissue water boils and gas formation results. The gas blocks the propagation of the ultrasound beam and significantly modifies the energy deposition pattern.

Advantages and Disadvantages of Focused Ultrasound

The main advantages of using focused ultrasound are that it is noninvasive and that it can be focused. This allows deep targets to be destroyed without any damage to the overlying or surrounding tissue. These characteristics also make it possible to deliver the energy rapidly, thus minimizing the effects of perfusion and thermal conduction; these factors result in sharp temperature gradients and accurate tissue coagulation.

The main disadvantages of focused ultrasound are its strong attenuation in bone, and its reflection at gas interfaces, which limits the use of ultrasound to sites with a soft tissue window for beam propagation. In addition, the sharp focusing of ultrasound makes the treatment time long when large tumors are treated.

Lynn et al (26) investigated the potential surgical application of focused ultrasound (FUS) over six decades ago. Since then, therapeutic ultrasound has been tested extensively for noninvasive surgery both in animals and humans (27–29). During the past two decades, clinical trials using focused ultrasound for noninvasive surgery of the prostate and other sites have been conducted with diagnostic ultrasound for localization and targeting (30). Although the use of FUS for ablation of malignant tumors has been shown to be promising (31,32), its widespread acceptance has been limited because of the lack of precise target definition and the difficulty in controlling the focal spot position and beam dosimetry without a temperature-sensitive imaging method.

Magnetic resonance imaging (MRI) can satisfy these requirements for FUS therapy (33–37). It has excellent anatomic resolution for targeting, high sensitivity for localizing tumors, and temperature sensitivity for online treatment monitoring. Several MRI parameters are temperature sensitive; the one based on the proton resonance frequency allows relatively small temperature elevations to be detected prior to any irreversible tissue damage (38). Thus, the location of the focus can be detected at relatively low powers, and the accuracy of targeting can be verified. In addition, using calibrated temperature-sensitive MRI sequences, focal temperature elevations and effective thermal doses may be estimated (39,40). Such thermal quantificaton allows for online feedback to ensure that the treatment is safe, by assuring that the focal heating is confined to the target volume and below the level for boiling. Thermal assessment predicts effectiveness by assuring that the temperature history is sufficient to ensure thermal coagulation.

The technical feasibility of performing MRI-guided focused ultrasound surgery utilizing MRI both to guide and monitor the therapy has been established in animal experiments (40–42). Clinical feasibility has been demonstrated on benign and malignant tumors of the breast (43–45). Adequacy of treatment of target volumes can be substantiated not only by intraprocedural, temperature-sensitive MRI, but also by using postprocedural T1- and T2-

weighted imaging, which reveals signal intensity changes in the treated tissue (46–48). Occlusion of the microvasculature within sonicated tissue can be detected by posttreatment MRI with intravenous contrast agent administration (47,49).

Uterine Leiomyomas

Leiomyomas are very common and cause a range of clinical symptoms, from severe bleeding to minor discomfort (50). Treatment options include hysterectomy, myomectomy, uterine artery embolization, and hormonal therapy. Thermal ablation of uterine leiomyomas by percutaneous interstitial laser therapy or cryoablation has been investigated as a potential minimally invasive treatment (51–53). Focused ultrasound, which delivers the thermal energy without the need to insert a probe, has the potential to become a fully noninvasive choice for selected patients. We designed a study to test the feasibility and safety of MRI-guided FUS for treatment of benign leiomyomas of the uterus.

Uterine leiomyomas, or myomas or fibroids, are the most common pelvic neoplasm in women; they occur in 20% to 50% of women over 30 years of age (50). Their clinical importance is that they are the leading indication for hysterectomy (54). They are treated by less invasive surgical options including myomectomy and uterine artery embolization (55,56). Fibroids account for significant morbidity in terms of both pelvic pressure and heavy menstrual bleeding (57).

The incidence of fibroids is increased in black women (58,59). This population of women develops more advanced disease by the time of surgical intervention, and has surgery at a younger age (60).

Pathologically, fibroids are smooth muscle tumors composed of whorls of muscle fibers arranged in circular fashion. They are well-defined focal masses that occur either intramurally in the myometrium, or are submucosal, subserosal, or pedunculated from the uterine surface. Rarely, fibroids arise in extrauterine locations such as the broad ligament or ovary, or on the peritoneal surface in a diffuse manner know as leiomyomatosis.

Uterine leiomyomas do not always require treatment. Although many authors recommend treatment with drugs such as birth control pills, there is little evidence to support this practice (61). Thus, the bulk of treatment options for fibroids is surgical.

Numerous factors influence treatment options, including the size, number, and location(s) of the myomas, the presenting symptoms, age, and reproductive desires of the woman.

Surgical Therapies

Abdominal myomectomy has been the traditional alternative to hysterectomy, since it preserves the uterus and allows childbearing (62). However, it does have morbidity, similar to that of hysterectomy, and it entails the significant possibility that subsequent surgery may be needed (63–65). For some fibroids, an endoscopic approach is possible with either laparoscopic or hysteroscopic myomectomy (55). However, the size, location, and number of fibroids eliminate this option for many women.

Uterine artery embolization (UAE) is increasingly the first-line alternative to hysterectomy for women with bulk-related symptoms and no desire for future pregnancy. It decreases menorrhagia and bulk-related symptoms in most women (66,67). Serious complications are rare, but appear to be increased when there is a single large myoma (68–71).

There also appears to be an age-related risk of ovarian failure that limits its use for women desiring fertility (67).

Magnetic Resonance Imaging of Uterine Leiomyomas

One of the most important roles of MRI in the body is imaging the female pelvis, as MRI has well-defined and established roles in imaging many diseases of the female pelvis. These roles range from evaluating congenital anomalies to staging gynecologic neoplasms, such as cervical cancer. One of the earliest applications was in the definition of pelvic masses that could not be diagnosed and characterized by ultrasound. Magnetic resonance imaging of the pelvis is performed, irrespective of magnet field strength, using a combination of T1- and T2-weighted sequences. The female genital organs vary in position and orientation, and thus multiplanar imaging is essential.

Leiomyomas vary both pathologically and on imaging. They vary in size, location, internal tissue character, and behavior. Their wide variety in appearance can explain, in part, their varied symptoms. On imaging they are classically large well-defined masses in the uterus. In many situations, a bulky uterus is often classified as "fibroid". Magnetic resonance provides the most accurate imaging of myomas currently. It can provide a full detailed assessment of each and every myoma in the uterus. This typically includes the number, sizes, and locations of all myomas in the uterus. However, there are many other features that require more attention and detailed examination. As focal ablative treatments for leiomyomas are investigated, the baseline imaging characteristics must be well understood, before intervening for new treatment. These focal therapies include uterine artery embolization, laser, and focused ultrasound surgery.

Location

Location of leiomyomas can be assessed in three dimensions, which is critical for treatment planning. Uterine artery embolization is not felt to be effective for large pedunculated myomas. For planning FUS, it is essential to define the location of the myoma, and most importantly its relationship to surrounding tissue. The locations of the bladder, bowel, and spine are important, as will be detailed in the procedure description below. To classify myomas by their symptoms, it is important to define their location, for example, submucosal ones are more likely to cause bleeding and anemia, while subserosal myomas typically have "bulk" symptoms, such as pressure on the bladder. Although it is difficult to assign specific symptoms to individual myomas, it is important to document the details of each prior to focal therapy.

Size/Volume

Magnetic resonance imaging obtains the truest measurement of in vivo size and volume. Ultrasound can provide the accurate size of the uterus and estimates of individual myomas. For treatment monitoring, three-dimensional (3D) MR volumetric assessment before and after therapy is a useful way to assess response.

Tissue Characteristics

Magnetic resonance imaging can demonstrate six patterns in uterine leiomyomas:

1. Classic
2. Hypercellular
3. Cystic degeneration
4. Hemorrhagic/carneous or "red" degeneration
5. Necrotic
6. Lipoleiomyomas

The typical signal intensity pattern of each of these is listed in Table 21.1. It is important to

TABLE 21.1. Typical signal intensity patterns of uterine leiomyomas.

Type	T1-weighted signal	T2-weighted signal	Postgadolinium
Classical	Isointense	Low signal	Homogeneous enhancement
Hypercellular	Isointense	High signal	Homogeneous enhancement
Cystic degeneration	Iso–low signal	Hyperintense areas with surrounding low signal	No enhancement in hyperintense areas
Carneous degeneration	Hyperintense	Mixed, low signal	Nonenhancing
Necrotic	Low signal	Hyperintense	Nonenhancing
Lipoleiomyomas	High signal	High signal	Nonenhancing

classifiy the myoma type prior to treatment because it is unlikely that an ablative treatment or embolization will be effective on necrotic or degenerated myomas. The effects of these therapies based on myoma type is not well understood.

Magnetic Resonance–Guided Focused Ultrasound Surgery for Uterine Leiomyomas

This procedure is being evaluated in the standard fashion with phase I, II, and III trials. Currently, we are in the latter stages of a phase III trial. The feasibility and safety of this method were assessed in multicenter, multinational phase I and II trials. In these trials, all women who were enrolled were scheduled for hysterectomy for their symptomatic uterine leiomyomas. They agreed to undergo FUS treatment 1 week prior to surgery.

The eligibility criteria for treatment in the protocol included: (1) patient was eligible for MRI, and had no pacemaker, claustrophobia, or other contraindication to MRI; (2) patient had no midline abdominopelvic scars; (3) the size of the uterus was 20 cm or less; (4) the size of the myomas was 10 cm or less; (5) patient had no intervening bowel or bladder between the transducer and the myoma.

Treatment Planning

All patients underwent screening in the clinic, and questionnaires were administered to document symptoms. All women had pretreatment MRI scans using a standardized protocol that included T1- and T2-weighted images before and after administration of intravenous (IV) gadolinium. The MR images defined the leiomyomas by size, volume, and location, and demonstrated enhancement after IV gadolinium contrast. Magnetic resonance imaging also was used to plan the beam path by ensuring that each targeted leiomyoma was in an accessible location.

As FUS is delivered through the anterior abdominal wall with the patient in the prone

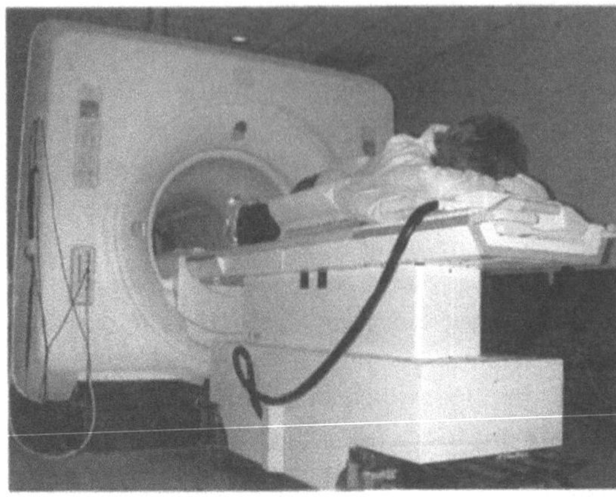

FIGURE 21.2. Patient in a magnetic resonance imager lying on the focused ultrasound (FUS) system table.

position, it was important to evaluate the images for possible obstacles to treatment such as bowel loops between the leiomyoma and the anterior abdominal wall. MRI images were used to determine which leiomyomas could be treated safely. If there were multiple leiomyomas in safe locations, the largest one was selected. The goal of this phase of the trial was to deliver a treatment that could safely induce thermocoagulation that was demonstrable pathologically.

All MRI examinations were performed on a 1.5-T standard whole-body system (Signa, GE Medical System) with the patient lying prone (Fig. 21.2). Standard T2-weighted fast spin echo (FSE) images were obtained in three planes through the uterus, using either a body coil or an external multicoil array. Initial localizer large field-of-view T2-weighted images were acquired to localize the transducer, uterus, and leiomyomas (Fig. 21.3). Typical parameters used for the T2-weighted FSE sequence were field of view (FOV) 160 to 250 mm, matrix size 256 × 192, TR 4 to 5000 ms, TE 90 to 120 ms, three data acquisitions, slice thickness 4 mm, with a 1-mm gap, BW = 16 Hz. Then T1-weighted SE sequences were obtained: FOV 160–250, matrix size 256 × 128, TR/TE = 600/20 ms, four data acquisitions, slice thickness 4/1 mm. For contrast-enhanced images, T1-weighted spoiled gradient recalled echo

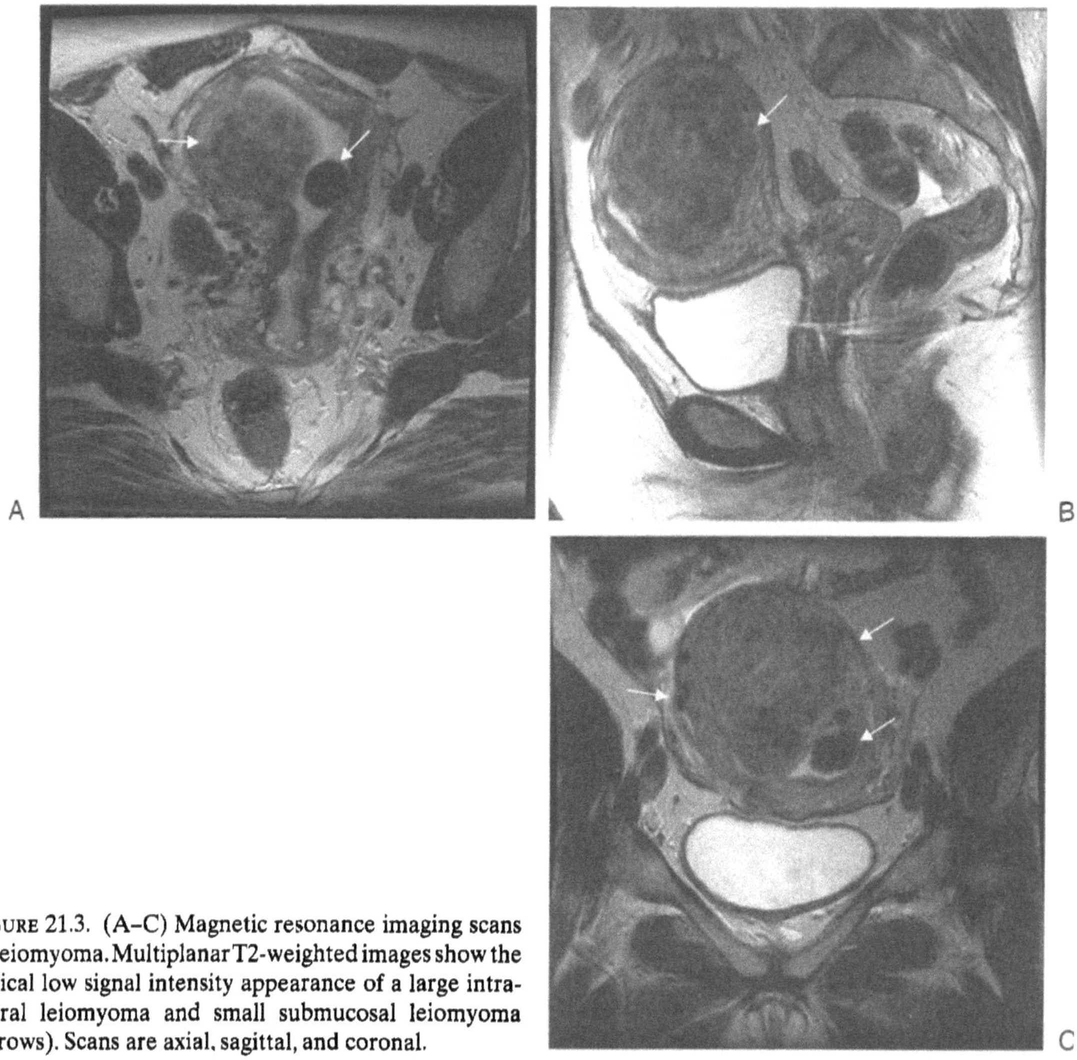

FIGURE 21.3. (A–C) Magnetic resonance imaging scans of leiomyoma. Multiplanar T2-weighted images show the typical low signal intensity appearance of a large intramural leiomyoma and small submucosal leiomyoma (arrows). Scans are axial, sagittal, and coronal.

(SPGR) imaging started very soon after IV injection of the gadolinium-based contrast agent (dose 0.1 mmol/kg body weight, Magnevist, Berlex Laboratories, Wayne, NJ). Pretreatment and posttreatment follow-up MRIs were obtained according to the same protocol. Gadolinium serves two purposes: (1) to assess perfusion of the myomas and the uterus, and (2) to provide information regarding location of the leiomyoma and its relationship to adjacent structures. All patients were imaged in the prone treatment position and on the treatment table containing the FUS transducer (Fig. 21.4A–C).

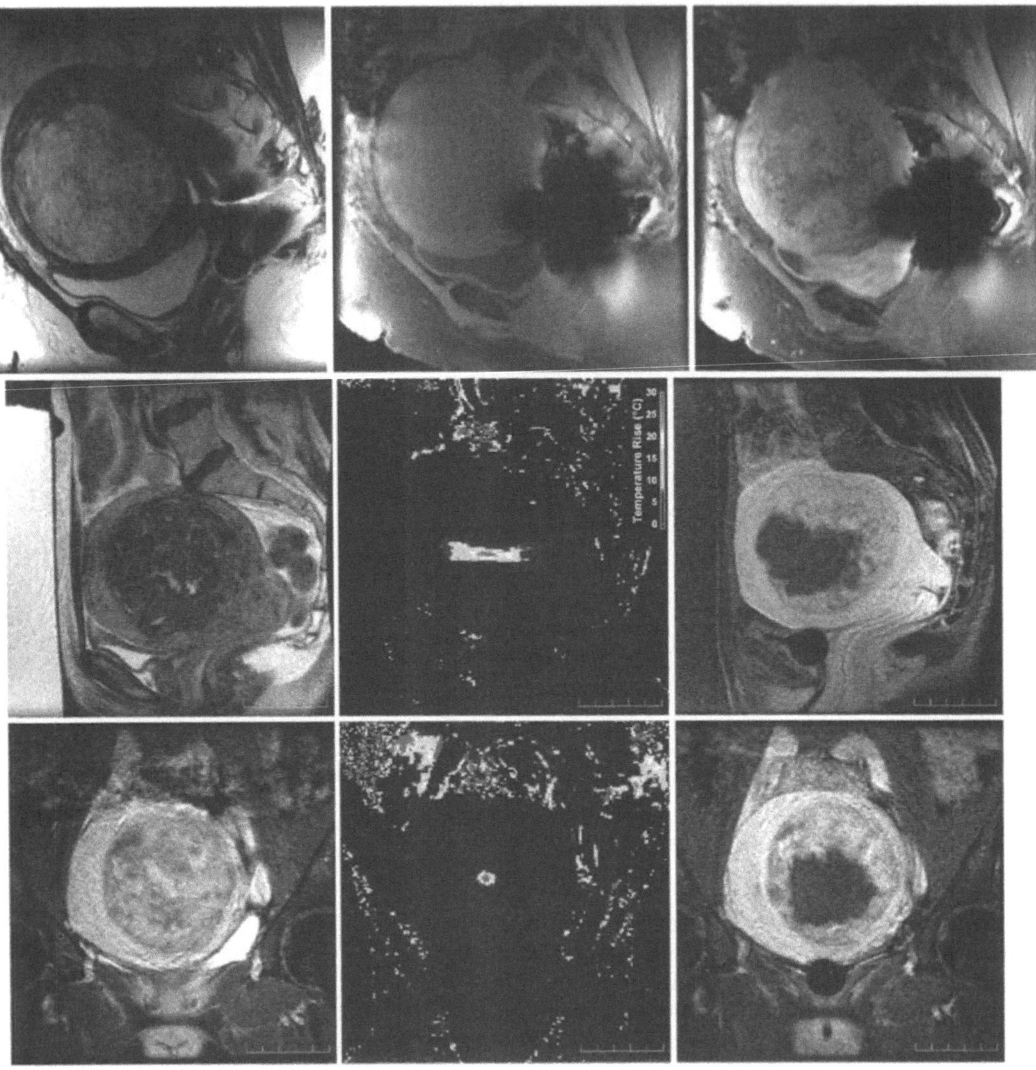

A–C

D

FIGURE 21.4. Atypical hypercellular leiomyoma on MR. (A) Woman with history of prior cervical cancer presents with large pelvic mass. Sagittal T2-weighted image shows large, well-defined high signal intensity mass in the myometrium. (B) Sagittal pregadolinium T1-weighted fat-saturated image shows homogeneously low signal intensity mass. (C) After the bolus IV injection of 20cc of gadolinium, the mass shows heterogeneous enhancement. (D) Left: T2-weighted (top left) and contrast-enhanced T1-weighted (bottom left) MR images acquired before the treatment. The contrast-enhanced image shows that the entire fibroid was perfused before the ultrasound treatment. Center: Temperature maps acquired during two focused ultrasound exposures. Multiple ultrasound exposures at overlapping locations were delivered to treat a volume in the fibroid. These maps were used to guide the treatment; they ensured that the ultrasound was focused in the correct location, and they verified that the heating was sufficient. Right: Contrast-enhanced images acquired after the treatment showing the treated area, which appears as a dark region. The image in the top row was acquired in a sagittal plane, which is parallel to the direction of the ultrasound beam. The image in the bottom was acquired in the coronal plane, and is perpendicular to the direction of the ultrasound beam.

MRg Focused Ultrasound Equipment

All treatments have been performed using an MRg FUS system (ExAblate 2000, InSightec-TxSonics, Haifa, Israel). A focused, piezoelectric transducer with a 120-mm diameter and operating frequency of 1.0 to 1.5 MHz generates the ultrasound field. It is located in the MR table, surrounded by a water bath. It can electronically control the location of the focal spot and the volume of the coagulated tissue. A thin plastic membrane window covers the water tank and allows the ultrasound to propagate into the patient's pelvis. All elements, cables, parts, and components have been manufactured to be MR compatible and function in an MR environment. The system operates inside a 1.5-T magnet (GE Signa, General Electric Medical Systems, Milwaukee, WI).

Patient Preparation

The night before the procedure the patient shaves all hair from the pubic bone upward to allow optimal skin coupling with the treatment transducer. The patient gets an IV for conscious sedation to reduce pain and prevent motion. This is achieved using either oral antianxiolytics, such as diazepam, or conscious sedation with IV fentanyl and Versed. Patients who receive conscious sedation are monitored during the procedure by a nurse, with routine heart rate, blood pressure, and oxygen saturation level measurements. The decision to use concious sedaton is based on the patient's level of comfort when lying prone during the initial MRI, and on whether she has complaints of joint pain, such as shoulder or neck pain. During the procedure the patient is asked to report any symptoms, especially pain or heat. These are reported to the nurse in the room and the radiologist at the treatment console outside the room.

Pretreatment Imaging

The patient is positioned prone in the magnet on the transducer with the water bath surrounding the transducers and providing skin coupling. Pretreatment imaging is performed with T2-weighted FSE images in three orthogonal planes. The radiologist outlines the volume to be treated in the leiomyoma, based on selected slices from the coronal T2-weighted images, using the system software. The target is visualized in two imaging planes, usually coronal and sagittal. The computer software in the system allows display of the ultrasound beam overlying all tissues through which it will pass. This permits evaluation of all tissues or structures in the beam path (Fig. 21.4D).

The T2-weighted images allow assessment of the beam path and determine if a safe treatment can be delivered. Care is taken to avoid contact with bowel loops, and there must be no bowel in the beam path. If necessary, the beam can be repositioned or even tilted to optimize the path. The entire beam path must be assessed, including the posterior path. It is best to avoid the beam directly passing through the spine, as bone absorbs a significant amount of the energy and can cause local bone pain.

After an appropriate volume is selected, the sonication plan is developed in the computer. This initial plan places equally spaced overlapping focal volumes such that the entire target can be covered. The positioning of the focal sonications is selected so that the induced tissue coagulation induces complete coverage in the selected volume. The volume to be treated is calculated by measuring the volume of the sonication cylinder, which is based on the size of the focal spot; the latter ranges from 4.5 to 6.0 mm, and the spot length ranges from 18.0 to 28.0 mm.

The locations of the planned sonications can be modified during the treatment by the operator to obtain accurate MRI thermometry-derived thermal dose and complete coverage of the target volume. In each treatment, all of the sonications are at the same depth (i.e., only one plane is sonicated). The T2-weighted images are used to outline and define the actual target for therapy manually in the treatment planning software. The total number of sonications is calculated and the plan confirmed.

Treatment

Before the therapy-level sonications, low-energy test pulses are aimed within the target volume. The power is increased, until the location of the focus is visible on the temperature-sensitive images. These sonications are below the level for thermal tissue damage, and rather are used to align the coordinates of the FUS system with the MR coordinates. When the test pulse is located in the planned position, the complete target volume is sonicated with a series of higher power pulses such that adequate temperature and thermal dose are reached. The pulse duration typically is 16 seconds. The interval between pulses is about 3 minutes. This allows for cooling of the tissues between each thermal treatment. During each treatment the number of sonications delivered is recorded, as is the number of visible MR temperature maps, the power used, and the temperature changes.

Thus, initial sonications are delivered at low power, followed by slow power increases to ensure that the patient is comfortable and that the thermal imaging demonstrates precise treatment location. Using phase maps, each sonication can be visualized directly as it is being delivered. Thus, not only can the actual temperature change be measured directly, but its precise location can be mapped. This occurs for every sonication delivered during the entire treatment. In a recent study, we found that 100% of visualized sonications were mapped.

The procedure continues with multiple sonications being delivered under direct MR guidance and with real-time MR thermometry. After a therapeutic dose has been delivered to the target volume, postprocedural imaging with two planes of T2-weighted images is obtained. The patient is then taken from the room and observed for 1 to 2 hours, and then discharged with an escort or family member to drive her home. Success of treatment in this phase of the protocol is judged on safety and feasibility. To date, early experience indicates that the procedure meets both criteria.

Ultimately the success of MRg FUS of uterine fibroids will be judged based on improvement of the patient's symptoms when this treatment modality is applied as a single treatment. To this end, a second study follows women with symptomatic fibroids before and after treatment, using a quality of life tool to measure treatment effect.

Conclusion

Clinical trials using FUS or MR-guided FUS are under way in many sites, with various clinical applications. Focused ultrasound of uterine fibroid tumors is feasible and safe in initial trials. This form of noninvasive treatment has the potential to become a major ablative method that may well have broad appeal to patients and their physicians.

References

1. Fry WJ, Barnard JW, Fry EJ. Ultrasonic lesions in the mammalian central nervous system. Science 1955;122:517–518.
2. Fry WJ, Fry FJ. Fundamental neurological research and human neurosurgery using intense ultrasound. IRE Trans Med Electron 1960;ME-7:166–181.
3. Coleman D, Lizzi FL, Driller J. Therapeutic ultrasound in the treatment of glaucoma. Ophthalmology 1985;92:339–346.
4. Sanghvi NT, Fry FJ, Bihrle R. Noninvasive surgery of prostate tissue by high-intensity focused ultrasound. IEEE Trans Ultrason Ferroelectr Freq Contr 1996;43:1099–1110.
5. Chapelon JW, Ribault M, Vernier F. Treatment of localised prostate cancer with transrectal high intensity focused ultrasound. Eur J Ultrasound 1999;9(1):31–38.
6. Vallancien G, Harouni M, Veillon B. Focused extracorporeal pyrotherapy: feasibility study in man. J Endourol 1992;6:173–180.
7. Sanghvi NT, Hynynen K, Lizzi FL. New developments in therapeutic ultrasound. IEEE Biomed Eng 1996;15:83–92. High intensity focused ultrasound. Exp Invest Endosc 1996;1994;4:383–395.
8. Hiller R, Weninger K, Putterman SJ. Effect of noble gas doping in single-bubble sonoluminescence. Science 1994;266:248–250.
9. ter Haar G. Ultrasound focal beam surgery. Ultrasound Med Biol 1995;21(9):1089–1100.
10. Crum LA, Hynynen K. Sound therapy. Physics World 1996;9:28–33.
11. Lehmann JF, DeLateur BJ, Warren CJ. Heating produced by ultrasound in bone and soft tissue. Arch Phys Med Rehabil 1967;48:397–401.

12. Hutchinson EB, Hynynen K. Intracavitary phased arrays for non-invasive prostate surgery. IEEE Trans Ultrason Ferroelectr Freq Contr 1996;43:1032–1042.
13. Hunt JW. Principles of ultrasound used for generating localized hyperthermia. In: Field SB, Franconi C, eds. Physics and Technology of Hyperthermia. Boston: Martinus Nijhoff, 1987: 354–389.
14. Fjield T, Hynynen K. The combined concentric-ring and sector-vortex phased array for MRI guided ultrasound surgery. IEEE Trans Ultrason Ferroelectr Freq Contr 1997;44:1157–1167.
15. Dorr LN, Hynynen K. The effect of tissue heterogeneities and large blood vessels on the thermal exposure induced by short high power ultrasound pulses. Int J Hyperthermia 1992;8(1): 45–59.
16. Yang R, Sanghvi NT, Rescorla FJ. Liver cancer ablation with extra-corporeal high-intensity focused ultrasound. Eur Urol 1993;23:15–22.
17. Kolios MC, Sherar MD, Hunt JW. Blood flow cooling and ultrasonic lesion formation. Med Phys 1996;23:1287–1298.
18. Moritz AR, Henriques FC Jr. Studies of thermal injury. II. The relative importance of time and surface temperature in the causation of cutaneous burns. Am J Pathol 1947;23:695–720.
19. Crile G. The effect of heat and radiation on cancers implanted on the feet of mice. Cancer Res 1963;23:372–380.
20. Sapareto SA, Dewey WC. Thermal dose determination in cancer therapy. Int J Radiat Oncol Biol Phys 1984;10(6):787–800.
21. Landry J, Marceau N. Rate-limiting events in hyperthermic cell killing. Radiol Res 1978;75: 573–585.
22. Delon-Martin C, Vogt C, Chigner E. Venous thrombosis generation by means of high-intensity focused ultrasound. Ultrasound Med Biol 1995;21(1):113–119.
23. Hynynen K, Colucci V, Chung A. Noninvasive artery occlusion using MRI-guided focused ultrasound. Ultrasound Med Biol 1996;22(8): 1071–1077.
24. Vaezy S, Marti R, Mourad P. Hemostasis using high intensity focused ultrasound. Eur J Ultrasound 1999;9(1):79–87.
25. Moonen C, Madio P, de Zwart J. MRI-guided focused ultrasound as a potential tool for control of gene therapy. Eur Radiol 1997;7:1165.
26. Lynn JG. A new method for the generation and use of focused ultrasound in experimental biology. J Gen Physiol 1942;179–193.
27. Fry WJ, Barnard JW, Fry FJ. Ultrasonically produced localized selective lesions in the central nervous system. Am J Phys Med 1955;34(3):413–423.
28. Lele PP. A simple method for production of trackless focal lesions with focused ultrasound: physical factors. J Physiol 1962;160:494–512.
29. Heimburger RF. Ultrasound augmentation of central nervous system tumor therapy. Indiana Med 1985;78(6):469–476.
30. Gelet A, Chapelon JY, Bouvier R. Urology Department, Edouard Herriot Hospital and INSERM Unite 28, Lyon, France.
31. Hill CR, ter Haar G. Review article: high-intensity focused ultrasound—potential for cancer treatment. Br J Radiol 1996;68:1296–1303.
32. Gianfelice DC. MR guided focused ultrasound ablation of primary breast neoplasms: works in progress. Radiology 1999;213:106–107.
33. Jolesz FA, Jakab PD. Acoustic pressure wave generation within an MR imaging system: potential medical applications. J Magn Reson Imaging 1991;1(5):609–613.
34. Cline HE, Schenck JF, Hynynen K. MR-guided focused ultrasound surgery. J Comput Assist Tomogr 1992;16(6):956–965.
35. Hynynen K, Darkazanli A, Unger E, Schenck JF. MRI-guided noninvasive ultrasound surgery. Med Phys 1993;20(1):107–115.
36. Cline HE, Schenck JF, Watkins RD. Magnetic resonance-guided thermal surgery. Magn Reson Med 1993;30(1):98–106.
37. Jolesz FA, Hynynen K. Magnetic resonance image-guided focused ultrasound surgery. Cancer J 2002;8(Suppl 1):S100–112.
38. Hynynen K, Vykhodtseva NI, Chung AH. Thermal effects of focused ultrasound on the brain: determination with MR imaging. Radiology 1997;204(1):247–253.
39. Chung AH, Jolesz FA, Hynynen K. Thermal dosimetry of a focused ultrasound beam in vivo by magnetic resonance imaging. Med Phys 1999; 26(9):2017–2026.
40. McDannold NJ, King RL, Jolesz FA. Usefulness of MR imaging-derived thermometry and dosimetry in determining the threshold for tissue damage induced by thermal surgery in rabbits. Radiology 2000;216(2):517–523.
41. McDannold NJ, Hynynen K, Wolf D. MRI evaluation of thermal ablation of tumors with focused ultrasound. J Magn Reson Imaging 1998;8(1):91–100.
42. Hazle JD, Stafford RJ, Price RE. Magnetic resonance imaging-guided focused ultrasound

thermal therapy in experimental animal models: correlation of ablation volumes with pathology in rabbit muscle and VX2 tumors. J Magn Reson Imaging 2002;15(2):185–194.
43. Hynynen K, Pomeroy O, Smith DN. MR imaging-guided focused ultrasound surgery of fibroadenomas in the breast: a feasibility study. Radiology 2001;219(1):176–185.
44. Huber PE, Jenne JW, Rastert R. A new noninvasive approach in breast cancer therapy using magnetic resonance imaging-guided focused ultrasound surgery. Cancer Res 2001;61(23): 8441–8447.
45. Tempany CM, Stewart EA, McDannold N. MR imaging-guided focused ultrasound surgery of uterine leiomyomas: a feasibility study. Radiology 2003;226:897–905.
46. Chen L, Bouley D, Yuh E. Study of focused ultrasound tissue damage using MRI and histology. J Magn Reson Imaging 1999;10(2):146–153.
47. Hynynen K, Darkazanli A, Damianou CA. The usefulness of a contrast agent and gradient-recalled acquisition in a steady-state imaging sequence for magnetic resonance imaging-guided noninvasive ultrasound surgery. Invest Radiol 1994;29(10):897–903.
48. Graham SJ, Stanisz GJ, Kecojevic A, Bronskill MJ, Henkelman RM. Analysis of changes in MR properties of tissues after heat treatment. Magn Reson Med 1999;42(6):1061–1071.
49. Rowland IJ, Rivens I, Chen L. MRI study of hepatic tumours following high intensity focused ultrasound surgery. Br J Radiol 1997;70:144–153.
50. Stewart EA. Uterine fibroids. Lancet 2001;357: 293–298.
51. Law P, Gedroyc WM, Regan L. Magnetic resonance-guided percutaneous laser ablation of uterine fibroids. J Magn Reson Imaging 2000; 12(4):565–570.
52. Law P, Gedroyc WM, Regan L. Magnetic resonance guided persutaneous laser ablation of uterine fibroids. Lancet 1999;354:2049–2050.
53. Sewell PE, Arriola RM, Robinette L. Real-time IMR-imaging—guided cryoablation of uterine fibroids. J Vasc Interv Radiol 2001;12:891–893.
54. Carlson KJ, Nichols DH, Schiff I. Indications for hysterectomy. N Engl J Med 1993;328(12): 856–860.
55. ACOG practice bulletin. Surgical alternatives to hysterectomy in the management of leiomyomas. Int J Gynaecol Obstet 2001;73(3):285–293.
56. Spies JB, Ascher SA, Roth AR. Uterine artery embolization for leiomyomata. Obstet Gynecol 2001;98(1):29–34.
57. Cote I, Jacobs P, Cumming D. Work loss associated with increased menstrual loss in the United States. Obstet Gynecol 2002;100(4):683–687.
58. Marshall LM, Spiegelman D, Barbieri RL. Variation in the incidence of uterine leiomyoma among premenopausal women by age and race. Obstet Gynecol 1997;90(6):967–973.
59. Baird D, Dunson D, Hill M. Cumulative incidence of uterine leiomyoma in black and white women: ultrasound evidence. Gen Obstet Gynecol 2003;188(1):100–107.
60. Kjerulff KH, Langenberg P, Seidman JD. Uterine leiomyomas. Racial differences in severity, symptoms and age at diagnosis. J Reprod Med 1996; 41(7):483–490.
61. Myers ER, Barber MD, Gustilo-Ashby T. Management of uterine leiomyomata: what do we really know? Obstet Gynecol 2002;100(1):8–17.
62. Bonney V. The technique and results of myomectomy. Lancet 1931;1:171–177.
63. Ecker JL, Foster FS, Friedman AJ. Abdominal hysterectomy or abdominal myomectomy for symptomatic leiomyoma: a comparison of preoperative demography and postoperative morbidity. J Gynecol Surg 1995;11(1):11–18.
64. Iverson RE Jr, Chelmow D, Strohbehn K. Relative morbidity of abdominal hysterectomy and myomectomy for management of uterine leiomyomas. Obstet Gynecol 1996;88(3):415–419.
65. Stewart EA, Faur AV, Wise LA. Predictors of subsequent surgery for uterine leiomyomata after abdominal myomectomy. Obstet Gynecol 2002;99(3):426–432.
66. Spies JB, Roth AR, Jha RC. Leiomyomata treated with uterine artery embolization: factors associated with successful symptom and imaging outcome. Radiology 2002;222(1):45–52.
67. Pron G, Bennett J, Common A. The Ontario uterine fibroid embolization trial part 2. Uterine fibroid reduction and symptom relief after uterine artery embolization for fibroids. Fertil Steril 2003;79(1):120–127.
68. Goodwin SC, Walker WJ. Uterine artery embolization for the treatment of uterine fibroids. Curr Opin Obstet Gynecol 1998;10(4):315–320.
69. Vashisht A, Studd J, Carey A. Fatal septicaemia after fibroid embolisation. Lancet 1999;354 (9175):307–308.
70. Godfrey CD, Zbella EA. Uterine necrosis after uterine artery embolization for leiomyoma. Obstet Gynecol 2001;98(5 Pt 2):950–952.
71. Spies JB, Spector A, Roth AR. Complications after uterine artery embolization for leiomyomas. Obstet Gynecol 2002;100(5 Pt 1):873–880.

22
New Technologies in Tumor Ablation

Bradford J. Wood, Ziv Neeman, and Anthony Kam

The technology and engineering of tumor ablation are evolving more rapidly than the clinical validation. Technical descriptions risk being obsolete by publication time. General principles and developing technical paradigms provide a simplified framework to practice and study radiofrequency ablation (RFA). This chapter reviews the general limitations of tissue ablation methods, the optimization of ablation in the radiofrequency range, and several emerging technologies and paradigms feasible in the laboratory and possibly translatable to clinical practice.

General Principles

Most efforts in the early development of ablation systems focused on altering the needle configuration, tissue properties, or treatment algorithms to optimize volume of tumor kill. Early technical developments reflected efforts to improve relatively similar RFA systems. These modifications include deployable probes, hypertonic saline infusion, multiprobe synergy, chilled electrodes, and current pulsing. Although vendors describe various benefits of their respective systems in marketing, temperature and impedance control are highly interrelated and similar. As temperature approaches boiling (100°C), tissue charring, vaporization, and a coalescence of organic microbubbles at the electrode surface all interact to insulate the electrode and limit energy deposition. Both temperature and impedance reflect this process. The logarithmic increase in impedance that accompanies early overcooking and charring is accompanied by an automated drop in current to allow tissue to cool (pulsing). This avoids the "char-broiled burger effect," in which the tissue in immediate contact with the electrode is overcooked, but the meat further from the heat source is raw. The goal should be to cook as evenly as possible to allow uniform thermal conduction throughout the soft tissues.

The limitations of various ablation methods can be divided into three categories: ablation volume, ablation shape, and lesion targeting. The first of these has received 95% of attention to date. The theme of the first decade of RFA for tumors, the 1990s, was "bigger is better." Most of the developments had the goal of larger tissue destruction in shorter times. This was largely successful, with 7-cm shapes being attained in tens of minutes. However, the predictability and reproducibility of ablation size and shape have received little attention. In reality, the shapes of the thermal lesions are not spherical or completely predictable. This complicates geometric overlapping, increases risk for collateral damage, and worsens outcomes. The different systems create different shapes: oval, teardrop, or disk-like (Fig. 22.1). Custom shaping of the thermal lesion with microwave, bipolar RFA, or multiprobe systems may be the next large technical development in tissue ablation. Custom thermal lesion shaping might lead to improved outcomes, with less collateral damage to normal structures.

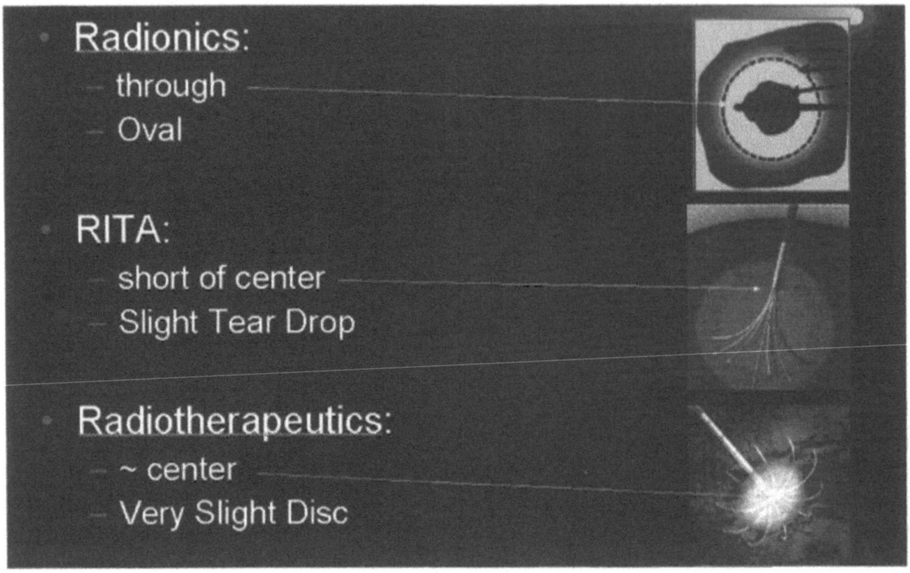

FIGURE 22.1. Thermal lesion size and shape in relation to needle geometry is an area that needs further clarification. Precise needle placement in relation to resulting thermal lesion shape and tumor geometry varies significantly among vendors [Radionics (Radionics Inc, Burlington, MA), RITA (RITA Medical Inc., Mountain View, CA), RadioTherapeutics (Boston Scientific, Natick, MA)].

Other Ablation Technologies

Tumor size is the most important factor in determining complete response rates for the various local or regional cancer therapies. This has led to the principle that for ablation volume, bigger is better. In alcohol ablation, the ablation volume is determined by the amount of alcohol that is injected. Although there is no safe cut-off volume of alcohol that can be injected, in practice, this volume is limited by systemic and local toxicity. In radiofrequency and laser ablation, direct heating takes place within a few millimeters of the electrode or fiber; heating at a distance from the electrode or fiber occurs via conduction. The probe itself does not heat up primarily, but does so secondarily from heat conducted from adjacent tissue. The ablation volume is primarily limited by cooling from tissue perfusion. Microwave ablation shares this limitation except that direct heating extends deeper into tissue. Thus, microwave ablation has the advantage of being less dependent on thermal conduction, since a large volume of tissue receives energy rapidly, and unlike RFA, does not depend on a narrow source of heat to propagate peripherally within a thermal lesion. This mechanism may overcome the "heat-sink effect", as tissue perfusion has less time to cool down adjacent tissue.

In high-intensity focused ultrasound (HIFU), each application of an ultrasound pulse produces a unit coagulation volume similar in size to a grain of rice. The ablation volume is dependent on the ability to overlap these unit volumes, the length of the procedure, and respiratory and patient motion. Although there are many choices for electromagnetic energy deposition in tissue, future ideal tissue ablation technology will have to surpass RFA in ease of use, convenience, cost, safety, accuracy, predictability, reproducibility, practicality, and efficacy.

Heat Transfer

Much early work in tissue ablation focused on optimization of heat transfer: increasing energy deposition, improving tissue heat conduction, and minimizing heat loss. This is within the framework of the oversimplified view of Penne's classic bioheat equation: coagulation necrosis is equal to energy deposited minus heat lost. The bioheat equation is more useful if it is quantitatively solved to predict ablation volumes and shapes for various clinical situations. Deciding where to place a probe or exactly when to use an occlusion balloon in a specific clinical situation may be helped by these developing mathematical models. For instance, if a 3-mm vessel lies within 5 mm of a tumor, modeling may be helpful to decide if balloon occlusion of the vessel is necessary to ablate the tumor.

Tumor modeling requires knowledge of the input parameters of the bioheat equation that include density, specific heat, thermal conductivity, electrical conductivity, and perfusion of tissue. These values are not available for most tumors. Instead, the values from the organ in which the tumor resides are extrapolated. Also, the values used in the various models are at body temperature. The temperature coefficient of tissue electrical conductivity above 40°C is substantially different from the coefficient below 40°C at frequencies used in RFA. Current modeling is based on false assumptions using constants that are true at body temperature, but are not true for tissue in the 50° to 100°C range. Finally, when blood vessels are modeled, it has been assumed that the temperature of blood is body temperature. This may not be valid for small blood vessels. The utility of validated models will be immense as more complex and larger tumors are considered for RFA.

Analysis of reflected versus absorbed power could shed light on the variability of RFA. Finite element modeling has been applied to various electrodes in an attempt to better understand and predict tissue effects (1). Personalized treatment planning and automated probe placements are being integrated into RFA treatments. There is a poor understanding of the nonlinear function of thermal and electrical conductivities in the clinical range (50° to 100°C near 500 kHz). Heat transfer is by conduction in solids, and by convection in fluids or flowing blood. Radiofrequency ablation works by alternating current; thus there is a complex interaction between electrical and thermal forces. The mathematical description of the perfusion effect (loss of heat due to convection) is complicated by the relative effects of small and large vessels, flow rates, and countercurrent heat exchange of warmed vessels.

Tissue Dielectrics

The dielectric correlates of specific tumor and organ histologies also are poorly characterized. Few data are published that differentiate organ and tumor effects. Identical RFA algorithms and parameters may result in surprisingly disparate ablation volumes in different locations, independent of perfusion (Fig. 22.2). Adrenocortical carcinoma, lymphoma, and chordoma are three cell types we have noticed that repeatedly heat quicker than usual, for example. The easier RFA of hepatocellular carcinoma versus same-size colorectal liver metastases also can be explained partially by differing dielectrics. Identifying the thermal and electrical conductivities of certain organs or tumors within clinical ranges of temperature and frequency could lead to tissue-specific and organ-specific algorithms that could improve outcomes. For example, a different algorithm and set of rules are used for kidney tumor ablation. The resulting volumes are predictably smaller than for liver, although this is largely perfusion-dependent. Ablation generators may be made with removable tissue and organ-specific modules that reprogram treatment algorithms for specific tissue and organ types.

Tumor Environment

The effects on RFA of high interstitial pressures within a tumor center, or an acidic or hypoxic environment are unknown. Radiofrequency ablation likely is less affected by the rugged environment in the typically poorly perfused tumor center. As such, RFA is an ideal candidate for combination therapies with blood-borne adjuvants like intravenous (IV) chemotherapy, IV liposomal vectors, chemoembolization, or directly injected adjuvants like polymerized drug depots or chemotherapy gels. Intravenous chemotherapy works on rapidly dividing cells at the tumor periphery where there is good blood supply, and RFA works on the highly pressurized and devascularized center of a tumor. Combination therapies like

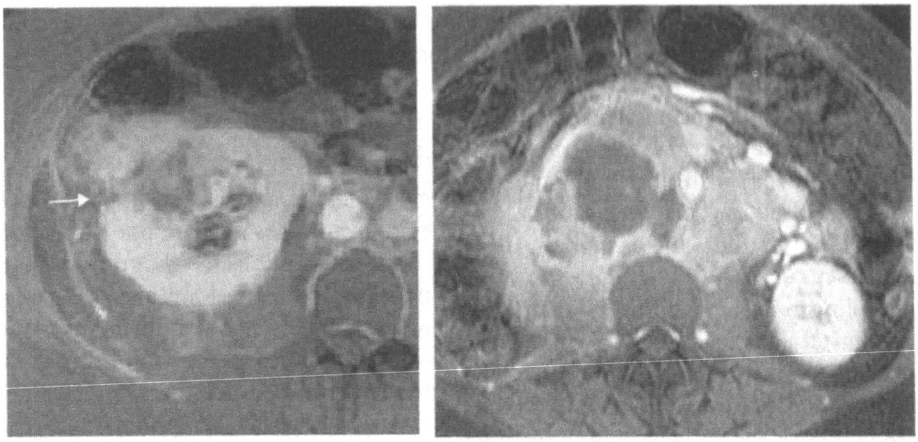

FIGURE 22.2. Radiofrequency ablation (RFA) burn variability. The smaller renal cell carcinoma burn on the left (arrow) was made by 24 minutes of treatment, and the larger burn on the right by 3 minutes with similar parameters and same histology. We know little about the tissue effects of RFA, and it is not as predictable as marketed.

RFA plus chemoembolization or balloon occlusion take advantage of such complementary effects; however, they likely add risk. The exact timing, sequence, and indications for these combination therapies have not been defined or optimized.

Technology for Optimization of Treatment Planning and Monitoring

Imaging

Imaging also is an imperfect surrogate for tumor margins with indistinct, irregular, or infiltrating edges. Better imaging with ultrasound contrast agents, three-dimensional ultrasound, multiplanar reconstruction, image processing, elastic fusion, dynamic MR, computed tomography (CT), fluoroscopy, noninvasive thermography, and MR thermometry also have been the subject of intense research.

Equipment

The rapid rate of technical developments has fueled the revolution in tissue ablation. Recent developments include a flexible probe that can fit into a CT gantry, MR-compatible probes, coaxial probes, and tissue-specific probes (bone). Further refinements could include biodegradable tapered tips to prevent capsule coring, and spring deployment to ensure complete deployment and avoid "kick-back" of the outer cannula that can result in misshaped deployments. Special probes could be developed to optimize the heat profiles for specific combination therapies. Specifically, new probes could leverage the benefits of heat activated drug delivery, drug depot polymers, or enhanced permeability (patents pending).

Radiofrequency Ablation and Thermometry

Percutaneous image-guided RFA risks thermal damage to nearby normal tissues. For tumors near sensitive anatomy, there is a trade-off between aggressive treatment that risks complications and undertreatment (which risks residual tumor). Thermometry may help the operator negotiate this trade-off. The exact thermal lesion margin remains somewhat unpredictable. Therefore, when temperature-sensitive structures (such as bowel and nerves) are nearby, direct (mounted on the RF needle) or indirect (remote or independent) thermometry could further increase the safety of RFA.

To date, thermometry has been described with a multitude of low-temperature hyperthermia systems, as well as with prostate ablation. Different tissues have variable thermal thresholds. This underscores the importance of real-time intraprocedural thermometry near adjacent, susceptible organs. For example, the temperature threshold for bowel injury when ablating the prostate is 45°C; myocardial injury occurs at 50°C; and nerve pain fiber ablation occurs at 45°C. We routinely use remote thermistors to protect adjacent organs during RFA, and we often modify the energy delivered or the treatment duration to limit risk to collateral structures.

Direct (Dependent) Thermistors

Some available RFA systems incorporate thermistors to evaluate tissue temperatures at the tip of the active RFA probe during post-RFA cooling such as Radionics (Radionics, Inc., Burlington, MA), or near the margin and in between active tips such as RITA (RITA Medical Inc., Mountain View, CA). The downside of this technique is that the thermistors cannot be deployed separately from the probe itself. Although these thermistors are directed to the target tissue, they cannot provide precise temperature information about adjacent nearby nontarget tissue.

Indirect (Independent) Thermistors

There are remote thermistor systems available. Radionics makes a 25-gauge accessory thermistor that acts as a stylet inside a 22-gauge SMK pole needle, with a digital TCA-2 monitor. The advantage is independent placement and positioning of the thermistors between the RFA probe and collateral, at-risk structures.

Magnetic Resonance Thermometry

Another way to monitor real-time temperature changes during RFA is by MR thermometry. This method gives three-dimensional volumetric data, and thus more reliably indicates temperature changes in the entire tissue of interest, not just from one point. Magnetic resonance thermometry may provide noninvasive, real-time monitoring of coagulation during HIFU, microwave, hot saline, laser, and RFA procedures. This is possible because of the temperature dependence of spin-lattice relaxation time, proton resonance frequency, and diffusion. The disadvantages are inaccurate temperature monitoring of moving targets due to respiration, scarce availability, switching back and forth from MR RF pulses to RFA, and the cost of MRI-compatible RFA systems. Also, the most robust sequences [proton resonance frequency (PRF)] are also very susceptible to breathing motion artifact.

Robotics

Robotics is being applied rapidly to RFA to assist needle placement. For percutaneous image-guided procedures, the main advantage of robotics is that it facilitates the use of a large amount of quantitative data from imaging; consequently, it allows a greater accuracy and precision in needle placement. A secondary advantage is that for CT or x-ray fluoroscopic-guided interventions, robotics can eliminate radiation exposure to the interventionalist (2). Machines are more accurate than humans when it comes to planning and enacting multiple overlapping treatments. Robotics also may facilitate translation of needle-based technologies into the community setting.

Defining robotic language will help one understand how these machines will soon transform how needles are placed. Bloom et al (3) describe fundamental robotics terminology as follows: A robotic arm consists of links that are connected by joints. At the distal end, there is an end-effector that performs the action of the robot. The axes through which an arm can translate or rotate define the degrees of freedom for the arm. For instance, since there are three degrees of translational freedom (x,y, and z axes) and three degrees of rotational freedom around those axes (pitch, roll, and yaw), an end-effector that has six degrees of freedom can take any position and any orientation. The terms *active* and *passive* have different meanings depending on whether they refer to a section of a robot or to the entire robot. A passive section is one that has to be moved manually; an active section is one that is self-propelled. For the entire robot, *active* and *passive* refer to the degree of autonomy. Active robots perform a task according to a program and without human assistance. Semiactive robots require human interaction to perform a task. Passive robots do not perform any task, but supply information.

A group at Johns Hopkins constructed a robotic arm for percutaneous interventions (2,4). Called PAKY-RCM (percutaneous access to the kidney–remote center of motion), this robot consists of a passive arm with seven degrees of freedom. Attached to this arm is an active remote center of motion that pivots a needle about its tip. An active needle driver holds the needle. The system can be operated as a semiactive robot (a surgeon manipulates a joystick to drive the needle), an active robot (completely computer-controlled with the robot indirectly registered to the CT image), or in combination. The Hopkins' group has shown that the number of attempts, time to access, and safety of robotic percutaneous access using PAKY-RCM and standard manual percutaneous access of renal calyces under fluoroscopy were comparable. For CT-guided interventions involving the kidney, liver, neobladder, spine, lung, and muscle, this group has achieved success at hitting the target without human intervention in 75% of patients. The remaining 25% were successful after fine adjustments with the joystick. Georgetown has developed a spinoff robot for fluoroscopic-guided needle interventions driven by a joystick (Fig. 22.3).

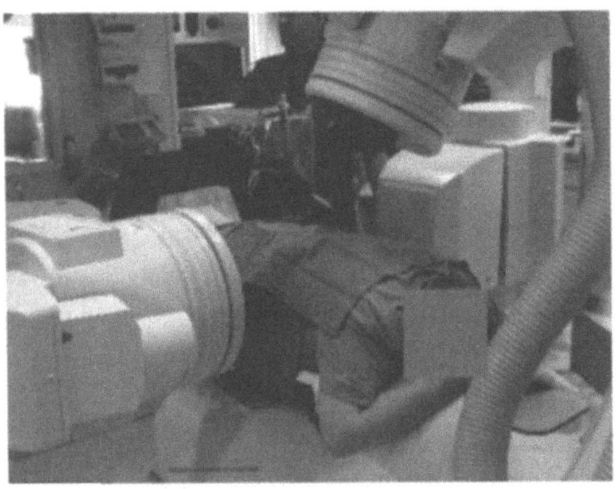

FIGURE 22.3. Table-mounted robot integrated with biplane fluoroscopy. Needle is driven using joystick controlled by physician. (Courtesy of Kevin Cleary, PhD, Georgetown University.)

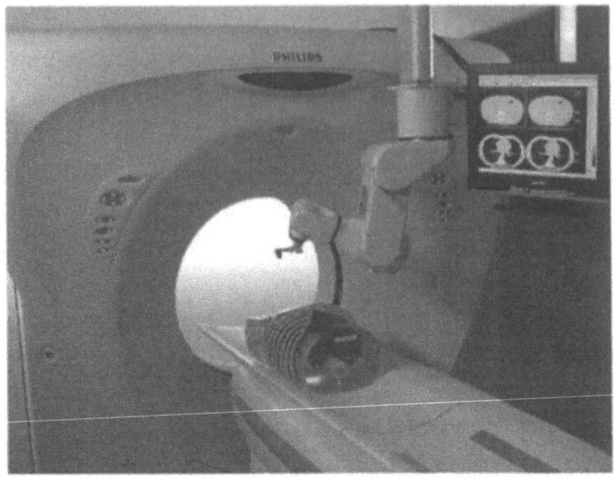

FIGURE 22.4. Active robot prototype demonstrating seamless direct integration of CT and robot by mechanically registering the robot to the CT coordinates using a gantry frame. (Copyright Jeff Yanof, PhD, Philips Medical Systems, Cleveland, OH.)

We are helping to design an interventional suite with a robot prototype mechanically registered to CT using a mechanical frame and arm (Philips Medical Systems, Cleveland, OH) (Fig. 22.4). During the first attempt with the prototype, a 1-mm BB was hit with a 22-gauge needle on a complex oblique path 15 cm deep in the dome of a phantom liver without CT fluoroscopy (5). Free-hand cannot be as accurate and precise.

Navigation, Needle Tracking, Image Fusion

Seamless integration with the imaging data set is a necessity for successful robotic-assisted RFA. Safety issues, respiratory motion, and organ shift during procedures remain the largest obstacles to robotic deployment for organs other than the brain, spine, prostate, and bone. The same obstacles limit utility of navigation and augmented reality systems to guide RFA. Magnetic tracking may be the most promising navigational tool for RFA (Figs. 22.5 to 22.7). A weak magnetic field is generated

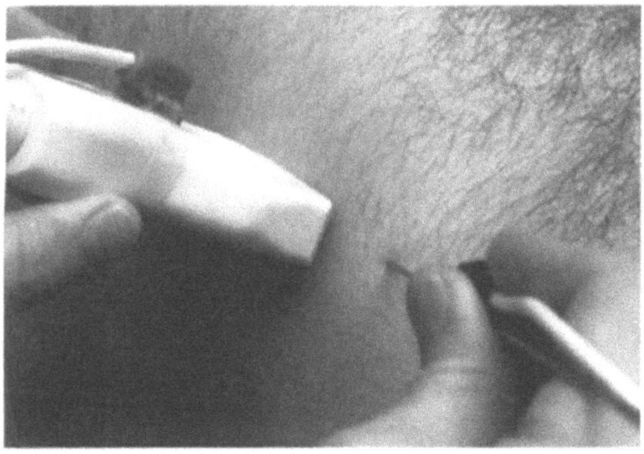

FIGURE 22.5. Conventional magnetic tracking device with clips on the ultrasound and the needle shaft.

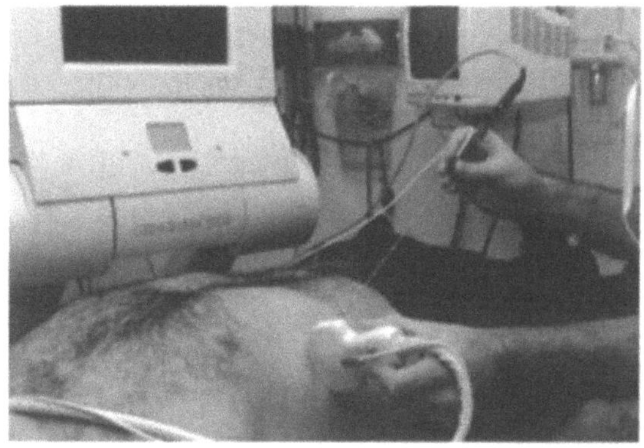

FIGURE 22.6. Conventional magnetic tracking device showing out of plane needle navigation with ultrasound.

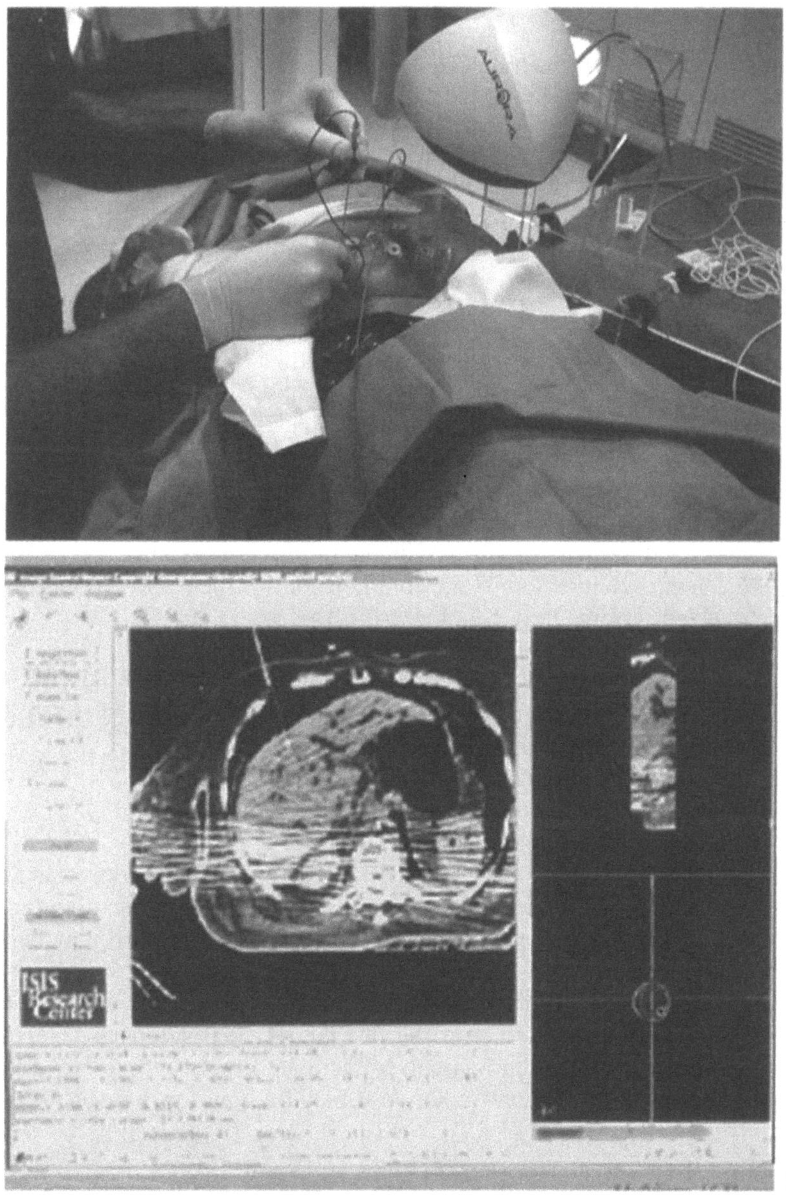

FIGURE 22.7. (A) Magnetic field generator for interstitial magnetic tracking with small sensors inside needle shaft. (B) Graphical user interface for magnetic tracking and sphere-packing for planning and navigating RF ablation. (Courtesy of Kevin Cleary, PhD, Georgetown University.)

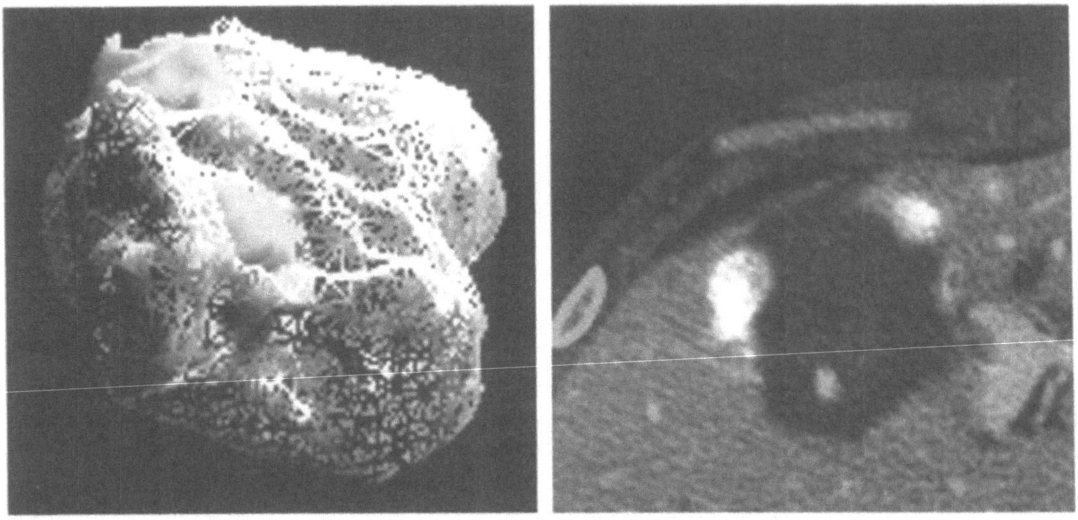

FIGURE 22.8. (A) Volumetric display of fused pre- and post-RFA images shows residual tumor and its spatial relationship to thermal lesion. (B) Rigid image fusion shows positron emission tomography (PET)-positive tissue at the edge of the thermal lesion 1 month post-RFA to define targets of residual tumor for next RFA. (Courtesy of Frederik Geisel, Hendrik von Tengg-Kobligk, Matt McAuliffe, and Medical Image Processing and Visualization Program, NIH.)

and small sensors may be placed on the ultrasound transducer, the RFA needle, as well as the patient. The exact *x,y,z* position in space and the projected pathway are displayed to assist needle placement. Major shortcomings thus far have been related to the position of the needle-based sensor, which is clipped to the needle shaft/hub junction in one common commercialized system (Figs. 22.5 and 22.6). This is prone to misregistration with bending of the needle, organ shift, or respiratory variation. Efforts are under way to optimize the use of interstitial sensors within stylets or RFA probes or internalized fiducials to optimize position information (Fig. 22.7) (patent pending).

The difficulties of organ shift and respiratory motion also complicate multiparametric image display or image fusion as guides for RFA. Image fusion may take advantage of off-line modalities during a CT-guided RFA. Pretreatment CT, MR, or positron emission tomography (PET) may be fused with the procedural imaging or the follow-up imaging to facilitate early detection of residual tumor so it may be re-treated before becoming geometrically unfavorable. Using a computer with Java-based image processing software, RFA can be performed with online real-time semiautomated image fusion to define targets and identify residual untreated neoplastic tissue (Fig. 22.8). Combined PET-CT scanners are popularizing the same process for diagnostic purposes.

Emerging Paradigms: Radiofrequency Ablation as Adjuvant Therapy?

Gene Therapy

Gene therapy has a long way to go to be clinically relevant and mainstream. However, when it arrives, it may be combined with heat, either as an adjuvant or as heat-activated gene delivery. This could be accomplished with a heat-activated particle or with a heat-upregulated gene promoter. The heat shock protein promoter has been used in animal studies to deliver genes locally to heated tissue. Gene delivery is verified by reporter gene (green fluorescent protein) imaging (6). Cleavable linkers also may be heat activated, releasing the active moiety upon exposure to heat (7). DNA may be engineered in the laboratory to manipulate tumor biology or the cellular response to therapies like heat and chemotherapy. Genes under investigation for cancer include therapeutic genes, oncogenes, suppressor genes, suicide genes, antisense genes, reporter genes, plasmid DNA, co-stimulatory genes, and genes coding for drug resistance, cytokines, antigens, drug efflux pump, and immunomodulation, to name but a few. The main obstacles to in vivo gene therapy have been specific and efficient delivery, transfer, and expression of the vector. Toxicity and inadequate targeting are related impediments.

Other forms of electromagnetic energy outside the 500-kHz range may be more effective at promoting gene transfection or altering local permeability. Ultrasound may augment gene transfection efficiency in vivo (8). The effects of sublethal RFA upon gene transfection are undefined. By the time gene therapy has moved beyond the mouse, in an effective clinical trial, tissue ablation systems will likely be completely different from the way they are currently.

Immunotherapy

Thermal ablation with microwaves has been shown to stimulate a tumor-specific immune response remote from the heated tissue (9). Radiofrequency ablation may act in a similar fashion, and may improve the function of dendritic cells or the presentation of tumor antigens to the immune system, as it recruits macrophages to the periphery of the thermal lesion in the sublethal zone (7). This immune response may be redirected to fight circulating tumor in remote locations. High-intensity focused ultrasound may hypothetically be the best antigen-presenting technology, given the violence inherent in cavitation, whereby tumor antigens may be presented suddenly and forcefully. Preclincial work needs to be done to answer these questions.

Radiation and Radiofrequency Ablation

Hyperthermia is a useful adjunct to radiotherapy for the local control of advanced malignancies. Low-temperature hyperthermia may be the most effective cellular radiosensitizer known. Heat acts via several pathways. Heat alone independently kills radioresistant cells (s-phase and hypoxic cells). Heat also potentiates the adverse effects of radiation on the cell's ability to repair radiation-induced DNA damage (10). These effects occur throughout the entire cell cycle, but most prominently at the s phase.

Although the exact timing and sequence remain to be optimized for human RFA plus radiation, there is much to be learned from prior experience in lower temperature hyperthermia plus radiation. In rodent studies, the highest level of radiosensitization was achieved when hyperthermia was applied simultaneously with radiation (with a radiosensitization half-life of 20 to 30 minutes). In humans, there is likely a 4-hour window (radiosensitization half-life of 100 to 120 minutes).

The synergistic effects of radiation plus hyperthermia have been supported by several recent reports, with various successful randomized clinical trials, including recurrent advanced breast cancer, recurrent or metastatic melanoma, head and neck cancer, non–small-cell lung cancer, glioblastoma multiforme, and intrapelvic malignancies (bladder, uterine cervix, and rectum). Ex-vivo studies suggest that most cell lines are sensitive to this synergistic combination therapy.

While the additive effects of hyperthermia and radiation have been well studied at low temperatures (40–44°C), there is sparse information regarding radiation and the RFA temperature range (60–100°C). Heat may improve the complex relationship among local perfusion, interstitial pressure, and oxygen tension in the center of an irradiated tumor. Radiation effects on perfusion could reduce heat sink convection during RFA, which could augment ablation volumes. The synergism between RFA and radiotherapy needs further clarification.

Drug Delivery

Radiofrequency ablation is one of several ways to deliver heat, with the advantage of selectivity by allowing heat to be delivered more specifically to the local tumor. Also, RFA may prove to be a tool broadly used for drug delivery or therapy augmentation. In this paradigm, RFA debulks the tumor and potentiates the local or regional effects of the combination therapy. Antiangiogenic targeted therapies may inhibit and repress a tumor without complete cell death. In this fashion, some cancers in the future may be kept from growing or metastasizing without complete eradication. Given that cancer may be considered a chronic disease in the future, RFA debulking also may evolve into a more accepted and standard rational practice. However, this may require translation of antiangiogenic therapies from the bench to the bedside. Debulking theoretically may allow other therapies to work better against smaller volumes of disease, although this is controversial in the oncology community, and largely depends on the cell type and clinical scenario.

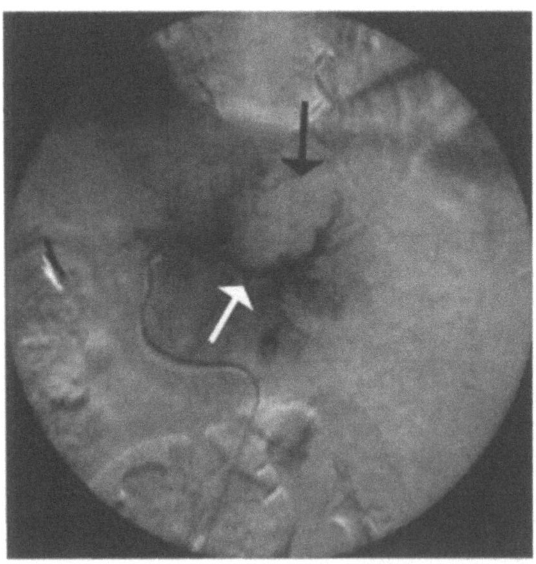

FIGURE 22.9. Selective hepatic artery angiography shows hypervascular rim (white arrow) around thermal lesion (black arrow) immediately following RFA.

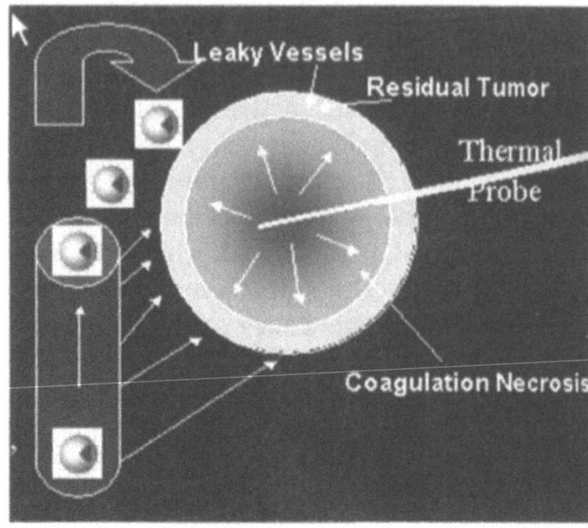

FIGURE 22.10. A combination of therapies, delivery systems, and strategies may be more effective than single therapy. RFA plus chemoembolization, injectables, gene therapy, molecular targeted drugs, liposomes, or immunotherapy should open doors to more broad clinical applications for thermal ablation in the future. (Courtesy of Jay Patti, MD.)

Aggressive debulking is more commonly being performed when the natural history of a neoplasm has proven itself to be less aggressive over time.

Selective drug delivery in cancer has met with limited success thus far due to a combination of problems. These include getting to the cell, getting inside the cell, staying there, avoiding natural defense systems, and minimizing systemic toxicity and effects on normal tissue. Radiofrequency ablation may be used to augment drug delivery via heat-activated particles or by simple increased permeability from sublethal heating (Figs. 22.9 and 22.10).

Drug Depot Effect

Tumor cell microenvironment may be made favorable for drug uptake or effect. Cryotherapy increases bleomycin uptake in tumors (11). Cryotherapy also increases membrane permeability. Any ablation technology potentially increases drug dwell time due to devascularization and vascular stasis. Radiofrequency ablation may further facilitate the drug depot effect, where the devascularized zone of coagulation necrosis holds on to the drug for much longer than in perfused tissue. In this model, the drug slowly seeps out of the coagulation necrosis sponge over time, resulting in lasting drug dwell time. Drug washout by perfusion is overshadowed by drug diffusion into surrounding tissues. This concept has been postulated by Haaga's group (12) with implanted doxorubicin-eluting polymer implants in rabbit liver following RFA. Drug-eluting millirod polymers combined with RFA could represent a winning combination that warrants further resources and study.

Electroporation

Drug, gene, particle, or protein delivery to the cell may be facilitated with electroporation or sonoporation. Electroporation therapy is the more mature of the two. In this technique, pulsed electric fields are used to temporarily increase the permeability of cell membranes by creating transient pores (13). Extracellular macromolecular therapeutic agents like drugs, proteins, or genes that normally have difficulty crossing cell membranes can enter cells through these pores. Needle electrodes placed directly into the target tissue are used to apply the pulsed electric fields. As a method for drug or gene delivery for cells in vitro, electroporation is well established. Electroporation also prolongs retention of plasmid-mediated gene transfer in liver vasculature (14).

Electroporation-assisted gene therapy (electrogene therapy) currently remains in the preclinical stage; however, electroporation-assisted chemotherapy (electrochemotherapy) has reached the stage of clinical trials. One advantage of electrochemotherapy over standard chemotherapy is that side effects are minimized because a much lower dose of the drug is used. One group of such trials involves electrochemotherapy with bleomycin. In 50 patients with 291 cutaneous or subcutaneous malignant tumors treated with electroporation and bleomycin given interstitially or intravenously, Mir et al (15) reported a complete response in 56.4% of tumors and a partial response in 28.9% of tumors, with minimal side effects.

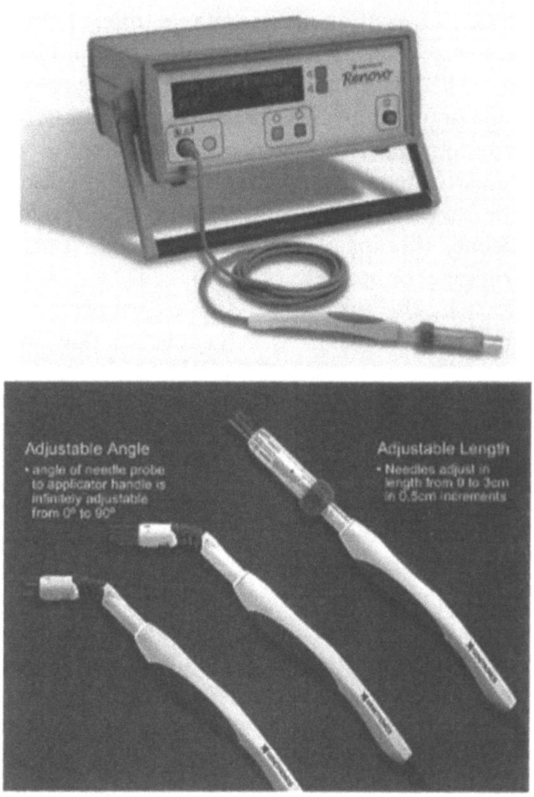

FIGURE 22.11. Intratumoral electroporation system for enhanced drug and gene delivery. (Photo printed with permission from Genetronics, Inc.)

Genetronics Inc. (San Diego, CA) is currently sponsoring a phase III clinical trial of electrochemotherapy with intratumoral bleomycin for head and neck cancers (Fig. 22.11). Sersa et al (16) reported a phase II trial involving electrochemotherapy with intratumoral cisplatin for malignant melanoma; 133 tumor nodules in 10 patients were divided as follows: 82 nodules were treated with electrochemotherapy, 27 nodules were treated with intratumoral cisplatin, two nodules were treated with electric pulses alone, and 22 nodules were not treated. After 4 weeks, objective (complete and partial) response was achieved in 78% of nodules in the electrochemotherapy group, whereas objective response was achieved in 38% of nodules in the intratumoral cisplatin group.

One barrier in the development and optimization of electroporation therapy in vivo is that currently there is no method to monitor the electroporation process in real time. Parameters for electric field pulses (amplitude, duration, duty cycle, and number) are typically based on preclinical work. For instance, microsecond pulses with high electric fields are used in electrochemotherapy, and millisecond pulses with lower electric fields are used in electrogene therapy (17). Necrosis and tumor shrinkage or expression of a gene are used to assess the efficacy of the electroporation process. Preclinical work has shown that for electrogene therapy with a fixed set of pulse parameters, transfection efficiency varies with the tumor type (17). Consequently, preclinical pulse parameters are not necessarily optimal for the clinical arena.

Recently, Davalos et al (18) proposed using electrical impedance tomography (EIT), a noninvasive method of imaging the impedance distribution inside the body, to monitor the electroporation process. Multiple electrodes are placed on the body surface. Current is then sourced at each electrode successively. Surface potentials are measured with each current source. The impedance image is obtained by solving Laplace's equation with the measured boundary values. The hypothesis of Davalos et al's proposal is that when pulsed electric fields are successful in creating pores in cell membranes, there will be a measurable change in tissue impedance.

Sonoporation

Another method of increasing the permeability of cell membranes transiently is ultrasound. Unlike HIFU, sonoporation is not a thermal injury. Although not well understood, sonoporation is believed to be mediated through cavitation. The evidence for this comes from a series of in vitro experiments showing that ultrasound contrast microbubbles enhance sonoporation (19,20). In an elegant experiment, Wu et al (21,22) have shown that microstreaming is responsible for sonoporation. Acoustic streaming is a steady flow in a liquid induced by an acoustic field. Microstreaming is a vortex-like streaming that occurs next to an oscillating bubble near a solid surface or next to a small solid vibrator. The microstreaming has a sharp velocity gradient that causes a shear stress on the solid surface or, in the present context, the cell membrane. The shear stress stretches the cell membrane outward and partially damages it.

Understanding the factors that affect cavitation is an area of active research. A few observations can be made. Cavitation requires the presence of cavitation nuclei in a media. In the absence of such nuclei, inertial or spontaneous cavitation occurs with a threshold of acoustic pressure. In contrast to electroporation, there has been less in vitro and preclinical work using sonoporation to enhance the delivery of drugs and genes (23,24). The frequencies used in these studies are typically much lower than the frequencies used in diagnostic ultrasound, on the order of kilohertz.

Shock Waves and Ultrasound-Released Particles

Shock waves may be used with similar goals. Shock waves are single pulses of pressure in which the speed of propagation is greater than the speed of sound. Shock waves have more pressure and are more localized than typical ultrasound. Shock wave poration causes increased chemotherapy uptake and increased membrane permeability. Ultrasound-mediated particle delivery systems have been developed in which the particle is burst locally by the ultrasound, which then locally deploys the payload in a fashion similar to some ultrasound contrast agents. Because ultrasound can be targeted and is noninvasive, ultrasonic technology for drug delivery warrants further development and is receiving much attention from the biotechnology industry currently.

Permeability

Sublethal thermal ablation enhances permeability and increases endothelial leakage, possibly widening endothelial gap junctions. Studies of hyperthermia (40° to 50°C) show increased selective drug uptake and decreased microvascular flow (less washout). A temperature of 41°C preferentially increases vascular permeability of tumor neovessels in a temperature-dependent fashion (25).

Radiofrequency ablation kills tissue in the center of a tumor where there are high interstitial pressures, ischemia, hypoxia, and poor perfusion. However, at the periphery of a thermal lesion, there remains a rind of hypervascular tissue (Fig. 22.9). This hypervascularity with leaky vessels should potentiate chemotherapy deposition to the cells that are most likely to be incompletely heated. This could allow for chemotherapy to reach residual viable actively dividing cells, where it may be most effective. Also, more cells in the periphery of a tumor generally will be undergoing cell division, and many chemotherapies work by this process.

Cryotherapy increases intracellular chemotherapy deposition in cells undergoing sublethal freezing, likely via increased membrane permeability and trapping of drug from vascular stasis. Radiofrequency ablation should have a similar drug depot effect, because there is increased membrane fluidity and increased endothelial leakage (26). Focused ultrasound also may prove useful for increasing drug delivery via a thermal effect as well as mechanical shaking of the tissue and vasculature with a high-amplitude subsecond pulsed wave (27).

Liposomes/Nanoparticles

Drug-laden liposomes take advantage of this altered permeability to improve drug deposition. First-generation liposomes have phospholipids that encapsulate drugs. Second-generation liposomes incorporate polyethylene glycol (PEG) to stabilize the particle and result in prolonged circulation and less phagocytosis or reticuloendothelial system uptake (Fig. 22.12). Early laboratory and clinical work suggest that such PEG-ylated liposomes encapsulating a payload of doxorubicin (Doxil/stealth liposome) may be potent adjuvants for RFA (28). Polymerization and polyvalency of liposomes can improve delivery of standard chemotherapy liposomes, with a high payload, low toxicity, and prolonged circulation. High heating of liposomes also may release cytotoxic free radicals that potentiate cytoreduction.

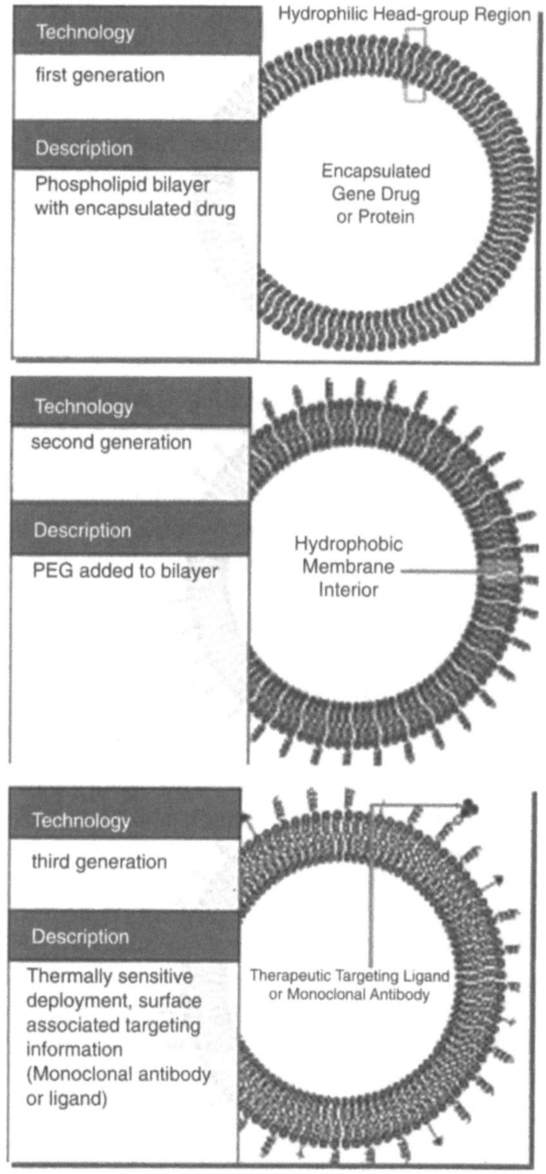

FIGURE 22.12. Evolution of liposome technology for drug delivery. Polyethylene glycol (PEG) coating results in prolonged circulation and avoidance of phagocytosis. Liposomes are a rational choice for RFA heat-activated therapeutics.

The dosing has not yet been optimized, however. Third-generation liposomes incorporate targeting ligands or monoclonal antibodies for specific delivery and local/regional effect (Fig. 22.12). Early laboratory studies suggest that a low-temperature–sensitive liposome engineered at Duke University (Durham, NC) may be advantageous for combining with RFA. This liposome deploys its cargo much faster than other liposomes (on the order of seconds) and then seals up after passing the heated tissue from RFA. It also is much more thermally sensitive than other conventional doxorubicin liposomes, deploying therapeutically at 39° to 42°C. This favorable thermal profile may facilitate drug deposition, allowing for more drug to deploy where needed with less systemic toxicity (29).

A nanoparticle that targets angiogenesis recently has been developed that uses the $\alpha_v \beta_3$ endothelial cell surface integrin as a target (Fig. 22.13). This integrin is upregulated and strongly expressed in tumor vessel endothelium, and may be better than vascular endothelial growth factor (VEGF). Polyvalency also may allow more specific targeting. This nanoparticle also can kill tumors by delivering genes selectively to growing blood vessels on tumor-bearing mice (30). Expression of this integrin may be imaged by PET or MR via a monoclonal antibody attached to paramagnetic contrast. Molecular imaging may provide a surrogate marker for incomplete tumor ablation, thus facilitating follow-up, prognosis, response, and early interventions before becoming geometrically unfavorable for repeat treatment. However, the effects of heat on angiogenesis are likely variable and complex.

Each method of targeting may allow for a higher order of specificity, so heat activation may augment local delivery rationales for many engineered drugs with molecular targeting. Defining the genomics and proteomics of tumor heating may classify upregulated genes that could be used to improve heat-mediated cell targeting or local gene delivery or transfection.

Selective local/regional drug delivery also will become more relevant in the future as patient-specific molecular targets are identified. Definition of temporal and spatial heterogeneities of specific tumors will lead to patient-specific drug cocktails to be administered at specific times, according to molecular imaging–defined guidelines. Radiofrequency ablation has the attractive features of debulking part of the tumor burden, and simultaneously increasing drug deposition via an increased permeability effect in the sublethally heated residual tumor. Many pharmaceutical treatments will be combined with thermal ablation to improve pharmacokinetics and efficacy (Fig. 22.10).

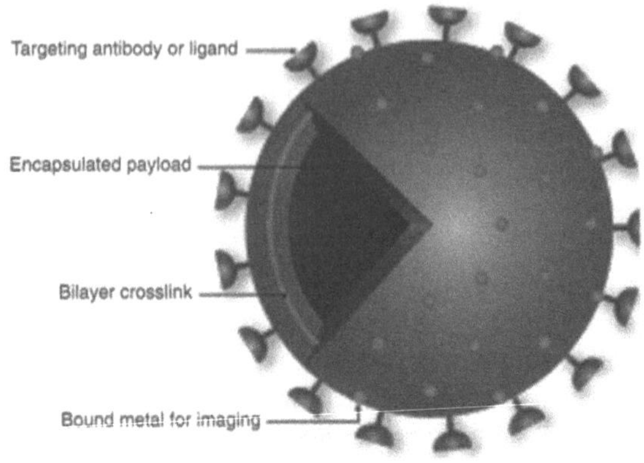

FIGURE 22.13. Nanoparticle delivered in the bloodstream with specific tumor targeting may be an ideal combination treatment for image-guided electromagnetic energy therapy like RFA.

Conclusion

One can envision the day when the treatment plan will be constructed by a computer program that decides where the best entry point is and the best needle position to avoid heat sink. The RFA treatment planning program also will calculate thermal dosimetry similar to radiation therapy planning. It will tell you whether balloon occlusion or the Pringle maneuver is required. The entry points and targets will be clicked with a mouse, and electromagnetic focusing needles will be placed by a robot, with physician assistance. Magnetic tracking within the needle will provide navigation using multimodality image fusion for deploying a predetermined treatment plan based on patient-specific anatomic and perfusion data with a dielectric feedback loop to optimize the tissue-specific treatment algorithm. The organ-specific module will be plugged into the generator and the tissue will be cooked, at which point image fusion will automatically identify areas of residual tumor. Augmented reality will display the anatomy below the skin when the needle is pointed toward the target before the needle is physically placed. Needle-based sensors will use optical spectroscopy to characterize chromatin density and identify tumor margins. An intravenous or local intraarterial injection of a molecularly targeted liposome will be performed to turn local RFA into regional or systemic therapy. Radiofrequency ablation, electroporation, or sonoporation will increase therapeutic gene transfection of the liposome payload. The physician pilot will be drinking coffee in the control room to make sure he stays awake.

References

1. Tungjitkusolmun S, Staelin ST, Haemmerich D, et al. Three-dimensional finite-element analyses for radio-frequency hepatic tumor ablation. IEEE Trans Biomed Eng 2002;49:3–9.
2. Solomon SB, Patriciu A, Bohlman ME, Kavoussi LR, Stoianovici D. Robotically driven interventions: a method of using CT fluoroscopy without radiation exposure to the physician. Radiology 2002;225:277–282.
3. Bloom MB, Salzberg AD, Krummel TM. Advanced technology in surgery. Curr Probl Surg 2002;39:733–830.
4. Su LM, Stoianovici D, Jarrett TW, et al. Robotic percutaneous access to the kidney: comparison with standard manual access. J Endourol 2002; 16:471–475.
5. Wood BJ, Banovac F, Friedman M, et al. CT-integrated programmable robot for image-guided procedures: comparison of free-hand and robot-assisted techniques. J Vasc Intervent Radiol 2003;14:S62.
6. Vekris A, Maurange C, Moonen C, et al. Control of transgene expression using local hyperthermia in combination with a heat-sensitive promoter. J Gene Med 2000;2:89–96.
7. Kruskal JB, Goldberg SN. Emerging therapies for hepatocellular carcinoma: opportunities for radiologists. J Vasc Intervent Radiol 2002;13: S253–S258.
8. Schratzberger P, Krainin JG, Schratzberger G, et al. Transcutaneous ultrasound augments naked DNA transfection of skeletal muscle. Mol Ther 2002;6:576–583.
9. Zhang J, Dong B, Liang P, et al. Significance of changes in local immunity in patients with hepatocellular carcinoma after percutaneous microwave coagulation therapy. Chin Med J (Engl) 2002;115:1367–1371.
10. Kampinga HH, Dikomey E. Hyperthermic radiosensitization: mode of action and clinical relevance. Int J Radiat Biol 2001;77:399–408.
11. Mir LM, Rubinsky B. Treatment of cancer with cryochemotherapy. Br J Cancer 2002;86:1658–1660.
12. Gao J, Qian F, Szymanski-Exner A, Stowe N, Haaga J. In vivo drug distribution dynamics in thermoablated and normal rabbit livers from biodegradable polymers. J Biomed Mater Res 2002;62:308–314.
13. Weaver JC, Chizmadzhev YA. Theory of electroporation: a review. Bioelectrochem Bioenergetics 1996;41:135–160.
14. Liu F, Huang L. Improving plasmid DNA-mediated liver gene transfer by prolonging its retention in the hepatic vasculature. J Gene Med 2001;3:569–576.
15. Mir LM, Glass LF, Sersa G, et al. Effective treatment of cutaneous and subcutaneous malignant tumours by electrochemotherapy. Br J Cancer 1998;77:2336–2342.
16. Sersa G, Stabuc B, Cemazar M, Miklavcic D, Rudolf Z. Electrochemotherapy with cisplatin: clinical experience in malignant melanoma patients. Clin Cancer Res 2000;6:863–867.
17. Cemazar M, Sersa G, Wilson J, et al. Effective gene transfer to solid tumors using different non-viral gene delivery techniques: electroporation, liposomes, and integrin-targeted vector. Cancer Gene Ther 2002;9:399–406.
18. Davalos RV, Rubinsky B, Otten DM. A feasibility study for electrical impedance tomography as a means to monitor tissue electroporation for molecular medicine. IEEE Trans Biomed Eng 2002;49:400–403.
19. Miller DL, Quddus J. Sonoporation of monolayer cells by diagnostic ultrasound activation of contrast-agent gas bodies. Ultrasound Med Biol 2000;26:661–667.
20. Ward M, Wu J, Chiu JF. Experimental study of the effects of Optison concentration on sonoporation in vitro. Ultrasound Med Biol 2000;26: 1169–1175.
21. Wu J, Ross JP, Chiu JF. Reparable sonoporation generated by microstreaming. J Acoust Soc Am 2002;111:1460–1464.
22. Wu J. Theoretical study on shear stress generated by microstreaming surrounding contrast agents attached to living cells. Ultrasound Med Biol 2002;28:125–129.
23. Anwer K, Kao G, Proctor B, et al. Ultrasound enhancement of cationic lipid-mediated gene

transfer to primary tumors following systemic administration. Gene Ther 2000;7:1833–1839.
24. Husseini GA, Runyan CM, Pitt WG. Investigating the mechanism of acoustically activated uptake of drugs from Pluronic micelles. BMC Cancer 2002;2:20.
25. Gnant MF, Noll LA, Terrill RE, et al. Isolated hepatic perfusion for lapine liver metastases: impact of hyperthermia on permeability of tumor neovasculature. Surgery 1999;126:890–899.
26. Kruskal JB, Oliver B, Huertas JC, Goldberg SN. Dynamic intrahepatic flow and cellular alterations during radiofrequency ablation of liver tissue in mice. J Vasc Intervent Radiol 2001; 12:1193–1201.
27. Bednarski MD, Lee JW, Callstrom MR, Li KC. In vivo target-specific delivery of macromolecular agents with MR-guided focused ultrasound. Radiology 1997;204:263–268.
28. Goldberg SN, Kamel IR, Kruskal JB, et al. Radiofrequency ablation of hepatic tumors: increased tumor destruction with adjuvant liposomal doxorubicin therapy. AJR 2002;179:93–101.
29. Kong G, Braun RD, Dewhirst MW. Characterization of the effect of hyperthermia on nanoparticle extravasation from tumor vasculature. Cancer Res 2001;61:3027–3032.
30. Hood JD, Bednarski M, Frausto R, et al. Tumor regression by targeted gene delivery to the neovasculature. Science 2002;296:2404–2407.

23 Combination Therapy for Ablation

Allison Gillams and William R. Lees

Radiofrequency ablation (RFA) is most effective for small tumors. In metastases, complete treatment has been reported in 91% of tumors <2cm, 88% of tumors <3cm, and 53% of 3 to 4.5cm tumors (1,2). In hepatocellular carcinoma (HCC), RFA achieved complete necrosis in 90% of lesions <3cm and 71% of lesions 3.1 to 5.0cm in diameter (3). In our practice, most patients present with larger lesions.

Many patients develop new disease following successful ablation of colorectal metastases; 50% develop new metastases elsewhere in the liver (4) and 40% develop extrahepatic disease (5). For HCC, the 5-year recurrence rate in the liver following successful resection varies from 67.6% to 100% (6). The vast majority of these patients eventually succumb to their disease. Therefore, combination therapies are required not only to increase the local ablative efficacy for larger lesions, but also to reduce the incidence of new lesions and extrahepatic disease.

Combination Therapies to Improve Local Ablation Efficacy

Vascular Occlusion and Radiofrequency Ablation

Normal liver, like other tissues, responds to thermal injury with an increase in arterial perfusion. This change has been quantified using contrast-enhanced computed tomography (CT). A mean 3.2-fold increase in hepatic arterial perfusion was observed in normal liver immediately adjacent to the area of ablation in a cohort of 32 patients (7). Tissue perfusion-mediated cooling, or the "heat-sink effect," restricts the volume of ablation that can be achieved. The relationship between tissue perfusion and the volume of necrosis has been elegantly demonstrated using pharmacologic manipulation. For example, a halothane-induced 46% reduction in blood flow resulted in a doubling of the diameter of the area of necrosis (8). Further experiments with occlusion of the hepatic artery, portal vein, or both vessels in animals produced increased amounts of necrosis (9). In one study, hepatic arterial occlusion increased the area of necrosis 2.5-fold, portal venous occlusion by 1.5 times, and occlusion of both vessels by 5.7-fold (10). In a second study, using a different RFA system, the volume of necrosis was increased 1.8-fold by hepatic arterial occlusion, twofold by portal venous occlusion, and 2.9-fold by occlusion of both vessels (11).

Balloon occlusion is practiced in some centers, particularly for the treatment of large HCCs (12). At surgery, the vascular pedicle can be clamped. It must be remembered that while vascular occlusion increases the volume of necrosis, it also removes the protective effect of cooling blood, and there is a predictable increase in bile duct injury (10). This could be important for treatment adjacent to the main bile ducts.

Another option for patients undergoing treatment under general anesthesia is "hypotensive anesthesia". This technique, employed in liver resection, is the controlled reduction of the systolic blood pressure to approximately 80 mmHg. In one study, this maneuver resulted in a 44% increase in necrosis volume (13).

Surgery and Radiofrequency Ablation

At Open Laparotomy

Radiofrequency ablation can be performed in conjunction with surgical resection (14). In some patients, the size and distribution of their metastases make this the optimal approach. Radiofrequency ablation can be used to increase the number of patients who are eligible for an ablative procedure. Advantages of the open surgical approach include better staging and improved detection of very small liver metastases with intraoperative ultrasound (US). Disadvantages of this approach include the invasiveness, complication rate, expense, and the lack of CT and magnetic resonance imaging (MRI) monitoring of the procedure. Intraoperative RFA, therefore, is indicated only when another procedure is required, for example, liver or bowel resection. Cryotherapy has been used to successfully reduce the incidence of edge recurrence following resection in patients with inadequately treated margins; RFA could be used in a similar fashion (15). It has also been used to produce a zone of dessication at the resection margin with a reported reduction in blood loss (16).

Laparoscopic Approach

Laparoscopic RFA is useful when contiguous structures that may be damaged by the ablation need to be moved away from the area to be treated. This is particularly important for bowel, stomach, or diaphragm. Some centers use percutaneous injection of sterile water both to separate important structures from the ablation area and to improve ultrasound visualization of the diaphragmatic surface of the liver. Laparoscopic RFA has been recommended for HCCs that are poorly visualized transcutaneously, or for large HCCs that require multiple electrode placements that confer the potential for hemorrhage (17). Theoretically, the laparoscopic approach could combine the advantage of reduced invasiveness offered by the percutaneous approach and better staging inherent in the surgical approach. However, the use of laparoscopic US to guide treatment is difficult and requires substantial skill. A comparison of open and laparoscopic approaches for ablation in an animal model using 1-cm target lesions showed a higher positive margin rate, 33%, with the laparoscopic approach vs. 9% with the open approach (18).

Intratumoral Injection and Radiofrequency Ablation

Ethanol

Injection of 100% ethanol into the tumor has been used in conjunction with thermal ablation to increase ablation efficacy. The postulated mechanism is vasoconstriction of tumor vessels that reduces the heat-sink effect. Our study in 19 patients treated with laser demonstrated a small (mean 5.4%) increase in the volume of necrosis.

Saline

Several groups have explored the use of saline to increase the volume of necrosis (19). The saline is thought to act as a wet electrode by increasing the effective electrode surface and hence the flux of RF current. The effect increases with the concentration of saline (20). Saline infusion can be performed as an adjunctive technique, and also has been incorporated into electrode design. Ex vivo and in vivo experiments with "wet electrodes" have shown larger areas of necrosis, but also a more irregular necrosis (21).

Hepatocellular Carcinoma vs. Liver Metastases

Intratumoral injection usually is more effective in HCC in which the injectate remains localized within a well-defined lesion. Injection into scirrhous metastases can be difficult, and extravasation of the injectate often is seen on US. We no longer use saline infusion on grounds of safety.

Radiofrequency Ablation and Systemic Therapies

Chemotherapy

Systemic Chemotherapy for Colorectal Liver Metastases

There have been exciting developments in the treatment of colorectal liver metastases with chemotherapy. For the first time, a significant, if small, improvement in survival has been achieved with irinotecan (22). Another new regime, Oxaliplatin and 5-fluorouracil (5-FU), has been shown to have higher response rates, as much as 53%, compared to 5-FU and folinic acid, in which the response rate was 28% (23). Trials are in progress evaluating these new agents alone and in conjunction with 5-FU, as first- or second-line therapy.

Neoadjuvant Chemotherapy

Surgical resection has been performed effectively in patients who have been downstaged by chemotherapy (24,25). Similarly, our results with RF have shown that chemoresponders can benefit from ablation (26). The survival from the diagnosis of liver metastases in chemoresponders was 39 months, compared to 42 months for patients who had either not received chemotherapy or had not been downstaged by it. With more efficacious first-line agents becoming available, many more patients will become suitable for ablative procedures, either surgical or RFA.

Adjuvant Chemotherapy

Radiofrequency ablation does not preclude chemotherapy as a concurrent treatment. Intraarterial chemotherapy has been used following both cryotherapy and in a small group of patients post-RFA (27,28). In the cryotherapy group, for those patients who managed to complete more than 3 months of chemotherapy, the median survival was 582 days compared to 331 days for those treated with cryotherapy alone. For patients on systemic chemotherapy, RFA treatment needs to be scheduled to avoid periods of bone marrow suppression with attendant thrombocytopenia and neutropenia. Central lines, in place for the administration of chemotherapy, are a common source of bacteremia and secondary infection of the necrotic ablation area in the liver, and are associated with a high morbidity. As a result of this additional comorbidity, we have tended to avoid concurrent systemic chemotherapy; we prefer to use chemotherapy prior to RFA to downstage patients with more extensive disease than is amenable to RFA alone.

Chemoembolization and Radiofrequency Ablation for Liver Metastases

Although chemoembolization is not a well-accepted therapy for metastatic disease, there are several reports that show response rates varying between 25% and 100%, with median survival between 7 and 23 months (29). The response is transient, but if a reduction in size is achieved, then it is feasible that this could be followed by RFA. We are currently exploring the role of chemoembolization followed by RFA for larger (>5 cm) metastases (Fig. 23.1).

Systemic Chemotherapy in Breast Liver Metastases

Radiofrequency ablation has been used successfully in patients with limited liver metastases (30). Some of these patients have had extrahepatic disease, often considered a contraindication to local ablative therapy. However, there is evidence that treated bony and mediastinal nodal metastases can be stabilized for long periods of time, such that RFA for localized liver metastases becomes a reasonable consideration.

Neuroendocrine Metastases

Radiofrequency ablation, cryotherapy, and surgery have been used to increase the efficacy of somatostatin analogues in patients who have developed uncontrolled hormone-secretion–related symptoms, despite optimal medical therapy (31).

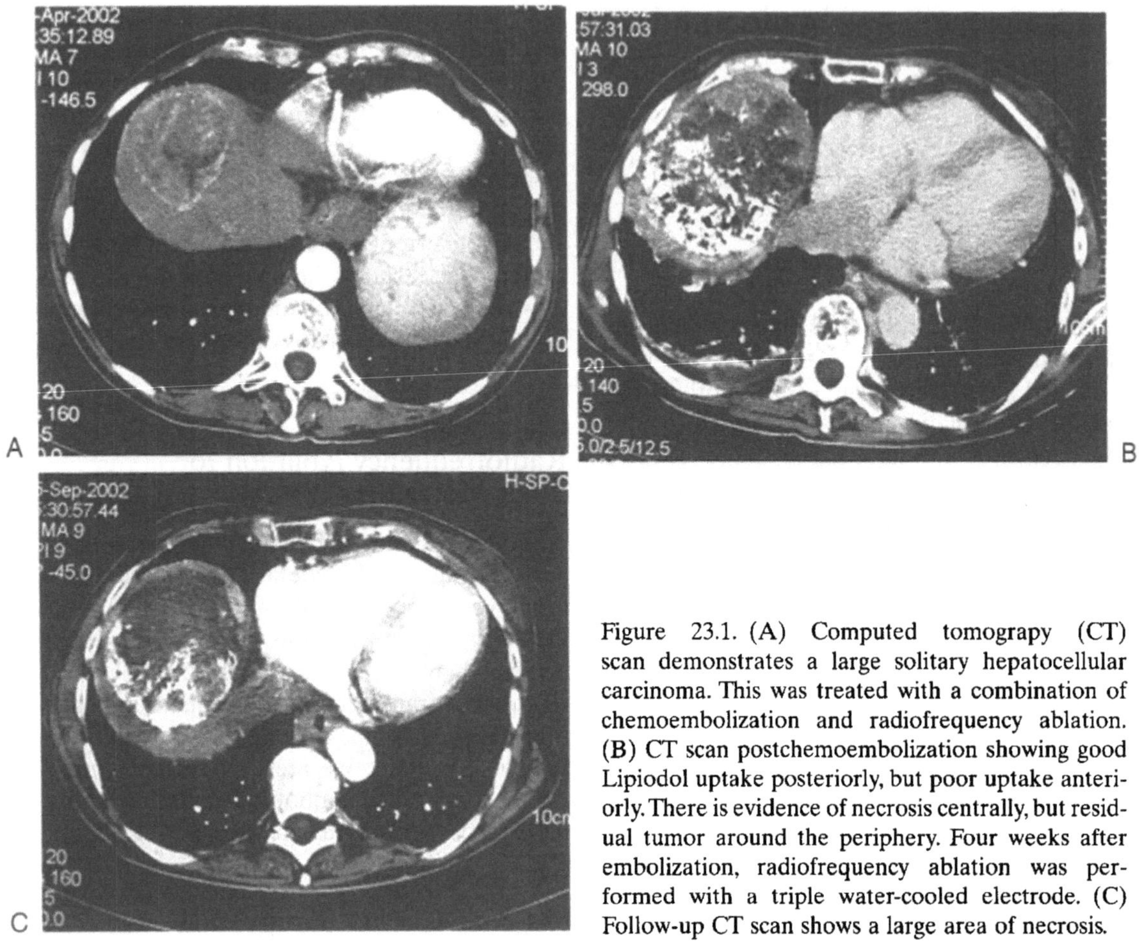

Figure 23.1. (A) Computed tomograpy (CT) scan demonstrates a large solitary hepatocellular carcinoma. This was treated with a combination of chemoembolization and radiofrequency ablation. (B) CT scan postchemoembolization showing good Lipiodol uptake posteriorly, but poor uptake anteriorly. There is evidence of necrosis centrally, but residual tumor around the periphery. Four weeks after embolization, radiofrequency ablation was performed with a triple water-cooled electrode. (C) Follow-up CT scan shows a large area of necrosis.

Radiotherapy/Chemotherapy and Radiofrequency Ablation–Induced Hyperthermia

Radiofrequency ablation requires temperatures in excess of 55°C to produce cell death. Lower temperatures, 42° to 46°C, so-called hyperthermia, result in reversible cell damage, but if used in conjunction with radiotherapy or chemotherapy will produce necrosis. Animal experiments in a rat breast tumor model have demonstrated an improved volume of necrosis when RFA was used in conjunction with chemotherapy (32). In an early clinical study in 10 patients with various liver tumors, a single bolus of IV liposomal doxorubicin 24 hours prior to RFA resulted in good areas of necrosis with extension of the necrotic areas over the ensuing 30 days. The downside of this approach is the inability to predict the final result at the time of treatment. Undoubtedly there will be a role for this type of therapy, but the exact role is still to be defined.

Chemotherapy/Prevention in Hepatocellular Carcinoma

Combination Transcatheter Arterial Chemoembolization /Ablation

Transcatheter arterial chemoembolization (TACE) alone results in complete necrosis in only 38% of lesions <3 cm in diameter (33). It has been combined with percutaneous ethanol injection (PEI) and has been shown to be superior to PEI alone, in reducing both the incidence of local residual disease as well as the number of new foci of HCC that arise in previously normal liver (34). Survival was not affected.

Radiofrequency ablation is effective in treating HCC up to 4.5 cm. However, in the absence of screening programs, many patients present with larger lesions. Chemoembolization has been used in conjunction with thermal ablation, both laser and RF, for large (5–8 cm) HCCs. Different techniques have been implemented, for example, laser ablation followed by TACE after an interval of 30 to 90 days, or RFA with balloon occlusion, followed immediately by selective embolization (35,36). Using laser followed by TACE, Pacella et al (35) reported a 90% rate of complete necrosis in large (mean 5.2 cm) HCCs.

Prevention

Several agents have been explored to attempt to reduce the incidence of HCC in high-risk patients. Immunopreventions, such as interferon and glycyrrhizin, have been used to suppress the development of HCC. Interferon prevents HCC in two groups—in those patients with long-term elimination of the hepatitis C virus (15–35% of patients), and in those with sustained normalization of serum transaminases (an additional 10%). Interferon has been shown to reduce recurrence after surgery (37). Glycyrrhizin, on the other hand, has no antiviral activity, but acts by reducing liver inflammation as indicated by suppressed transaminases (38).

The chemopreventive agent polyprenoic acid an acyclic retinoid, induces the disappearance of serum lectin reactive α-fetoprotein, which suggests a clonal deletion of minute premalignant cells. It has been shown to reduce the incidence of recurrent or new HCC postcurative resection 27% vs. 49% at 38 months (39).

Finally, another technique that had more modest success in reducing the incidence of recurrence postresection was a single dose of intraarterial ^{131}I Lipiodol. This resulted in a recurrence rate of 28.5% vs. 59% at a median follow-up of 34.6 months (40). In the future, a combination of immuno- and chemopreventions will be explored.

Conclusion

While the development of thermal ablation represents an exciting advance in the treatment of liver cancer, it is likely that a combination of different therapeutic modalities will be required for most patients.

References

1. Solbiati L, Livraghi T, Goldberg SN, et al. Percutaneous radiofrequency ablation of hepatic metastases from colorectal cancer: long-term results in 117 patients. Radiology 2001;221:159–166.
2. de Baere T, Elias D, Dromain C, et al. Radiofrequency ablation of 100 hepatic metastases with a mean follow-up of more than 1 year. AJR 2000;175:1619–1625.
3. Livraghi T, Goldberg SN, Lazzaroni S, et al. Hepatocellular carcinoma: radiofrequency ablation of medium and large lesions. Radiology 2000;214:761–768.
4. Gillams AR, Lees WR. Radiofrequency ablation of colorectal metastases in 167 patients. Eur Radiol 2004;14(12):2261–2267.
5. Chopra S, Dodd GD III, Chintapalli KN, et al. Tumor recurrence after radiofrequency thermal ablation of hepatic tumors: spectrum of findings on dual-phase contrast-enhanced CT. AJR 2001; 177:381–387.
6. Izumi N, Asahina Y, Noguchi O, et al. Risk factors for distant recurrence of hepatocellular carcinoma in the liver after complete coagulation by microwave or radiofrequency ablation. Cancer 2001;91:949–956.
7. Gillams AR, Lees WR. Thermal ablation induced changes in hepatic arterial perfusion. Radiology 1999;213P;382.
8. Goldberg S, Hahn P, Halpern E, Fogle R, Gazelle GS. Radiofrequency tissue ablation: effect of pharmacological modulation of blood flow on coagulation diameter. Radiology 1998; 209:761–767.
9. Germer CT, Isbert C, Albrecht D, et al. Laser-induced thermotherapy combined with hepatic arterial embolization in the treatment of liver tumors in a rat tumor model. Ann Surg 1999; 230:55–62.
10. Denys A, de Baere T, Mahe C, et al. Radiofrequency tissue ablation of the liver: effects of vascular occlusion on lesion diameter and biliary

and portal damages in a pig model. Eur Radiol 2001;11:2102–2108.
11. Chinn SB, Lee FT, Kennedy GD, et al. Effect of vascular occlusion on radiofrequency ablation of the liver: results in a porcine model. AJR 2001; 176;789–795.
12. Yamasaki T, Kurokawa F, Shirahashi H, et al. Percutaneous radiofrequency ablation therapy with combined angiography and CT assistance for patients with hepatocellular carcinoma. Cancer 2001;91:1342–1348.
13. Lees WR, Schumillian C, Gillams AR. Hypotensive anesthesia improves the effectiveness of radiofrequency ablation in the liver. Radiology 2000;217:228.
14. Wood TF, Rose DM, Chung M, Allegra DP, Foshag LJ, Bilchik AJ. Radiofrequency ablation of 231 unresectable hepatic tumors: indications, limitations and complications. Ann Surg Oncol 2000;7:593–600.
15. Gruenberger T, Jourdan JL, Zhao J, King J, Morris DL. Reduction in recurrence risk for involved or inadequate margins with edge cryotherapy after liver resection for colorectal metastases. Arch Surg 2001;136:1154–1157.
16. Weber JC, Navarra G, Jiao LR, Nicholls JP, Jensen SL, Habib I. New technique for liver resection using heat coagulation necrosis. Ann Surg 2002;236(5):560–563.
17. Montorsi M, Santambrogio R, Bianchi P, et al. Radiofrequency interstitial thermal ablation of hepatocellular carcinoma in liver cirrhosis: role of the laparoscopic approach. Surg Endosc 2001; 15:141–145.
18. Scott DJ, Fleming JB, Watumull LM, et al. Accuracy and effectiveness of laparoscopic vs. open hepatic RF ablation. Surg Endosc 2001;15: 135–140.
19. Miao Y, Ni Y, Yu J, Marchal G. A comparative study on validation of a novel cooled-wet electrode for radiofrequency liver ablation. Invest Radiol 2000;35:438–444.
20. Goldberg SN, Ahmed M, Gazelle GS, et al. Radio-frequency thermal ablation with NaCl solution injection: effect of electrical conductivity on tissue heating and coagulation-phantom and porcine liver study. Radiology 2001;219: 157–165.
21. Livraghi T, Goldberg N, Monti F, et al. Saline enhanced radiofrequency tissue ablation in the treatment of liver metastases. Radiology 1997; 202:205–210.
22. Douillard JY, V303 Study Group. Irinotecan and high dose fluorouracil/leucovorin for metastatic colorectal cancer. Oncology 2000;14:51–55.
23. Giacchetti S, Perpoint B, Zidani R, et al. Phase III multicenter trial of oxaliplatin added to chronomodulated fluorouracil-leucovorin as first line treatment of metastatic colorectal cancer. J Clin Oncol 2000;18:136–147.
24. Bismuth H, Adam R, Levi F, et al. Resection of nonresectable liver metastases from colorectal cancer after neoadjuvant chemotherapy. Ann Surg 1996;224:509–522.
25. Shankar A, Leonard P, Renaut AJ, et al. Neoadjuvant therapy improves resectability rates for colorectal cancer. Ann R Coll Surg Engl 2001;83: 85–88.
26. Gillams A, Lees W. Should thermal ablation be offered to patients with colorectal liver metastases downstaged by chemotherapy? Radiology 2000;217(P):539.
27. Preketes A, Caplehorn J, King J, et al. Effect of hepatic artery chemotherapy on survival of patients with hepatic metastases from colorectal carcinoma treated with cryotherapy. World J Surg 1995;19:768–771.
28. Kainuma O, Asano T, Aoyama H, et al. Combined therapy with radiofrequency thermal ablation and intra-arterial infusion chemotherapy for hepatic metastases from colorectal cancer. Hepatogastroenterology 1999;46:1071–1077.
29. Tellez C, Benson A, Lyster M, et al. Phase II trial of chemoembolization for the treatment of metastatic colorectal carcinoma to the liver and review of the literature. Cancer 1998;82:1250–1259.
30. Livraghi T, Goldberg N, Solbiati L, et al. Percutaneous radiofrequency ablation of liver metastases from breast cancer: initial experience in 24 patients. Radiology 2001;220:145–149.
31. Chung MH, Pisegna J, Spirt M, et al. Hepatic cytoreduction followed by a novel long-acting somatostatin analogue: a paradigm for intractable neuroendocrine tumors metastatic to the liver. Surgery 2001;130:954–964.
32. Goldberg SN, Saldinger P, Gazelle GS, et al. Percutaneous tumor ablation: increased necrosis with combined radiofrequency ablation and intratumoral doxorubicin in a rat breast tumor model. Radiology 2001;220:420–427.
33. Higuchi T, Kikuchi M, Okazaki M. Hepatocellular carcinoma after transcatheter hepatic arterial embolization. A histopathological study of 84 resected cases. Cancer 1994;72:2259–2267.
34. Koda M, Murawaki Y, Mitsuda A, et al. Combination therapy with transcatheter arterial chemoembolization and percutaneous ethanol injection compared with percutaneous

ethanol injection alone for patients with small hepatocellular carcinoma. Cancer 2001;92:1516–1524.

35. Pacella CM, Bizzarri G, Cecconi O, et al. Hepatocellular carcinoma: long-term results of combined treatment with laser thermal ablation and transcatheter arterial chemoembolization. Radiology 2001;219:669–678.
36. Lencioni R, Cioni D, Donati F, Bartolozzi C. Combination of interventional therapies in hepatocellular carcinoma. Hepatogastroenterology 2001;48:8–14.
37. Ikeda K, Arase Y, Saitoh S, et al. Interferon beta prevents recurrence of hepatocellular carcinoma after complete resection or ablation of the primary tumor. Hepatology 2000;32:228–232.
38. Okuno M, Kojima S, Moriwaki H. Chemoprevention of hepatocellular carcinoma: concept progress and perspectives. J Gastroenterol Hepatol 2001;16:1329–1355.
39. Muto Y, Moriwaki H, Ninomiya M, et al. Prevention of second primary tumors by an acyclic retinoid, polyprenoic acid in patients with HCC. N Engl J Med 1996;334:1561–1567.
40. Lau WY, Leung TWT, Ho S, et al. Adjuvant intra-arterial iodine-131 labelled lipiodol for resectable hepatocellular carcinoma: a prospective randomized trial. Lancet 1999;353:797–801.

Section V
Organ System Tumor Ablation

24
Ablation of Liver Metastases

Luigi Solbiati, Tiziana Ierace, Massimo Tonolini, and Luca Cova

Metastatic liver disease represents one of the most common clinical problems in oncology practice. Multiple treatment options are available including hepatic resection, chemoembolization, intraarterial and systemic chemotherapy, cryotherapy, and radiofrequency ablation (RFA) (1,2).

Over the past few years, advances in diagnostic imaging modalities such as contrast-enhanced ultrasound, single- and multidetector helical computed tomography (CT) and magnetic resonance imaging (MRI) with hepatobiliary and reticuloendothelial-specific contrast agents have achieved early detection and accurate quantification of hepatic metastatic involvement (3–10). As a result, correct selection of patients for different treatment options is usually possible.

When feasible, surgical resection of hepatic metastases is the accepted standard therapeutic approach in patients with colorectal cancer. Surgery also offers potential for cure in selected patients with other primary tumors (2,11–28).

Percutaneous radiofrequency thermal ablation is an established therapeutic option for liver metastases, which may obviate the need for a major surgery and result in prolonged survival and chance for cure. Extensive operators' experience and technical advances provide larger coagulation volumes and therefore allow safe and effective treatment of medium- and even large-size metastases. Results of RFA in terms of global and disease-free survival currently approach those reported for surgical metastasectomy. Furthermore, in published series this technique demonstrated significant advantages including (a) feasibility of treatment in previously resected patients and nonsurgical candidates due to extent of metastatic involvement, age, and comorbidity; (b) repeatability of treatment when incomplete and when local recurrence or development of metachronous lesions occur; (c) combination with systemic or regional chemotherapy; (d) minimal invasiveness with limited complications rate and preservation of liver function; (e) limited hospital stays and procedure costs (29–42).

Pathology of Metastatic Liver Disease

After regional lymph nodes, the liver is the organ most commonly involved with metastatic disease, usually from primary cancers of the gastrointestinal tract, breast, and lung. The presence of a dual blood supply (from the arterial system and the portal/splanchnic venous system) and the discontinuous endothelium of the hepatic sinusoids (allowing communication with the extracellular space) account for the high incidence of metastatic spread to the liver.

Morphologic features of liver metastases as well as their localization and number may be extremely variable on gross pathology. Histopathology explains the lack of the peculiar "oven effect" observed and understood during experience with RFA of hepatocellular carcinoma (HCC). During treatment of HCC, the tumor capsule and the surrounding fibrotic, poorly vascularized cirrhotic parenchyma prevent thermal conduction outside the treated lesion; therefore, optimal heat diffusion is maintained in the softer, usually well-circumscribed tumoral nodule (34). Liver metastases are not encapsulated and tend to infiltrate the surrounding well-vascularized liver tissue that limits tumor heating (32,33).

Analysis of surgical series demonstrated that after resection of liver metastases, local recurrence is frequent if a surgical margin of 1 cm of normal hepatic tissue surrounding the tumor is not removed (15). Similarly, RFA of liver metastases should aim to ablate a 0.5- to 1.0-cm-thick "safety margin" of peritumoral liver tissue to kill infiltrating tumor undetectable by currently available imaging modalities, thus reducing the risk of recurrence (30).

Therefore, adequate RFA treatment of liver metastases often requires the creation of large volumes of coagulation necrosis. Recent technical innovations including internally cooled electrodes (43), cluster electrodes (44), pulsed RF energy application (45), and peritumoral saline injection prior to or during energy deposition (46) enable better energy deposition and increase coagulation necrosis volumes, thus allowing extended indications for RFA.

More recently, further improvements in induced coagulation have been achieved. These include decreasing blood flow during ablation using balloon occlusion of a hepatic vein or segmental portal branch (47), by adopting strategies of precise overlapping of subsequent electrode placements (48), or by adjuvant IV injection of doxorubicin in liposome carriers before the procedure (49).

Patient Selection and Indications for Treatment

In the early phase of our experience with RFA, treatment was performed in patients with new metastases or local recurrences after previous hepatic resection and in patients refusing or not eligible for surgery for technical or general health reasons. Currently, increasing awareness by referring oncologists of the reported results and of the minimal invasiveness of RFA make this technique a valid therapeutic option for local treatment of patients with limited metastatic liver disease.

Radiofrequency ablation is applicable to patients with one to five metachronous liver metastases up to 3.5 to 4 cm in largest diameter from previous radically treated colorectal or other primary cancer, in whom surgery is not feasible, contraindicated, or not accepted. Some patients with large lesions or more than five nodules may undergo RFA after successful tumor debulking by means of chemotherapy (Table 24.1).

We consider the presence of active extrahepatic disease a contraindication to RF treatment, with the exception of bone or lung metastases in breast cancer patients if they are responding or unchanged with systemic chemotherapy (30). Exclusion criteria include the presence of severe coagulopathy, renal failure, or jaundice. Informed consent of the

Table 24.1. Indications for radiofrequency (RF) ablation treatment of patients with liver metastases.

Primary tumor (most frequently colorectal or breast cancer) previously treated radically with surgery, radiotherapy, and without adjuvant chemotherapy
No evidence of active extrahepatic disease: possible exception for breast cancer metastases in the lung or bone showing regression or stability over time on hormonal or chemotherapy
Liver metastasis (cyto/histologically confirmed, compatible with primary tumor)
Residual tumor after previous treatment with RF ablation or other treatment
Local recurrence after surgical resection, RF ablation, or other treatment
Metachronous new metastasis after previous resection, RF ablation, or other treatment
Up to 4 to 5 lesions, each 4 cm or less in maximum diameter; lesions over 4 cm may be treated after debulking by systemic or regional chemotherapy
Metastases visible with B-mode and/or contrast-enhanced ultrasound
Feasible and safe percutaneous access (not abutting the hepatic hilum, the gallbladder, or the colon)
Adequate coagulation, hepatic and renal function
Informed consent obtained

patient is obtained after explanation of the procedure, the expected results, and the possible complications.

Accurate assessment of the extent of metastatic liver disease is crucial to optimal patient selection. Intraoperative ultrasound (IOUS) is still considered the "gold standard" for detection of focal liver lesions. At our institution, candidates for RFA of hepatic metastases undergo pretreatment diagnostic workup that includes laboratory tests, tumor markers, conventional and contrast-enhanced liver ultrasound, and single- or multidetector helical CT examinations. Tumor staging usually is completed by thoracic CT and radionuclide bone scan to exclude distant tumor dissemination.

Whereas ultrasound is the most commonly used imaging modality in screening for metastatic spread, the sensitivity of unenhanced (B-mode) ultrasound is significantly affected by the operator's experience as well as the patient's body habitus and presence of bowel gas distention. Sonography is further limited in enlarged, grossly hyperechoic livers due to steatosis, fibrosis, chronic liver disease, and postchemotherapeutic changes. The detection of isoechoic and subcentimeter lesions is particularly difficult: in our personal experience a 20% sensitivity rate is not surprising. Contrast-specific ultrasound software with the use of first-generation (in the late liver-specific phase) or second-generation contrast agents facilitates an increase in detection rate, particularly for small lesions, as well as better characterization of focal lesions (5–9). Precise staging of hepatic neoplastic disease may require the use of a contrast-enhanced ultrasound (CEUS) examination to overcome limitations of conventional B-mode ultrasound and to maximize detection of metastatic lesions, possibly modifying the therapeutic approach (8).

Multiphase contrast-enhanced helical CT currently constitutes the mainstay of hepatic imaging, providing overall staging of liver disease and accurate assessment of resectability. Sensitivity of CT was estimated at 85% in surgically controlled series, and missed lesions average 0.7 mm in diameter (3,4). In some institutions hepatic staging is obtained by means of dynamic gadolinium-enhanced MRI; the use of reticuloendothelial and liver-specific MR contrast agents may allow even higher sensitivity rates (3).

Procedure

In our department RFA treatment sessions are carried out in a dedicated operating room under general anesthesia using endotracheal intubation and mechanical ventilation. Some other centers adopt conscious sedation.

A 200-W, 480-kHz RF generator system (Radionics, Burlington, MA) with an automated pulsed-RF algorithm is used together with single or cluster internally cooled electrodes. Usually percutaneous RFA is performed under contrast-enhanced ultrasound guidance. In some patients CT guidance is preferred when sonographic targeting is not possible, with significantly increased procedure time. The choice of the electrodes is based on the size of the target nodule: for lesions smaller than 2 cm, a single insertion of a 3-cm exposed tip single electrode is sufficient. Lesions 2 to 3 cm in size can be treated with a single insertion of a cluster electrode or with multiple insertions of a 3-cm exposed tip electrode. Lesions exceeding 3 cm can be treated only with one to two insertions of a cluster electrode and one to two single electrode insertions.

The applied energy is variable, and usually reaches 1600 to 1800 mA for single electrodes and 1800 to 2000 mA for cluster electrodes. Each application of energy lasts 12 minutes, and total procedure time ranges from 12 to 15 minutes for small solitary lesions to 45 to 60 minutes for large or multiple ablations.

B-mode and color/power Doppler ultrasound are not reliable to assess the size and completeness of induced coagulation necrosis at the end of the energy application; furthermore, additional repositioning of the electrode is usually made difficult by the hyperechogenic "cloud" that appears around the distal probe. Therefore, we routinely use contrast-enhanced ultrasound performed at the presumed end of the treatment, with the patient still under anesthesia, to enable rapid assessment of the extent of achieved tumor ablation and to discover viable tumor that requires additional immediate treatment (50).

Patients receive antibiotic prophylaxis with ceftriaxone 2 gr prior to the treatment and also antiemetic and analgesic drugs as needed post-procedurally. Hospitalization lasts for 48 hours after the treatment; discharge follows documentation of necrosis and exclusion of complications by means of 24-hour contrast-enhanced CT scan.

In our experience, patients usually experience mild to moderate pain in the right abdomen that lasts for 2 to 5 days and is particularly severe in patients with subcapsular lesions. Pericapsular and subcapsular injection of long-acting anesthetic drug (ropivacaine) is performed at the end of the treatment to reduce postprocedure pain. Fever may be present for the first 2 to 3 days after treatment and recedes with antipyretic drugs (acetaminophen). No impairment in liver function tests has been observed. Morbidity encountered in a large series of patients treated with RFA is discussed in the chapter on complications.

Initial cross-sectional examinations serve to assess completeness of treatment and provide a basis for imaging follow-up. However, given the

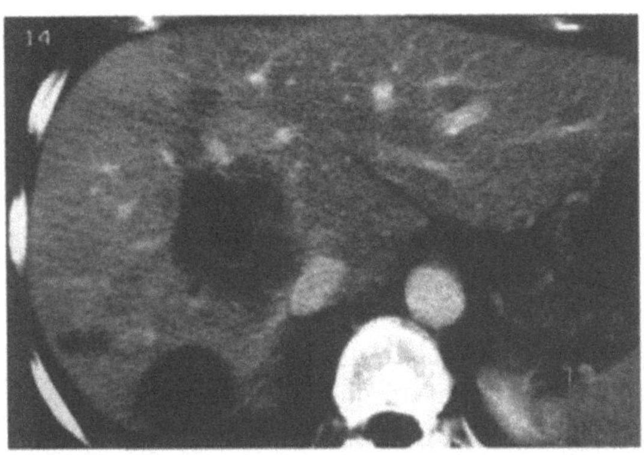

FIGURE 24.1. Contrast-enhanced helical computed tomography (CT) scan of patient underwent radiofrequency (RF) ablation of two metastases at segments VII and VIII from colorectal adenocarcinoma, 9 months before. The area of thermal coagulation at segment VII is well demarcated and does not show signs of local recurrence. Oppositely, along the medial margin of the area of coagulation at segment VIII, a slightly hypodense oval area due to recurrence is visualized. Furthermore, new tiny metastases at segments VII, VIII, and II are demonstrated.

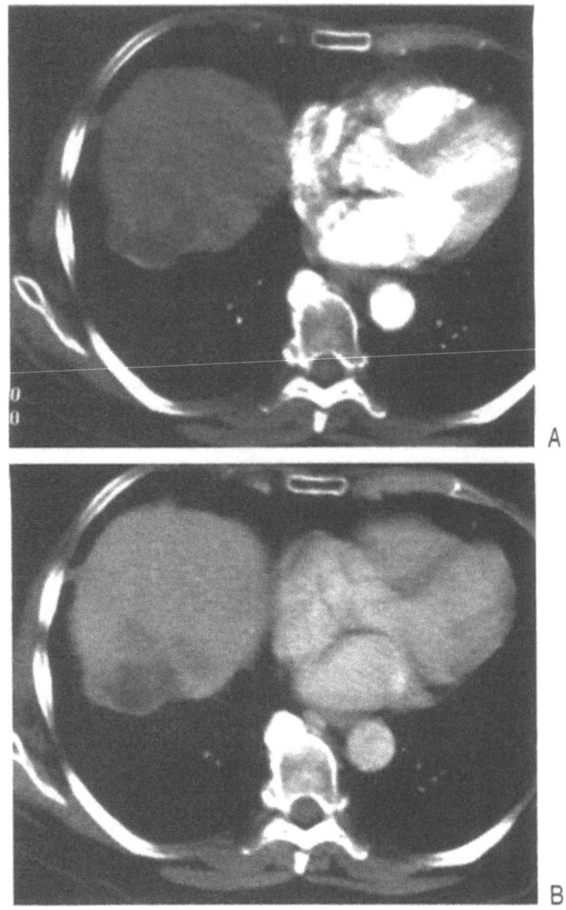

FIGURE 24.2. A 71-year-old patient with history of solitary colorectal metastasis at segment VII, treated with RFA 4 years before. (A) Biphasic CT scan shows thick, mildly hypodense peripheral rim located anteriorly to the coagulation area. (B) Local RFA retreatment has been subsequently performed.

resolution and accuracy of current imaging techniques, residual microscopic foci of malignancy at the periphery of a treated lesion may sometimes go undetected and give rise to local recurrence.

Contrast-enhanced helical CT and MRI are used in the long-term assessment of therapeutic response, allowing confident discrimination between ablated and residual viable tumor (Figs. 24.1 and 24.2). Cross-sectional imaging studies obtained at 3 to 4 months intervals are correlated with serum carcinoembryonic antigen (CEA) levels to detect local or distant recurrences. Imaging findings on follow-up examinations with patterns of complete necrosis and of local recurrences are discussed elsewhere in this book.

In our experience, CEUS has proved valuable in the follow-up setting for the detection or confirmation of local recurrences and new metastases and for contrast-guided re-treatment (48).

Fluorodeoxyglucose (FDG)-labeled positron emission tomography (PET) offers great potential in the evaluation of treatment response and is synergistic, and is perhaps superior to cross-sectional imaging modalities in the surveillance of treated patients. Areas of abnormal FDG uptake following ablative procedures have been reported to represent disease relapse or residual viable tumor with a high degree of sensitivity (50,51).

Combination Therapy

The decision to administer simultaneous chemotherapy is determined by the referring oncologist based on the patient's risk of recurrence, as in patients with poorly differentiated or node-positive primary tumors. Thanks to its minimal invasiveness RFA may be used as a first-choice local therapy instead of surgery. Use of RFA does not prevent the simultaneous or subsequent use of other, potentially synergistic, treatments.

Hormonal therapy, systemic chemotherapy, and intraarterial infusional chemotherapy each can be given prior to or after RFA, according to oncologists' preferences and practice guidelines. If recurrence or development of new lesions is detected, additional RF treatment sessions may be performed when technically feasible after a consensus decision between the radiologist, the oncologist, and the patient.

Results: Colorectal Cancer Metastases

The liver is the first, most common, and often unique site of metastasis of colorectal cancer. Approximately 50% of patients with colorectal cancer develop recurrent disease that involves the liver during the course of their diseases.

Surgical resection is a potentially curative treatment for colorectal liver metastases, but metastatic liver involvement is often multifocal, so that only 20% to 25% of patients have resectable disease. Moreover, surgery may be excluded due to older age and associated pathologic conditions that increase anesthesiologic risk, and is associated with prolonged hospital stays, significant perioperative morbidity, and a 2% to 8% mortality rate.

Survival rates for resected patients range from 25–28% to 35–40% at 5 years in most series, but many successfully resected patients develop recurrence in the liver and/or extrahepatic sites, and repeat resection can be performed in only a minority of them (11–20). Prognostic factors include stage of primary tumor, biologic factors (CEA level, differentiation, ploidy), number of hepatic lesions, size of dominant lesion, and infiltration of resection margins.

Regional therapies such as RFA can be offered to patients with limited but unresectable liver metastases and no extrahepatic disease, whereas chemoembolization and hepatic intraarterial chemotherapy are applicable to patients with extensive liver involvement not suitable for ablation (12,18). Radiofrequency ablation increases the possibilities of curative treatment in patients with liver recurrence after hepatectomy from 17% to 26%, and is preferred over repeat surgery because it is less invasive (52).

Several published series report promising results with RFA of liver metastases; however, these early reports had only short-term follow-up and included patients with both primary and metastatic liver tumors (37–41).

At our institution 166 patients have been treated with RFA during a 7-year span; 12% had previous surgery for liver neoplastic involvement, and repeat resection was considered unfeasible or too invasive. One to five metastases (mean 2.28) were ablated in each patient for a total of 378 treated lesions; 64.5% of the treated lesions were 3 cm or less in size, and 35.5% were larger than 3 cm.

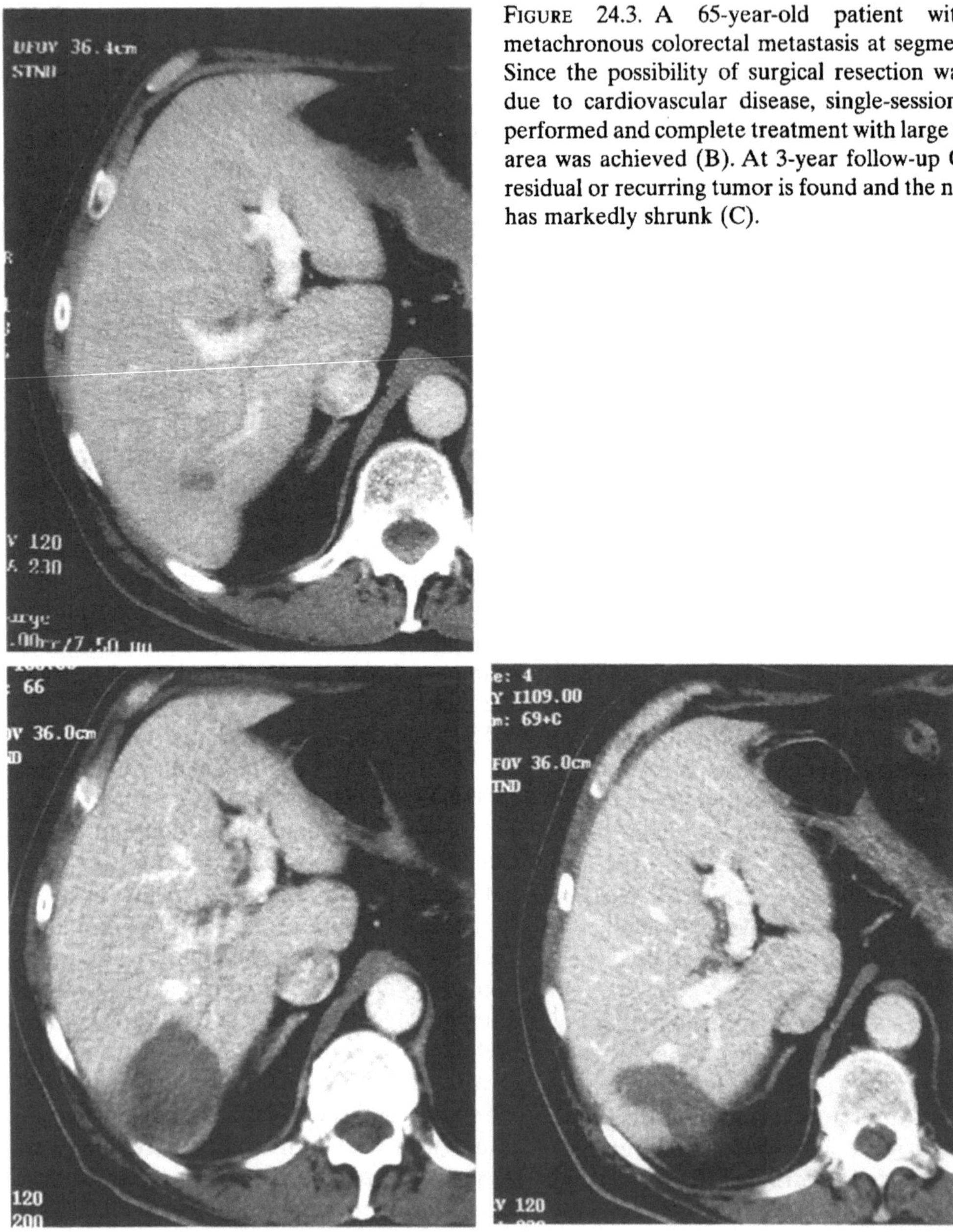

FIGURE 24.3. A 65-year-old patient with solitary metachronous colorectal metastasis at segment VII (A). Since the possibility of surgical resection was excluded due to cardiovascular disease, single-session RFA was performed and complete treatment with large coagulation area was achieved (B). At 3-year follow-up CT scan, no residual or recurring tumor is found and the necrotic area has markedly shrunk (C).

In our series, local tumor control was achieved in 71.4% of lesions (Figs. 24.3 and 24.4), whereas local recurrence occurred in the remaining 28.6% (see Figs. 24.1 and 24.2). In the largest published analysis of treated patients with colorectal cancer liver metastases with follow-up of more than 3 years, including our group, local recurrence was observed overall in 39.1% of lesions. The incidence of recurrence was significantly related to the original size of the treated metastasis: effective local tumor control was achieved in 78% of tumors up to 2.5 cm, 47% of tumors >2.5 to 4 cm, and 32% of tumors larger than 4 cm (36). In another series reported by De Baere and coworkers (42), the percutaneous approach allowed local

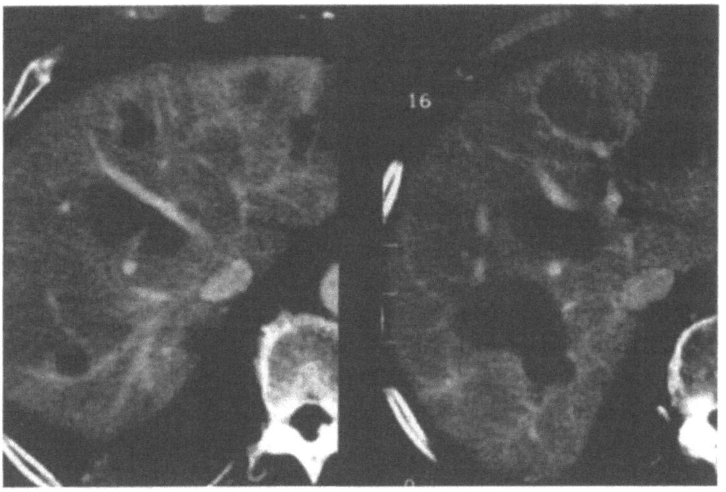

FIGURE 24.4. A 4-year follow-up CT scan of patient with history of sigmoid adenocarcinoma and many metachronous liver metastases, subsequently developing during the follow-up period. Each metastasis was treated with cool-tip RFA. No evidence of residual or recurrent disease is currently apparent.

control of 90% of treated lesions after 1 year of follow-up, but the mean diameter was significantly smaller than in our series. The time of recurrence was related to lesion size: local relapse occurred almost always during the first 12 months (36). In our patients the median time to local recurrence was 6 months. Repeated RFA treatment was carried out in 37.6% of metastases with progressive local tumor growth. Including repeat treatments, one to four sessions were performed in each patient, for a total of 197 sessions (mean 1.18).

Distant, metachronous metastases developed at follow-up in 36% of our patients. The estimated median time until detection of new metastases was 10 months in our patients, 12 months in the published analysis, and not significantly related to the original number of treated lesions (36).

In our series, Kaplan-Meier survival analysis included overall survival rates at 1, 2, 3, 4, and 5 years of 96.2%, 64.2%, 45.7%, 36.9%, and 22.1%, respectively; estimated median survival was 33 months (Fig. 24.5). The issue of disease-free survival has been evaluated in the cooperative group and rates were calculated as 49% and 35% at 1 year and 2 years; interestingly, time to death was not related to the number of metastases or to the size of the dominant metastasis (36).

Recently, the "test of time" approach has been proposed by surgeons to delay resection of liver metastases to allow additional, still undetected lesions to develop and become identifiable. This limits the number of resections carried out in patients who will ultimately develop more metastases. The use of RFA in this setting can decrease the number of resections required by obtaining complete tumor control in some patients without major surgery. At the same time, RFA is better accepted by patients than a simple "wait and see" approach and allows an interval for those who are destined to develop aggressive, disseminated disease. In a recent analysis metastasectomy was spared in 98% of patients with complete ablation with radiofrequency including 43% of

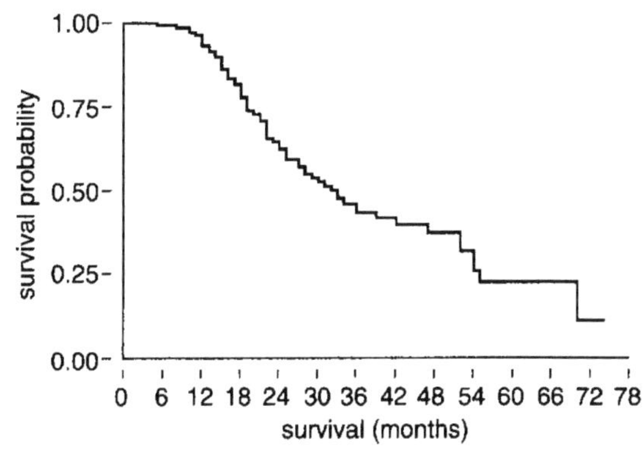

FIGURE 24.5. The 5-year survival curve of patients treated with RFA for colorectal metastases.

those in whom prior incomplete tumor control was now achieved by RFA (53).

Breast Cancer Metastases

Whereas the vast majority of RFA treatments address liver metastases from colorectal primaries, a significant subset of secondary hepatic tumors occurs in patients with breast cancer (30). Breast cancer, histologically usually ductal adenocarcinoma, is the most frequent neoplasm in women and often metastatizes to the liver.

Metastatic breast cancer traditionally has been considered the expression of systemic disease that requires chemotherapy; however, liver-only metastatic disease occurs in 5% to 12% of breast cancer patients and they may be eligible for surgical metastasectomy. Early reports demostrated improved survival (18–24% at 5 years' follow-up) in patients undergoing resection of limited hepatic metastases from breast cancer (21–23). More recent reports yielded even superior survival rates with 51% with disease-free interval with stage of primary as prognostic factor (24).

Therefore, surgery may allow long-lasting benefit and be potentially curative; patients with hepatic resection as the first and sole site of relapse have a threefold greater median survival than patients treated with standard nonsurgical treatment.

With this background, we used percutaneous RFA to achieve local control of liver metastases in patients with breast cancer (30). Twenty-four patents were treated for 64 liver metastases: complete necrosis was obtained with a single treatment session in 92% of lesions. Interestingly, the rate of complete necrosis was superior to that obtained with colorectal metastases of comparable size (96% for lesions less than 3 cm and 75% for 3- to 5-cm lesions). These figures suggest that occult invasion of surrounding liver tissue may be absent or less pronounced in breast tumors (30).

Over half of the patients (58%) developed new metastases during follow-up, but 63% of 16 patients with liver-only metastatic breast cancer were disease-free 4 to 44 months after the treatment. Considering the natural history of the disease and its minimal invasiveness, RFA is an effective local therapeutic alternative to surgical resection of liver metastases in patients with breast cancer. Furthermore, RFA may be extremely useful for tumor recurrences after hepatectomy, since in over half of these patients the liver is the only involved site of relapse. Combination treatment with hormonal therapy or systemic or intraarterial infusion chemotherapy usually is required.

Metastases from Other Primary Tumors

Radiofrequency ablation has been performed in several patients with cancer histologies different from colorectal and breast carcinoma. In our experience RFA represents a useful treatment in patients with metastases from previously treated malignancies provided that local control of liver disease may be beneficial from the oncologic perspective in terms of improved survival or quality of life, and that size, number, and location allow adequately wide necrosis. In our institution patients with liver metastases from neuroendocrine, gastric, pancreatic, renal, pulmonary, uterine, and ovarian cancer and from melanoma have been treated successfully with RFA.

Under these conditions RFA has to be considered a less invasive therapeutic alternative to surgery. Indications for RFA of liver metastases from other primary cancers may follow those of surgical resection. Hepatectomy for liver metastases appears favorable in patients with gynecologic, gastric, and testicular primary tumors, with survival rates over 20%; unfortunately, no definite selection criteria have been reported in the literature (22,26,27).

Particular consideration is reserved for patients with neuroendocrine tumors, which commonly metastasize to the liver. In cases with metastatic disease, combinations of surgical debulking and medical treatment usually are used. In patients with limited metastases, surgery is considered a treatment option. Liver metastasectomy from endocrine primary tumors is followed by long survival in a substantial proportion of patients with 56% to 74% 5-year survival rates (22,25–27). Interesting results have been reported with RFA, used alone or in combination with surgery, for local control of metastases from neuroendocrine tumors: disease eradication was obtained in 28.5% of patients treated with curative intent (29).

References

1. Bhattacharya R, Rao S, Kowdley KV. Liver involvement in patients with solid tumors of nonhepatic origin. Clin Liver Dis 2002;6:1033–1043.
2. Nordlinger B, Rougier P. Nonsurgical methods for liver metastases including cryotherapy, radiofrequency ablation and infusional treatment: what's new in 2001? Curr Opin Oncol 2002;14:420–423.
3. Sica GT, Ji H, Ros PR. CT and MR imaging of hepatic metastases. AJR 2000;174:691–698.
4. Valls C, Andia E, Sanchez A, et al. Hepatic metastases from colorectal cancer: preoperative detection and assessment of resectability with helical CT. Radiology 2001;218:55–60.
5. Harvey CJ, Blomley MJK, Eckersley RJ, et al. Hepatic malignancies: improved detection with pulse-inversion US in the late phase of enhancement with SHU 508A—early experience. Radiology 2000;216:903–908.
6. Albrecht T, Hoffmann CW, Schmitz SA, et al. Phase-inversion sonography during the liver specific late phase of contrast enhancement: improved detection of liver metastases. AJR 2001;176:1191–1198.
7. Quaia E, Bertolotto M, Forgacs B, et al. Detection of liver metastases by pulse inversion harmonic imaging during Levovist late phase: comparison with conventional ultrasound and helical CT in 160 patients. Eur Radiol 2003;13:475–483.
8. Solbiati L, Tonolini M, Cova L, et al. The role of contrast-enhanced ultrasound in the detection of focal liver lesions. Eur Radiol 2001;11:E15–E26.
9. Albrecht T, Blomley MJ, Burns PN, et al. Improved detection of hepatic metastases with pulse-inversion US during the liver-specific phase of SHU 508A: multicenter study. Radiology 2003;227:361–370.
10. Semelka RC, Helmberger TC. Contrast agents for MR imaging of the liver. Radiology 2001;218:27–38.
11. Geoghegan JG, Scheele J. Treatment of colorectal liver metastases. Br J Surg 1999;86:158–169.
12. Yoon SS, Tanabe KK. Surgical treatment and other regional treatments for colorectal cancer liver metastases. Oncologist 1999;4:197–208.
13. Taylor M, Forster J, Langer B, et al. A study of prognostic factors for hepatic resection for colorectal metastases. Am J Surg 1997;173:467–471.
14. Nordlinger B, Guigner M, Vaillant JC, et al. Surgical resection of colorectal carcinoma metastases to the liver. A prognostic scoring system to improve case selection based on 1568 patients, Association Francaise de Chirurgie. Cancer 1996;77:1254–1262.
15. Elias D, Cavalcanti A, Sabourin JC, et al. Resection of liver metastases from colorectal cancer: the real impact of the surgical margin. Eur J Surg Oncol 1998;24:174–179.
16. Cady B, Jenkins RL, Steelde GD, et al. Surgical margin in hepatic resection for colorectal metastasis: a critical and improvable determinant of outcome. Am Surg 1998;227:566–571.
17. Holm A, Bradley E, Aldrete JS. Hepatic resection of metastases from colorectal carcinoma. Morbidity, mortality and patterns of recurrence. Ann Surg 1989;209:428–434.
18. Fong Y, Salo J. Surgical therapy of hepatic colorectal metastasis. Semin Oncol 1999;26:514–523.
19. Liu LX, Zhang WH, Jiang HC. Current treatment for liver metastases from colorectal cancer. World J Gastroenterol 2003;9:193–200.
20. Hugh TJ, Kinsella AR, Poston GJ. Management strategies for colorectal liver metastases—part I. Surg Oncol 1997;6:19–30.
21. Elias D, Lasser PH, Montrucolli D, Bonvallo S, Spielmann M. Hepatectomy for liver metastases from breast cancer. Eur J Surg Oncol 1995;21:510–513.
22. Elias D, Cavalcanti A, Eggenspieler P, et al. Resection of liver metastases from a noncolorectal primary: indications and results based on 147 monocentric patients. J Am Coll Surg 1998;187:487–493.
23. Raab R, Nussbaum KT, Behrend M, et al. Liver metastases of breast cancer: results of liver resection. Anticancer Res 1998;18:2231–2234.
24. Maksan SM, Lehnert T, Bastert G, et al. Curative liver resection for metastatic breast cancer. Eur J Surg Oncol 2000;26:209–212.

25. Chen H, Hardacre JM, Uzar A, et al. Isolated liver metastases from neuroendocrine tumors: does resection prolong survival? J Am Coll Surg 1998;187:88–93.
26. Berney T, Mentha G, Roth AD, et al. Results of surgical resection of liver metastases from non-colorectal primaries. Br J Surg 1998;85:1423–1427.
27. Lindell G, Ohlsson B, Saarela A, et al. Liver resection of noncolorectal secondaries. J Surg Oncol 1998;69:66–70.
28. Maksan SM, Lehnert T, Bastert G, Herfarth C. Curative liver resection for metastatic breast cancer. Eur J Oncol 2000;26:209–212.
29. Hellman P, Ladjevardi S, Skogseid B, et al. Radiofrequency tissue ablation using cool tip for liver metastases of neuroendocrine tumors. World J Surg 2002;26:1052–1056.
30. Livraghi T, Goldberg SN, Solbiati L, et al. Percutaneous radiofrequency ablation of liver metastases from breast cancer: initial experience in 24 patients. Radiology 2001;220:145–149.
31. Goldberg SN, Gazelle GS, Mueller PR. Thermal ablation therapy for focal malignancy. A unified approach to underlying principles, techniques, and diagnostic imaging guidance. AJR 2000;174: 323–331.
32. Solbiati L, Goldberg SN, Ierace T, et al. Hepatic metastases: percutaneous radio-frequency ablation with cooled-tip electrodes. Radiology 1997; 205:367–373.
33. Solbiati L, Ierace T, Goldberg SN, et al. Percutaneous US-guided radiofrequency tissue ablation of liver metastases: treatment and follow-up in 16 patients. Radiology 1997;202:195–203.
34. Livraghi T, Goldberg SN, Lazzaroni S, et al. Small hepatocellular carcinoma: treatment with radiofrequency ablation versus ethanol injection. Radiology 1999;210:655–661.
35. Livraghi T, Goldberg SN, Lazzaroni S, et al. Hepatocellular carcinoma: radio-frequency ablation of medium and large lesions. Radiology 2000; 214:761–768.
36. Solbiati L, Livraghi T, Goldberg SN, et al. Percutaneous radiofrequency ablation of hepatic metastases from colorectal cancer: long-term results in 117 patients. Radiology 2001;221: 159–166.
37. Curley SA, Izzo F, Delrio P, et al. Radiofrequency ablation of unresectable primary and metastatic hepatic malignancies: results in 123 patients. Ann Surg 1999;230:1–8.
38. Jiao LR, Hansen PD, Havlik R, et al. Clinical short-term results of radiofrequency ablation in primary and secondary liver tumors. Am J Surg 1999;177:303–306.
39. Lencioni R, Goletti O, Armillotta N, et al. Radiofrequency thermal ablation of liver metastasis with cooled-tip electrode needle: results of a pilot clinical trial. Eur Radiol 1998;8:1205–1211.
40. Rose DM, Allegra DP, Bostick PJ, et al. Radiofrequency ablation: a novel primary and adjunctive ablative technique for hepatic malignancies. Am Surg 1999;65:1009–1014.
41. Rossi S, Buscarini E, Garbagnati F, et al. Percutaneous treatment of small hepatic tumors by an expandable RF needle electrode. AJR 1998; 170:1015–1022.
42. De Baere T, Elias D, Dromain C, et al. Radiofrequency ablation of 100 hepatic metastases with a mean follow-up of more than 1 year. AJR 2000; 175(6):1619–1625.
43. Goldberg SN, Gazelle GS, Solbiati L, et al. Radiofrequency tissue ablation: increased lesion diameter with a perfusion electrode. Acad Radiol 1996;3:636–644.
44. Goldberg SN, Solbiati L, Hahn PF, et al. Large-volume tissue ablation with radiofrequency by using a clustered, internally cooled electrode technique: laboratory and clinical experience in liver metastases. Radiology 1998;209:371–379.
45. Goldberg SN, Stein MC, Gazelle GS, et al. Percutaneous radiofrequency tissue ablation: optimization of pulsed-radiofrequency technique to increase coagulation necrosis. J Vasc Interv Radiol 1999;10:907–916.
46. Livraghi T, Goldberg SN, Monti F, et al. Saline-enhanced radiofrequency tissue ablation in the treatment of liver metastases. Radiology 1997; 202:205–210.
47. De Baere T, Bessoud B, Dromain C, et al. Percutaneous radiofrequency ablation of hepatic tumors during temporary venous occlusion. AJR 2002;178:53–59.
48. Rhim H, Goldberg SN, Dodd GD III, et al. Essential techniques for successful radiofrequency thermal ablation of malignant hepatic tumors. Radiographics 2001;21(spec. no.):S17–35.
49. Goldberg SN, Kamel IR, Kruskal JB, et al. Radiofrequency ablation of hepatic tumors: increased tumor destruction with adjuvant liposomal doxorubicin therapy. AJR 2002;179:93–101.
50. Akhurst T, Larson SM. Positron emission tomography imaging of colorectal cancer. Semin Oncol 1999:26(5):577–583.
51. Anderson GS, Brinkmann F, Soulen MC, et al. FDG positron emission tomography in the sur-

veillance of hepatic tumors treated with radiofrequency ablation. Clin Nucl Med 2003;28:192–197.

52. Elias D, De Baere T, Smayra T, et al. Percutaneous radiofrequency thermoablation as an alternative to surgery for treatment of liver tumour recurrence after hepatectomy. Br J Surg 2002;89:752–756.

53. Livraghi T, Solbiati L, Meloni F, et al. Percutaneous radiofrequency ablation of liver metastases in potential candidates for resection: the "test of time" approach. Cancer 2003;97:3027–3035.

25 Ablation for Hepatocellular Carcinoma

Maria Franca Meloni and Tito Livraghi

Hepatocellular carcinoma (HCC) is the fifth most common cancer in the world, and it represents more than 5% of all cancers (1). It usually coexists with underlying chronic liver disease, and according to the stage, one disease will prevail over the other. The stage of HCC at the time of diagnosis is very important to decide the type of treatment—possibly curative when the diagnosis is early, palliative or no treatment when the diagnosis is late.

In countries in which ultrasound (US) screening of the population at risk is practiced, early diagnosis of HCC is possible. Elsewhere, the diagnosis is not made until the disease is already advanced. Because HCC is an organ pathology, the first nodule detected is only a prelude to others; thus HCC needs multistep detection and treatment.

The survival studies of untreated patients with HCC that usually are taken as points of reference fall into four conventional and gross groups: (1) the disease is at an early stage (single HCC <5 cm, or up to three lesions <3 cm) and therefore likely to be amenable to cure; (2) the disease is considered intermediate, that is, without an invasive tumor pattern (absence of portal thrombosis or extrahepatic spread), and asymptomatic; (3) the disease is advanced (between intermediate and terminal stage); and (4) terminal (PST stage 3 or 4 or Okuda stage III). A similar staging has been used for practical purposes in many centers, but was only recently codified by the Liver Unit of Barcelona (2).

The range of treatment options is fairly wide, and the choice is not always easy, given the number of variables to be assessed. The options today are surgery (liver transplantation and partial resection); percutaneous ablation techniques (ethanol injection, thermal ablation); intraarterial techniques including transarterial embolization and transarterial chemoembolization (TAE-TACE); radiation; and systemic therapies. Most of them have not been validated with randomized controlled studies, that is, versus the natural history or versus other therapies, but are applied only on the basis of local control of the tumor.

The only therapy likely to afford a definitive cure in selected patients is liver transplantation (LT). However, the shortage of donors, high costs, advanced technology, and ethical reasons limit this option. Surgical resection can achieve complete ablation of the first nodule (also of peripheral satellites if anatomic resection is carried out). According to the Japanese Nationwide Survey in 2001, re-resection is performed for only 1.6% of new lesions (3).

In the majority of studies, the survival rates after surgery were roughly comparable with those obtained with percutaneous ethanol injection therapy (PEIT) (4,5). A more recent trial also documented similar results (6). In this latter study, 97 comparable patients with HCC <3 cm in diameter and three or fewer in number were treated, 39 with PEI and 58 with surgical resection, respectively, during the same period. Their 3- and 5-year survival was 82% and 59% in the PEIT group, and 84% and 61% in the surgery group. These results probably reflect a balance between the advantages and disadvantages of the two therapies. Moreover, the results of surgery have been hampered by an incorrect selection of patients, with some undergoing resection, even though they have adverse prognostic factors. PEIT survival curves are always better than those of resected patients who present with adverse prognostic factors.

Another confirmation of such an interpretation comes from the report of the Liver Cancer Study Group of Japan. Three- and 5-year survival in Child's class A patients with a single HCC <5 cm was 67% and 49% respectively, in the previous report of 1982–89 when PEIT was not available. Survival was 77% and 59% in the report of 1988–95 (75% and 46% with PEIT) because of better patient selection (perioperative mortality remained substantially unchanged) and the probable shift to PEIT of some patients who, before the advent of PEIT, would have been treated surgically (7).

After the introduction of other percutaneous techniques, mainly radiofrequency ablation (RFA), a question that remains is the choice between PEIT and RFA. We consider these techniques complementary as well as selective TACE. We use them according to the features of the disease, most notably number, location of tumor(s), presence of satellites, portal thrombosis, and response to prior treatment. This approach means a tailored strategy for every patient, that is, a multistep multimodality image-guided local treatment. For instance, multifocal HCC can be treated with only one, all, or a combination of the techniques. Most lesions are treated with RFA, since RFA obtains both a higher rate of necrosis than PEIT and a higher rate of necrosis and fewer side effects than TACE (8,9). But PEIT is preferable in tumors at risk for RFA, such as those adjacent to main biliary ducts because of the possibility of stricture, and those juxtaposed to gastrointestinal structures because of the possibility of perforation (10,11), or for treating segmental portal thrombosis. Selective TACE is used for lesions not recognizable at ultrasound, in lesions not completely necrosed and not re-treatable by RFA or PEIT, and in the presence of peripheral satellites after complete necrosis of the dominant lesion.

Rationale for Percutaneous Interventional Procedures in HCC

The following are reasons for use of percutaneous interventional procedures for tumor ablation:

1. They do not have the disadvantage of loss of or damage to nonneoplastic hepatic parenchyma. The underlying chronic hepatic disease, generally of viral origin, accompanies the neoplastic disease in its different stages. Percutaneous therapies should not worsen liver function.

2. They are low-risk procedures. In published series, the mortality rates are extremely low: 0.09% in the largest study of PEIT (12), ranging between 0.3% and 0.5% in the largest studies of RFA (11,13), and no mortality due to selected TAE (14,15).

3. They can be easily repeated when new lesions appear, as occurs in most patients within 5 years. Hepatocellular carcinoma is considered an organ disease, since it has been proven to be multicentric over time. A recent study demonstrated that multicentricity is already present in 50% of early stages, and that 93% of resected patients with a single small HCC developed other lesions within 5 years (16). Since new lesions reflect the natural history of the disease, the patient should be followed frequently so that the new lesions can be treated as they are detected. An advantage is that the patient can be followed by the same physician in the diagnostic as well as therapeutic phase.

4. The low cost and easy availability of the necessary material (particularly as regards PEIT) and the simplicity of these techniques make it possible to perform them even in peripheral centers. Patients with small HCCs generally are treated as outpatients, and most patients quickly return to normal daily life. In Italy, the cost of one PEIT cycle is about $1000, partial resection about $30,000, and liver transplantation about $125,000 (17). In Japan, an

average cost is $759 for outpatient PEIT, and $27,105 for resection (18). Since every year the number of patients who develop the disease is about 25,000 in Japan and 10,000 in Italy, the problem of cost is an essential consideration (17). The cost of RF generators ranges from $12,000 to $30,000. Nonreusable needle electrodes cost $500 to $1000. The cost of TACE is about $1000 per session (19).

Percutaneous Interventional Procedures

Percutaneous interventional techniques can be performed using an approach directly through the liver parenchyma or through the hepatic artery. Interstitial local ablation therapies are those treatment modalities that allow the introduction of a damaging agent directly into the neoplastic tissue. Local ablation therapies may be based on destroying the tissue chemically, such as with ethyl alcohol (PEIT) or acetic acid, or physically, as with laser, radiofrequency (RF), or microwave. The range of indications for local ablation treatments is becoming wider than for surgery or intraarterial therapies.

Percutaneous Ethanol Injection

Local-regional therapies may be based on destroying the tissue chemically, such as with ethyl alcohol (PEIT). It was the first percutaneous treatment to be used (20). For some years, only patients with up to three small (<5 cm) lesions were treated, and this guideline still applies at many centers. With the introduction of the "single-session" procedures under general anesthesia (21), even patients with lesions greater in number or larger in size are now treated. Percutaneous ethanol injection therapy spreads rapidly, thanks to its ease of execution, safety, low cost, repeatability, and therapeutic efficacy. Survival rates are comparable to those of surgical resection (4,18,22). Today PEIT is one of the treatments most frequently offered to patients detected by US screening to have HCC.

Other Injectable Therapies

Honda et al (23) treated 20 patients with 23 lesions less than 3 cm in diameter with hot saline solution therapy. No complications occurred. Therapeutic efficacy was evaluated with CT, histopathologic examination, and serum marker levels.

Ohnishi et al (24) treated 91 patients with small HCCs using percutaneous injection of acetic acid (from 15% to 50% concentration) under US guidance. No major complications were reported. No evidence of local recurrence was found 6.5 years later. Survival at 1, 2, 3, 4, and 5 years was 95%, 87%, 80%, 63%, and 49%, respectively. The disease-free survival at 1, 2, 3, 4, and 5 years was 83%, 54%, 50%, 37%, and 29%. A second study reported from the same group, using percutaneously injected 50% acetic acid in 25 patients with HCC, demonstrated shrinkage of all lesions (25). No viable tumor was found at follow-up by biopsy, CT, or surgical wedge resection (two cases).

A comparison among PEIT, acetic acid, and hot saline injection has not been reported.

Radiofrequency Ablation (RFA)

Thermoablation with RFA exploits the conversion of energy of an electromagnetic wave into heat. The most widely used instruments are made by three companies: Radiotherapeutics, Sunnyvale, CA; RITA Medical Systems, Mountain View, CA; and Radionics, Burlington, MA (26,27). Each of the devices uses a different needle design, wattage, and algorithms. The first two use an expandable electrode that is 1.9 mm in diameter, which, once positioned in the tumor, opens out into seven to 10 retractable curved electrodes around the target, like an umbrella. These systems produce a reproducible area of necrosis about 3 to 4 cm in diameter. To increase the necrotic area with the aforementioned techniques, interruption of the arterial supply to the tumor by means of occlusion of the hepatic artery with a balloon catheter or the feeding arteries with gelatin sponge particles can be performed (28).

The third device utilizes a cold perfusion electrode with a diameter of 1.2 mm, and an exposed tip of 2 to 3 cm (29). By avoiding early increments of impedance linked to carbonization, these electrodes permit application of a greater power than conventional electrodes. To obtain cooling, a physiologic solution brought to 2° to 5°C is circulated within two coaxial lumens that are situated in the electrode. The technique produces a reproducible area of necrosis of 2.4 cm in diameter. A recently constructed electrode with three cooled tips that permits a higher current deposition yields greater than 4.5 cm diameter of coagulation necrosis (30).

Unexpectedly, it has been observed that in HCCs of about 3 cm in diameter, the area and shape of the necrosis reproduced that of the original tumor like a mold. Such an effect was designated the "oven effect". It was believed that the surrounding cirrhotic tissue with its high fibrotic component and poor vascularization was a poor conductor and thus functioned as an insulating material. These factors resulted in higher deposition of energy within the neoplastic tissue (8).

Studies have been published on the treatment of HCC with RFA on local therapeutic efficacy. The first was carried out using a hooked expandable electrode on 23 patients with HCC up to 3.5 cm in diameter. With an average of 1.4 sessions, a complete response was reported in all tumors and no complications were observed (31). The second study was controlled and prospective; it compared PEIT and RFA on 86 patients with 112 HCCs that measured up to 3 cm in diameter. A complete response was achieved in 90.3% with RFA and in 80.0% with PEIT. These results were obtained with an average of 1.2 sessions for RFA and 4.8 sessions for PEIT. However, there were more complications with RFA, that is, one severe (hemothorax that required drainage) and four minor, compared to none with PEIT (8). The third study was prospective, and it compared PEIT and RFA on 119 patients with a single HCC that measured up to 3 cm in diameter. Complete tumor necrosis was achieved in 100% of the RFA group, and in 94% of the PEIT group, with the same local recurrence rate. But RFA required an average of only 1.5 sessions, whereas PEIT required an average of 4.0 sessions (32).

Benefiting from the "oven effect," a fourth study, on the treatment of larger HCCs, was performed (33). In 114 patients with 80 medium-diameter (3.0–5.0 cm) or 40 large HCCs (5.1–9.0 cm diameter), complete necrosis was attained in 60 lesions (47.6%) and nearly complete necrosis (90–99%) in 40 other lesions (31.7%). Medium and non-infiltrating tumors were treated successfully (71%) more often than large and infiltrating tumors (23%). Two major complications (death from septic shock due to peritonitis in an obese patient with diabetes and hemorrhage that required laparotomy) and five minor complications were observed (11). The results of the study supported the importance of the "oven effect". However, the oven effect also may explain the limited success in treating satellite nodules that remain a limitation for RFA or PEIT ablation, despite continued technical improvements. Probably, the fibrotic tissue that is interposed between the main tumor and the satellites limits heat diffusion. A longer follow-up is needed to determine the prognostic improvement that results from treatment of the main tumor alone. However, in some cases, when the location of satellites is favorable, RFA can obtain satisfying results.

Microwave

Microwave therapy was devised by a Japanese team in 1986 (34). It is the next thermal therapy used for interstitial percutaneous ablation. The equipment consists of a microwave generator and an 18-gauge reusable needle electrode that is 25 cm long. The electrode is placed through a 14-gauge styleted access needle. The microwave needle functions as an antenna for externally applied energy at 1000 to 2450 MHz (35).

Saitsu et al (36) published the first report on intraoperative microwave coagulation treatment in 21 patients with HCCs less than 5 cm in diameter. Recurrence of disease occurred in 23.8% of the lesions. Twenty patients survived to a maximum of 39 months. Several studies with good clinical results from treatment of liver tumors with microwave have been published (37–41). The results of 60 patients with

69 small HCCs treated by microwave and studied by dynamic CT demonstrated a complete response in 72%, and incomplete necrosis or tumor recurrence in 28%. The mean disease-free period was 24.2 months. The survival rates at 1 and 2 years were 83.1% and 68.7%, respectively. Major complications were ascites in three patients, pleural effusion in two, intraperitoneal abscess in one, and seeding in two (38,39).

Interstitial Laser Photocoagulation

Interstitial laser photocoagulation is another thermotherapy that induces coagulation necrosis in tumor cells (42). The first studies on liver tumors (hepatoma and metastases) with laser therapy were reported by Hashimoto et al (43) and Steger et al (44).

Laser therapy is performed with US- or CT-guided imaging, using conscious sedation and local lidocaine anesthesia. Laser fibers are inserted through a cannula and attached to a neodymium:yttrium-aluminum-garnet (Nd:YAG) laser, which is excited at 2 to 4W for 5 to 15 minutes.

Several reports have been published on the use of laser coagulation to treat liver tumors (45–50). Lees and Gillams's group (19) reported on patients with inoperable colorectal metastases to the liver. They had a 5-year survival rate of 26%, and a median survival of 27 months; these results were comparable to patients who had been operated and had a median survival of 33 months and a 5-year survival rate of 30%. In 500 patients, major complications have included segmental infarction in five patients, abscesses in three patients, pleural effusion in one patient, tumor seeding in six patients, pain, and one death from a spontaneous hepatic infarction that occurred 6 days after treatment. A recent study in 74 patients with 92 small HCCs demonstrated complete ablation in 97% of lesions, with local recurrence rates (1–5 years) from 1.6% to 6%. One-, 3-, and 5-year survival rates were 99%, 68%, and 15%, respectively. No major complications occurred (50). Interstitial laser photocoagulation is a safe therapy for small HCCs.

Cryoablation

Cryoablation is the oldest interstitial thermotherapy to treat liver tumors (51). It uses intraoperative cooled probes that measure 3mm in diameter to freeze and destroy large areas of tumor tissue (52). This technique has recently became adapted for percutaneous use (53).

Selective Transarterial Chemoembolization

For many years, TAE or TACE of the whole liver was the most widely used therapeutic option for patients with intermediate HCC. The rationale for this approach is that in contrast with normal liver tissue, HCCs receive almost the totality of their blood supply through the hepatic artery. Transarterial embolization and TACE have marked antitumoral effect, although only in encapsulated lesions. However, recent randomized controlled trials did not show any statistically significant difference in survival between treated and untreated patients (54–56). Treated patients have slower tumor progression and even a decrease in the incidence of portal vein invasion; however, cancer-related complications or liver decompensation was no different compared to untreated patients. This is probably due to a counterbalance between local tumor control and damage to nonneoplastic tissue, which hastens liver insufficiency, even though a study particularly dedicated to this problem failed to demonstrate such an interconnection (57).

In a study by the Liver Unit of Barcelona, 2- and 4-year survival was 49% and 13% after TAE, and 50% and 27% after no treatment (56). A more recent randomized controlled trial (58) demonstrated improved survival in stringently selected patients with intermediate-stage HCC: 3-year survival was 29% in the treated group and 0% in the untreated group. Thus, the current trend is to use TAE or TACE with lobar disease by selective catherization because it does not cause deterioration of liver function, compared to the whole-liver technique, and with a better tumor response being achieved (59). A recent meta-analysis study demonstrated that chemoembolization improves survival of patients with unresectable HCC, and may become a standard treatment (60).

Evaluation of Therapeutic Efficacy

To evaluate therapeutic response means to determine whether a tumor has become completely necrotic or whether areas of neoplastic tissue remain. Measures to assess response include a combination of investigations and serum assays for tumor markers. These metrics are the same as those used during initial staging. We prefer to use spiral CT with triphasic technique (4–5 mL/sec; 20, 60, and 300 seconds after the injection of contrast medium), and US with first- and second-generation ultrasound contrast agents (USCAs) (Levovist, Shering, Berlin, Germany; SonoVue, Bracco, Milan, Italy). A recent study demonstrated that the sensitivity of pulse inversion harmonic ultrasound imaging (83.3%) with Levovist was significantly greater ($p < .05$) for detecting residual nonablated tumor after radiofrequency treatment compared to conventional contrast-enhanced power Doppler sonography (61). Solbiati et al (62) reported that the routine use of contrast-enhanced harmonic US (SonoVue) reduces costs by decreasing the number of percutaneous ablations and follow-up examinations.

Other imaging examinations (MRI, PET) or biopsy are performed only in cases of doubt about partial or complete response. If the areas of viable tissue are very small, beyond the present powers of imaging resolution, they will obviously not be recognizable. Some authors find it difficult to recognize viable tissue from coagulation necrosis when the target is small, and consequently there is uncertainty about retreatment (63). However, residual tumor will be more easily identified during follow-up imaging examinations as zones of increased enhancement at CT or of increased growth of enhanced tumor. The response is considered complete on imaging when CT scans show total disappearance of contrast enhancement within the neoplastic tissue, or when the same picture is confirmed with ultrasound contrast media examination, and on scans performed on successive follow-up visits. The absence of contrast media enhancement means the absence of blood flow due to necrosis and fibrotic effects. Even with such characteristics, after the treatment, necrotic tumor occupies space and remains visible in place of the tumor, but reduces in size over time. Ultrasound with contrast agents can be useful, but should not be used as the only test to establish the result, because it is less sensitive than CT in detecting vascularity of small residual tumor areas (61).

Different degrees of Lipiodol uptake after TAE-TACE are a good indicator of therapeutic efficacy, and its labeling can be checked during follow-up by CT scans (64). Re tumor markers, we use α-fetoprotein (AFP) and des-gamma-carboxy-prothrombin (DCP), which often are complementary. Nevertheless, their assay is useful only if levels initially are high. When imaging techniques show a complete response that is not corroborated by reduction in AFP or DCP levels, it means that neoplastic tissue is not detected or is growing elsewhere outside the liver. Moreover, an increase in levels during follow-up always suggests a local recurrence or the appearance of new lesions. Follow-up with ultrasound alone, or with contrast agents, with CT, and serum assay of tumor markers is done a month after treatment and then every 4 to 6 months.

Multistep Modality Image-Guided Local Treatment: Why and When

The large number of patients enrolled in US screening programs has created a demand for effective, safe, repeatable, and economical treatment that can be made available in many centers. In the absence of randomized trials, it is and will be difficult to find agreement on indications of the respective therapeutic options. In our opinion, the only course at this time is to extrapolate from retrospective comparative studies and from reports on prognostic factors the unequivocal information that can prevent useless or even damaging therapies. Moreover, economic resources and the expertise that is available at each center are other factors that have a role in the choice of treatment.

In our opinion, multistep modality image guidance of local treatment is indicated as the treatment of choice for most patients who are followed by ultrasound screening, excluding those candidates for partial resection, and who have (1) favorable factors: Child's A class, (2) transaminases <3× normal values, (3) younger than 75 years, (4) no portal hypertension, (5) normal bilirubin, (6) no portal thrombosis, (7) single lesion (also with peripheral satellites), (8) feasibility of anatomic operation, and (9) skilled operators assuring perioperative mortality of less than 2%. However, we prefer to perform RFA in single HCCs <2 cm, since the possibility of peritumoral microinvasion is low, and the rate of complete ablation approaches 100%. Furthermore, in these cases, the management of patients following the rationale of the "test of time" (based on survival benefit from hepatic resection) is determined by the biologic features of the tumor, rather than by early detection. Resection could be performed in patients whose tumors are incompletely treated with the multimodality approach, and who do not develop additional tumors during follow-up.

Conclusions

The tailored combination of RFA, PEIT, and selective TACE is indicated as the treatment of choice for most patients enrolled by US screening, excluding those candidates for liver transplantation and for partial surgical resection. Unfortunately, transplantation is available for few patients in Western countries because of the shortage of donors, in poorer countries because of the lack of advanced technology, and in Japan because of ethical reasons. Candidates for partial resection should not have adverse prognostic factors (7,65,66).

It is still controversial whether a complex resection is an appropriate choice for a patient who does not have adverse prognostic factors and a tumor less than 2 cm in diameter, when the possibility of peritumoral microinvasion is low, and the comparative rate of complete ablation with percutaneous ablation techniques is probably 100%.

The best strategy to follow might be early detection of HCCs by means of US surveillance in an at-risk population, treatment with percutaneous interventional techniques, follow-up with imaging methods and tumor markers, and further treatment of any new lesions.

References

1. Parkin DM, Bray F, Ferlay J, Pisani P. Estimating the world cancer burden: GLOBOCAN 2000. Int J Cancer 2001;94:153–156.
2. Llovet JM, Bru C, Bruix J. Prognosis of hepatocellular carcinoma: the BCLC staging classification. Semin Liver Dis 1999;19:329–339.
3. Arii S, Teramoto K, Kawamura T, et al. Characteristics of recurrent hepatocellular carcinoma in Japan and our surgical experience. J Hepatobiliary Pancreat Surg 2001;8:397–403.
4. Livraghi T, Bolondi L, Buscarini L, et al. No treatment, resection and ethanol injection in hepatocellular carcinoma: a retrospective analysis of survival in 391 patients with cirrhosis. J Hepatol 1995;22:522–526.
5. Ryu M, Shimamura Y, Kinoshita T, et al. Jpn J Clin Oncol 1997;27:251–257.
6. Yamamoto J, Okada S, Shimada K, et al. Treatment strategy for small hepatocellular carcinoma: comparison of long-term results after percutaneous ethanol injection therapy and surgical resection. Hepatology 2001;34:707–713.
7. The Liver Cancer Study Group of Japan. Predictive factors for long-term prognosis after partial hepatectomy for patients with hepatocellular carcinoma in Japan. Cancer 1994;74:2772–2780.
8. Livraghi T, Goldberg N, Lazzaroni S, Meloni F, Solbiati L, Gazelle S. Small hepatocellular carcinoma: treatment with radio-frequency ablation versus ethanol injection. Radiology 1999;210:655–661.
9. Livraghi T, Meloni F, Corso R, Rampoldi A. Comparison between RF ablation and TACE in the treatment of multifocal hepatocellular carcinoma: preliminary experience. Radiology 2000;217:287–288.
10. Meloni MF, Goldberg SN, Moser V, Piazza G, Livraghi T. Colonic perforation and abscess fol-

lowing radiofrequency ablation treatment of hepatoma. Eur J Ultrasound 2002;15(1–2):73–76.
11. Livraghi T, Solbiati L, Meloni F, Gazelle GS, Halpern EF, Goldberg SN. Percutaneous radiofrequency ablation: complications encountered in a multicenter study of the treatment of focal liver tumors. Radiology 2003;226:441–451.
12. Di Stasi M, Buscarini L, Livraghi T, et al. Percutaneous ethanol injection in the treatment of hepatocellular carcinoma: a multicenter survey of evaluation practice and complication rates. Scand J Gastroenterol 1997;32:1168–1173.
13. Mulier S, Mulier P, Ni Y, et al. Complications of radiofrequency coagulation of liver tumors. Br J Surg 2002;89:1206–1222.
14. Matsui O, Kadoja M, Yoshikawa J, Gabata T, Takashima T, Demachi H. Small hepatocellular carcinoma: treatment with subsegmental arterial embolization. Radiology 1993;188;78–93.
15. Uchida H, Matsuo N, Nishimine K, Nishimine Y, Sakaguchi H, Ohishi H. Transcatheter arterial embolization for hepatoma with lipiodol. Hepatic arterial and segmental use. Semin Intervent Radiol 1993:10:19–26.
16. Nakashima O, Kojiro M. Recurrence of hepatocellular carcinoma: multicentric occurrence or intrahepatic metastasis? A viewpoint in terms of pathology. J Hepatobiliary Pancreat Surg 2001; 8:404–409.
17. Livraghi T, Giorgio A, Marin G, et al. Hepatocellular carcinoma and cirrhosis in 746 patients: long-term results of percutaneous ethanol injection. Radiology 1995;197:101–108.
18. Kotoh K, Sakai H, Sakamoto S, et al. The effect of percutaneous ethanol injection therapy on small solitary hepatocellular carcinoma is comparable to that of hepatectomy. Am J Gastroenterol 1994;89:194–198.
19. Dodd GD III, Soulen MC, Kane RA, et al. Minimally invasive treatment of malignant hepatic tumors: the threshold of a major breakthrough. Radiographics 2000;20(1):9–27.
20. Livraghi T, Festi D, Monti F, Salmi A, Vettori C. US-guided percutaneous alcohol injection of small hepatic and abdominal tumors. Radiology 1986;161:309–312.
21. Livraghi T, Vettori C, Torzilli G, Lazzaroni S, Pellicano S, Ravasi S. Percutaneous ethanol injection of hepatic tumors: single session therapy under general anesthesia. AJR 1993;160: 1065–1069.
22. Onodera H, Ukai K, Nakano N, et al. Outcomes of 116 patients with hepatocellular carcinoma. Cancer Chemother Pharmacol 1994;33:103–108.
23. Honda N, Guo Q, Uchida H, Ohishi H, Hiasa Y. Percutaneous hot saline injection therapy for hepatic tumors: an alternative to percutaneous ethanol injection therapy. Radiology 1994;190(1): 53–57.
24. Ohnishi K, Ohyama N, Ito S, Fujiwara K. Small hepatocellular carcinoma: treatment with US-guided intratumoral injection of acetic acid. Radiology 1994;193(3):747–752.
25. Ohnishi K, Normura F, Ito S, Fujiwara K. Prognosis of small hepatocellular carcinoma (less than 3 cm) after percutaneous acetic acid injection: study of 91 cases. Hepatology 1996;23(5): 994–1002.
26. Gazelle GS, Goldberg SN, Solbiati L, Livraghi T. Tumor ablation with radiofrequency energy. Radiology 2000;217:633–646.
27. McGahan JP, Dodd GD III. Radiofrequency ablation of the liver: current status. AJR 2001; 176:3–16.
28. Rossi S, Garbagnati F, Lencioni R, et al. Percutaneous radiofrequency ablation of nonresectable hepatocellular carcinoma after occlusion of tumor blood supply. Radiology 2000;217:119–126.
29. Goldberg SN, Gazelle GS, Solbiati L, Rittman WJ, Müeller PR. Radiofrequency tissue ablation: increased lesion diameter with a perfusion electrode. Acta Radiol 1996;3:636–644.
30. Goldberg SN, Solbiati L, Hahn PF, et al. Large volume tissue ablation with radiofrequency by using a clustered, internally cooled electrode technique: laboratory and clinical experience in liver metastases. Radiology 1998;209:371–379.
31. Rossi S, Buscarini E, Garbagnati F. Percutaneous treatment of small hepatic tumors by an expandable RF needle electrode. AJR 1998;170:1015–1022.
32. Ikeda M, Okada S, Ueno H, Okusaka T, Kurijama H. Radiofrequency ablation and percutaneous ethanol injection with small hepatocellular carcinoma: a comparative study. Jpn J Clin Oncol 2001;31:322–326.
33. Livraghi T, Goldberg SN, Lazzaroni S, et al. Hepatocellular carcinoma: radiofrequency ablation of medium and large lesions. Radiology 2000;214:761–768.
34. Tabuse Y, Tabuse K, Mori K, et al. Percutaneous microwave tissue coagulation in liver biopsy: experimental and clinical studies. Nippon Geka Hokan 1986;55:381–392.
35. King RWP, Shen LC, Wu TT. Embedded insulated antenna for communication and heating. Electromagnetics 1981;1:51–172.

36. Saitsu H, Mada Y, Taniwaki S, et al. Investigation of microwave coagulo-necrotic therapy for 21 patients with small hepatocellular carcinoma less than 5 cm in diameter. Nippon Geka Gakkai Zasshi 1993;94(4):359–365.
37. Seki T, Wakabayashi M, Nakagawa T, et al. Ultrasonically guided percutaneous microwave coagulation therapy for small hepatocellular carcinoma. Cancer 1994;74(3):817–825.
38. Murakami R, Yoshimatsu S, Yamashita Y, Matsukawa T, Takahashi M, Sagara K. Treatment of hepatocellular carcinoma: value of percutaneous microwave coagulation. AJR 1995;164:1159–1164.
39. Matsukawa T, Yamashita Y, Arakawa A, et al. Percutaneous microwave coagulation therapy in liver tumors: a 3-year experience. Acta Radiol 1997;38:410–415.
40. Yamanaka N, Tanaka T, Oriyama T, Furukawa K, Tanaka W, Okamoto E. Microwave coagulonecrotic therapy for hepatocellular carcinoma. World J Surg 1996;20:1076–1081.
41. Dong BW, Liang P, Yu XL, et al. Sonographically guided microwave coagulation treatment of liver cancer: an experimental and clinical study. AJR 1998;171:449–454.
42. Amin Z, Brown SG, Lees WR. Liver tumor ablation by interstitial laser photocoagulation: review of experimental and clinical studies. Semin Intervent Radiol 1993;10:88–100.
43. Hashimoto D, Takami M, Idezuki Y. In depth radiation therapy by YAG laser for malignant tumors in the liver under ultrasonic imaging. Gastroenterology 1985;88:1663.
44. Steger AC, Lees WR, Walmsley K, Brown SG. Interstitial laser hyperthermia: a new approach to local destruction of tumours. BMJ 1989; 299:362–365.
45. Nolsoe CP, Torp-Pedersen S, Burcharth F, et al. Interstitial laser hyperthermia of colorectal liver metastases with a US-guided Nd-YAG laser with a diffuser tip: a pilot clinical study. Radiology 1993;187:333–337.
46. Vogl TJ, Muller PK, Hammerstingl R, et al. Malignant liver tumors treated with MR imaging-guided laser-induced thermotherapy: technique and prospective results. Radiology 1995;196:256–257.
47. Amin Z, Bown SG, Lees WR. Local treatment of colorectal metastases: a comparison of interstitial laser photocoagulation (ILP) and percutaneous alcohol injection (PAI). Clin Radiol 1993; 48:166–177.
48. Pacella CM, Bizzarri G, Ferrari FS, et al. Interstitial photocoagulation with laser in the treatment of liver metastases. Radiol Med 1996; 92:438–447.
49. Vogl TJ, Mack MG, Roggan A, et al. Internally cooled power laser for MR-guided interstitial laser-induced thermotherapy of liver lesions: initial clinical results. Radiology 1998;209: 381–385.
50. Pacella CM, Bizzarri G, Magnolfi F, et al. Laser thermal ablation in the treatment of small hepatocellular carcinoma: results in 74 patients. Radiology 2001;221(3):712–720.
51. Cooper IS. Cryogenic surgery: a new method of destruction or extirpation of benign or malignant tissues. N Engl J Med 1963;268:743–749.
52. Kane RA. Ultrasound-guided hepatic cryosurgery for tumor ablation. Semin Intervent Radiol 1993;10:132–142.
53. Mala T, Edwin B, Tillung T, Kristian Hol P, Soreide O, Gladhaung I. Percutaneous cryoablation of colorectal liver metastases: potentiated by two consecutive freeze-thaw cycles Cryobiology 2003;46(1):99–102.
54. Group d'Etude et de Traitment de Carcinome Hepatocellulaire. A comparison of lipiodol chemoembolization and conservative treatment for unresectable hepatocellular carcinoma. N Engl J Med 1995;332;1256–1261.
55. Pelletier G, Ducreux M, Gay F. Treatment of unresectable hepatocellular carcinoma with lipiodol chemoembolization: a multicenter randomized trial. J Hepatol 1998;29:129–134.
56. Bruix J, Llovet JM, Castells A, et al. Transarterial embolization versus symptomatic treatment in patients with advanced hepatocellular carcinoma. Results of a randomised controlled trial in a single institution. Hepatology 1998;27:1578–1583.
57. Caturelli E, Siena D, Fusilli S, et al. Transcatheter arterial chemoembolization for hepatocellular carcinoma in patients with cirrhosis: evaluation of damage to nontumorous liver tissue. Radiology 2000;215:123–128.
58. Llovet JM, Real MI, Montana X, for the Barcellona Clinic Liver Cancer Group. Arterial embolization or chemoembolization versus symptomatic treatment in patients with unresectable hepatocellular carcinoma: a randomised controlled trial. Lancet 2000;359:1734–1739.
59. Matusani S, Sasak Y, Imaoka S, et al. The assessment of preoperative transcatheter arterial embolization for hepatocellular carcinoma: the comparison between "whole-liver" TAE and

"lobar or segmental" TAE (in Japanese) Nippon Shokakibyo Gakkai Zasshi 1991;88: 2757–2762.
60. Llovet JM, Bruix J. Systematic review of randomised trials for unresectable hepatocellular carcinoma: chemoembolization improves survival. Hepatology 2003;37(2):429–442.
61. Meloni MF, Goldberg SN, Livraghi T, et al. Hepatocellular carcinoma treated with radio frequency ablation: comparison of pulse inversion contrast-enhanced harmonic sonography, contrast-enhanced power-Doppler sonography and helical CT. AJR 2001;177(2):375–380.
62. Solbiati L, Martegani A, Leen E, Correas JM, Burns PN, Becker D. Contrast-Enhanced Ultrasound of Liver Disease. New York: Springer, Verlag Italia, 2003. pp 103–113.
63. De Baere T, Elias D, Dromain C, et al. Radiofrequency ablation of 100 hepatic metastases with a mean follow-up of more than 1 year. AJR 2000;175:1619–1625.
64. Murakami R, Yoshimatsu S, Yamashita Y, Sagsra K, Arakawa A, Takahashi M. Transcatheter hepatic subsegmental arterial chemoembolization therapy using iodized oil for small hepatocellular carcinoma. Correlation between lipiodol accumulation pattern and local recurrence. Acta Radiol 1994;35:576–580.
65. Bruix J, Castells A, Bosch J, et al. Surgical resection of hepatocellular carcinoma in cirrhotic patients: prognostic value of perioperative portal pressure. Gastroenterology 1996;3:1018–1022.
66. Noun R, Jagot P, Farges O, Sauvanet A, Belghiti J. High preoperative serum alanine transferase levels: effect on the risk of liver resection in Child grade A cirrhotic patients. World J Surg 1997;21:390–395.

26
Radiofrequency Ablation of Neuroendocrine Metastases

Thomas D. Atwell, J. William Charboneau, David M. Nagorney, and Florencia G. Que

Neuroendocrine tumors encompass a wide spectrum of neoplasms with a common origin in the neuroendocrine cell system. They share the capacity for hormone secretion that results in distinct clinical syndromes. Although neuroendocrine tumors can arise in organs such as the adenohypophysis, thymus, lung, thyroid, adrenal medulla/paraganglia, and skin (1), most familiar are the gastroenteropancreatic neuroendocrine tumors that include carcinoid and islet cell neoplasms. Given the high occurrence of hepatic metastases within this subgroup of neuroendocrine tumors, they are a model for the management of other hormonally active tumors.

Gastroenteropancreatic neuroendocrine neoplasms, which include the carcinoid and islet cell tumors, are a rare group of neoplasms, with an incidence of one to two cases per 100,000 people (2). They are relatively unique in that they typically are associated with an indolent rate of growth, and frequently are associated with tumor-specific hormone production and a secondary clinical syndrome.

Because these neoplasms have a unique pathophysiology, the treatment approach is different from the traditional management of hepatic metastases. Much of what we know about aggressive management has been learned through surgical experience, with interventional radiology providing insight into more palliative therapy. Radiofrequency ablation (RFA) will likely prove itself to be a valuable treatment modality for neuroendocrine hepatic metastases.

This chapter reviews carcinoid and islet cell tumors. Different treatment options traditionally incorporated into the management of hepatic metastases from these tumors include surgery and embolization. Radiofrequency ablation of neuroendocrine hepatic metastases is reviewed, including a brief review of the literature.

Carcinoid Tumor

Carcinoid tumors are slow-growing neoplasms that arise primarily from three sites in the gastrointestinal tract: the appendix, rectum, and small intestine. Small-bowel carcinoids are the most common (3), and probably the most significant clinically because of the symptoms of bowel ischemia that occur with mesenteric spread. In as many as 40% of patients, the carcinoid tumor is discovered incidentally during the evaluation of an unrelated clinical condition (4).

Metastatic disease is present in 45% of carcinoid patients at the time of diagnosis (3). These tumors are apt to metastasize to the liver over extended time, with metastases eventually occurring in up to 85% of patients (5). This slow rate of spread allows the liver to adapt to the bulky metastatic disease. Patients with both carcinoid and islet cell hepatic metastases classically present with a markedly enlarged liver, yet these patients are fully functional with minimal symptoms (6).

Carcinoid syndrome is a unique symptomatic manifestation of advanced carcinoid disease, characterized by flushing, diarrhea, asthma, and bronchospasm, and, in late disease, tricuspid valve regurgitation. Carcinoid syndrome is encountered in about 7% to 10% of all carcinoid patients, and in 35% to 50% of patients with hepatic metastases (4,7). The syndrome is typically associated with elevated levels of urine 5-hydroxyindoleacetic acid (5-HIAA).

Carcinoid tumors are notorious for having a slow, indolent disease course. Historically, surgery has been the standard of treatment, providing prolonged disease-free survival and cure in many patients. Among patients with limited disease treated for curative intent, 80% five-year survival has been achieved, although only 23% of the patients remained recurrence free at twenty-five years (6). Even with incurable metastatic disease to the liver, median survival time exceeds 3 years, and 5-year survival approaches 21% to 30% (6–8).

Islet Cell Neoplasms of the Pancreas

Pancreatic islet cell neoplasms are derived from neuroendocrine cells. Slightly greater than 50% of these tumors are considered functional because they produce various hormones (8). Such tumors often are named for the characteristic hormone produced; these include insulinoma, gastrinoma, glucagonoma, VIPoma, and so on. Occasionally, these tumors produce more than one hormone, which results in a mixed clinical picture or a change in the hormone syndrome over time. As with carcinoid and other neuroendocrine tumors, production of a specific hormone leads to characteristic syndromes that often result in substantial morbidity and mortality.

Hepatic metastases frequently occur in patients who have pancreatic islet cell neoplasms, eventually developing in up to 5% to 10% with insulinoma, 23% to 90% with gastrinoma, and 70% to 75% with glucagonoma (9). The unique hormonal syndrome associated with each tumor typically is proportional to the gross functional tumor burden. Despite the frequency of hepatic metastases, these tumors often behave in a protracted manner. In patients with metastatic disease to the liver, the 3-year survival is 56% and the overall survival rate is 42% (8). Death is often secondary to hepatic insufficiency related to tumor burden or complications from hormone production.

Treatment of Neuroendocrine Hepatic Metastases

The frequency of metastatic disease, the hormone production, and the protracted clinical course make gastroenteropancreatic neuroendocrine hepatic metastases responsive to multiple therapeutic modalities that include surgical resection, hepatic artery embolization, cryotherapy, and radiofrequency thermal ablation. The surgical experience has formed the foundation for the management of neuroendocrine hepatic metastases.

Surgery

The standard of care for patients with neuroendocrine cancer metastatic to the liver is now resection of the primary tumor mass and hepatic metastases when technically feasible. While bulky and often numerous, these metastases often are circumscribed, and they cause a simple mass effect on adjacent liver parenchyma, as opposed to invasion or encasement of adjacent structures. This allows for excision with optimal margins.

Patients considered for surgery include those with preoperative imaging studies that suggest resectability of primary and regional tumor, as well as resectability of 90% or more of the hepatic tumor volume (10). Such treatment has resulted in increased survival of patients, up to 73% to 93% at 4 years (10,11) and 61% to 73% at 5 years (12,13). Survival at 10 years is 35%, which emphasizes the indolent, yet relentless nature of this malignancy. There is no appreciable difference in 5-year survival between patients with carcinoid tumors and patients with islet cell tumors (13).

Perhaps more significant is the effect of resection on the control of symptoms. The degree of endocrinopathy is proportional to tumor volume. Thus, symptom control gained by debulking of hepatic metastases is significant. Relief of hormone-related symptoms occurs in 96% of patients following resection (13). Complete relief of symptoms is achieved in 86% of patients with carcinoid syndrome treated with palliative intent (14). The mean duration of symptom relief following resection of neuroendocrine metastases to the liver is 45 months, with recurrence of symptoms in 59% of patients at 5 years (13). Complete response is more prolonged when hepatic resection is performed for cure.

We have found no significant difference in the survival rates or initial symptomatic response between patients who had curative resection and patients who had palliative or incomplete resection of hepatic metastases from neuroendocrine cancer (10). With this in mind, the goal of cytoreductive surgery has evolved into either complete resection of the tumor mass or resection of greater than 90% of the tumor burden.

Despite these promising results of curative resection and cytoreduction, surgical resection of these metastases is possible in only 10% of patients (15). Bilobar liver disease is present in most patients (76%), and in approximately 50% of the patients the tumor involves more than 50% of the liver (13,16). In addition, the required surgery is often quite extensive and associated with significant perioperative risk. Major hepatectomy (excision of more than one lobe) may be required in more than half of the patients (13). In a review of 74 patients by Que et al (10), more than half of the patients had major or extended hepatic resections and concurrent intestinal and pancreatic resections. Perioperative mortality from such resections is 1.2% to 2.7% (13).

Consistent with the natural history of neuroendocrine malignancy, recurrence of disease occurs in a large majority of these patients. Recurrence following resection occurs in 84% of patients at 5 years and 94% at 10 years (13). It is very difficult to cure patients of this disease.

Hepatic Artery Embolization

Hepatic artery embolization, with or without combined intraarterial infusion of chemotherapeutic agents, is an effective alternative to surgical resection in patients with surgically unresectable metastases. This therapy makes use of the exclusive hepatic arterial supply of neuroendocrine metastases compared to the normal liver parenchyma, which receives nearly 75% of its blood supply from the portal vein. After establishing the hepatic arterial anatomy, either the right or left hepatic artery is selectively embolized using particles, absorbable gelatin, or iodinated oil. Only one lobe is embolized during a session to avoid hepatic insufficiency.

Both isolated particle embolization and chemoembolization have proven effective in treating neuroendocrine hepatic metastases. In a study of isolated particle embolization, the response rate was 96% with duration ranging from 6 to 18 months, depending on the clinical scenario (17). Other investigators have had less success with mid-gut carcinoid tumors, reporting a response rate of 52% and median duration of effect of 12 months (18). These same investigators reported a 50% response rate in patients with islet cell metastases to the liver, with the median duration of 10 months. With chemoembolization, the expected response rate is approximately 87% and the expected duration is 11 months (5).

In a study comparing patients who had hepatic artery occlusion with and without subsequent systemic chemotherapy, the patients who also received subsequent chemotherapy had a greater degree of objective tumor regression (80% compared to 60%), and a more prolonged response (18.0 months compared with 4.0 months) (19).

Cryotherapy

Cryotherapy has been incorporated in the treatment of neuroendocrine hepatic metastases (20–22). Cryoablation systems deliver liquid nitrogen or argon gas to the tip of a thin probe after it has been placed into the metastasis, commonly under ultrasound guidance. A series of freeze-thaw cycles is performed, destroying the tumor. Cryotherapy is effective in alleviating symptoms and reducing tumor markers in more than 90% of patients (20–22).

In a study by Seifert et al (20), 52 neuroendocrine metastases in 13 patients were treated with intraoperative cryotherapy. Five of the seven symptomatic patients had complete alleviation of symptoms; the remaining two had partial relief. A significant reduction in levels of serum tumor markers also was observed among patients for whom data were available. Morbidity occurred in four of the 13 patients: coagulopathy necessitated reoperation in two carcinoid patients, and acute renal failure and pulmonary embolism occurred in one patient each.

Bilchik et al (22) summarized their results for using intraoperative cryotherapy to palliate disease in 19 symptomatic patients with neuroendocrine metastases to the liver. Estimated tumor destruction during the surgery was 70% to 90% of the total tumor bulk. Several patients had concurrent resection of the primary tumor or hepatic metastases. All the patients had a transient coagulopathy that was treated with fresh frozen plasma or platelets. All 19 patients were symptom free following surgery, and 18 of the 19 had a reduction in tumor markers.

Cozzi et al (21) described six patients who had hepatic metastases from neuroendocrine tumors treated with intraoperative cryotherapy. All six patients were treated successfully with no local recurrence at median follow-up of 24 months. The four symptomatic patients had complete relief of symptoms. Levels of tumor markers decreased by more than 89% in the three patients with positive markers. Coagulopathy requiring additional surgery occurred in two of the three patients with carcinoid.

Radiofrequency Ablation

Perhaps the most important lesson from the surgical literature is that both complete and near-complete excision of hepatic metastases can have a significant impact on both patient symptoms and survival. Therefore, RFA can be expected to accomplish two objectives in the management of gastroenteropancreatic neuroendocrine hepatic metastases: (1) In our experience, the most frequent application for RFA is the debulking of hepatic metastases to palliate symptoms and increase survival (Fig. 26.1). (2) Treatment with RFA may be used with the goal of cure in patients who have a limited number of hepatic metastases.

Currently, specific indications for RFA in treating neuroendocrine hepatic metastases are for patients who: (1) need intraoperative ablation as an adjunct to resection (Fig. 26.2), (2) have limited hepatic disease, but are not operative candidates, (3) are inoperable and unresponsive to embolization treatments, or (4) have recurrence after resection (Fig. 26.3).

Dedicated studies of RFA of neuroendocrine hepatic metastases are limited. The largest study to date reported results from using laparoscopic RFA to treat 34 patients with 234 neuroendocrine hepatic metastases (23). Relief of symptoms was achieved in 95% of the patients, including complete relief in 63%. Mean duration of response was 10 months. Data from 32 of the patients showed local recurrence at 3% of the treated metastases, documented between 6 and 12 months following RFA. New liver metastases developed in 28% of the patients at a mean follow-up of 1.6 years. After the treatment, 65% of the patients had a decrease in the level of at least one hormonal marker. Two complications occurred, including transient atrial fibrillation and a hepatic abscess, the latter treated by percutaneous drainage.

Hellman et al (24) reported 21 patients who had 43 neuroendocrine hepatic metastases treated with either percutaneous or intraoperative RFA. Fifteen of these patients were treated with curative intent, that is, an attempt was made to ablate all lesions. The authors used a cooled-tip electrode to treat lesions that ranged in size from 2 to 7 cm (mean, 2.0 cm). At follow-up (mean, 2.1 years), 41 lesions had no evidence of local recurrence; this resulted in a success rate of 95%. Local recurrence developed in only two treated lesions, each at 6 months following treatment. Absence of residual disease was documented in only four of the 15 patients treated with curative intent. There were two non–life-threatening complications. The authors also showed that monitoring levels

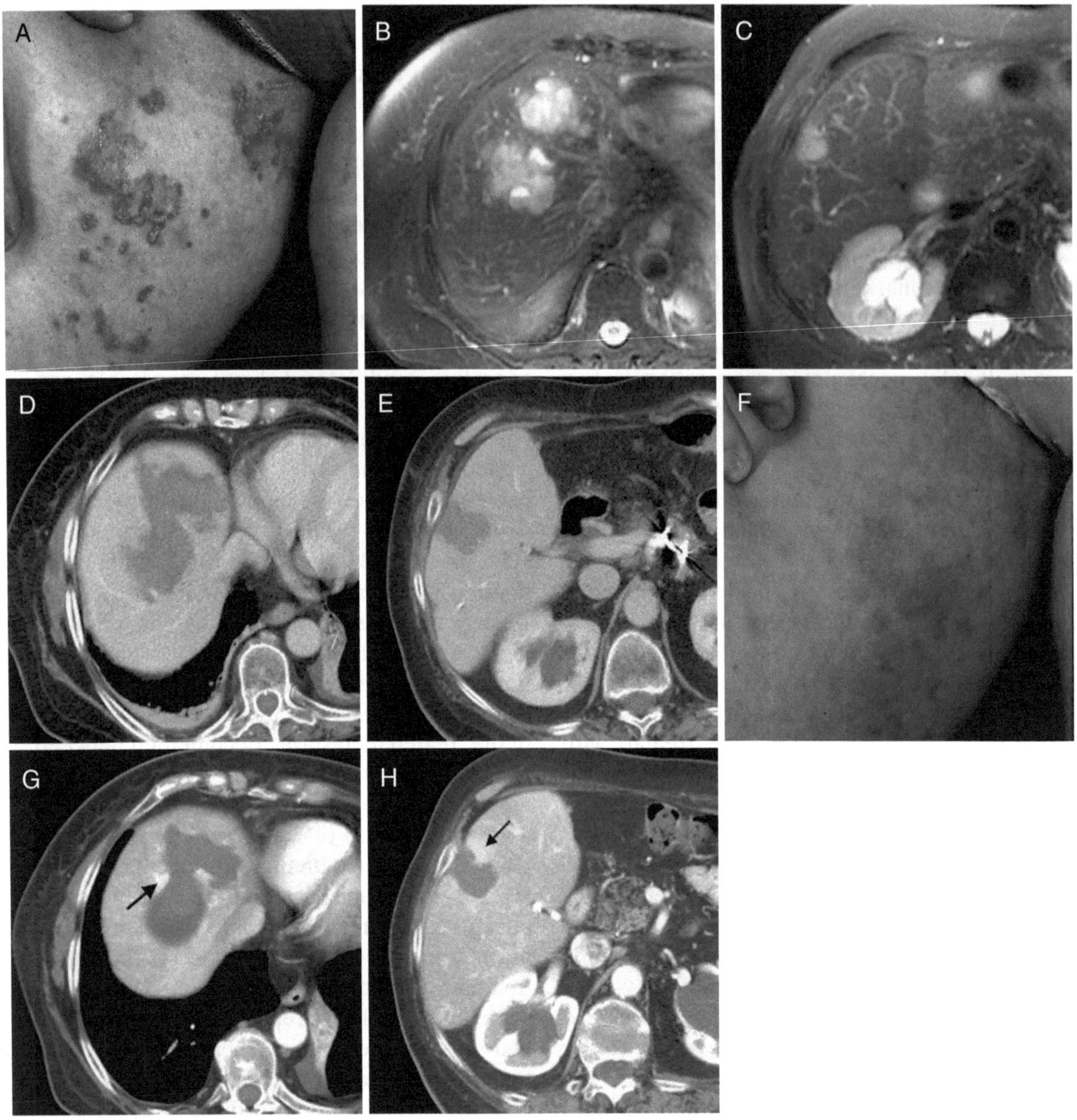

FIGURE 26.1. Radiofrequency ablation (RFA) of metastatic glucagonoma causing symptomatic erythema. A 67-year-old woman who had prior wedge resections of hepatic metastases, presented with worsening symptomatic rash, compatible with characteristic necrolytic migratory erythema (A), and elevated serum glucagon of 16,000 pg/mL. Magnetic resonance imaging showed multiple hepatic metastases, with three dominant lesions (B,C). Percutaneous ultrasound-guided RFA was performed on these three largest metastases for debulking and symptom control. Contrast-enhanced computed tomography (CT) performed hours after the RFA shows large corresponding ablation defects in the liver parenchyma (D,E). The patient's rash resolved within days of the RFA. At the 2-month follow-up, the patient was asymptomatic, the rash had healed (F), and the serum glucagon was 3700 pg/mL. Contrast-enhanced CT at this follow-up visit showed that the bulk of tumor remained destroyed with only small nodular recurrences (arrows) at the ablation sites (G,H).

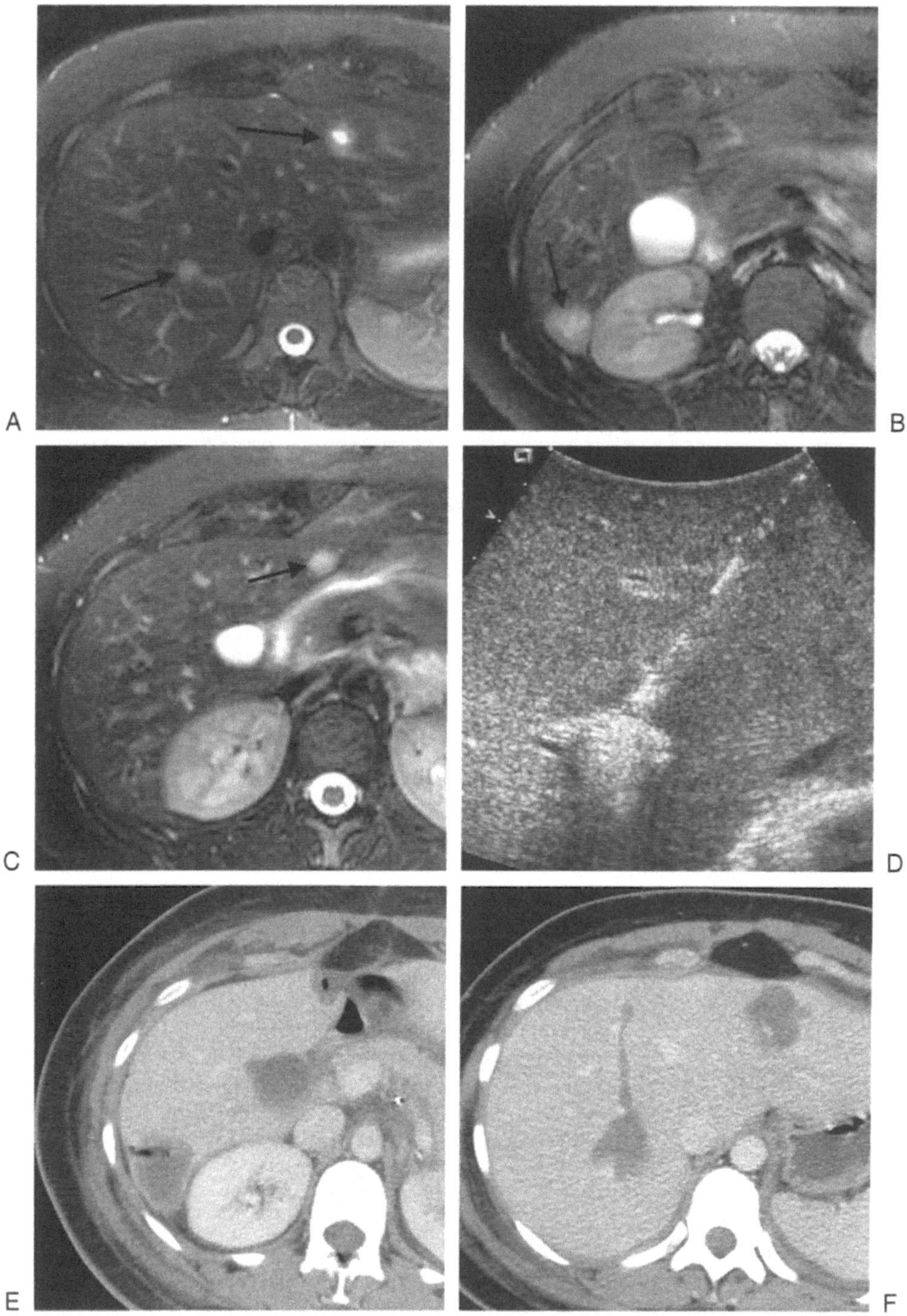

FIGURE 26.2. Intraoperative RFA of metastatic functional pheochromocytoma. A 22-year-old woman presented with a history of pheochromocytoma and worsening palpitations and hypertension that required therapy with multiple antihypertensive medications. Magnetic resonance imaging (MRI) showed recurrence of tumor in the left adrenal bed and four hepatic metastases (arrows) (A–C). At operation, the superficial metastases were resected and intraoperative ultrasound-guided RFA was performed on the two deeper lesions (D). CT obtained 3 days following ablation showed both the surgical wedge defects (E) and the RFA ablation defects (F). The patient's hypertension resolved, and she was discharged from the hospital without antihypertensive medication.

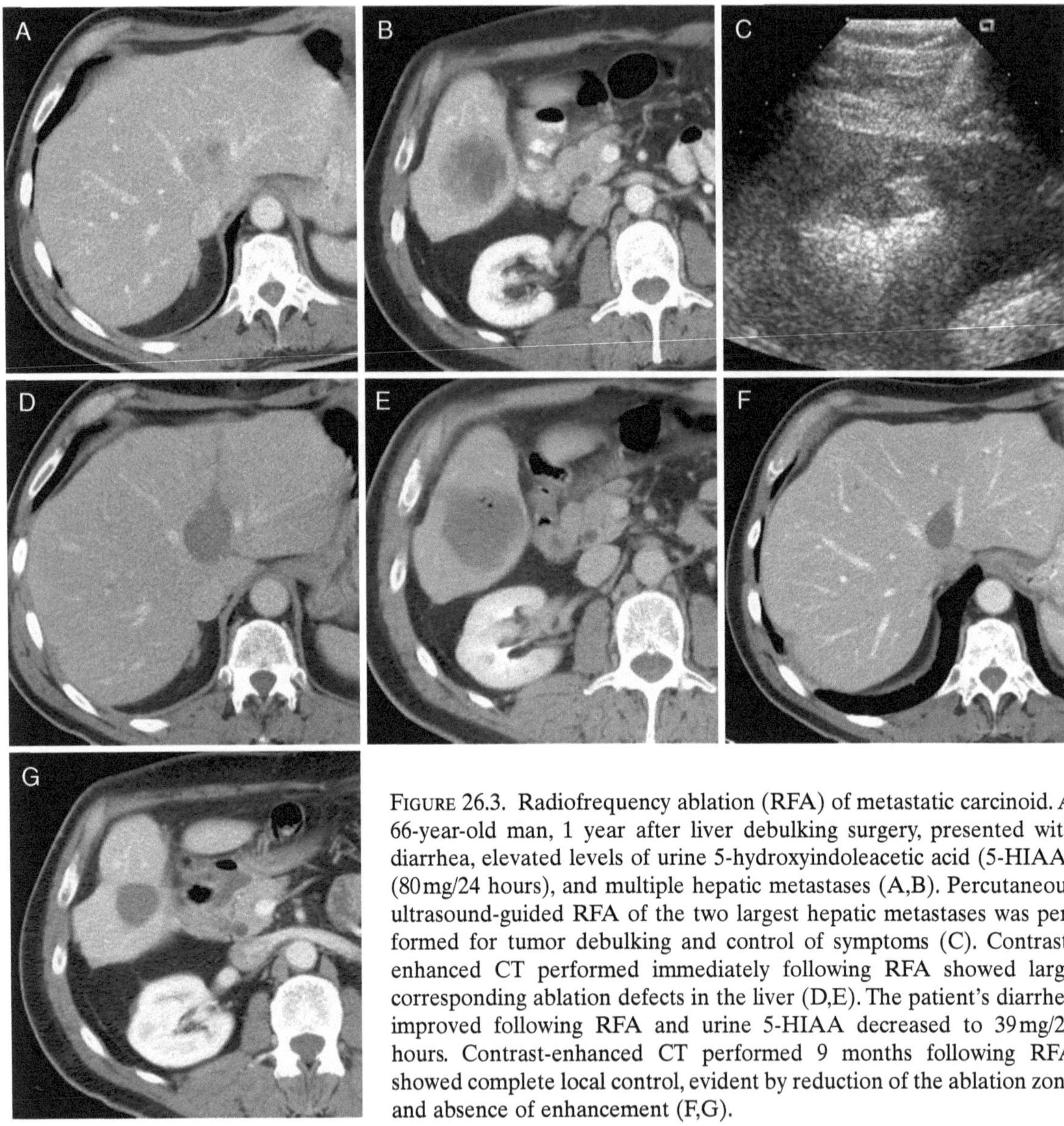

FIGURE 26.3. Radiofrequency ablation (RFA) of metastatic carcinoid. A 66-year-old man, 1 year after liver debulking surgery, presented with diarrhea, elevated levels of urine 5-hydroxyindoleacetic acid (5-HIAA) (80 mg/24 hours), and multiple hepatic metastases (A,B). Percutaneous ultrasound-guided RFA of the two largest hepatic metastases was performed for tumor debulking and control of symptoms (C). Contrast-enhanced CT performed immediately following RFA showed large corresponding ablation defects in the liver (D,E). The patient's diarrhea improved following RFA and urine 5-HIAA decreased to 39 mg/24 hours. Contrast-enhanced CT performed 9 months following RFA showed complete local control, evident by reduction of the ablation zone and absence of enhancement (F,G).

of tumor markers after treatment is difficult due to the presence of disease elsewhere in the abdomen.

Wessels and Schell (25) reported the use of intraoperative RFA in three patients for treatment of carcinoid hepatic metastases refractory to hepatic artery embolization (24). All three patients suffered from malignant carcinoid syndrome. In all three, symptoms improved after RFA treatment, the dosage of octreotide therapy was decreased, and tumor size was smaller on follow-up computed tomography (CT) scans. There were no complications.

Results of these studies show that RFA relieves symptoms in patients who have neuroendocrine tumors. Although the cure of neuroendocrine malignancy is challenging, RFA provides a relatively safe method of tumor debulking, and the rate of local recurrence is low.

Summary

Neuroendocrine malignancies are rare neoplasms frequently associated with characteristic hormonal syndromes. Gastroenteropancreatic neuroendocrine tumors frequently develop hepatic metastases. Their biologic behavior affords multiple treatment options. If surgically feasible, resection of metastases is the best option for the patient. Hepatic artery embolization is also effective in nonsurgical patients, and provides at least short-term palliation.

Radiofrequency ablation is evolving into an effective method of tumor destruction, and it can improve patient symptoms. As demonstrated in the surgical literature, removal of the bulk of neuroendocrine hepatic metastases improves patient survival. On the basis of this surgical experience, we expect a similar effect on patient survival with RFA.

Probably the most significant contribution of RFA will be as adjunctive treatment intraoperatively and postoperatively. Coordination of surgical and ablation techniques during the course of surgery allows optimal treatment of the neuroendocrine malignancy through surgical excision of both the primary tumor and accessible hepatic metastases, as well as concurrent ablation of deep-seated lesions in the liver. This affords the surgical option to a larger percentage of patients who have metastases that were previously deemed unresectable. Following surgery, RFA allows minimally invasive treatment of the almost inevitable recurrence of disease in the remaining liver.

References

1. DeLellis RA, Tischler AS. The dispersed neuroendocrine system. In: Kovacs K, Asa SL, eds. Functional Endocrine Pathology. Malden, MA: Blackwell Science, 1998:529–549.
2. Oberg K. State of the art and future prospects in the management of neuroendocrine tumors. Q J Nucl Med 2000;44:3–12.
3. Modlin IM, Sandor A. An analysis of 8305 cases of carcinoid tumors. Cancer 1997;79:813–829.
4. Shebani KO, Souba WW, Finkelstein DM, et al. Prognosis and survival in patients with gastrointestinal tract carcinoid tumors. Ann Surg 1999; 229:815–821; discussion 822–823.
5. Proye C. Natural history of liver metastasis of gastroenteropancreatic neuroendocrine tumors: place for chemoembolization. World J Surg 2001; 25:685–688.
6. Moertel CG. Karnofsky memorial lecture. An odyssey in the land of small tumors. J Clin Oncol 1987;5:1502–1522.
7. Moertel CG, Sauer WG, Dockerty MB, Baggenstoss AH. Life history of the carcinoid tumor of the small intestine. Cancer 1961;14:901–912.
8. Thompson GB, van Heerden JA, Grant CS, Carney JA, Ilstrup DM. Islet cell carcinomas of the pancreas: a twenty-year experience. Surgery 1988;104:1011–1017.
9. Carty SE, Jensen RT, Norton JA. Prospective study of aggressive resection of metastatic pancreatic endocrine tumors. Surgery 1992;112: 1024–1031; discussion 1031–1032.
10. Que FG, Nagorney DM, Batts KP, Linz LJ, Kvols LK. Hepatic resection for metastatic neuroendocrine carcinomas. Am J Surg 1995;169:36–42; discussion 42–43.
11. Grazi GL, Cescon M, Pierangeli F, et al. Highly aggressive policy of hepatic resections for neuroendocrine liver metastases. Hepatogastroenterology 2000;47:481–486.
12. Chen H, Hardacre JM, Uzar A, Cameron JL, Choti MA. Isolated liver metastases from neuroendocrine tumors: does resection prolong survival? J Am Coll Surg 1998;187:88–92; discussion 92–93.
13. Sarmiento JM, Heywood G, Rubin J, Ilstrup DM, Nagorney DM, Que FG. Surgical treatment of neuroendocrine metastases to the liver: a plea for resection to increase survival. Journal Amer Coll Surgeons 2003;197(1):29–37.
14. Que FG, Heywood GM. Hepatic surgery for metastatic gastrointestinal neuroendocrine tumors. In: Blumgart LH, Fong Y, Jarnagin W, eds. Hepatobiliary Cancer. American Cancer Society and B.C. Dekker, 2000;97–116.
15. McEntee GP, Nagorney DM, Kvols LK, Moertel CG, Grant CS. Cytoreductive hepatic surgery for neuroendocrine tumors. Surgery 1990;108: 1091–1096.
16. Chamberlain RS, Canes D, Brown KT, et al. Hepatic neuroendocrine metastases: does intervention alter outcomes? J Am Coll Surg 2000; 190:432–445.
17. Brown KT, Koh BY, Brody LA, et al. Particle embolization of hepatic neuroendocrine metastases for control of pain and hormonal symptoms. J Vasc Intervent Radiol 1999;10:397–403.

18. Eriksson BK, Larsson EG, Skogseid BM, Lofberg AM, Lorelius LE, Oberg KE. Liver embolizations of patients with malignant neuroendocrine gastrointestinal tumors. Cancer 1998;83:2293–2301.
19. Moertel CG, Johnson CM, McKusick MA, et al. The management of patients with advanced carcinoid tumors and islet cell carcinomas. Ann Intern Med 1994;120:302–309.
20. Seifert JK, Cozzi PJ, Morris DL. Cryotherapy for neuroendocrine liver metastases. Semin Surg Oncol 1988;14:175–183.
21. Cozzi PJ, Englund R, Morris DL. Cryotherapy treatment of patients with hepatic metastases from neuroendocrine tumors. Cancer 1995;76: 501–509.
22. Bilchik AJ, Sarantou T, Foshag LJ, Giuliano AE, Ramming KP. Cryosurgical palliation of metastatic neuroendocrine tumors resistant to conventional therapy. Surgery 1997;122:1040–1047; discussion 1047–1048.
23. Berber E, Flesher N, Siperstein AE. Laparoscopic radiofrequency ablation of neuroendocrine liver metastases. World J Surg 2002; 26:985–990.
24. Hellman P, Ladjevardi S, Skogseid B, Akerstrom G, Elvin A. Radiofrequency tissue ablation using cooled tip for liver metastases of endocrine tumors. World J Surg 2001;26:1052–1056.
25. Wessels FJ, Schell SR. Radiofrequency ablation treatment of refractory carcinoid hepatic metastases. J Surg Res 2001:95:8–12.

27 Tumor Ablation in the Kidney

Debra A. Gervais and Peter R. Müeller

The interventional radiologist who establishes a percutaneous tumor ablation program will likely become skilled in liver tumor ablation before attempting to treat renal cell carcinoma. Liver tumors are more common than primary renal tumors, and most patients with liver tumors are not surgical candidates. Thus, a steady influx of patients eligible for percutaneous ablation of hepatic tumors can be expected in many centers. In contrast, surgical removal remains the standard therapy for small renal cell carcinomas, and most patients can undergo resection (1). Nevertheless, with the incidence of renal cell carcinoma (RCC) increasing and with the aging population in the United States, the number of patients with small RCCs who are not good surgical candidates is expected to increase (2–4). Thus, from time to time, the radiologist experienced in percutaneous tumor ablation can expect to encounter patients for whom percutaneous treatment of RCC is the only option or the most reasonable one.

In current practice, the least expensive, most readily available, and most straightforward percutaneous therapeutic option is radiofrequency ablation (RFA). Most RFA educational symposia or syllabi are devoted predominantly to liver ablation with all of its nuances. Renal tumors, if they are discussed at all, are often included under the rubric "extrahepatic" ablation. This overarching categorization includes ablation of tumors of the lung, head and neck, adrenals, spleen, and miscellaneous abdominal and pelvic tumors, thereby leaving little attention to the details specific to ablation of RCC. This chapter reviews the current clinical management of RCC, and the clinical and technical considerations in performing RFA for renal tumors. In addition, postablation imaging findings are reviewed, along with the associated challenges inherent in imaging follow-up.

Renal Cell Carcinoma: Staging, Prognosis, and Current Therapies

Staging and Prognosis

Staging systems for RCC have undergone several revisions over the years. Each revision represents an attempt to improve the correlation of staging with prognosis. In 1997 the American Joint Committee on Cancer established the current staging system for RCC that is summarized in Table 27.1 (5). As we shall see, the limitations of tumor size for which there is a reasonable chance to achieve local control with RFA is well within 7 cm, the size criterion that the American Joint Committee on Cancer (AJCC) staging system designates as the demarcation between stage I and stage II for RCCs that have not spread beyond the kidney (5–7). Thus, the radiologist who performs RFA of RCC will be focused predominantly on stage I tumors. While the search for the perfect prognostic tool continues, tumor staging remains the most reliable and thus the most important parameter (8).

Other tumor features have been studied for their prognostic utility. Among the most famil-

TABLE 27.1. Renal cell carcinoma TNM classification and staging system of the American Joint Committee on Cancer (AJCC).

TNM Definitions

Primary tumor (T)	
T1	Tumor 7 cm or less, limited to kidney
T2	Tumor more than 7 cm, limited to kidney
T3	Tumor extends into major veins or invades adrenal or perinephric tissues, but not beyond Gerota's fascia
T3a	Tumor invades adrenal or perinephric tissues, not beyond Gerota's fascia
T3b	Tumor grossly extends into renal vein(s) or IVC below diaphragm
T3c	Tumor grossly extends into renal vein(s) or IVC above diaphragm
T4	Tumor invades beyond Gerota's fascia
Regional lymph nodes (N)	
NX	Nodes cannot be assessed
N0	No lymph nodes
N1	Metastasis in a single regional node
N2	Metastases in more than one regional node
Distant metastases (M)	
MX	Metastases cannot be assessed
M0	No metastases present
M1	Metastases present

Staging

Stage I	T1, N0, M0
Stage II	T2, N0, M0
Stage III	T1, N1, M0
	T2, N1, M0
	T3a, N0, M0
	T3a, N1, M0
	T3b, N0, M0
	T3b, N1, M0
	T3c, N0, M0
	T3c, N1, M0
Stage IV	T4, N0, M0
	T4, N1, M0
	Any T, N2, M0
	Any T, Any N, M1

Note: For T3 tumors, adrenal involvement refers to direct invasion only, not to hematogenous metastatic spread. IVC, inferior vena cava.

iar are grading and tumor histology (9,10). Grading of renal cell carcinoma is based on nuclear characteristics, whereas histology is based on tissue architecture. In North America, the Fuhrman grading system, which consists of four grades, is the most commonly utilized system (9). However, the prognostic utility has proven variable when evaluated by different investigators. In addition, grading can be subjective among pathologists. For these reasons, grading remains of secondary importance to staging for practical clinical applications.

With respect to histology, there are four types of renal cell carcinoma (10). The most common type is clear cell carcinoma, also known as conventional RCC. Clear cell carcinoma accounts for approximately 70% of solid renal masses in surgical series. The next most common histologic type of RCC is papillary, or chromophil, RCC, which accounts for 10% to 15% of solid renal masses. Some investigators have reported a more favorable prognosis than for clear cell, whereas other investigators have shown a worse prognosis. The prognosis of papillary RCC compared to clear cell RCC remains controversial and further studies regarding cytogenetics and molecular markers may clarify this issue.

Rarer RCCs are the chromophobe type (5%) with a favorable prognosis compared to clear cell RCC (10). On the other hand, collecting duct RCCs (<1%) are aggressive and metastasize early. In large part, the remainder of renal masses are tumors that cannot be subtyped into one of these four categories, either because of features of more than one type or due to sarcomatoid changes. Sarcomatoid change is not a unique subtype, as it can be seen in any of the underlying histologic types (10). However, it carries a universally poor prognosis, regardless of the underlying histologic type of RCC. Other terminology that may be encountered in the clinical evaluation of renal masses includes papillary adenoma, metanephric adenoma, and oncocytoma. These are generally considered benign tumors.

Finally, there are several new promising prognostic features that currently are being evaluated; these include cytogenetic and molecular markers (11). For the time being, these remain experimental and have yet to enter widespread clinical use.

Current Therapy

The treatment for RCC in the absence of distant metastases is surgical resection (1). The conventional procedure has been radical nephrectomy, a procedure that carries a 1% to 2% mortality risk and 15% to 30% morbidity (1,12,13). Although it may not always be feasible, nephron-sparing surgery (partial nephrectomy) allows for preservation of renal function and has proven equally effective. Developments in laparoscopic resection have reduced recovery times for patients in whom the this method is appropriate (1). Nevertheless, despite the diminished morbidity and mortality associated with these less invasive options, an even less invasive procedure may be indicated in selected patients such as those with existing comorbid conditions that make anesthesia or surgery highly risky, those patients with multiple tumors such as occur in von Hippel–Lindau (VHL) disease, or the elderly. These patients might tolerate a percutaneous procedure better than a laparoscopic resection, and they are the impetus for new clinical developments in tumor ablation.

Indications/Contraindications for Percutaneous Radiofrequency Ablation

Ideal Tumor

The limits on the volume of coagulation necrosis that can be achieved with a single application of RFA and the basic science underlying this limitation are discussed elsewhere in this volume. Based on experimental observations, one can reasonably expect to achieve complete coagulation necrosis of most RCCs that are 3cm or less (14). In addition, one can reasonably expect to achieve complete necrosis of tumors up to 5cm, but some of these may require more ablation sessions (6,14). These hypothetical expectations have been confirmed by initial clinical reports of RFA of RCC (6). While absolute size limits are difficult to establish, one is likely to encounter a rapid decline in rates of complete coagulation necrosis as tumor size increases beyond 5cm. This has been confirmed for liver tumors and by initial results for kidney tumors (7,15).

Tumor location is also likely to influence RFA success. Exophytic tumors, partially surrounded by perinephric fat, are favorable for RFA. The fat serves as an insulator that facilitates maintenance of high temperatures within the tumors, thereby enhancing necrosis (6,7). This phenomenon has been termed the *oven effect* by Livraghi et al (16), who described improved coagulation necrosis in encapsulated, and hence insulated, hepatomas. On the other hand, central tumors with extensions into the renal sinus are more difficult to treat with RFA (6,7). This increased difficulty is related to perfusion-mediated tissue cooling, the *heat-sink effect*, mediated by the large central blood vessels (17). The constant inflow of blood at body temperature results in cooling of the portions of tumor adjacent to large blood vessels. This limits both the peak temperatures and the duration of these temperatures in regions of tumor that as a consequence may undergo inadequate coagulation necrosis (17).

Thus, the ideal tumor for percutaneous RFA is a 3cm or less exophytic tumor without direct contiguity to vital structures such as bowel or ureter (7). Tumors up to 5cm are also reasonable candidates. Small central tumors (those with a component in the renal sinus) can undergo successful RFA, but proximity to large renal arteries or veins is almost guaranteed as the tumor size enlarges. The cooling effect of the large vessels may preclude successful ablation, or may result in the need for additional ablation sessions to achieve complete tumor necrosis (7).

Finally, when assessing a tumor for possible RFA, staging relies on imaging and clinical evaluation. Although not a common occurrence, metastases can occur even with small primary RCCs. Thus, review of an abdominal computed tomography (CT) or magnetic resonance imaging (MRI) exam of a renal mass for potential RFA includes assessment of the retroperitoneal lymph nodes, inferior vena cava, liver, lung bases, bones, and contralateral kidney for metastases or synchronous tumors.

Patient Selection

Despite promising results following percutaneous RFA of RCCs with up to 4 years of follow-up available in a few patients, RFA remains a relatively new procedure to treat stage I RCC (6,7,18,19). In the treatment of RCC, the historical standard to which new techniques have been compared is open radical nephrectomy (1). Newer less invasive procedures such as partial nephrectomy and laparoscopic nephrectomy have been required to demonstrate similar rates of 5-year survival and disease-free survival for the results to be considered equivalent. Using this benchmark, partial nephrectomy has proven as effective as complete nephrectomy, and initial reports on 5-year results following laparoscopic resection likewise show results similar to open resection (1). The currently available clinical experience with RFA of RCC is limited to several series of 25 to 50 patients with mean postablation periods of approximately 1 to 1.5 years (6,7,18,19).

Until long-term data are available, we are limiting RFA for the treatment of RCC to select patients. The primary patients are those who are unable to undergo nephrectomy because of comorbid diseases that make the surgical risk of morbidity and mortality excessively high. Typically, these comorbid diseases include cardiovascular or pulmonary conditions as well as other malignancies (6). In addition, patients with less than a 10-year life expectancy based on comorbid conditions or advanced age are reasonable candidates for percutaneous ablation (6). We do require that there be a reasonable likelihood of at least 1 year of life expectancy, as any patient with a condition with expected mortality within a year is not likely to experience any deleterious effect on health from a stage I RCC. Patients for whom surgical resection would risk or guarantee a dependency on dialysis also are candidates for RFA. These include patients with solitary kidneys and patients with predisposition to multiple RCCs, such as occur in VHL disease or in familial cases of RCC (6,7,18).

Finally, in selecting patients for percutaneous RFA, we have found collaboration with a urologist to be indispensable (6). The involvement of the urologist ensures thorough assessment of all therapeutic options for the patient. In patients for whom resection may be difficult and for whom percutaneous ablation is deemed unsafe due to proximity to adjacent ureter or bowel, laparoscopic mobilization of these adjacent structures may facilitate ablation if the patient is a suitable candidate for anesthesia and if the tumor cannot be removed. The optimal technique in these situations is to combine the laparoscopic expertise of the urologist with that of image-guided ablation of the radiologist. Finally, in the unlikely event of a complication that requires retrograde ureteral stent placement, a urologist familiar with the patient is most appropriate.

Planning Radiofrequency Ablation of Renal Cell Carcinoma

Based on the tumor and patient criteria defined above, an algorithm for triaging patients can be implemented. The first of two critical questions to answer is this: Is the patient a good candidate for surgical resection based on the evaluation of a urologist? If so, then, proceed to resection. If not, the second question follows: Is percutaneous image-guided RFA technically safe and feasible? Review of available imaging is mandatory to begin to answer this question. These first two steps allow rapid screening of patients who are not suitable for RFA, either because they can have surgery or because the tumor size, location, or proximity to other structures makes RFA impossible or unsafe.

Once a stage I RCC is deemed suitable for percutaneous RFA, the next step is to assess the adequacy of the available imaging. The role of imaging for RFA is not only to screen the case for suitability, but also four other important functions:

- To choose a modality for procedure guidance
- To define preablation margins—the whole target for RFA
- To serve as a baseline for postablation imaging
- To plan the ablation approach—percutaneous or laparoscopic

If any of these functions is not adequately served by available imaging or if imaging is not recent, then additional cross-sectional imaging should be performed to address all of these issues. At a minimum, a contrast-enhanced CT or MRI is needed before RFA since these are the imaging modalities that will be used to monitor the result. Ideally, the modality that is used for postablation imaging is available at baseline to facilitate comparison. In current practice, CT remains the modality of choice; MRI is used only for patients who cannot receive intravenous (IV) contrast material because of renal insufficiency or prior anaphylaxis.

The choice of imaging modality to guide RFA is limited in clinical practice to ultrasound or CT. When compared to CT guidance, ultrasound is generally more readily available and allows real-time assessment of the needle tip position that facilitates and expedites needle adjustments. However, depending on body habitus and tumor location, ultrasound visualization of a given tumor may be suboptimal to guide ablation. Furthermore, while ultrasound may demonstrate a portion of the RCC, all of the tumor must be well-visualized with ultrasound to allow accurate needle and electrode placement for overlapping (or even single) ablations to achieve complete coagulation necrosis. If the tumor cannot be assessed completely with ultrasound, then CT may be a better choice for guidance. Magnetic resonance guidance has shown promising results, with clear advantages of both accurate intraprocedural monitoring of the necrosis margins and imaging guidance of the needle electrode in off-axial planes of imaging (20). However, in North America, there are no commercially available MR-compatible RF generators and needle electrode systems. Thus, at present MR guidance remains in the realm of researchers with dedicated equipment.

Accurate delineation of the tumor extent is critical, both for achieving complete coagulation necrosis when performing RFA and for serving as a baseline comparison for postablation imaging. Tumor margins can be obscured by the kidney if available CT is not contrast enhanced or if the timing of the contrast bolus is suboptimal for renal mass evaluation.

Finally, in cases of RCC in direct contiguity with bowel or ureter, percutaneous ablation may not be safe. However, if the patient is a suitable candidate for anesthesia, such as in a relatively young patient with VHL disease and multiple RCCs, then laparoscopic mobilization of these structures may allow RFA. If laparoscopic ablation is performed, imaging guidance in the form of operating room ultrasound still is needed to ensure optimal electrode positioning for complete tumor necrosis.

Preablation Biopsy

The role of needle biopsy of renal masses remains controversial and is evolving. Standard urology practice is to remove solid renal masses without biopsy (1). For most patients with solid renal masses, this approach is not likely to change soon. However, there are many patients for whom a biopsy diagnosis may be desirable prior to surgery or other invasive therapy. For example, in the setting of another primary malignancy, active or in remission, biopsy may be prudent (1,21). Wood et al (21) found in his series that 12 of 24 patients with primary malignancies other than RCC had solid renal masses that were metastases, not RCC. Furthermore, management changed in 32 of 79 (41%) cases based on biopsy results.

In patients with another primary malignancy, biopsy should be considered before proceeding with RFA. In some patients, biopsy may not be necessary. For example, Pavlovich et al (18) did not perform preablation renal mass biopsy in their series of 24 tumors since all patients had VHL disease or hereditary RCC. In the Pavlovich series, all masses were enhancing on CT and had shown growth on serial CT. Radiofrequency ablation of an enhancing enlarging solid renal mass is reasonable regardless of the results of the needle biopsy, and we have occasionally performed ablation of such a mass in the setting of a nondiagnostic or negative needle biopsy. However, our practice is to perform preablation biopsy since urologists at our institution manage biopsy-proven oncocytomas as benign neoplasms that are followed closely by imaging, and not resected in older patients. This particular management of oncocytoma is not universal practice, as there is a divergence of opinion among urologists on this issue (1).

We have adopted the practice pattern of our local urologists and do not perform RFA of oncocytomas. Thus, needle biopsy prior to ablation serves to triage solid renal masses. Because there remains regional variability in the approach to oncocytomas, the radiologist undertaking RFA of renal masses should be familiar with the preferred management of local urologists and plan accordingly.

Performing Radiofrequency Ablation of Renal Cell Carcinoma

Sedation

Most patients are able to tolerate percutaneous RFA as an outpatient procedure performed with IV sedation (6,7). Since the duration of the procedure is longer than for a typical biopsy or drainage procedure, the recovery from the IV sedation also can be slightly longer. For these reasons, RFA is best performed early enough in the day to allow sufficient time for the procedure and recovery the same day. Medically complex patients may require overnight observation following RFA (7). In some cases, the patient is admitted the day prior to the procedure to allow adequate hydration, to achieve blood pressure control, and/or to correct a coagulopathy if needed. Rare patients may require assistance of an anesthesiologist who may administer sedation or general anesthesia as appropriate.

Intravenous sedation regimens vary among institutions, and must be kept within established institutional guidelines (22). In our practice, we have achieved adequate sedation and analgesia in almost all cases with a combination of midazolam (2–5 mg), fentanyl (100–300 mg), and meperidine (25–50 mg) (6,7). Our initial cases received droperidol as the third agent both for its antiemetic and calming effects, but droperidol is no longer available (6). Thus, we have added meperidine for most patients for its longer analgesic action. We are currently giving ondansetron (4 mg IV) as an antiemetic as needed.

Optimizing Ablation: Choice of Systems and Performing Overlapping Ablations

Since the major focus of preclinical and early clinical work in RFA of soft tissue tumors has been the liver, generator design and ablation protocols for commercially available systems for soft tissue tumor ablation have been optimized for ablation of liver tumors. Experimental preclinical work on RFA for renal tumors is more limited, and in practice, most radiologists use the same ablation parameters for renal tumors as prescribed for liver tumors (6,7,23,24). The kidney is similar to the liver in that it too is a very vascular parenchymal organ. Nevertheless, the electrical and thermal characteristics are likely different from liver, given the different electrolyte milieu. Critics of rapid assimilation of RFA into clinical use for extrahepatic soft tissue tumors have suggested that the use of system parameters optimized for liver tumors may not be optimal for the treatment of renal tumors. While further experimental work may shed new insights into the features unique to the renal response to thermal ablation, these features may or may not translate into the need for changes in ablation protocols. Given the gross similarities between the two organs, the results of early clinical experience and the current knowledge regarding renal response to thermal ablation, the current clinical approach appears justified (6,7,18,19).

The available RF generator systems and their compatible needle electrodes are reviewed in detail elsewhere in the book. Each available generator system has prescribed end points for terminating a given ablation using one of three parameters: rapid rise in impedance (Radiotherapeutics, Boston Scientific, Natick, MA), target temperature (RITA, Mountain View, CA), or time (Radionics, Burlington, MA). If an umbrella array electrode is chosen, the diameter should be similar to the tumor size. If the tumor is larger than the largest available electrode, then overlapping ablations will be needed. The straight needle electrodes come in single or clustered arrangements (Radionics) with electrically active tips of 2.0 and 3.0 cm for the single electrodes and 2.5 cm for the cluster electrodes. For small tumors up to 2.5 cm, a single 2- or 3-cm active tip is adequate. For tumors 2.5 cm or larger, a cluster electrode provides more rapid necrosis of the tumor, although one can achieve coagulation necrosis of masses 2.5 to 4.0 cm with multiple overlapping ablations with a single electrode.

Tumor ablation requires more meticulous technique than needle biopsy. Biopsy requires needle placement within a tumor. Once diagnostic cells are obtained, the procedure is over. Needle repositioning is needed only if rapid cytologic or frozen-section evaluation fails to identify diagnostic material. Tumor ablation, however, requires induction of cell death throughout the entire three-dimensional volume of the target tumor (25). This task requires strategic needle electrode placement whether for a single ablation or for multiple overlapping ablations (14,25). In theory, umbrella array systems create thermal lesions in the shape of spheres, and perfectly overlapped ablation spheres create a larger composite thermal lesion with the narrowest diameter at the surface indentations of the three-dimensional composite (25). In theory, straight needle electrodes create cylindrical thermal lesions of varying diameter, dependent on single or cluster arrangement, and slightly longer than the electrically active shaft (14).

In practice, however, a different picture usually emerges. The reality is that the shapes of the thermal lesions can be irregular, of variable diameters, and difficult to predict. Furthermore, the diameters of overlapping thermal lesions created by the same needle electrode during the same session and in the same tumor may vary. Thus, decision making during RFA regarding positioning of electrodes is based in part on empirical science, but a large part of the practical application of RF ablation of soft tissue tumors remains an art.

For small tumors that require a single ablation, the needle electrode must be positioned as near to perfectly central as possible so as to avoid peripheral residual viable tumor. If this central positioning is not readily achieved and if an eccentric ablation is performed, then additional ablations can be performed to compensate for any anticipated regions of viable tumor. In reality, multiple overlapping ablations are needed for most tumors based not only on size, but also on tumor geometry. Even if needle electrodes could produce perfectly predictable and reproducible thermal lesions, tumors do not come in perfect spheres or cylinders. They may have an oval shape or irregular projections that necessitate special attention to achieve complete tumor necrosis. Whereas a simple eccentric projection of a tumor can be anticipated to require a dedicated eccentric needle electrode placement and ablation, the more difficult issue is how to predict optimal needle electrode placement to achieve thermal lesions that completely overlap a 4- to 5-cm tumor (Figs. 27.1 and 27.2).

Computed tomography and ultrasound findings do not predict the margins of necrosis accurately during RFA. Thus, the positioning of electrodes in performing overlapping ablations is made by the operator, based on size and geometry of the tumor, expected size and shape of the thermal lesions from the electrode system in use, and any anticipated effects from tumor surroundings such as perfusion-mediated tissue cooling from large vessels at any edge of the tumor (7). In addition, tissue temperature may provide some insight into whether the thermal lesion is at the larger or smaller end of the range that can be achieved. For internally cooled systems, the ideal temperature response following cessation of cooling and of electrical current at 12 minutes is a rapid rise in temperature to well over 60°C and slow return to less than 60°C. A temperature less than 60°C will achieve coagulation necrosis in a smaller volume of tissue. For the temperature controlled system (RITA), the computer chip alerts the operator to check the temperature at 30 seconds after termination of the ablation. A rapid decrease in temperature

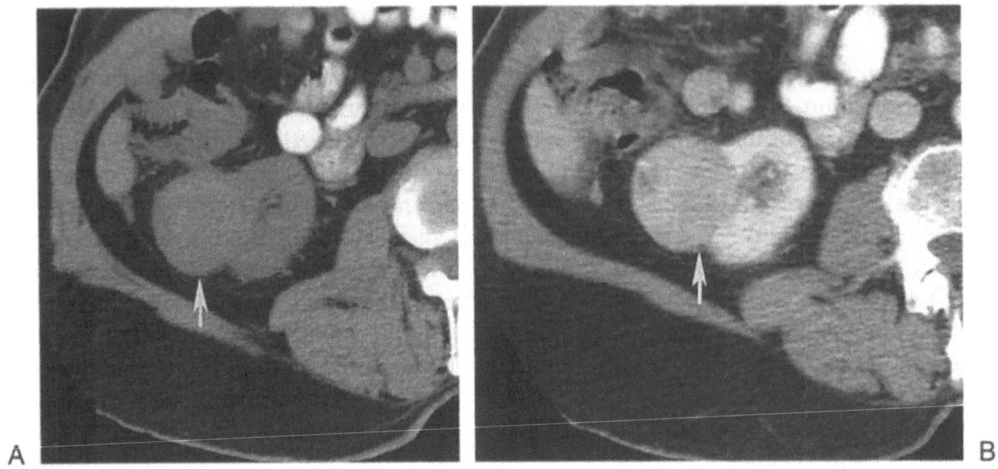

FIGURE 27.1. Computed tomography (CT) scan in an 81-year-old man with a solitary kidney and a 4.2-cm biopsy-proven renal cell carcinoma (RCC) (arrow). (A) CT scan without IV contrast material shows an exophytic RCC that measures 48 Hounsfield units. (B) CT scan following IV contrast material again shows the RCC now with a better determination of the medial margin. The RCC enhanced to 139 Hounsfield units.

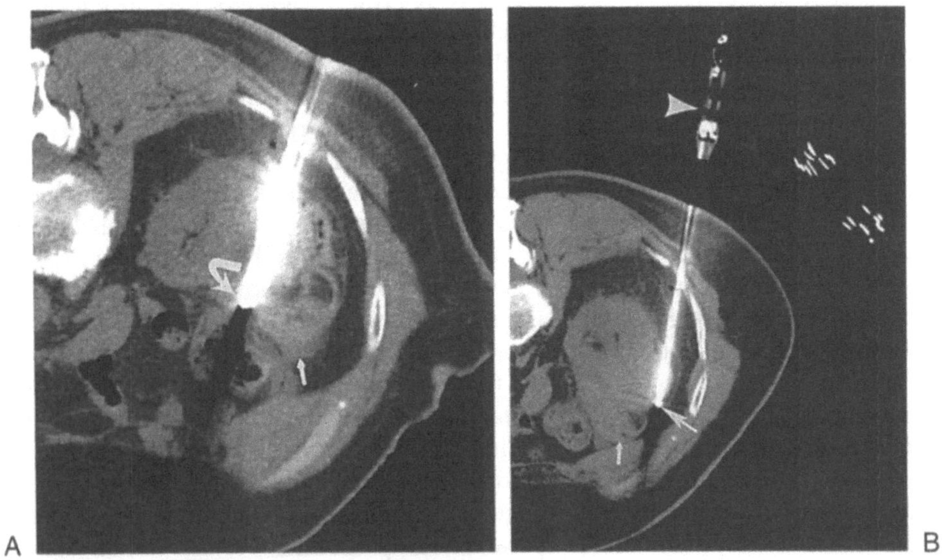

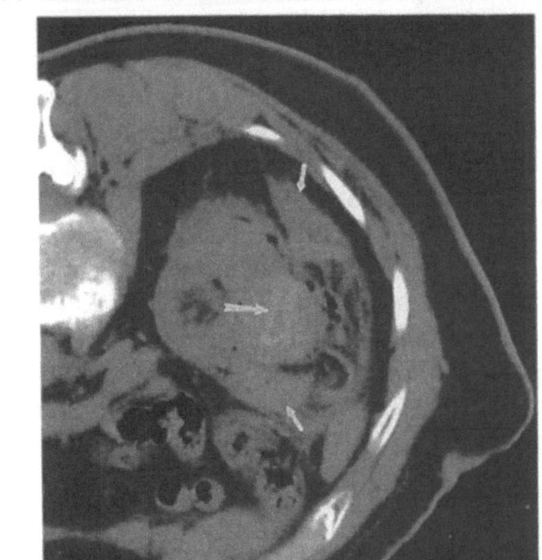

FIGURE 27.2. CT scan during and immediately following radiofrequency ablation (RFA). (A) CT scan with the patient prone shows cluster needle electrode (curved arrow) near the medial margin of the tumor. Note that a small amount of hemorrhage (small arrow) displaces the tumor from the colon. (B) CT scan shows the cluster electrode (arrow) repositioned into the lateral and inferior aspects of the tumor. Again seen is a small amount of hemorrhage (small arrow) anteriorly. The electrode handle (arrowhead) is demonstrated. When positioning the patient for CT-guided RFA, the operator must leave enough room for the patient and the electrode handle to fit within the CT gantry. (C) CT scan performed after final removal of the electrodes and a total of four overlapping ablations shows hemorrhage anterior and posterior to the kidney (small arrows). There is scattered air adjacent to the tumor. Note the linear bands of increased density (arrow) within the tumor. This finding is thought to be from desiccation related to RFA.

indicates fast tissue cooling and suggests the thermal lesion will not be at the large end of the range. If rapid cooling is encountered, the umbrella device can be redeployed in the exact same location following rotation of the tines so as to deploy them in different locations within the tumor. The straight needle system can be repositioned more closely than might be the case if high temperatures are achieved and maintained. In addition, once a straight needle is repositioned, the temperature reading over 60°C suggests that it is in an area already treated by the prior ablation. Although no single parameter allows accurate prediction of the final ablation margins, with experience the operator can integrate all of this information and perform overlapping ablations accordingly (Fig. 27.2).

For exophytic tumors, some authors have suggested that the first ablation be strategically performed at the interface between tumor and normal kidney so as to limit blood flow to the remainder of the tumor and thereby facilitate coagulation necrosis for the remaining overlapping ablations (26). When easily achievable, this is a reasonable approach. However, depending on the location and orientation of the tumor–kidney interface, percutaneous placement of a straight needle electrode directly at the interface may not be possible due to intervening structures. Indeed, tumors have been treated successfully with RFA in our experience with a needle electrode approach perpendicular to the tumor–kidney interface.

Ablation sessions are terminated once the operator has performed overlapping ablations from which complete coagulation necrosis is anticipated (7). For very large tumors, more than one session can be anticipated. The maximum ablation that can be achieved in any session usually is based on the duration of adequate analgesia and sedation determined by limits set by institutional protocol (7).

Ideally, for patient convenience and for cost minimization, a strategy that achieves complete tumor treatment in a single session is desirable. Tumors 3 cm or smaller are almost all treated with a single session. However, for tumors 3 cm or larger, a significant minority of patients in our experience has required second ablation sessions to achieve complete necrosis (7). Although multiple sessions are less than ideal, for some patients who are unable to have surgery, a second session is not unreasonably onerous if it can achieve complete tumor necrosis.

Complications and Postablation Syndrome

The most commonly reported major complication associated with percutaneous RFA of RCC is hemorrhage (6,7,18,19). In all reported cases, hemorrhage and its treatment resulted in no prolonged deleterious outcomes. Other reported complications include ureteral strictures (7). Although not yet reported, injury to other organs or structures such as bowel, adrenal gland, spleen, lung, or pancreas is possible. Skin burns at the grounding pad sites also can occur. To date, there have been no reports of procedure-related mortality.

The postablation syndrome, described as flu-like symptoms, consisting of generalized aches, malaise, and fevers to 103°F can occur after RFA, although we have not seen this syndrome as commonly with RCC as with liver tumors. Although anecdotally felt to be more common following larger volume ablations, the incidence of this syndrome and the predisposing factors are not well known, especially with respect to ablation of RCC.

Postablation Imaging

Since necrotic tumor is left in situ, imaging remains the only effective means of evaluation of the entire tumor volume, and thus plays a critical role in the evaluation of patients following RFA. The key determinant of residual viable tumor following RFA ablation is the uptake of contrast material administered intravenously (6,7,18,27). Portions of tumor that do not enhance reflect regions of coagulation necrosis (Fig. 27.3). Regions that demonstrate persistent enhancement reflect residual disease. This interpretation of imaging findings is extrapolated from radiologic-pathologic corre-

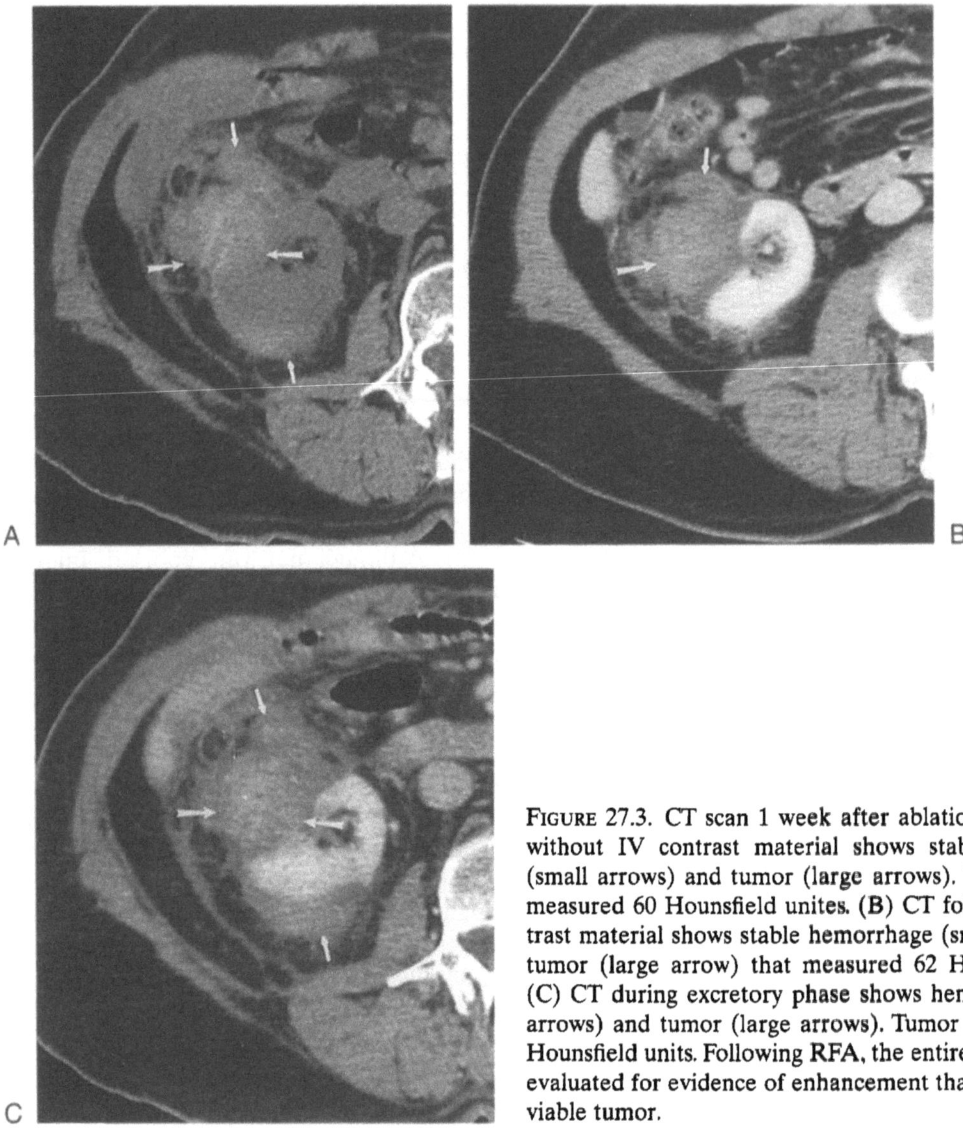

FIGURE 27.3. CT scan 1 week after ablation. (A) CT scan without IV contrast material shows stable hemorrhage (small arrows) and tumor (large arrows). The tumor now measured 60 Hounsfield unites. (B) CT following IV contrast material shows stable hemorrhage (small arrow) and tumor (large arrow) that measured 62 Hounsfield units. (C) CT during excretory phase shows hemorrhage (small arrows) and tumor (large arrows). Tumor remained at 62 Hounsfield units. Following RFA, the entire tumor must be evaluated for evidence of enhancement that would suggest viable tumor.

lation work performed in hepatic tumors (27). Goldberg et al (27) were able to confirm coagulation necrosis that corresponded to areas of nonenhancement to within 2mm. Persistent peripheral nodular enhancement correlated pathologically with viable tumor. Ongoing clinical experience supports the use of this CT interpretation scheme for postablation imaging of renal tumors.

On postablation CT, the tumor typically does not disappear. A decrease in maximum diameter by 1 to 5mm is common (7,18). Nonenhancing regions of adjacent renal parenchyma may be seen following RFA (18,28). Although CT is the modality used for assessment of RFA in most patients, for patients who cannot receive IV contrast material because of renal insufficiency or prior anaphylactoid reaction, MRI, without and with gadolinium-chelate enhancement may be useful (6,7).

Imaging generally is performed at more frequent intervals in the early postablation period. Generally, we have been assessing patients within approximately 1 month, 3 months, and 6 months (6,7). Once the 1-year CT is reached, and no viable tumor has been demonstrated, then CT scans can be performed at 1-year intervals.

Clinical Experience to Date

While only a few reports have appeared in the literature, the delays from manuscript preparation to publication guarantee a larger cumulative experience than the approximately 90 cases reported thus far. The total cumulative experience of most of the large centers performing RFA of RCC is now likely to be well over many hundreds of patients. The reported series provide strong support for the use of RFA for small tumors, less than 3.0 cm. For exophytic tumors up to 5.0 cm, our experience has been that up to 30% of these patients may require a second ablation session, but complete coagulation necrosis can be achieved in all cases (7).

Review of published series must take into account changes in technology that evolved rapidly over the middle to late 1990s. Generator systems have become more powerful so that early preclinical or clinical suboptimal results need to be reevaluated with the more powerful modern systems. Several early reports were based on work with 50-W generators. An early study that compared the three available systems found that the most powerful created the largest lesion, suggesting that power output might be a factor that limited the size of thermal lesions with less strong generators (29). With most generator systems now in clinical use in the 150- to 250-W range, further increases in power are not likely to further augment the volume of a single ablation.

Several developments in RFA of RCC are likely in the foreseeable future. Radiofrequency ablation systems are readily available and relatively inexpensive. Thus, in the near future, the use of RFA ablation to treat RCC is likely to continue to grow as the technology continues to disseminate. To emphasize a point made previously, a more thorough evaluation of outcomes compared to surgical resection can be performed once 5-year results are available. These data are likely to be available in the next 2 to 3 years. In addition, RFA may be useful in a limited number of patients with small foci of isolated metastatic RCC that appear after nephrectomy. Reports of successful treatment of isolated lung nodules and lymph nodes have already appeared (30,31).

Conclusions

Radiofrequency ablation of kidney tumors has shown encouraging early results using modern RF-generator systems designed for soft tissue tumor ablation. While 5-year data are pending, limitation of this therapeutic option to patients who are not good candidates for surgical resection of RCC is prudent. Postablation imaging is critical for assessment of ablation success, and radiologists must be familiar with the appearance of necrotic tissue and viable tumor.

References

1. Novick AC, Campbell SC. Renal tumors. In: Walsh PC, ed. Campbell's Urology. 8th ed. Philadelphia: WB Saunders, 2002:2672–2731.
2. Greenlee RT, Murray T, Bolden S, Wingo PA. Cancer statistics 2000. CA Cancer J Clin 2000; 50:7–33.
3. Jayson M, Sanders H. Increased incidence of serendipitously discovered renal cell carcinoma. Urology 1998;51:203–205.
4. Chow WH, Devesa SS, Warren JL, Fraumeni JF. Rising incidence of renal cell cancer in the United States. JAMA 1999;281:1628–1631.
5. Kidney. In: American Joint Committee on Cancer: AJCC Cancer Staging Manual. 5th ed. Philadelphia: Lippincott-Raven, 1997:231–234.
6. Gervais DA, McGovern FJ, Wood BJ, Goldberg SN, McDougal WS, Mueller PR. Radio-frequency ablation of renal cell carcinoma: early clinical experience. Radiology 2000;217:665–672.
7. Gervais DA, McGovern FJ, Arellano RS, McDougal WS, Mueller PR. Radiofrequency ablation of renal cell carcinoma: clinical experience and technical success in 42 tumors. Radiology 2003;226(2):417–424.
8. Gettman MT, Blute ML. Update on pathologic staging of renal cell carcinoma. Urology 2002; 60:209–217.
9. Medeiros LJ, Jones EC, Aizawa S, et al. Grading of renal cell carcinoma. Cancer 1997;80:990–991.

10. Storkel S, Eble JN, Adlakha K, et al. Classification of renal cell carcinoma. Cancer 1997;80: 987–989.
11. Swanson DA, Rothenberg HJ, Boynton AL, et al. Future prognostic factors for renal cell carcinoma. Cancer 1997;80:997–998.
12. Uzzo RG, Novick AC. Nephron sparing surgery for renal tumors: indications, techniques and outcomes. J Urol 2001;166:6–18.
13. Reddan DN, Raj GV, Polascik TJ. Management of small renal tumors: an overview. Am J Med 2001;110:558–562.
14. Goldberg SN, Gazelle GS, Mueller PR. Thermal ablation therapy for focal malignancy: a unified approach to underlying principles, techniques, and diagnostic imaging guidance. AJR 2000;174: 323–331.
15. Livraghi T, Goldberg SN, Lazzaroni S, et al. Hepatocellular carcinoma: radiofrequency ablation of medium and large lesions. Radiology 2000;214:761–768.
16. Livraghi T, Goldberg SN, Lazzaroni S, Meloni F, Solbiati L, Gazelle GS. Small hepatocellular carcinoma: treatment with radiofrequency ablation versus ethanol injection. Radiology 1999;210: 655–661.
17. Goldberg SN, Hahn PF, Tanabe KK, et al. Percutaneous radiofrequency tissue ablation: does perfusion mediated tissue cooling limit coagulation necrosis? J Vasc Intervent Radiol 1998;9: 101–111.
18. Pavlovich CP, Walther MM, Choyke PL, et al. Percutaneous radio frequency ablation of small renal tumors: initial results. J Urol 2002;167: 10–15.
19. Mayo-Smith WW, Dupuy DE, Ridlen MS, Cronan JJ. Radiofrequency ablation of solid renal masses: results of 26 consecutive treatments in 22 patients. AJR 2003;180(6):1503–1508.
20. Lewin JS, Connell CF, Duerk JL, et al. Interactive MRI-guided radiofrequency interstitial thermal ablation of abdominal tumors: clinical trial for evaluation of safety and feasibility. J Magn Reson Imaging 1998;8:40–47.
21. Wood BJ, Khan MA, McGovern F, Harisinghani M, Hahn PF, Mueller PR. Imaging guided biopsy of renal masses: indications, accuracy and impact on clinical management. J Urol 1999;161:1470–1474.
22. American Society of Anesthesiologists Task Force on Sedation and Analgesia by Non-Anesthesiologists. Practice guidelines for sedation and analgesia by nonanesthesiologists. Anesthesiology 1996;84:459–470.
23. Zlotta AR, Wildschutz T, Raviv G, et al. Radiofrequency interstitial tumor ablation (RITA) is a possible new modality for treatment of renal cancer: ex vivo and in vivo experience. J Endourol 1997;11:251–258.
24. Zlotta AR, Schulman CC. Ablation of renal tumors in a rabbit model with interstitial saline-augmented radiofrequency energy. Urology 1999;54:382–383.
25. Dodd GD III, Frank MS, Aribandi M, Chopra S, Chintapalli KN. Radiofrequency thermal ablation: computer analysis of the size of the thermal injury created by overlapping ablations. AJR 2001;77: 777–782.
26. Dupuy DE, Mayo-Smith WW, Cronan JJ. Image-guided biopsy and radiofrequency ablation of renal masses. Semin Intervent Radiol 2000;17: 373–380.
27. Goldberg SN, Gazelle GS, Compton CC, Mueller PR, Tanabe KK. Treatment of intrahepatic malignancy with radiofrequency ablation: radiologic-pathologic correlation. Cancer 2000; 88:2452–2463.
28. Gervais DA, O'Neill MJ, Arellano RS, McGovern FJ, McDougal WS, Mueller PR. Peritumoral CT changes associated with radiofrequency (RF) ablation of focal renal lesions: description, incidence, and significance. Radiology 2001;221(P):180.
29. de Baere T, Denys A, Kuoch V, Elias D, Vilgrain V, Roche A. Radio-frequency tissue ablation of the liver: in vivo and ex vivo experiments with four different systems. Eur Radiol 2003;13(10): 2346–2352.
30. Zagoria RJ, Chen MY, Kavanagh PV, Torti FM. Radiofrequency ablation of lung metastases from renal cell carcinoma. J Urol 2001;166: 1827–1828.
31. Gervais DA, Arellano R, McDougal WS, McGovern FJ, Mueller PR. Radiofrequency (RF) ablation of metastatic soft tissue tumors of the genitourinary system: indications, results, and the role of RFA after failed conventional therapies. Radiology 2001;221(P):261.

28 Radiofrequency Ablation for Thoracic Neoplasms

Sapna K. Jain and Damian E. Dupuy

Lung cancer statistics in the United States estimate that 171,900 people in 2003 were diagnosed with lung cancer (1). As the leading cause of cancer death among men and women in the United States, the associated death rate for lung cancer is 28%, surpassing mortality rates of colon, prostate, and breast cancer combined (1). This startling fact underscores the importance of improved methods to treat this aggressive form of cancer. Its ominous prognosis is reflected by the overall 5-year survival rates for previously untreated patients with primary non–small-cell lung cancer (NSCLC) after surgical treatment (according to pathologic stage): 63% to 67% in stage IA, 46% to 57% in IB, 52% to 55% in IIA, 33% to 39% in IIB, and 19% to 23% in IIIA (2,3).

With NSCLC, 30% of patients present with disease confined to the parenchyma, 30% with spread to intrathoracic lymph nodes, and 40% with metastatic disease (4). In cases of regional disease, a combination of surgery, chemotherapy, and external beam radiation therapy [x-ray therapy (XRT)] prevails as standard treatment. For patients with localized disease not invading the mediastinum, surgical resection remains the best treatment option. Surgery is not the primary treatment when there are coexistent morbid medical conditions or advanced stage of the disease. In these patients who are not surgical candidates, the treatment options rely primarily on XRT, with or without chemotherapy. In small-cell lung cancer and in other cases in which radiotherapy cannot be administered, chemotherapy may be administered solely. The best current therapies result in an overall 5-year survival rate, for all stages combined, of only 15% (1). The poor response of lung cancer to current treatment methods necessitates the use of alternative modalities.

Less invasive therapies that can accomplish tumor destruction or complete eradication without the use of general anesthesia may complement, improve, or replace existing therapies. One such ablative tumor therapy that may add to the treatment regimen in this complex group of patients is radiofrequency ablation (RFA). Percutaneous image-guided tumor RFA is an expanding minimally invasive modality for the local treatment of solid malignancies. First reported in 2000 (5), RF ablation of human lung tumors may be a promising treatment option for nonsurgical candidates, given the suboptimal outcomes with current treatment. The insertion of an RF electrode into the defined tumor bed and establishment of an electric field to a reference electrode that oscillates with generated alternating RF currents ultimately create a conduit for frictional heating (6). This tissue heating consequently induces coagulative necrosis and cell death in a controlled and predictable manner (6). The surrounding air in the normal parenchyma of the lung acts as an insulator and concentrates RF energy in the targeted tissue, thereby requiring less energy deposition (7). The high vascular flow of the lung results in a "heat-sink" effect that dissipates heat away from normal adjacent tissue and concentrates the effective energy deposition within the solid component of the lesion. This chapter discusses the clinical rationale, technique, potential applications, and early clinical experience in thoracic RFA.

Clinical Scenarios

General

Lung neoplasms are a heterogeneous group of tumors. Primary lung cancer can be categorized into several different cell types: squamous cell carcinoma, adenocarcinoma (including bronchoalveolar), large cell carcinoma, and small cell carcinoma. These different cell types have different biologic properties; thus the disease presentation and treatment may differ accordingly. For example, the effective response rate to XRT in cases of lung cancer metastatic to bone varies with cell type: 80% for small cell carcinoma, 72% for adenocarcinoma, and 40% for squamous cell carcinoma (8). As stated earlier, stage at presentation is a critical determinant of the treatment strategy. Stage IV (metastatic disease) is quite variable in its clinical course and outcome. Certain metastatic histologies such as osteosarcoma tend to be isolated to the lungs, have an indolent growth pattern similar to renal cell carcinoma or colorectal carcinoma (9), and therefore are more likely to respond to a local form of therapy.

New minimally invasive treatments must bring new benefits for patients. A shotgun approach could be detrimental to the patient, as well as hinder research and acceptance of any new treatment modality. As with the application of any new treatment, utilization of a multidisciplinary team ensures a prudent clinical approach with the patient's interests paramount. Pulmonary tumor boards or general oncology tumor boards are excellent venues for educational exchange and should be attended by anyone engaged in the treatment of lung neoplasms.

Metastatic Disease

Surgical treatment of metastatic lung cancer is controversial, given the lack of randomized controlled clinical trials comparing surgery with nonoperative treatments, but its use is becoming more widely accepted (10,11). Pulmonary metastasectomy for isolated pulmonary metastases of different tumor types results in an overall 5-year survival rate of approximately 36% (12), and is associated with a mortality rate of <2% (11). Indications for surgery include exclusion of other distant disease, no tumor at the primary site, probability of complete resection, and adequate cardiopulmonary reserve to withstand the operation. However, there are several clinical scenarios in which local therapy via surgery or alternative treatment modalities may improve survival or provide palliation when these indications are not met. Cited 5-year survival rates range are as follows for pulmonary metastasectomy: osteogenic sarcoma, 20% to 50%; soft tissue sarcoma, 18% to 28%; head and neck carcinoma, 40.9% to 47%; colon carcinoma, 21% to 48% (13), breast carcinoma, 31% to 49.5% (11); and renal cell carcinoma, 20% to 44% (14). Repeat resection is supported in select patients who are free of disease at the primary location, but have recurrent metastatic disease to the lung (15,16).

Palliative Care

Given that many patients with lung neoplasms present with advanced disease and that the majority of patients with lung cancer (86%) will die from their disease (17,18), one can deduce that at least one of the following symptoms/problems will clinically manifest itself during the course of the disease: pain, dyspnea, cough, hemoptysis, metastases to the central nervous system or musculoskeletal system, tracheoesophageal fistula, or obstruction of the superior vena cava (18). Symptomatic palliation, therefore, becomes an important part of treatment, yet the current medical literature reports failure to do so (19), with 50% of patients dying without adequate pain relief (20). Approximately 5% of lung cancers extend beyond the lung to invade the pleura, soft tissues, or osseous structures of the chest wall (21).

Three main causes of malignancy-related pain in lung cancer are osseous metastatic disease (34%), Pancoast tumor (31%), and chest wall disease (21%) (22). Mechanisms that result in pain include tumor progression and related pathology (e.g., periosteal inflammation, nerve damage), side effects of radiation or chemotherapy, infection, and muscle aches secondary to limited physical capability. Approximately 70% to 90% of patients with advanced cancer have pain, and effective palliation can be achieved in 90% (18,19).

The management of cancer pain is addressed by the clinical practical guidelines from the Agency for Health Care Policy and Research (AHCPR) (23, now not current according to its Web site, but referenced in the literature). Various strategies and potential disadvantages include analgesic medications (nonsteroidals, acetaminophen, morphine) that may impair mental function; palliative radiation that may fail to affect insensitive tumors, damage normal tissue, and/or be limited by maximum tolerated doses; antineoplastic therapies (with the goal of reducing tumor burden); nerve blocks that have short-lived effects; and palliative invasive surgery.

Conventional treatment of osseous metastatic disease involves XRT and chemotherapy. X-ray therapy has been shown to palliate respiratory symptoms and improve quality of life in patients with NSCLC (24). Current recommendations by the AHCPR for bone metastases include pharmacologic use to control pain, followed by XRT to control localized pain. The use of systemic corticosteroids (prednisone, 20–40 mg/d), bisphosphonates, calcitonin, and radiopharmaceuticals (e.g., ethylenediamine tetramethylene phosphonic acid or strontium-89 chloride) may be used with or without XRT. The results, however, are poor to fair, with a small to moderate net benefit. Furthermore, extension of tumor into the chest wall and osseous metastatic disease can be limited and difficult to treat with XRT, since prior treatment fields may have encompassed the symptomatic region. Current treatment thus is often ineffective in complex patients (25–27). Because up to 70% of patients have disease that is too advanced for resection (28), newer alternatives such as percutaneous ethanol injection, embolization of bone tumor vasculature, and RFA may be considered salvage methods by providing, at minimum, palliative relief to patients who fail conventional modalities. Utilization of RFA in the treatment of pain due to trigeminal neuralgia and osteoid osteoma has been documented (29,30).

Chest Wall Invasion

Cited 5-year survival rates for NSCLC with chest wall invasion treated surgically range from 15% to 38% (31). When microscopically incomplete or gross residual disease after attempted resection is present, overall 5-year survival rate declines to 4% (21). Survival rates are dependent on the extent of nodal involvement, depth of invasion, and the completeness of resection (21). Incomplete resections, even if leaving only microscopic disease, offer no chance for cure for the patient (21).

Technique

Patients referred for lung tumor RFA initially are evaluated in a clinic setting where the patient history and pertinent imaging studies are reviewed. At this time, the appropriateness for RFA, risks and benefits of the procedure, and any additional preprocedural studies are discussed and planned. This preprocedural evaluation is similar to a surgical evaluation, whereby any possible risks of bleeding or serious cardiopulmonary issues are addressed. Side effects from this procedure, such as postprocedural pyrexia secondary to conductive local heating of tissue and circulatory systemic heating through the bloodstream (32) also are discussed. In general, virtually all patients healthy enough to undergo computed tomography (CT)-guided needle biopsy are good candidates for pulmonary RFA. Patients with only one lung can safely undergo pulmonary RFA, as long as provisions for rapid deployment of a chest catheter are made. Patients with severe emphysema who require supplemental oxygen also can be treated. However, it is important to remember that patients with emphysema who retain carbon dioxide may lose their respiratory drive when given higher percentages of supplemental oxygen under conscious sedation during an RFA procedure. Patients with underlying idiopathic pulmonary fibrosis should be considered poor candidates for pulmonary RFA, as exacerbation of the underlying disease may lead to serious respiratory failure and death after the procedure.

To reduce potential complications of sedation-induced nausea and aspiration of gastric contents, all patients fast overnight. Patients may take hypertension and cardiac medications in the morning with a small quantity of water. Insulin-dependent diabetic patients should administer half of their usual morning insulin dose. An abridged physical exam is performed outside the procedure suite and an intravenous line is placed. Thirty minutes prior to the commencement of the procedure, all patients are given 0.625 mg of droperidol intravenously for sedative and antiemetic effects. Patients with Parkinson's disease should not receive droperidol, as it may exacerbate symptoms.

Patients then are brought to the CT scanner where the technical staff places the appropriate grounding pads on the opposite chest wall from the skin entry site (e.g., anterior chest wall for patient lying prone) to direct the RF current and thus prevent damage to adjacent structures in the target area. After the initial scout images are taken, a skin mark is placed on the patient that corresponds to the entry site determined by the computer grid at the appropriate table position. Horizontal and vertical laser lights in the CT gantry correspond to the x- and y-axes from the computer grid on the screen, and a ruler can be placed to match the desired skin entry site as determined on the computer screen. The area is prepped and draped in sterile fashion, and local buffered lidocaine anesthesia is administered both intradermally and to the level of the pleura with a 25-gauge skin needle and a 22-gauge spinal needle, respectively. Computed tomography fluoroscopy is initiated, and an image is taken with the spinal needle in place to identify proper table position and needle angle. Repositioning can be performed with the spinal needle if necessary. A small skin incision is made at the correct skin entry site by a No. 11 scalpel blade 1 to 2 cm into the subcutaneous tissues.

The RF electrode is placed through the skin and pleura to a length that corresponds to one-half to two-thirds the distance to the target lesion. A CT-fluoroscopic image is obtained, and the RF electrode angle in the x, y, and z planes is corrected as necessary.

For pleural-based masses, a shorter RF electrode is used. Placement of the electrode within the target tumor in this situation may need to be performed without initial superficial positioning, since superficial placement from a lateral position may result in protrusion of the electrode that limits placement of the patient into the CT gantry. A coaxial guiding instrument also could be used in this situation, whereby the RF electrode is placed directly into the mass after the correct outer cannula position has been confirmed.

For lesions smaller than 2 cm in diameter, central and distal positioning of the RF electrode usually is adequate for the first ablation with subsequent tandem ablation zones performed during more proximal positioning. When at all possible, the target lesion should be entered along its longitudinal axis to allow for this type of sequential overlapping tandem ablations during electrode withdrawal. For lesions larger than 2 cm in diameter, larger electrodes or multiple overlapping ablation zones may need to be performed to ensure adequate thermocoagulation of the target lesion.

Ablation of the liver may be used as a comparison to the lung. Similar to liver tumor ablation, working around the periphery of larger tumors in the lung helps ensure adequate ablation of the soft tissue margins. Ablation of lung tumors, in contrast to tumors in the liver, tends to require less time and current to achieve adequate thermocoagulation. The baseline circuit impedance of small parenchymal masses surrounded by aerated lung may not allow the same amount of current deposition compared to a liver tumor ablation. Depending on the RF equipment employed, each ablation should be carried out according to the manufacturer's specifications regarding temperature and/or impedance.

Just prior to and during RF heating, patients are given intravenous conscious sedation with midazolam (1 mg doses) and fentanyl (50 μg doses) monitored by continuous vital signs and an electrocardiogram. The RF heating of small parenchymal masses away from the visceral pleura may require less sedation and may not produce any pain. On the other hand, pleural-based masses can be quite painful during RF heating. Given the somatic innervation of the parietal pleura (via the intercostal and phrenic nerves), irritation may result in pain felt either on the body wall or in the corresponding dermatomes, for which multiple doses of sedation during the procedure may be needed. Radiofrequency heating of central lesions adjacent to bronchi elicits a prominent cough response from patients that may require sedation to reduce patient motion. Occasionally, general anesthesia may need to be used in pediatric patients or patients who may not tolerate the RF heating with conscious sedation alone. Dual-lumen endotracheal (ET) tubes are not necessary as the pulmonary bleeding from RFA is not any different from that in a CT-guided biopsy and may be less, given the coagulating effect of the RF current.

After the target tumor is treated, the RF electrode is removed and a CT-fluoroscopic image is obtained to evaluate for a pneumothorax. Large pneumothoraces can be evacuated at this time with chest catheters and wall suction. Smaller asymptomatic pneumothoraces can be followed with chest radiographs. In the latter group, we put patients on 100% oxygen via a nonrebreathing mask and obtain an immediate chest radiograph, followed by a 2-hour chest x-ray. An increasing pneumothorax on this 2-hour follow-up typically necessitates chest catheter placement. Once a chest catheter has been placed and there is radiographic documentation of pneumothorax resolution, the patient may be discharged with a Heimlich valve that is placed on the end of the catheter. A 24-hour follow-up chest x-ray is formed. Hospitalization may be required because of pain or patient apprehension about outpatient chest catheter management. If the pneumothorax is resolved on follow-up chest x-ray, the tube is checked for an air leak by having the patient cough with the tube end in a container of sterile water. If no air bubbles are visualized, then the tube is removed with a petroleum jelly–based gauze to provide an airtight seal on removal. In patients with air leaks, prolonged chest catheter drainage may be required, which may include placement of a surgical chest tube that will require prolonged hospitalization. All patients are observed for at least 2 hours postprocedure, and interval follow-up imaging is scheduled at discharge.

Potential Applications and Early Clinical Experience

The application of radiofrequency energy to pulmonary neoplasms is a revolutionary concept whose clinical applications are just beginning to be developed. Unlike conventional therapies such as chemotherapy and XRT, multiple applications can be performed for local control without additional difficulty or morbidity. The safety is not significantly different from that of a lung biopsy. Almost all of our RF procedures are performed in an outpatient setting. Contraindications for RFA are few; they include uncorrectable bleeding disorders and recent use of anticoagulants. Potential complications include pneumothorax, hemorrhage, pleural effusion, pleurisy, damage to adjacent anatomic structures (low likelihood given the predictable nature of the procedure), skin burns secondary to grounding pads, and infection. The exact role of RFA for pulmonary neoplasms and its complementary applications with standard therapies remains to be elucidated. Early data are extremely encouraging, and continued clinical research will be necessary to define precisely which patients will benefit most from this novel therapy.

The most exciting application for RFA is the treatment of primary bronchogenic carcinoma, specifically NSCLC. With the overall 5-year relative survival rate for all stages less than 15% (1), newer treatment modalities are sorely needed. Since RFA is a local therapy, the clearest indication for its utilization would be in incidental or screen-detected stage I disease in which the tumor size is less than 3 cm in diameter and there is no evidence of regional or distant spread by staging CT or positron emission tomography (PET) scanning. The gold standard therapy for this group of patients is lobectomy, which has a 70% five-year survival (33). Studies report overall 5-year survival rates ranging from 53.8% to 82% when both anatomic (lobectomy) and nonanatomic (limited/wedge resection) are included (34–38). However, many patients with stage I tumors are poor surgical candidates due to severe underlying cardiopulmonary disease. In this group of patients, a limited local therapy such as RFA or radiotherapy may benefit survival compared to no treatment (Fig. 28.1).

In patients with localized disease who can be treated safely by RFA, tumor control can be achieved (25). We have just completed a phase II trial comparing combination therapy of primary RFA followed by conventional XRT to the known historical data of radiotherapy alone. Given the low sensitivity and specificity of CT to detect mediastinal lymph nodes, as well as the influence of lymph node metastases on prognosis, PET scanning was used to evaluate lymph nodes rather than primary tumor status. Tumor staging was done by PET scanning, and PET and CT are used to evaluate local progression (Fig. 18.2). Pulmonary toxicity was evaluated by pre- and posttherapy pulmonary function testing. In the 23 patients treated with this approach with a median follow-up of 16 months, there have been no local treatment failures. Four patients have died: one from a cerebrovascular accident 3 months after completion of therapy, two from early metastatic disease that was detected within 3 months of RFA, and one patient 18 months after therapy secondary to respiratory failure. No significant pulmonary toxicities have been observed. These early results are encouraging and we eagerly await the long-term results.

Pulmonary RFA alone for the treatment of primary lung cancer is not validated currently, given prospective surgical data that demonstrate a threefold increase (or 75% increase) and 2.4-fold increase in the locoregional recurrence rate with local treatment (wedge resection and segmental resection, respectively)

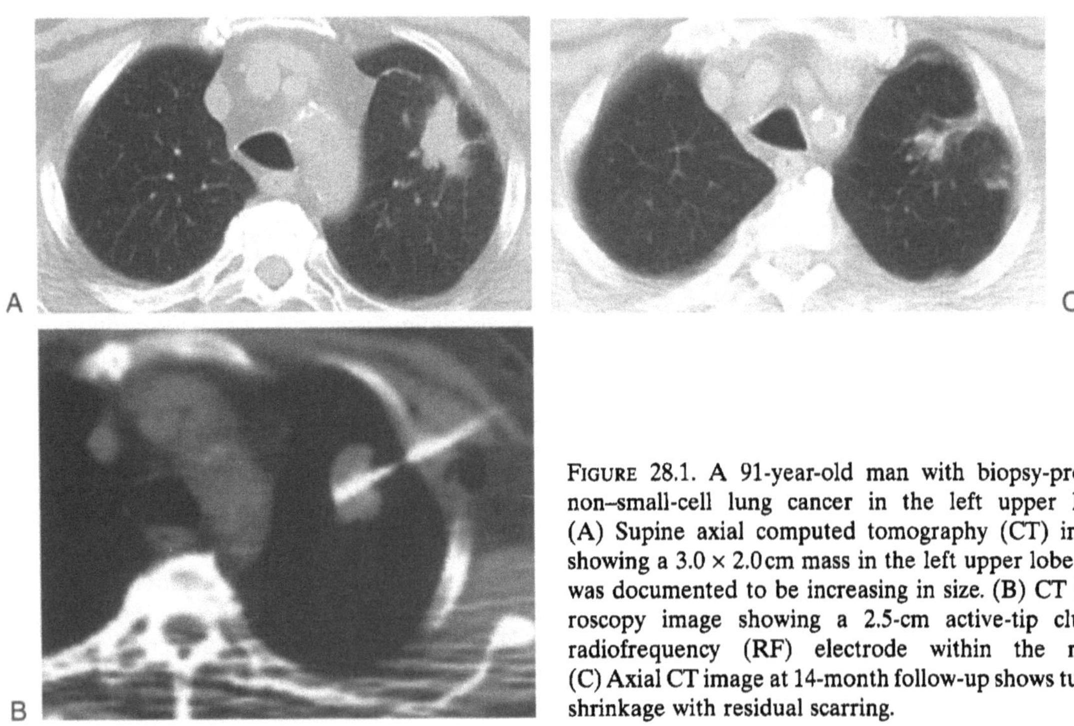

FIGURE 28.1. A 91-year-old man with biopsy-proven non–small-cell lung cancer in the left upper lobe. (A) Supine axial computed tomography (CT) image showing a 3.0 × 2.0 cm mass in the left upper lobe that was documented to be increasing in size. (B) CT fluoroscopy image showing a 2.5-cm active-tip cluster radiofrequency (RF) electrode within the mass. (C) Axial CT image at 14-month follow-up shows tumor shrinkage with residual scarring.

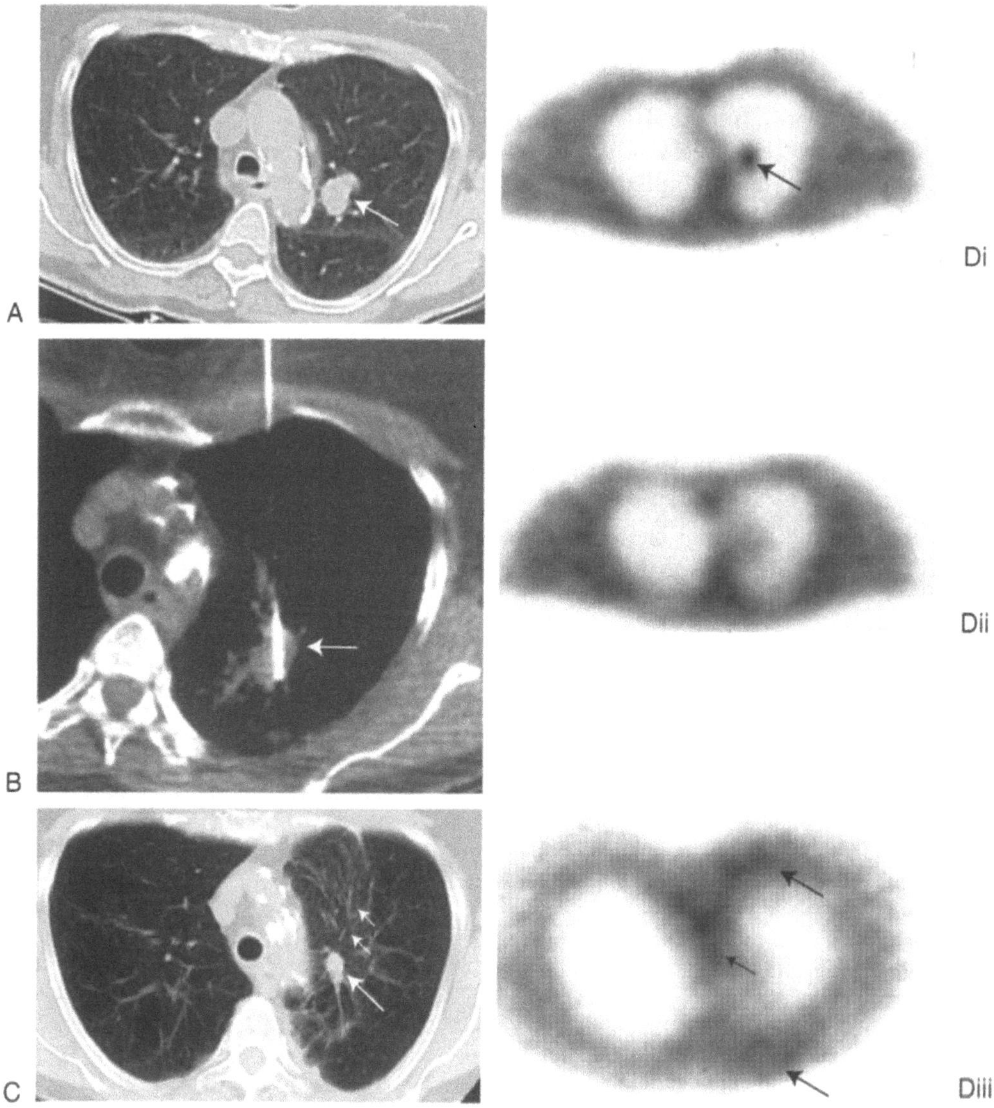

FIGURE 28.2. A 76-year-old woman with primary non–small-cell lung carcinoma (T1N0M0) of the left lung. (A) Axial CT showing a circumscribed 2-cm mass in the mid-aspect of the left upper lobe (arrow). (B) Radiofrequency ablation (RFA) of the tumor with the electrode (arrow) in the tumor bed. (C) Axial CT at 20 months follow-up status post–RFA and x-ray therapy (XRT) showing tumor contraction (large arrow), diffuse emphysematous changes, and scarring (small arrows) consistent with XRT. (D) Axial positron emission tomography (PET) images prior to RFA (i), 7 months status post–RFA and XRT (ii), and 16 months status posttreatment (iii). (i) Focal increased area of uptake in the left suprahilar region after 6.6 mCi of F-18 FDG (arrow). (ii) Previously noted focus of activity in left suprahilar region no longer seen. iii. Increased uptake in the superficial anterior and posterior thorax (large arrow) as well as minimum uptake in the left mediastinum (small arrow), likely secondary to radiation-related changes. No evidence of tumor recurrence is shown.

compared to lobectomy (17). Recurrences after a "complete" resection will develop over the next 5 years in 20% to 30% of patients with stage I disease, in 50% with stage II, and in 70% to 80% with stage III disease (39). More current studies that compare limited resection (segmentectomy) and lymph node assessment versus lobectomy in patients with stage IA NSCLC with tumor size less than 2 cm in diameter have shown equivalent rates for overall 5-year survival (87.1% vs. 93%) and local recurrence (40,41). Thus, in a properly selected patient population, wedge resection or segmentectomy may be superior to nonsurgical alternatives. Recurrence from residual microscopic disease may be delayed or prevented with neoadjuvant and adjuvant chemotherapy and XRT (4,42). External beam reirradiation also has been documented as a potential solution to recurrence in the current literature (43), but complications such as radiation pneumonitis, esophagitis, or myelopathy are potential hazards.

Explanations for recurrence include inadequate resection of the primary tumor and the presence of microscopic lymphatic disease within the lung and ipsilateral hilar nodes. Unfortunately, these microscopic deposits cannot be detected, and current RF technology does not allow the treatment region to extend far enough into normal aerated lung parenchyma. Yet for patients who are nonsurgical candidates due to comorbid conditions, poor cardiopulmonary reserve, or prior XRT with regrowth in the treatment field, RFA is an alternative (Fig. 28.3). Studies on repeated pulmonary metastasectomy for recurrent disease have reported 5-year survival rates of 48% (16).

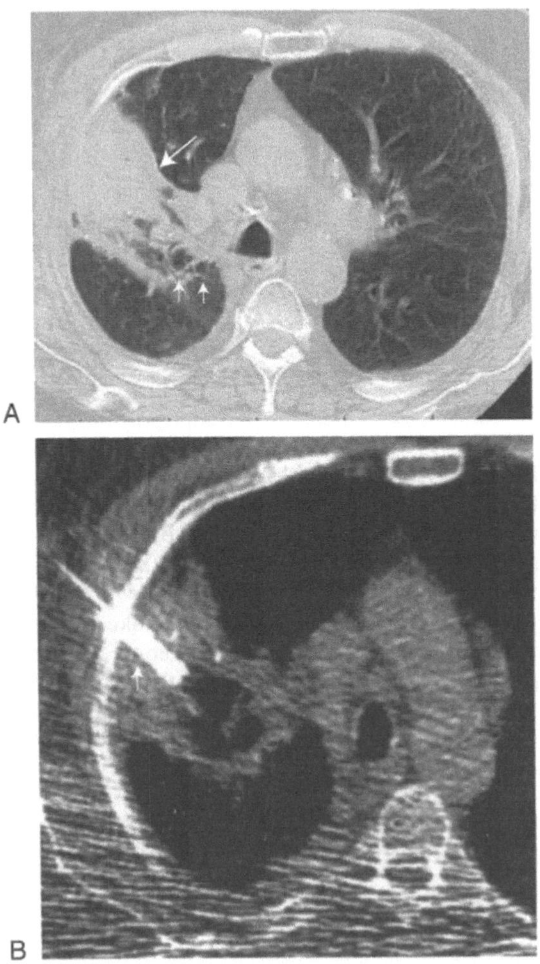

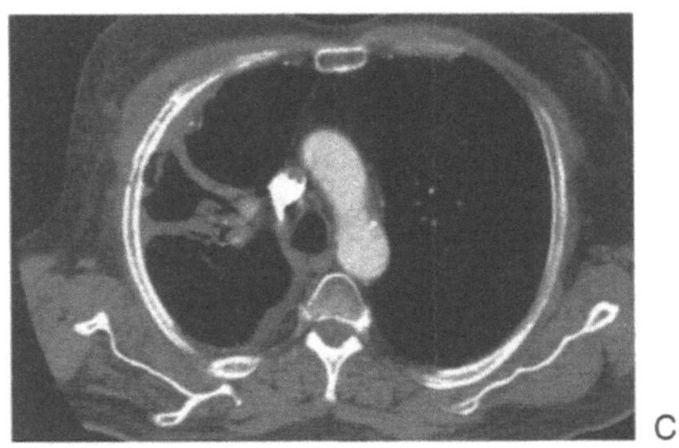

FIGURE 28.3. A 71-year-old man with non–small-cell lung carcinoma involving the right upper lobe status post–chemotherapy and radiation with regrowth within the radiation field. The patient was not a candidate for surgery or continued XRT. (A) Axial CT showing a 7.0 × 4.0 cm mass (large arrow) in the right upper lobe abutting the pleura. Secondary radiation changes of scarring and fibrosis are seen adjacent to the mass (small arrows). (B) CT fluoroscopy image showing RF electrode (arrow) within the tumor bed. (C) Axial CT at 6-month follow-up shows an air-filled cavity with no residual soft tissue.

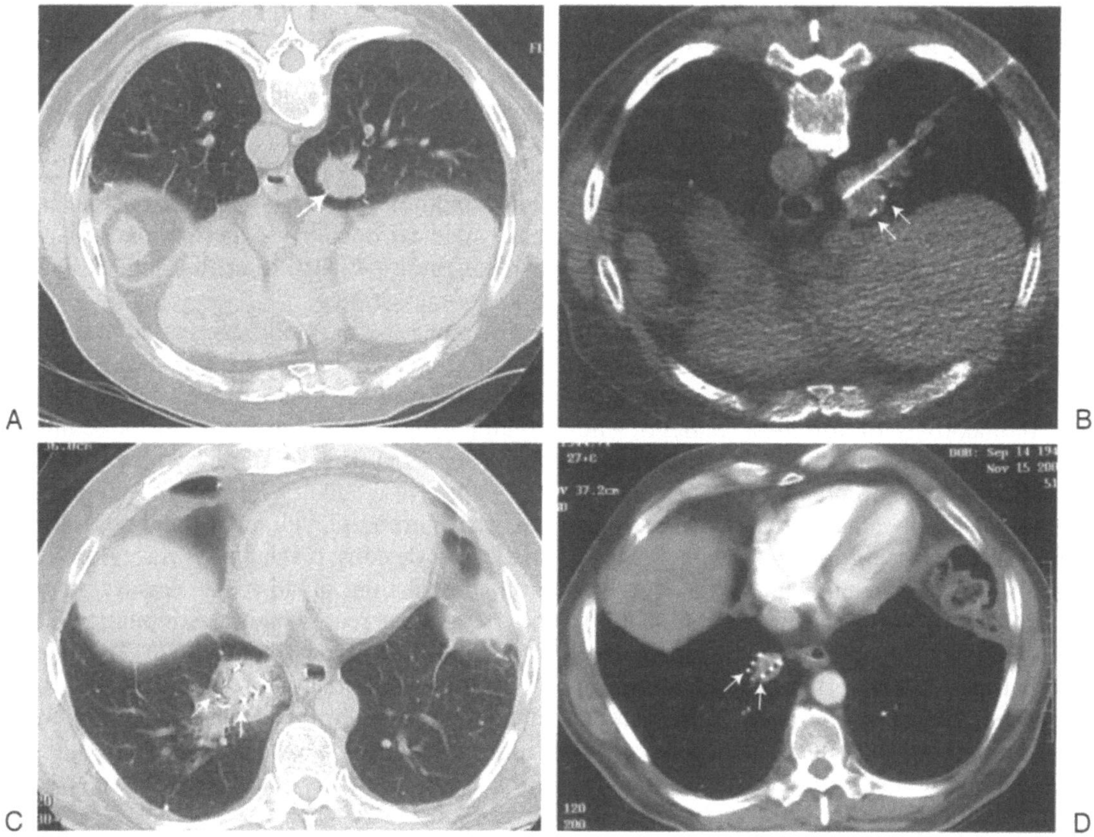

FIGURE 28.4. A 61-year-old man with metastatic renal cell carcinoma status post–bilateral pulmonary wedge resection and chemotherapy with new metastatic lesion in the right lower lobe. (A) Prone CT axial image shows a 3.5 × 2.5 × 2.0 cm mass (arrow) in the medial portion of the right lower lobe. (B) Following RFA, iodine-125 seeds were deposited in the tumor periphery (arrows) with the BRT catheter repositioned posteromedially for further seed placement. (C) Axial CT immediately after RFA. Note seeds along the periphery of the tumor bed (arrows). (D) Prone CT axial image at 1-year follow-up shows tumor contraction with more peripheral seed placement (arrows).

In addition to XRT, utilization of RFA with other treatment modalities is increasing. For larger asymptomatic parenchymal masses, combination therapy with brachytherapy implants (both high-dose and low-dose radioactive sources) may provide greater local control by magnifying cytoreduction and enhancing the radiation effect by destruction of centrally located hypoxic tumor (25; unpublished data). The benefits of concurrent brachytherapy with RFA are that the entire treatment can be accomplished in a single day, and the brachytherapy seeds can be placed under CT guidance after the RFA procedure (Fig. 28.4). If one analyzes the tumor histologies and their propensity for infiltrative growth, then tumors that tend to be more encapsulated and with a sharper tumor/lung interface (e.g., well-differentiated squamous cell carcinoma) may be better candidates for local therapy alone. If concurrent external beam radiotherapy is contraindicated, then high-dose radioactive (HDR) brachytherapy may provide improved local control in these patients.

Pulmonary metastatic disease tends to be an indicator of widespread systemic disease. However, in certain tumors and certain patients, pulmonary metastatic disease may exist in isolation. In these patients with a finite number of metastatic deposits in the lung from a tumor with favorable biologic characteristics (such as soft tissue sarcoma, renal cell carcinoma, colorectal carcinoma, and pulmonary carcinoma), resection is considered a viable treatment option that improves prognosis (depending on the nodule size, completeness of resection, and lymph node status) (44–49). In colorectal metastases, for example, studies have shown the overall 5-year and 10-year survival rates to increase from 22% to 62% and 42% to 47%, respectively, and a 3-year survival benefit after resection of pulmonary metastases (47,48). For patients at high risk for morbidity from thoracotomy or for those patients who refuse surgery, the only treatment alternatives are systemic chemotherapy or local therapy by external beam radiation. X-ray therapy as primary treatment in patients with stage I lung cancer results in an overall 5-year survival rate of 34% in the geriatric population (50). Radiofrequency ablation may be applied to these patients and to certain patients in whom a small number of slowly growing metastases are identified. In particular, metastases from renal cell carcinoma, sarcoma, and colorectal carcinoma are those that will benefit from this therapy (46,47). One-third of patients with renal cell carcinoma have pulmonary metastases [60% with metastasis in general (45)], and one-half of patients who have undergone nephrectomy for renal cell carcinoma will develop pulmonary metastases later (15). Data from several groups presented in abstract form (51) have shown early success with RFA for colorectal metastases. Tumor control has been achieved in approximately 90% in RFA of colorectal hepatic metastases (52). However, long-term outcome data are not available.

The exact size and number of lesions have yet to be defined, but it is not unreasonable to use similar parameters that have been applied to liver tumors (i.e., four or fewer metastases). The maximum size for effective treatment has not been established, but again, lesions less than 3 cm in size (as in the liver) are optimal candidates, given the treatment regions achievable with current RFA technology (Fig. 28.5). Histologic evidence of complete lethal thermal injury in pulmonary metastases by RFA has been shown (53,54). As with most cancers, early detection and staging are essential. In our experience, localized tumors over 3 cm in size may have early, undetected metastatic disease by current imaging and staging techniques. Invasive staging techniques (e.g., mediastinoscopy) are not options in these patients with medical comorbidities. Therefore, it may be beneficial to have medical oncology expertise early in the care of these patients, given the higher likelihood of metastases.

For palliation of symptoms related to a focal lesion, size is less important, and larger tumors with chest wall and osseous involvement can be treated with attention to the tumor/bone interface (Fig. 28.6). The current literature confirms the palliative results of RFA in musculoskeletal, gastrointestinal, pulmonary, and neurologic associated lesions presumably via cytoreduction, destruction of adjacent sensory neural fibers, and decreased neural stimulation secondary to debulking (27,29,55–57). The resultant improved quality of life illustrates the dynamic use of this procedure, but more controlled studies need to be done. Callstrom et al (57) have reported palliative effects within 1 week of RFA of osseous metastases, with increasing benefit and quality of life directly related to time.

Conclusion

The minimally invasive technique of RFA has a promising impact in the treatment of nonsurgical patients of lung tumors, provided that control of local disease will improve quality of life, survival, and overall prognosis. It may become a procedure for curative as well as palliative intent, either solely or as an adjunct to current standard modalities. Advantages of RFA include precise control, low cost, acceptable morbidity and mortality as well as complication rate, and use in the outpatient setting. The potential paradigm shift in standard treatment toward use of alternative methods such as RFA depends on precise scientific and clinical research/data to provide evidence-based medicine. Long-term follow-up elucidating the mechanism and effect of this procedure await further studies.

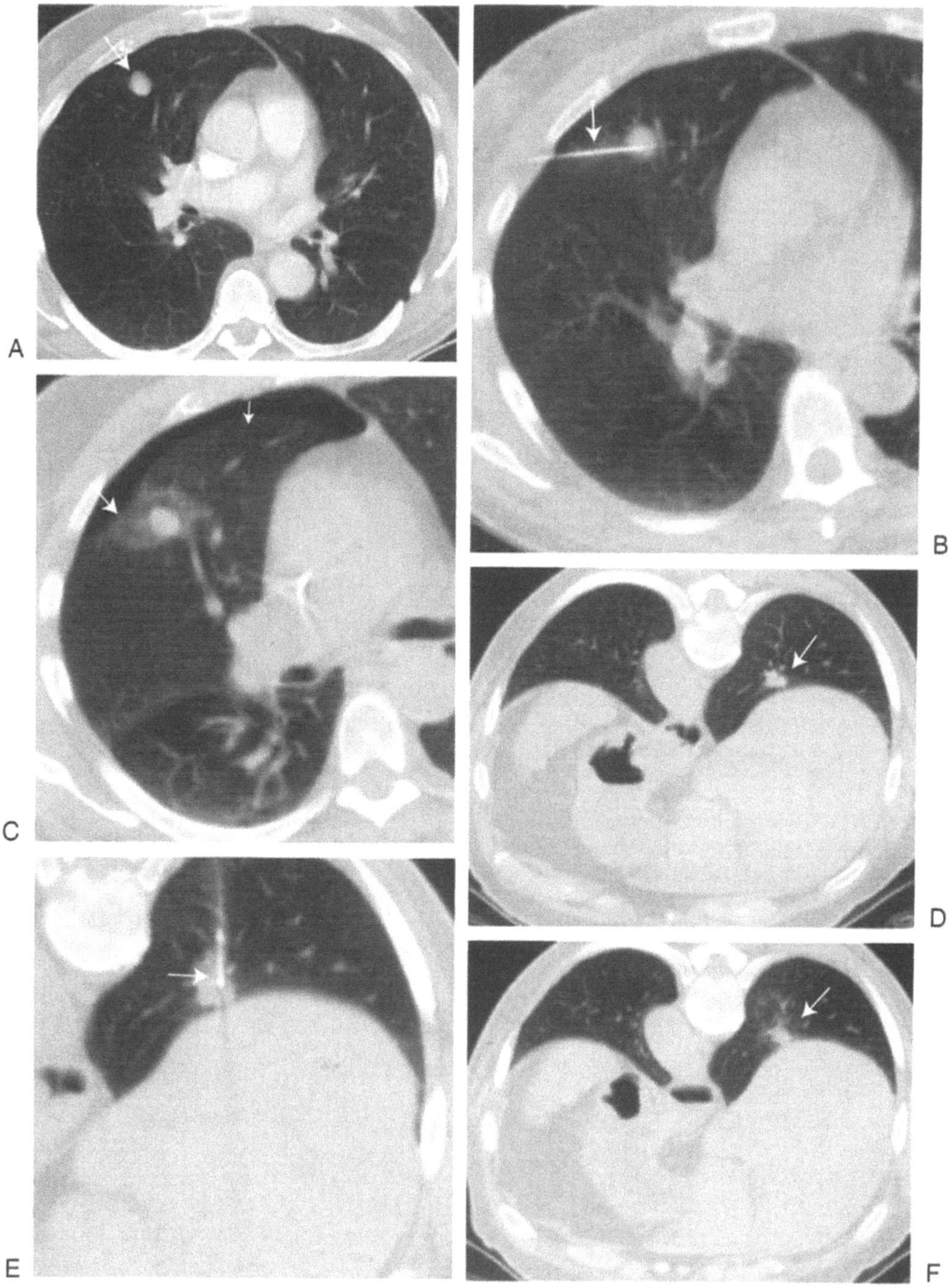

FIGURE 28.5. A 68-year-old man with metastatic renal cell carcinoma to the left kidney, brain, and lungs, status post–wedge resection. (A) Axial CT image showing a pulmonary nodule in the right upper lobe (arrow). (B) RFA of the tumor with the electrode (arrow) in the nodule. (C) Axial CT image immediately postprocedure revealed a small pneumothorax (small arrow) as well as hemorrhage and air space opacity (larger arrow) around the nodule. Both resolved without any intervention. (D) Axial CT image showing a 1.7-cm spiculated nodule in the right lower lobe (arrow). (E) RF electrode (arrow) within the tumor bed. (F) Axial CT image immediately postprocedure revealed a small pneumothorax as well as hemorrhage and air space opacity (arrow) around the nodule. Both resolved without any intervention.

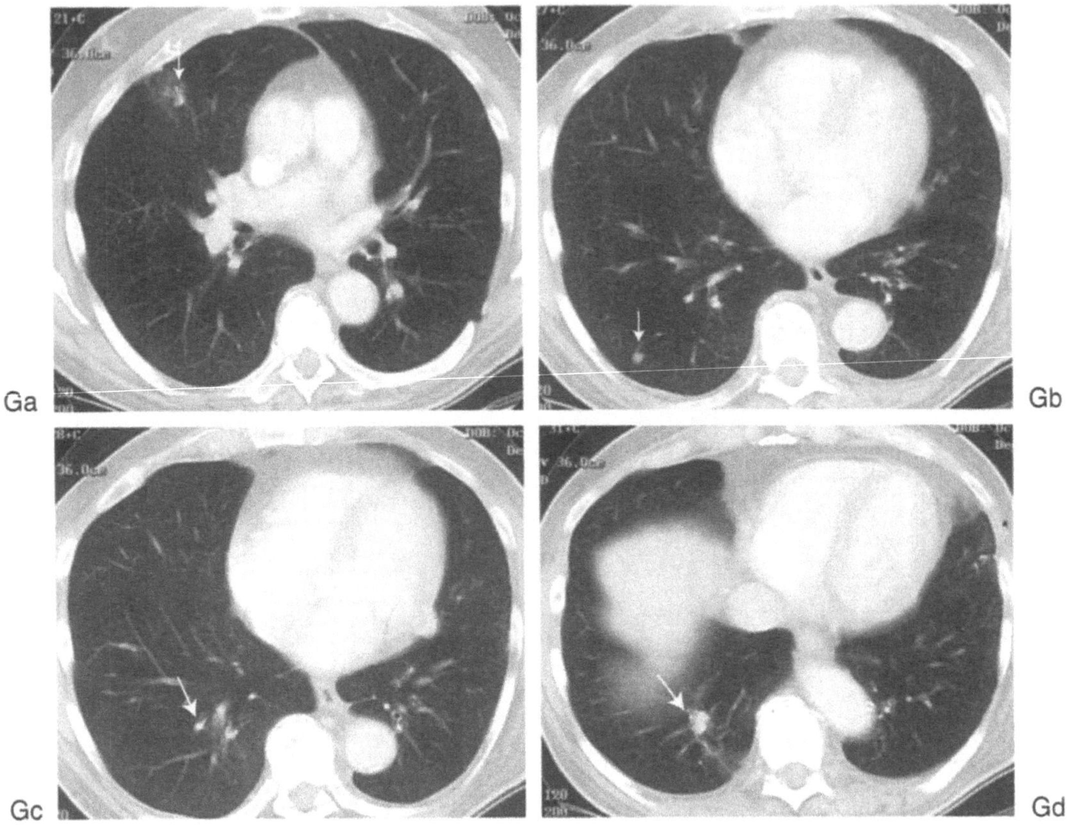

FIGURE 28.5. (G) Serial axial CT images at 3-year follow-up showing stable RFA site of lung metastases in the right upper and lower lobes (large arrow) with stable subcentimeter nodules (small arrows) in the right lung.

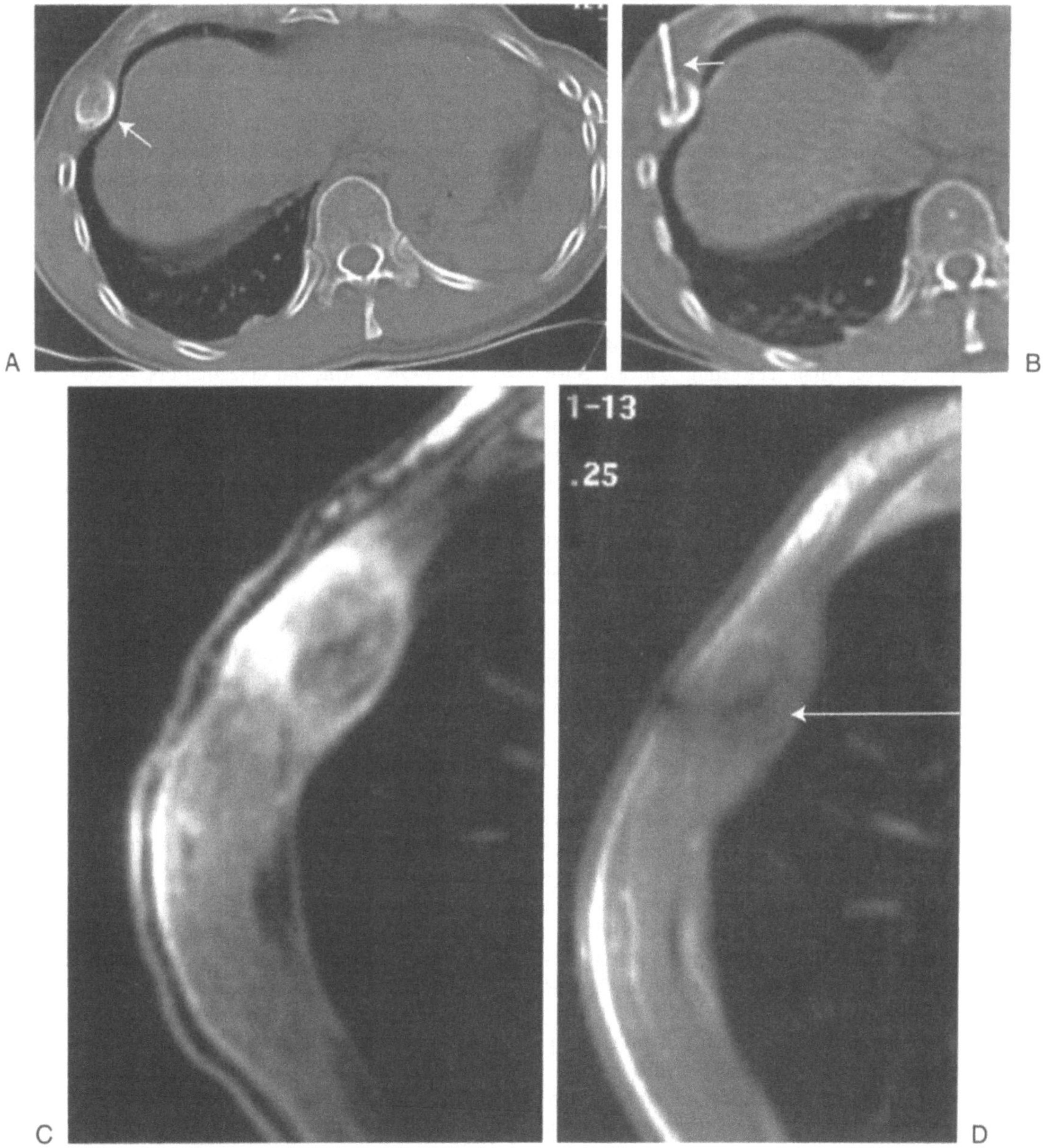

FIGURE 28.6. A 40-year-old man with metastatic lung cancer status post–left pneumonectomy with adjuvant chemotherapy and radiation referred for RFA for chest wall palliation. (A) A 4.0 × 2.0 × 2.2 cm expansile, mixed lytic and sclerotic rib metastasis in the right anterolateral rib cage (arrow). (B) RFA of the tumor. Arrow indicates the electrode within the lesion. (C,D) Follow-up magnetic resonance imaging. T1-weighted gradient echo postcontrast images at 1-month (C) and 3-month (D) follow-up. The latter (arrow) shows reduced enhancement in comparison to the former.

References

1. Cancer Facts and Figures 2003. Atlanta: American Cancer Society, 2003.
2. Mountain CF. Revisions in the International System for Staging Lung Cancer. Chest 1997; 111:1710–1717.
3. Van Rens M, de la Riviere AB, Elbers HRJ, et al. Prognostic assessment of 2,361 patients who underwent pulmonary resection for non-small cell lung cancer, stage I, II, and IIIA. Chest 2000; 117:374–379.
4. Rajdev L, Keller SM. Neoadjuvant and adjuvant therapy of non-small cell lung cancer. Surg Oncol 2002;11:243–253.
5. Dupuy DE, Zagoria RJ, Akerley W, Mayo-Smith W, Kavanagh PV, Safran H. Percutaneous radiofrequency ablation of malignancies in the lung. AJR 2000;174:57–59.
6. Goldberg SN, Dupuy DE. Image-guided radiofrequency tumor ablation: challenges and opportunities—part I. J Vasc Intervent Radiol 2001;12:1021–1032.
7. Dupuy DE, Goldberg SN. Image-guided radiofrequency tumor ablation: challenges and opportunities—part II. J Vasc Intervent Radiol 2001;12:1135–1148.
8. Murai N, Koga K, Nagamachi S, et al. Radiotherapy in bone metastases, with special reference to its effect on relieving pain. Gan No Rinsho 1989;35:1149–1152.
9. Highland AM, Mack P, Breen DJ. Radiofrequency thermal ablation of a metastatic lung nodule. Eur Radiol 2002;suppl 4:S166–S170.
10. Hoegler D. Radiotherapy for palliation symptoms in incurable cancer. Curr Probl Cancer 1997;21:129–183.
11. Todd TR. The surgical treatment of pulmonary metastases. Chest 1997;112:287S–290S.
12. Pastorino U, Buyse M, Friedel G, et al. Long-term results of lung metastasectomy: prognostic analyses based on 5206 cases. J Thorac Cardiovasc Surg 1997;113:37–49.
13. Sakamoto T, Tsubota N, Ivanaga K, et al. Pulmonary resection for metastases from colorectal cancer. Chest 2001;119:1069–1072.
14. Fourquier P, Regnard J, Rea S, et al. Lung metastases of renal cell carcinoma: results of surgical resection. Eur J Cardiothorac Surg 1997;11: 17–21.
15. Dekernion JB, Ramming KP, Smith RB. The natural history of metastatic renal cell carcinoma: a computer analysis. J Urol 1978;120: 148–152.
16. Kandioler D, Kromer E, Tuchler H, et al. Long-term results after repeated surgical removal of pulmonary metastases. Ann Thorac Surg 1998; 65:909–912.
17. Ginsberg RJ, Rubinstein LV. Randomized trial of lobectomy versus limited resection for T1 N0 non-small cell lung cancer. Lung Cancer Study Group. Ann Thorac Surg 1995;60:615–623.
18. Kvale RA, Simoff M, Prakash UBS. Palliative care. Chest 2003;123:284S–311S.
19. Griffin JP, Nelson JE, Koch KA, et al. End-of-life care in patients with lung cancer. Chest 2003;123: 312S–331S.
20. SUPPORT principal investigators. A controlled trial to improve care for seriously ill hospitalized patients. JAMA 1995;274:1591–1598.
21. Downey RJ, Martini N, Rusch V, et al. Extent of chest wall invasion and survival in patients with lung cancer. Ann Thorac Surg 1999;68:188–193.
22. Watson PN, Evans RJ. Intractable pain with lung cancer. Pain 1987;29:163–173.
23. Jacox A, Carr DB, Payne R, et al. Management of cancer pain: clinical practice guideline No. 9. Rockville, MD: Agency for Health Care Policy and Research, U.S. Department of Health and Human Services, Public Health Service, March 1994; AHCPR Publication No. 94-0592.
24. Langendijk JA, Ten Velde GPM, Aaronson NK, et al. Quality of life after palliative radiotherapy in non-small cell lung cancer: a prospective study. Int J Radiat Oncol Biol Phys 2000;47: 149–155.
25. Dupuy DE, Mayo-Smith WW, Abbott GF, DiPetrillo T. Clinical applications of radiofrequency tumor ablation in the thorax. RadioGraphics 2002;22:S259–S269.
26. Warzelhan J, Stoelben E, Imdahl A, et al. Results in surgery for primary and metastatic chest wall tumors. Eur J Cardiothorac Surg 2001;19:584–588.
27. Patti J, Neeman Z, Wood B. Radiofrequency ablation for cancer-associated pain. J Pain 2002; 3:471.
28. McCaughan B. Recent advances in managing non-small-cell lung cancer: 2. Med J Aust 1997; 166(suppl):S7–S10.
29. Dupuy DE, Safran H, Mayo-Smith WW, Goldberg SN. Radiofrequency ablation of painful osseous metastatic disease: scientific paper presented at RSNA annual meeting Chicago. Radiology 1998;209S:171S–172S.
30. Kapural L, Mekhail N. Radiofrequency ablation for chronic pain control. Current Pain Headache Rep 2001;5:517–525.

31. Elia S, Griffo S, Gentile M, et al. Surgical treatment of lung cancer invading chest wall: a retrospective analysis of 110 patients. Eur J Cardiothorac Surg 2001;20:356–360.
32. Sawada M, Watanabe S, Tsuda H, et al. An increase in body temperature during radiofrequency ablation of liver tumors. Anesth Analg 2002;94:1416–1420.
33. Landreneau RJ, Sugarbaker DJ, Mack MJ, et al. Wedge resection versus lobectomy for stage 1(T1 N0 M0) non-small cell lung cancer. J Thorac Cardiovasc Surg 1997;113:691–698.
34. Martini N, Bains MS, Burt ME, et al. Incidence of local recurrence and second primaries in resected stage I lung cancer. J Thorac Cardiovasc Surg 1995;109:120–129.
35. Mountain CF. A new international staging system for lung cancer. Chest 1986;89:225–233.
36. Naruke T, Goya T, Tsuchiya R, et al. Prognosis and survival in resected lung carcinoma based on the new international staging system. J Thorac Cardiovasc Surg 1988;96:440–447.
37. Shimizu J, Watanabe Y, Oda M, et al. Results of surgical treatment of stage I lung cancer. Nippon Geka Gakkai Zasshi 1993;94:505–510.
38. Williams DE, Pairolero PC, Danis CS, et al. Survival of patients surgically treated for stage I lung cancer. J Thorac Cardiovasc Surg 1981; 82:70–76.
39. Martini N. Surgical treatment of non-small cell lung cancer by stage. Semin Surg Oncol 1990;6: 248–254.
40. Kodama K, Doi O, Higashiymama M, et al. Intentional limited resection for selected patients with T1 N0 non-small cell lung cancer: a single-institution study. J Thorac Cardiovasc Surg 1997;114:347–353.
41. Okada M, Yoshikawa K, Hatta T, et al. Is segmentectomy with lymph node assessment an alternative to lobectomy for non-small cell lung cancer of 2cm or smaller? Ann Thorac Surg 2001;71:956–960.
42. Wright SE. Adjuvant chemotherapy and radiation therapy for elimination of residual microscopic non-small cell lung cancer. Int J Oncol 1999;14:347–351.
43. Okamoto Y, Murakami M, Yoden E, et al. Reirradiation for locally recurrent lung cancer previously treated with radiation therapy. Int J Radiat Oncol Biol Phys 2002;52:390–396.
44. Temple LK, Brennan MF. The role of pulmonary metastasectomy in soft tissue sarcoma. Semin Thorac Cardiovasc Surg 2002;14:35–44.
45. van der Poel HG, Roukema JA, Horenblas S, van Geel AN, Debruyne FM. Metastasectomy in renal cell carcinoma: a multicenter retrospective analysis. Eur Urol 1999;35:197–203.
46. Piltz S, Meimarakis G, Wichmann MW, et al. Long-term results after pulmonary resection of renal cell carcinoma metastases. Ann Thorac Surg 2002;73:1082–1087.
47. Okumura S, Kondo H, Tsuboi M, et al. Pulmonary resection for metastatic colorectal cancer: experience with 159 patients. J Thorac Cardiovasc Surg 1996;112:867–874.
48. Labow DM, Buell JE, Yoshida A, Rosen S, Posner MC. Isolated pulmonary recurrence after resection of colorectal hepatic metastases—is resection indicated? Cancer J 2002;8:342–347.
49. Hamy A, Baron O, Bennouna J, Roussel JC, Paineau J, Douillard JY. Resection of hepatic and pulmonary metastases in patients with colorectal cancer. Am J Clin Oncol 2001;24:607–609.
50. Gauden S, Tripcony L. The curative treatment by radiation therapy alone of stage I non-small cell lung cancer in a geriatric population. Lung Cancer 2001;32:71–79.
51. Glenn DW, Clark W, Morris DL, et al. Percutaneous radiofrequency ablation of colorectal pulmonary metastases. In: RSNA Conference 2001, November 25–30, Chicago (Abstract 391).
52. de Baere T, Elias D, Dromain C, et al. Radiofrequency ablation of 100 hepatic metastases with a mean follow-up of more than 1 year. AJR 2001;175:1619–1625.
53. Steinke K, Habicht JM, Thomsen S, Soler M, Jacob AL. CT-guided radiofrequency ablation of a pulmonary metastasis followed by surgical resection. Cardiovasc Intervent Radiol 2002;25: 543–546.
54. Miao Y, Yicheng N, Bosmans H, et al. Radiofrequency ablation for eradication of pulmonary tumor in rabbits. J Surg Res 2001;99:265–271.
55. Kishi K, Nakamura H, Sudo A, et al. Tumor debulking by radiofrequency ablation in hypertrophic pulmonary osteoarthropathy associated with pulmonary carcinoma. Lung Cancer 2002; 38:317–320.
56. Ohhigashi S, Nishio T, Watanabe F, et al. Experience with radiofrequency ablation in the treatment of pelvic recurrence in rectal cancer: report of two cases. Dis Colon Recum 2001;44:741–745.
57. Callstrom MR, Charboneau JW, Goetz MP, et al. Painful metastases involving bone: feasibility of percutaneous CT- and US-guided radiofrequency ablation. Radiology 2002;224:87–97.

58. Anderson BO, Burt ME. Chest wall neoplasms and their management. Ann Thorac Surg 1994; 58:1774–1781.
59. Pearson FG. Lung cancer: the past twenty-five years. Chest 1986;89 (4 suppl):200S–205S.
60. Wada H, Tanaka F, Yanagihara K. Time trends and survival after operations for primary lung cancer from 1976 through 1990. J Thorac Cardiovasc Surg 1996;112:349–355.
61. Flehinger BJ, Kimmel M, Melamed MR. The effect of surgical treatment on survival from early lung cancer: implications for screening. Chest 1992;101:1013–1018.

29
Soft Tissue Ablation

Sridhar Shankar, Eric vanSonnenberg, Stuart G. Silverman, Paul R. Morrison, and Kemal Tuncali

Overview

Over the past several years, percutaneous image-guided tumor ablation procedures have proliferated (1–7). Several new technologies, in addition to the previously available percutaneous injection of toxic substances (such as alcohol, hot saline, acetic acid), have been added to the interventional radiologist's armamentarium. These technologies include radiofrequency ablation (RFA), laser (laser interstitial tumor therapy, LITT), cryotherapy, microwave therapy, and high-intensity focused ultrasound (HIFU) therapy; all except HIFU are percutaneous techniques, and HIFU is transcutaneous (8). Several centers are now using these techniques clinically, and a large body of experience has accumulated. While most of these ablative techniques have been used predominantly for the treatment of malignant liver tumors, new sites and indications continue to emerge.

The impetus for treating tumors in extrahepatic sites is based mostly on clinical trials that have demonstrated percutaneous ultrasound (US) and computed tomography (CT) guidance, predominantly using RFA to be safe and effective in selected patients with liver lesions (4,9). Consequently, RFA is now being used as an alternative to conventional treatment (i.e., surgery, radiation, and chemotherapy) for tumors in several other organ systems, including lung, kidney, bone, and soft tissue, in certain select situations (10–13). Indeed, osteoid osteomas have been successfully treated percutaneously with CT-guided RFA for several years (14–16). More recently, ultrasound and CT-guided RFA has been suggested as a method for the palliation of painful metastases involving bone and soft tissues (7,17–20).

Definitions

Ablation of soft tissue tumors is not new; animal studies using tumor models (e.g., VX2 tumor model, rat breast cancer) use ablation of artificially induced soft tissue tumors to assess efficacy of various ablative techniques (21–24).

Soft tissue lesions comprise those that are situated in no particular organ system; the closest, perhaps, is the musculoskeletal system, although many lesions lie outside that system per se. Several lesions are inseparable from the underlying, or closely related bone; indeed, situations are common in which the lesion is part soft tissue and part bone. Many of these lesions can more properly be considered under the umbrella term *soft tissue and bone lesions*. Clinically the most important situation would likely be a malignant lesion, and examples include recurrent tumors in the resection bed of intraabdominal (including retroperitoneal tumors), pelvic, thoracic, extremity, and head and neck cancers. Some benign lesions such as arteriovenous malformations (11) also may be included in this category.

Indications

Most patients who are referred for percutaneous ablation of soft tissue tumors are candidates for palliation only. Commonly, referrals are for local tumor and/or pain control, and few patients realistically have the possibility for cure. Less common indications include interference with function of a limb or organ, and paraneoplastic symptoms that are believed to be secondary to humoral factors elaborated by the tumor (The referral in this case would be to debulk the tumor to control the paraneoplastic syndrome.). Most patients already have had surgical resection, with or without palliative radiotherapy, and many patients are either undergoing chemotherapy presently or have done so previously.

Sites of Application and Potential Complications

Moving sequentially from the head to the foot, soft tissue ablation has myriad current and potential applications:

Head and Neck

Several case reports and small series that detail percutaneous, intraoperative, and laparoscopic ablations in the head and neck region are available. Most of these detail the performance of ablation on a case-by-case basis (25,26). Alcohol injection has been successfully and safely performed in metastatic thyroid cancer to cervical lymph nodes (27). We recently palliatively injected alcohol into large cervical nodes in a patient with metastatic small-cell lung cancer for pain relief with successful short-term results (Fig. 29.1). Radiofrequency ablation of recurrent thyroid cancer also has been reported (28). The factor of overriding importance in these situations appears to be the care taken to avoid or minimize damage to adjacent critical structures, such as nerves and vessels that are present in the head and neck region. Intermittent intraprocedural neurologic examination during conscious sedation is one way to be forewarned of this possibility (29). Also, care must be taken to avoid damage to the skin, as many soft tissue tumors are located superficially (30,31).

Thorax

There are several published studies on ablation of lung and thoracic tumors; several of the ablated tumors extend beyond the confines of the lung, and invade the pleura, ribs, and adjacent soft tissues. Many of these procedures are performed for palliation of pain, and could be included under the purview of soft tissue tumor

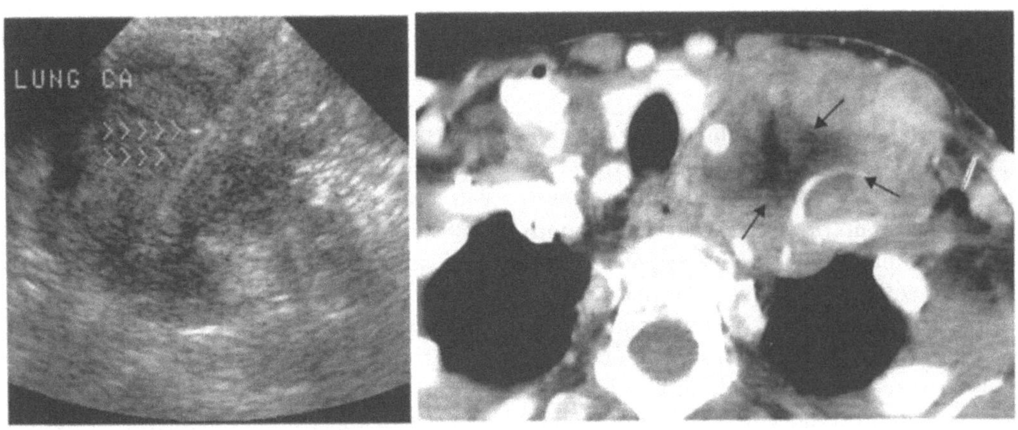

A B

FIGURE 29.1. A 70-year-old woman with metastatic small-cell lung cancer and bulky cervical lymphadenopathy. (A) A 22-gauge needle (arrowheads) within the left-sided supraclavicular nodal mass. (B) Immediate postprocedure contrast-enhanced computed tomography (CT) scan following injection of 20 cc of alcohol demonstrates low-density central necrosis (arrows).

ablation (32,33). Pain control usually is achieved by ablating the portion of the tumor that invades the chest wall; we have found adjunctive intercostal nerve block to be useful for pain control as well (32).

Abdomen

Retroperitoneal tumors comprise the commonest extravisceral site in this category. Representative tumors include leiomyosarcoma, usually recurrent following primary resection, transitional cell cancer, renal cell cancer, colon cancer, and metastatic and nodal disease from a variety of primaries (13,20). We have performed both alcohol injection and RFA (Fig. 29.2) in the retroperitoneum. Close to the pancreas, care should be taken not to cause alcohol leak or thermal injury that might result in pancreatitis.

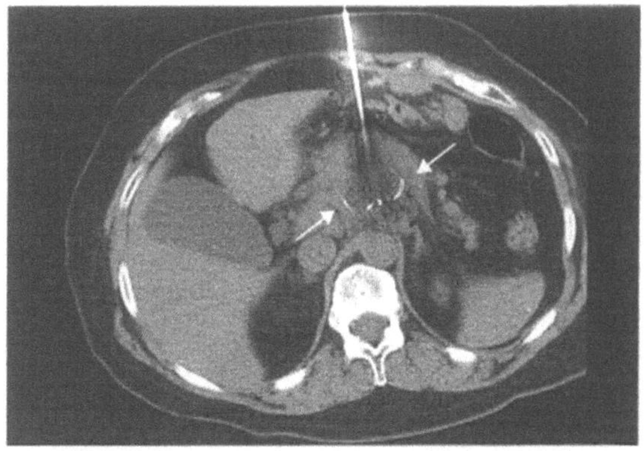

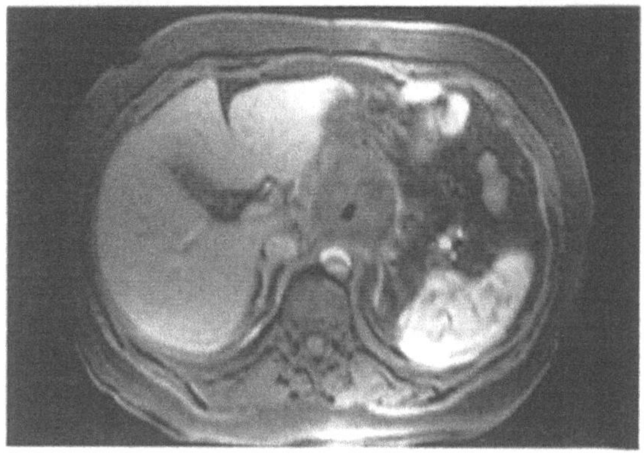

FIGURE 29.2. A 73-year-old woman with metastatic gastric cancer with a conglomerate lymph node mass in the retroperitoneum. (A) CT image during RFA; probe is seen positioned within the retroperitoneal nodal mass (arrows). Small specks of gas are seen surrounding the probe, a common finding. (B) Postprocedure contrast-enhanced MR image demonstrates a predominantly nonenhancing mass. Central low-intensity area is a susceptibility artifact.

Pelvis

A common situation for ablation is presacral recurrence of rectal cancer following abdominoperineal resection. It is a good practice to biopsy the lesion at a separate session prior to performing the ablation, even in the presence of fairly convincing imaging evidence of tumor recurrence. In our experience, some of these lesions have been shown to be of infectious, postsurgical scarring, or some other benign etiology, proven by percutaneous biopsy and imaging follow-up (Fig. 29.3).

Caution should be exercised when ablating lesions located in the inguinal region, as in many instances these lesions involve nerves that cannot be visualized using current imaging techniques. We have encountered an injury to the femoral nerve from ablation of a soft tissue sarcoma in the groin with RF. Indeed, it is essential that patients be informed about the potential for nerve injury and limb paralysis during the consent process.

Extremities and Other Sites

Many primary tumors of the extremities recur after local resection, and some of these patients are not candidates for re-resection for medical reasons or due to the presence of other metastases. Metastatic tumors from primary tumors such as lung and breast cancer to bone and soft tissues can be painful; percutaneous ablation of these lesions can be a worthwhile palliative treatment for these patients (17) (Figs. 29.4 and 29.5). We have performed palliative magnetic resonance imaging (MRI) guided cryoablation in a patient with metastatic mesothelioma to both the humerus and femur with good pain control achieved. Other sites include lesions involving, or close to, the vertebral column that are either painful or cause pressure symptoms on adjacent nerves (11,34).

Menendez et al (35) reported 12 cases of extremity sarcomas that they treated with intraoperative US-guided cryotherapy, and

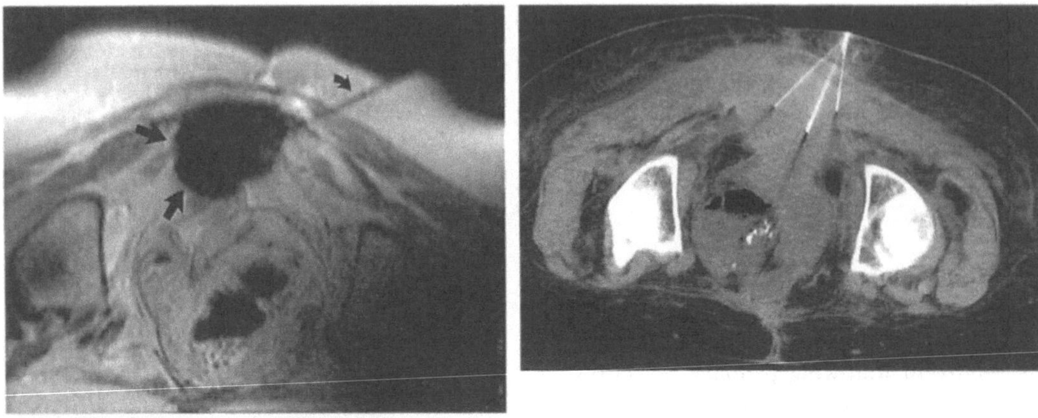

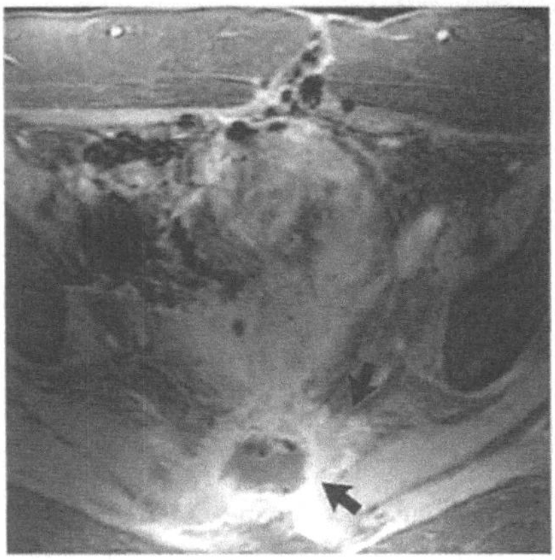

Figure 29.3. A 50-year-old woman with locally recurrent rectal cancer in the presacral area. She had undergone abdominoperineal resection of the primary tumor 6 years earlier. (A) MR-guided cryoablation of the presacral tumor—the iceball is seen as an exquisitely well-defined area of signal void in this prone axial scan (arrows). Note cryoprobe (curved arrow) entering from the right gluteal region. (B) Contrast-enhanced MR image of the pelvis obtained approximately 12 months following the procedure demonstrates irregular enhancing areas in the presacral region (arrows). The previously ablated area has decreased in size. (C) CT-guided fan biopsy of suspicious areas in the presacral region. Pathology revealed fibroconnective tissue with necrosis, acute inflammation, and granulation tissue, but no evidence of tumor.

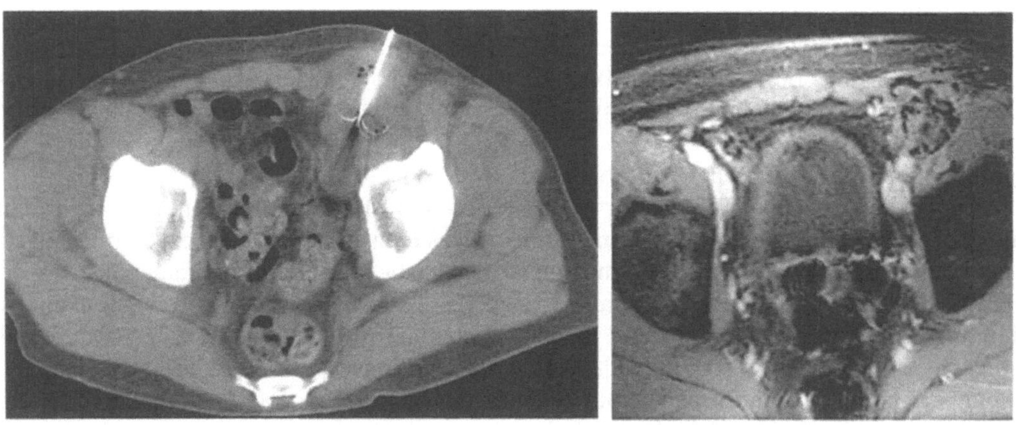

Figure 29.4. A 45-year-old man with locally recurrent, painful sarcoma in the left groin. (A) CT-guided RFA of the left groin tumor. (B) Eight-month follow-up contrast-enhanced MR exam demonstrates no enhancement in the treated tumor, and no evidence of local recurrence. The patient sustained injury to the femoral nerve with paresis of his quadriceps; he has slowly recovered with the aid of physical therapy.

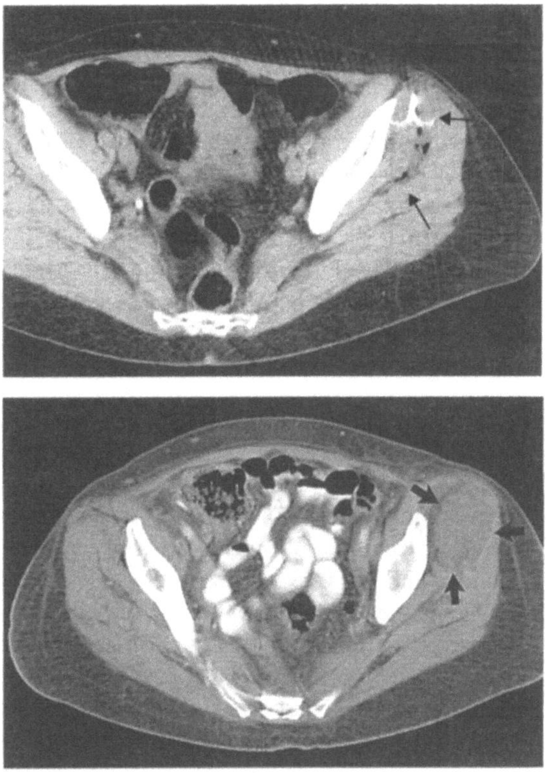

FIGURE 29.5. A 48-year-old woman with metastatic leiomyosarcoma to the left gluteal region. (A) CT-guided RFA of the left gluteal mass (arrows). (B) Postprocedure contrast-enhanced CT scan demonstrates the ablated area (arrows) to be nonenhancing.

concluded that the technique was safe and feasible. They encountered three patients with nerve palsy, all of whom recovered completely.

Special Situations and Adjunctive Procedures for Ablation

Tumors located adjacent to critical structures demand measures beyond customary caution to treat the lesion successfully. Thus, preprocedural ureteral stenting can help avoid damage to the ureter while treating lesions in proximity to it. The urologist performs the ureteral stenting cystoscopically, one day prior to or on the day of the procedure. Urethral warming catheters can be used to prevent injury to the urethra while treating lesions that invade the prostate (Fig. 29.6), bladder base, or are otherwise situated too close to the urethra; this is standard technique for prostate cryotherapy (36).

Percutaneously introduced saline, carbon dioxide (37,38), and possibly balloons or other mechanical devices may be helpful in moving structures such as the colon, kidney, or spleen out of the area to be treated, such that both complete ablation may be achieved and injury to bowel avoided.

Injury to overlying skin, if too close to the ablative site, may be prevented by using heated or cooled saline moistened gauze packs to prevent thermal injury. We use warm saline-soaked gauze packs routinely to keep the skin from freezing while treating lesions close to the surface with cryotherapy. Conversely, cool packs may also be useful for lowering the skin temperature during RFA of lesions close to the surface.

It may be worthwhile to remember that larger volumes of tumor necrosis with soft

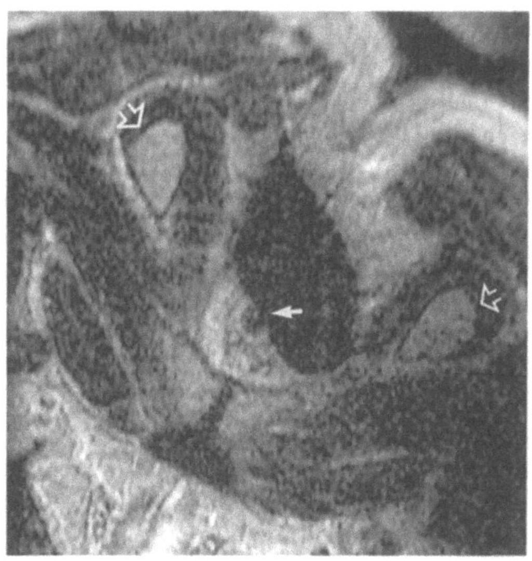

FIGURE 29.6. Locally recurrent rectal cancer invading the prostate gland. MR-guided cryotherapy with a urethral warming catheter within the urethra (prone oblique image). Note indentation of the iceball adjacent to the urethral warming catheter (arrow). The ischial tuberosities are seen on either side of the iceball (open arrows).

tissue lesions than tumors in the liver sometimes may be achieved with RFA. This is because most standard RF algorithms are created for the liver, which is liberally perfused. The larger lesion sizes achieved in soft tissue lesions may be secondary to these tumors being less well vascularized, differences in water content, or electrical and thermal conductivity of the tumor tissue (29,39).

Larger volumes of tissue necrosis also may be achieved by percutaneous injection of alcohol into the tumor prior to performing RFA (22). We have found this technique useful in obtaining significantly larger volumes of tumor necrosis in the liver (40).

Techniques, Guidance Modalities, and Follow-Up

In general, the techniques and guidance systems that are utilized elsewhere in the body can be directly extrapolated to soft tissue tumors. As discussed above, different body parts have different requirements in terms of precautions and ancillary measures. Computed tomography and US are the most commonly utilized modalities to target tumors and guide needle/probe placement. The major disadvantage with both imaging techniques is that they do not allow monitoring of the effects of RFA in sufficient detail to allow the operator to visualize the margins of the ablation. As a result, percutaneous US- or CT-guided RFA may be hazardous in patients with metastatic or recurrent tumors of soft tissue or bone situated adjacent to critical structures such as bowel, bladder, and nerves. Magnetic resonance imaging (MRI)-guided percutaneous cryotherapy may be the most elegant technique available in terms of visualization of tumor, guidance, treatment monitoring, and follow-up currently (41,42).

Follow-up of treated soft tissue tumors is performed by a combination of various imaging modalities. We utilize CT and MRI in the immediate postprocedure period, and CT, MRI, and positron emission tomography (PET) at baseline (preprocedure), and at approximately 12-week intervals to evaluate efficacy of treatment and tumor recurrence. The rationale for using multiple modalities for lesion assessment is that some tumors are poorly vascularized, and many lesions demonstrate irregular areas of intratumoral necrosis that may add to confusion while assessing the postprocedure thermal effect. Pain evaluation can be performed using the Wisconsin Brief Pain Questionnaire, which rates the patient's pain on a scale of 0 to 10, with 0 being no pain and 10 the worst pain the patient has ever experienced (43,44).

Conclusions

Many malignant tumors of soft tissues can be treated percutaneously using a variety of techniques and devices. These therapies may provide a means for the palliation of pain unresponsive to other therapies, in addition to local control of tumor. Care with structures either within (nerves, vessels) or juxtaposed to (bowel, urethra, ureter) these soft tissue tumors must be exercised, as these are distinct hazards in the treatment of these lesions.

References

1. Livraghi T, Goldberg SN, Lazzaroni S, et al. Hepatocellular carcinoma: radio-frequency ablation of medium and large lesions. Radiology 2000;214:761–768.
2. Livraghi T, Goldberg SN, Solbiati L, Meloni F, Ierace T, Gazelle GS. Percutaneous radiofrequency ablation of liver metastases from breast cancer: initial experience in 24 patients. Radiology 2001;220:145–149.
3. Curley SA, Izzo F. Radiofrequency ablation of primary and metastic liver tumors. Surg Technol Int 2002;10:99–106.
4. Gazelle GS, Goldberg SN, Solbiati L, Livraghi T. Tumor ablation with radio-frequency energy. Radiology 2000;217:633–646.
5. Gervais DA, McGovern FJ, Wood BJ, Goldberg SN, McDougal WS, Mueller PR. Radiofrequency ablation of renal cell carcinoma: early clinical experience. Radiology 2000;217:665–672.
6. Solbiati L, Goldberg SN, Ierace T, et al. Hepatic metastases: percutaneous radio-frequency ablation with cooled-tip electrodes. Radiology 1997; 205:367–373.

7. Wood BJ, Fojo A, Levy EB, Gomez-Horhez J, Chang R, Spies J. Radiofrequency ablation of painful neoplasms as a palliative therapy: early experience. 2000;11(S):207.
8. Hynynen K, Pomeroy O, Smith DN, et al. MR imaging-guided focused ultrasound surgery of fibroadenomas in the breast: a feasibility study. Radiology 2001;219:176–185.
9. Goldberg SN, Gazelle GS, Mueller PR. Thermal ablation therapy for focal malignancy: a unified approach to underlying principles, techniques, and diagnostic imaging guidance. AJR 2000;174: 323–331.
10. Wood BJ, Ramkaransingh JR, Fojo T, Walther MM, Libutti SK. Percutaneous tumor ablation with radiofrequency. Cancer 2002;94:443–451.
11. vanSonnenberg E, Hadjipavlou A, Chaljub G, Nolsoe C, Ko E. Therapeutic cryotherapy guided by MRI and ultrasound for vascular malformations in erector muscles of the back. Min Invas Ther Allied Technol 1997;6:343–348.
12. Nader R, Alford BT, Nauta HJ, Crow W, van-Sonnenberg E, Hadjipavlou AG. Preoperative embolization and intraoperative cryocoagulation as adjuncts in resection of hypervascular lesions of the thoracolumbar spine. J Neurosurg 2002;97:294–300.
13. Gervais DA, Arellano RS, Mueller PR. Percutaneous radiofrequency ablation of nodal metastases. Cardiovasc Intervent Radiol 2002;25: 547–549.
14. Rosenthal DI. Percutaneous radiofrequency treatment of osteoid osteomas. Semin Musculoskel Radiol 1997;1:265–272.
15. Rosenthal DI, Alexander A, Rosenberg AE, Springfield D. Ablation of osteoid osteomas with a percutaneously placed electrode: a new procedure. Radiology 1992;183:29–33.
16. Rosenthal DI, Hornicek FJ, Wolfe MW, Jennings LC, Gebhardt MC, Mankin HJ. Percutaneous radiofrequency coagulation of osteoid osteoma compared with operative treatment. J Bone Joint Surg [Am] 1998;80:815–821.
17. Callstrom MR, Charboneau JW, Goetz MP, et al. Painful metastases involving bone: feasibility of percutaneous CT- and US-guided radiofrequency ablation. Radiology 2002;224:87–97.
18. Dupuy DE, Safran H, Mayo-Smith WW, Goldberg SN. Radiofrequency ablation of painful osseous metastatic disease. Radiology 1998;209(P):389.
19. Gevargez A, Matysek M, Kriener PG, Siepmann G, Braun M, Gronemeyer DHW. CT guided percutaneous radiofrequency ablation of spinal tumors. European Congress of Radiology, 2001.
20. Shankar S, Tuncali K, vanSonnenberg E, Morrison PR, Kacher D, Silverman SG. MRI guided percutaneous cryotherapy of soft tissue and bone metastases. Radiology 2001;221(P): 558.
21. Hazle JD, Stafford RJ, Price RE. Magnetic resonance imaging-guided focused ultrasound thermal therapy in experimental animal models: correlation of ablation volumes with pathology in rabbit muscle and VX2 tumors. J Magn Reson Imaging 2002;15:185–194.
22. Goldberg SN, Kruskal JB, Oliver BS, Clouse ME, Gazelle GS. Percutaneous tumor ablation: increased coagulation by combining radiofrequency ablation and ethanol instillation in a rat breast tumor model. Radiology 2000;217: 827–831.
23. Monsky WL, Kruskal JB, Lukyanov AN, et al. Radio-frequency ablation increases intratumoral liposomal doxorubicin accumulation in a rat breast tumor model. Radiology 2002;224:823–829.
24. Ahmed M, Lobo SM, Weinstein J, et al. Improved coagulation with saline solution pretreatment during radiofrequency tumor ablation in a canine model. J Vasc Intervent Radiol 2002; 13:717–724.
25. Bui QT, Dupuy DE. Percutaneous CT-guided radiofrequency ablation of an adenoid cystic carcinoma of the head and neck. AJR 2002;179: 1333–1335.
26. Owen RP, Ravikumar TS, Silver CE, Beitler J, Wadler S, Bello J. Radiofrequency ablation of head and neck tumors: dramatic results from application of a new technology. Head Neck 2002;24:754–758.
27. Lewis BD, Hay ID, Charboneau JW, McIver B, Reading CC, Goellner JR. Percutaneous ethanol injection for treatment of cervical lymph node metastases in patients with papillary thyroid carcinoma. AJR 2002;178:699–704.
28. Dupuy DE, Monchik JM, Decrea C, Pisharodi L. Radiofrequency ablation of regional recurrence from well-differentiated thyroid malignancy. Surgery 2001;130:971–977.
29. Neeman Z, Patti JW, Wood BJ. Percutaneous radiofrequency ablation of chordoma. AJR 2002; 179:1330–1332.
30. Kanpolat Y, Savas A, Bekar A, Berk C. Percutaneous controlled radiofrequency trigeminal rhizotomy for the treatment of idiopathic trigeminal neuralgia: 25-year experience with

1600 patients. Neurosurgery 2001;48:524–532; discussion 532–534.
31. Onofrio BM. Radiofrequency of percutaneous Gasserian ganglion lesions. Results in 140 patients with trigeminal pain. J Neurosurg 1975; 42:132–139.
32. vanSonnenberg E, Shankar S, Tuncali K, Silverman SG, Morrison PR, Jaklitsch M. Initial clinical experience with RF ablation of lung tumors. Radiology 2002;225(P):291.
33. Dupuy DE, Mayo-Smith WW, Abbott GF, DiPetrillo T. Clinical applications of radiofrequency tumor ablation in the thorax. Radiographics 2002;22:S259–269.
34. Dupuy DE, Hong R, Oliver B, Goldberg SN. Radiofrequency ablation of spinal tumors: temperature distribution in the spinal canal. AJR 2000;175:1263–1266.
35. Menendez LR, Tan MS, Kiyabu MT, Chawla SP. Cryosurgical ablation of soft tissue sarcomas: a phase I trial of feasibility and safety. Cancer 1999;86:50–57.
36. Weider J, Schmidt JD, Casola G, vanSonnenberg E, Stainken BF, Parsons CL. Transrectal ultrasound-guided transperineal cryoablation in the treatment of prostate carcinoma: preliminary results. J Urol 1995;154:435–441.
37. Goodacre BW, Savage C, Zwischenberger JB, Wittich GR, vanSonnenberg E. Salinoma window technique for mediastinal lymph node biopsy. Ann Thorac Surg 2002;74:276–277.
38. Langen HJ, Jochims M, Gunther RW. Artificial displacement of kidneys, spleen, and colon by injection of physiologic saline and CO_2 as an aid to percutaneous procedures: experimental results. J Vasc Intervent Radiol 1995;6:411–416.
39. Dupuy DE, Goldberg SN. Image-guided radiofrequency tumor ablation: challenges and opportunities—part II. J Vasc Intervent Radiol 2001;12:1135–1148.
40. Shankar S, vanSonnenberg E, Silverman SG, Tuncali K, Morrison PR. Combined radiofrequency (RF) and direct alcohol infusion for percutaneous tumor ablation. AJR 2004;183:1425–1429.
41. Shankar S, vanSonnenberg E, Silverman SG, Tuncali K. Interventional radiology procedures in the liver. Biopsy, drainage, and ablation. Clin Liver Dis 2002;6:91–118.
42. Silverman SG, Tuncali K, Adams DF, et al. MR imaging-guided percutaneous cryotherapy of liver tumors: initial experience. Radiology 2000; 217:657–664.
43. Daut RL, Cleeland CS, Flanery RC. Development of the Wisconsin Brief Pain Questionnaire to assess pain in cancer and other diseases. Pain 1983;17:197–210.
44. Daut RL, Cleeland CS. The prevalence and severity of pain in cancer. Cancer 1982;50: 1913–1918.

30 Image-Guided Palliation of Painful Skeletal Metastases

Matthew R. Callstrom, J. William Charboneau, Matthew P. Goetz, and Joseph Rubin

Painful skeletal metastases are a common problem in patients with cancer. Autopsy studies have shown up to 85% of patients who die from breast, prostate, and lung cancer have evidence of bone metastases at the time of death (1). Skeletal metastases often result in complications such as pain, fractures, and decreased mobility that adversely affect a patient's quality of life, and ultimately reduce performance status. In addition, these complications can affect a patient's mood and lead to associated depression and anxiety (1, 2). Current treatment for patients with bone metastases is primarily palliative and includes the following: localized therapies (radiation and surgery), systemic therapies (chemotherapy, hormonal therapy, radiopharmaceuticals, and bisphosphonates), and analgesics (opioids and nonsteroidal antiinflammatory drugs).

The causes of pain in patients with bone metastases are not fully understood, and the presence of pain is not correlated with the type of tumor, location, number, or size of the metastases (2–4). Possible mechanisms of pain include: (1) stretching of the periosteum secondary to tumor growth, (2) fractures (both micro- and macro-), (3) cytokine-mediated osteoclastic bony destruction that results in stimulation of nerve endings in the endosteum (5–11), and (4) tumor growth into surrounding nerves and tissues.

External-beam radiation therapy (RT) is the standard of care for patients who present with localized bone pain. This treatment results in a reduction in pain for the majority of these patients; however, 20% to 30% of patients treated with this modality do not experience pain relief, and few options exist for these patients (12–17). Furthermore, patients who have recurrent pain at a previously irradiated metastatic site may not be eligible for further RT because of limitations in normal tissue tolerance. Unfortunately, skeletal disease in this patient population often is refractory to standard chemotherapy or hormonal therapy. Surgery, which is usually reserved for impending fracture, is not always an option when patients present with advanced disease and poor functional status. Radiopharmaceuticals, which have known benefit in patients with diffuse painful bony metastases, are not considered the standard of care for patients with isolated, painful lesions. For many patients with painful metastatic disease, analgesics remain the only alternative treatment option. Unfortunately, to obtain sufficient pain control for many of these patients, side effects such as constipation, nausea, and sedation can be significant.

Many patients with pain from metastatic disease exhaust the current conventional treatment options and have persistent poorly controlled pain. Because of the shortcomings of the currently available therapies, additional treatment options for palliation of focal pain due to metastatic disease would be helpful. Fortunately, many investigators currently are exploring alternative therapies. Described below are several reports that offer new image-guided percutaneous treatments for the palliation of pain from metastatic skeletal disease.

Percutaneous Therapies for Palliation of Painful Metastases

Several new strategies recently have been reported for the treatment of painful metastatic disease. All of these new methods are based on using percutaneous image-guided methods to deliver tissue-ablative devices into focal metastatic lesions. These methods include the use of ethanol, laser-induced interstitial thermotherapy (LITT), and percutaneous radiofrequency ablation (RFA).

Percutaneous Ethanol Administration

Gangi and coworkers (18) described the use of computed tomography (CT)-guided percutaneous administration of 95% ethanol for the palliation of pain from 27 metastatic bone lesions in 25 patients previously treated with radiotherapy and/or chemotherapy. Sixteen lesions received a single dose of ethanol, while 10 lesions received two doses and one lesion received three doses. The response of these patients to this treatment was assessed by the reduction in use of analgesic medicines 48 hours and 2 weeks following therapy. Complete relief of pain was achieved in four patients, and very good but incomplete relief (75% analgesic medicine reduction) in 11 patients. Seven patients received little or no relief with the treatment.

Percutaneous Laser-Induced Interstitial Thermotherapy

Groenemeyer and coworkers (19) reported the treatment of three patients with spinal metastases using a neodymium:yttrium-aluminum-garnet (Nd:YAG) laser with a wavelength of 1064 and a 400-μm fiber. With local anesthesia and CT guidance, a coaxial system was used via a transpedicular approach. Laser energy was applied at a power of 4 to 10W with a pulse length of 0.1 to 1.0 seconds at 1-second intervals. To achieve coverage greater than 7mm, the fiber was repositioned and the thermal treatment was repeated, allowing completion of the procedure in 60 to 90 minutes. Three months posttreatment, the patients had 30% to 45% pain reduction.

Percutaneous Radiofrequency Ablation

Recently, several case reports have appeared that describe the treatment of painful metastatic lesions with percutaneous RFA. Included below are descriptions of several of these case reports. Following this, we include results of an ongoing prospective clinical trial designed to determine the clinical magnitude and durability of the use of RFA for the treatment of painful metastatic bone disease.

Case Reports

As a prelude to treatment of spinal metastatic disease, Dupuy and coworkers (20) used a pig model to examine the temperature distribution within a vertebral body and the adjacent spinal canal with the RFA electrode placed within the vertebral body. They found decreased heat transmission in cancellous bone and an insulative effect of cortical bone. Importantly, temperature elevations in the epidural space were not high enough to cause injuries to the adjacent spinal cord. Subsequently, these workers reported the treatment of a woman with a painful osteolytic focal metastatic hemangiopericytoma lesion in an anterior lumbar vertebral body. Using local anesthesia and conscious sedation, the lesion was accessed from a lateral approach that passed through intact cortex with a 14-gauge Ackermann bone biopsy needle (Cook Inc., Bloomington, IN). Subsequently a 3-cm exposed tip Radionics radiofrequency electrode (Tyco Healthcare Group LP, Burlington, MA) was used to treat the lesion. The patient had improved pain control at 13-month follow-up.

Groenemeyer and coworkers (21) reported the RFA treatment of 10 patients with 21 unresectable painful spinal metastases using an expandable-type electrode (RITA Medical System, Inc., Mountain View, CA) and a 50-W generator. The patients were treated under local anesthesia only. Target temperature for the ablations was based both on the distance from the spinal cord and patient tolerance for the procedure. Four patients also were treated with vertebroplasty and received 3 to 5.5 mL of polymethylmethacrylate 3 to 7 days following RFA. At last follow-up, nine of the 10 patients reported reduced pain, with an average pain reduction of 74%.

Wood's group (22) reported the treatment of a patient with metastatic fallopian tube carcinoma with multiple painful subcutaneous masses. Using conscious sedation and local anesthesia, the lesions were treated for 10 minutes at a target temperature of 110°C with a model 70 electrode and 50-W generator. Immediately following treatment, the patient had no pain at the treated sites. She reported 1–3/10 pain 1 month later.

Ohhigashi and coworkers (23) reported the RFA treatment of painful recurrent rectal cancer in the pelvis. Notably, recurrent rectal cancer may produce local pain, rectal bleeding, or bowel obstruction with resultant poor quality of life. Although a curative approach such as total pelvic exenteration is possible, few patients are eligible (24). Unfortunately, radiation therapy is palliative only and of limited clinical benefit (25). These workers treated two patients with 4-cm and 6-cm diameter recurrent rectal carcinomas located anterior to the sacrum that had not responded to chemotherapy or radiation therapy. Using epidural catheter–mediated analgesia, a LeVeen RF electrode (Boston Scientific Corp., Natick MA.), was placed into the lesions using CT guidance. Both patients reported a decrease in pain following the treatment and a reduction in oral analgesic requirements.

Clinical Trial

Because of several reports that suggest the potential benefits of RFA for palliation of pain due to metastatic disease, we conducted a feasibility clinical trial to determine the safety and benefits of RFA in patients with painful metastatic lesions that involve bone (26, 27). Our preliminary data showed that this procedure was safe and resulted in significant relief of pain; therefore, the study was expanded to enroll patients from other centers in the United States and Europe. Here is a brief description of this ongoing prospective trial:

Method

In an ongoing prospective trial, we have treated 43 patients at five centers in the United States and Europe over the past two years. Patients who were included had ≥4/10 worst pain over a 24-hour period from ≤2 painful sites of metastases based on the Brief Pain Inventory (BPI) (28, 29). In the BPI, patients are asked to rate their worst, least, and average pain in the past 24 hours, with allowed responses ranging from 0 to 10 (0 = no pain, 10 = pain as bad as you can imagine). Relief of pain secondary to the RFA procedure or to pain medications is scored on a scale of 0% (no relief) to 100% (complete relief). Pain interference with daily living is evaluated with questions concerning general activity, mood, walking ability, normal work, relations with other people, sleep, and enjoyment of life, also on a 0 to 10 scale (0 = no interference, 10 = completely interference).

Patients were treated under conscious sedation or general anesthesia at the discretion of the individual investigator. We have found that an epidural catheter, placed prior to treatment of lesions, greatly improves patient pain control following the procedure when the lesion is located in the pelvis or lower extremities. Two dispersive electrodes (grounding pads) are placed on the patient at equidistant sites from the RF source, usually on the patient's thighs. To avoid skin burns from the ground pads, we place two monitoring temperature electrodes (Mallinckrodt Mon-a-therm Model 4070 with 700 series thermistor) on the corners of the leading edges (nearest the ablation location) of both grounding pads. If the skin temperature reaches 38°C, dry cold packs are applied over the grounding pads. All patients included in the study were treated with a Starburst XL model needle (RITA Medical Systems, Mountain View, CA), a 14-gauge/6.4-Fr device, with an active electrode trocar tip, and nine electrodes

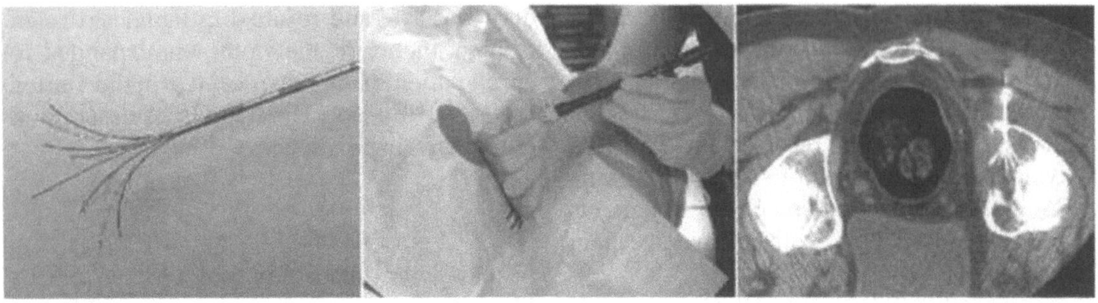

FIGURE 30.1. (A) Radiofrequency ablation (RFA) electrode with full deployment (Starburst XL electrode, RITA Medical Systems). (B) Percutaneous introduction of RFA electrode using intermittent computed tomography (CT) guidance. (C) CT image with RFA electrode deployed in an osteolytic lesion in the acetabular region.

spread in a ball-like fashion that generate up to a 5-cm-diameter zone of necrosis.

A single ablation typically is performed for lesions of ≤3 cm in diameter with a target temperature of 100°C maintained for a minimum of 5 minutes. For larger lesions, multiple systematic deployments are used with 3- to 5-cm deployments of the electrode with the 100°C target temperature maintained for 5 to 10 minutes. For lesions >5 cm in diameter, the entire lesion was often not completely treated; rather, the ablation treatments are focused on the margin of the bony lesion, with the goal of treating the soft tissue/bone interface. For full deployment of the electrode, a target temperature of 100°C was maintained for 5 to 15 minutes.

Figure 30.1 shows the needle fully deployed, typical CT-guided placement of the needle, and deployment of the tines into an osteolytic lesion in the periacetabular region. This figure illustrates that the electrode is advanced into the soft tissue portion of the lesion to be treated, and the tips of the tines of the electrode are placed against the soft tissue/bone interface. Figure 30.2 shows another example of an osteolytic lesion that involves the caudal aspect of the sacrum with associated partial destruction. The RF electrode is placed with the tines of the deployed electrode driven against the soft tissue/bone interface. Subsequent electrode deployments (not shown) are performed to completely treat the portion of bone involved in the destructive metastatic lesion. Electrode deployment diameters are chosen to adequately cover the metastatic lesion without damaging nearby normal, uninvolved tissues.

In other centers, some lesions have been treated with placement of the electrode into the center of the lesion with resultant debulking of the lesion, but with incomplete ablation of the soft tissue/bone interface. Figure 30.3 shows a large osteolytic metastatic lesion involving the sacrum 6 weeks following RFA. This image shows central low attenuation within the

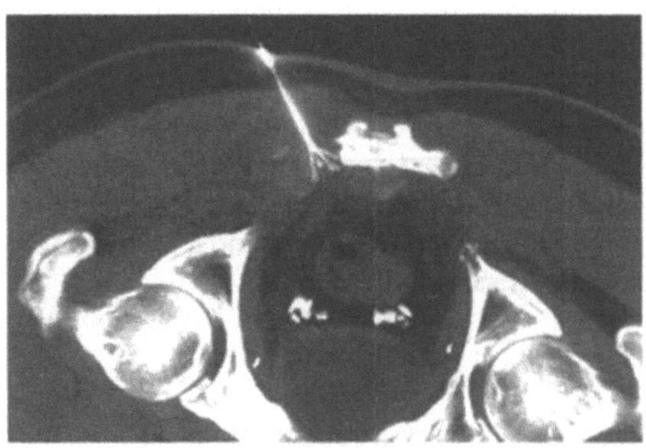

FIGURE 30.2. RFA treatment of the bone–tumor interface. Prone CT demonstrates an osteolytic mass involving the left caudal aspect of the sacrum. This mass causes destruction of the adjacent bone. The bone–tumor interface is a key site for electrode deployment to destroy nerve endings that were the likely cause of pain.

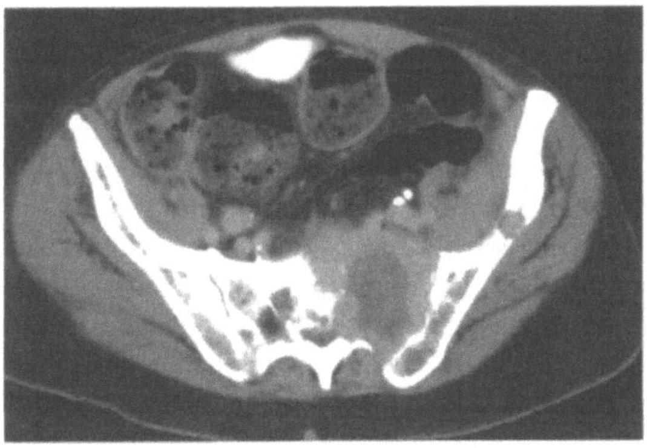

FIGURE 30.3. Failed palliation of pain due to RFA treatment of the central portion of a metastatic lesion without treatment of the tumor–bone interface. CT performed 6 weeks post-RFA demonstrates necrosis in the treated central portion of the tumor with moderate residual tumor that involves the sacrum and iliac bone. To be effective, the RFA treatment should be at the tumor–bone interface. Debulking of the central portion of metastatic lesions is not effective to reduce pain.

metastatic lesion consistent with necrosis from the RFA procedure. Residual tumor is clearly present along the medial aspect of the sacrum and against the adjacent iliac bone. Following this treatment, the patient failed to derive reduction in pain and had no clear benefit from the procedure.

We have found that it is critically important to examine each patient prior to the RFA treatment to determine if the patient's pain corresponds to an identifiable lesion on CT, magnetic resonance imaging (MRI), or ultrasound (US) imaging. Figure 30.4 shows a prone CT image of a metastatic osteolytic lesion that involves the mid sacrum. We examined the patient and placed a metallic marker on the skin overlying the site of greatest pain. As shown in Figure 30.4 the site of pain corresponded to a sacral fracture on the side opposite of the destructive sacral lesion. Because the patient's pain likely resulted from the underlying sacral fracture, we did not treat the adjacent destructive sacral lesion.

Figure 30.5 shows CT images of the pelvis of a woman with metastatic endometrial carcinoma. A large destructive lesion involves both pubic bones with osteolytic destruction, most marked on the left. On examination, the patient described 8/10 pain from the left pubic bone lesion with minimal pain to the right of midline. The left pubic bone lesion was treated with several overlapping deployments. Four weeks following treatment, the patient's pain dropped from 8/10 to 0/10. The patient died 12 weeks posttreatment with 3/10 pain at the treated site.

We have treated several patients with recurrent or residual metastatic rectal carcinoma centered anterior to the sacrum in the presacral space, often with associated osteolytic destruction of the underlying sacrum. Figure 30.6 shows a typical lesion in a 38-year-old man that measured approximately 3 cm in diameter and was located at the level of the coccyx with 8/10 pain. The patient's pain was reduced to 2/10 at week 4, and the patient reports 1/10 pain at the treated site at the latest follow-up interview, 11 months following treatment.

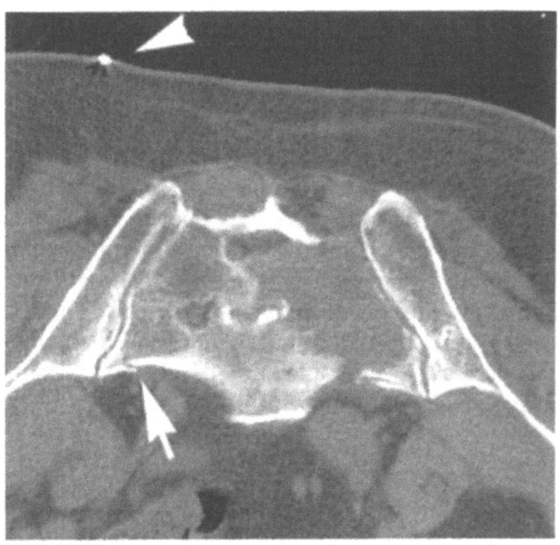

FIGURE 30.4. Pain due to sacral fracture rather than osteolytic tumor. Prior to prone CT examination, the patient was examined and a metallic marker was placed on the skin overlying the site of focal pain. CT imaging at this level shows an osteolytic destructive lesion involving the right side of the sacrum. The metallic marker (arrowhead) overlies a left sacral fracture (arrow). This lesion was not treated because the patient's pain was due to the sacral fracture rather than the adjacent osteolytic lesion.

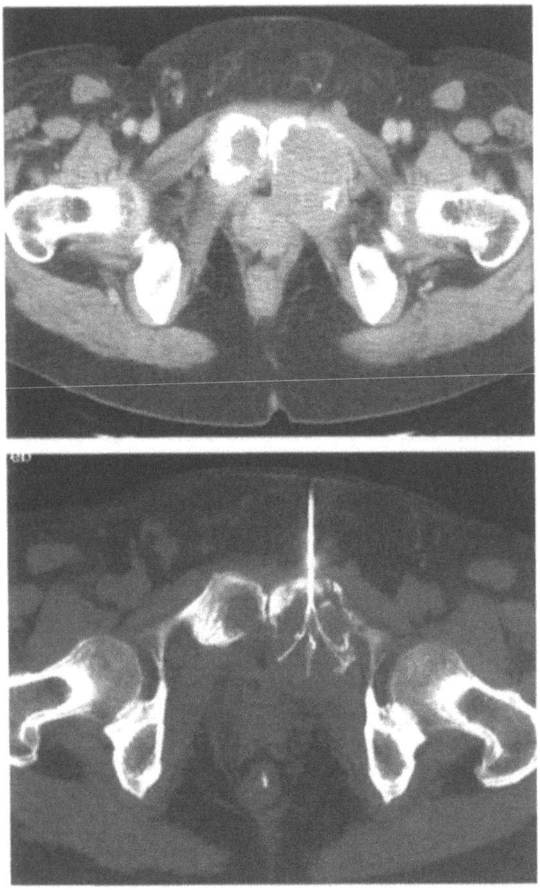
A
B

FIGURE 30.5. RFA of a pubic symphysis metastasis. (A) CT scan demonstrates osteolytic destructive lesions involving both pubic bones due to metastatic endometrial carcinoma. The lesion on the patient's left caused severe pain in spite of prior treatment with chemotherapy and radiation therapy. (B) RF electrode deployed in the osteolytic lesion. Patient's pain decreased from 8/10 before RF ablation to 3/10 4 weeks posttreatment.

Large painful lesions may be treated effectively with RFA. Figure 30.7 shows a portion of a destructive infiltrative metastatic rectal carcinoma lesion that involves the sacrum. This lesion measured approximately 11 cm in diameter and involved a majority of the sacrum. Figure 30.7A is a CT image at the level of the lower sacrum that shows the large destructive lesion. This patient was unable to sit or lie on his back due to severe pain (8/10). Prior treatment included resection of the rectum with a diverting colostomy. The patient had reduced bladder function with difficulty initiating voiding and incomplete emptying of his bladder. Because of the desire to retain the patient's bladder function, we systematically treated the lesion in two stages, 6 weeks apart, with a total of 14 electrode deployments; the initial treatment focused on the caudal aspect of the sacrum. Figure 30.7B shows one of the seven RFA electrode deployments in the first stage of the treatment. Following the initial treatment, the patient was able to sit in bed the same day,

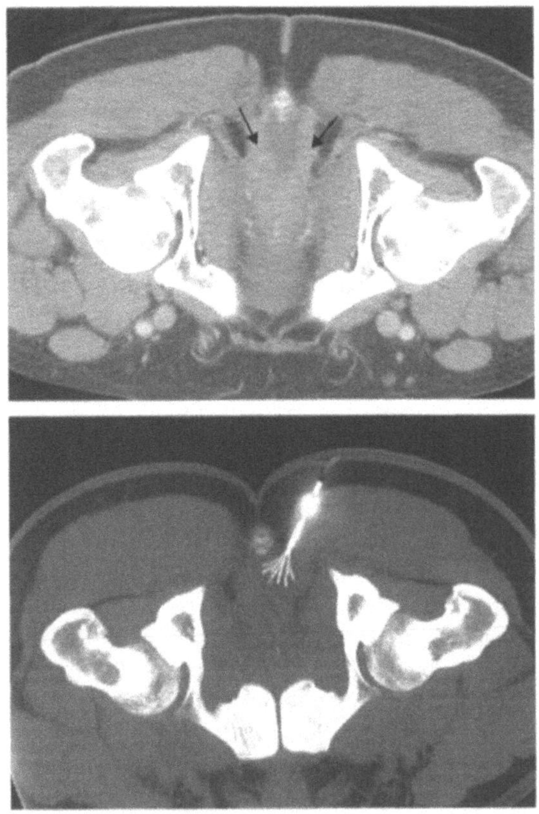
A
B

FIGURE 30.6. Metastatic presacral rectal carcinoma. (A) Prone contrast-enhanced CT demonstrates an oval peripherally enhancing soft tissue mass anterior to the coccyx (arrows). (B) Prone CT demonstrates the RFA electrode deployed within the mass. Patient's pain decreased from 8/10 to 1/10 4 weeks posttreatment. The patient continues to report 1/10 pain at this site 11 months posttreatment.

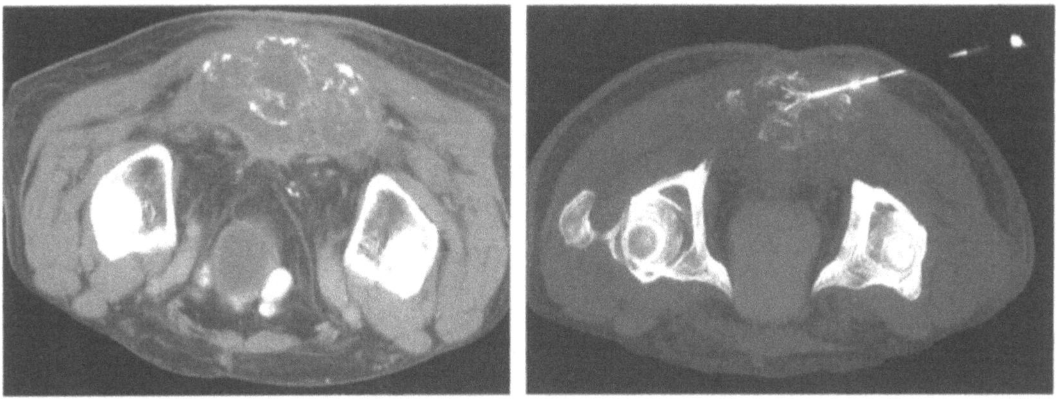

FIGURE 30.7. RFA of a large sacral metastasis. (A) Prone CT demonstrates near-complete replacement of the sacrum by metastatic rectal carcinoma. (B) RFA electrode deployed to 5 cm. This was one of seven electrode placements during the first stage of treatment for the ablation of much of the caudal aspect of the osteolytic lesion. The second stage was performed 6 weeks later. Patient was unable to sit prior to treatment and had resting pain of 8/10. One day following the ablation, the patient was able to sit. His pain decreased to 3/10.

and described 3/10 pain in the treated region 4 weeks following the procedure. Because of the patient's desire for greater pain relief, and with the understanding that further RFA could lead to loss of bladder function, we treated the superior portion of the lesion up to the level of the S2 neural foramina. Within 4 weeks, his pain was reduced to 0/10 at the treated region. Fortunately, his bladder function was not disturbed by the treatment.

Radiofrequency ablation of painful paraspinal metastatic lesions also is possible. Extreme caution must be used when metastatic lesions have destroyed the vertebral body with resultant loss of the insulative effect of the adjacent bone (20). Figure 30.8A is a CT image of a large metastatic colorectal carcinoma lesion that involves a rib, vertebral body, and pleural surface. To avoid thermal damage to the spinal cord, we placed a passive thermocouple along the lateral aspect of the destroyed pedicle (Fig. 30.8B,C). We subsequently treated the lesion with three electrode deployments along the involved rib. With the electrode deployed in the nearest paraspinal location (Fig. 30.8D), we discontinued further treatment when the passive thermocouple reached 40°C. This patient reported a reduction in pain from 10/10 prior to the treatment to 3/10 4 weeks after the RFA procedure.

Immediate postprocedural pain has been treated with epidural or intravenous (IV) opioid analgesics. Depending on the size of the treated lesion and the degree of postoperative pain, patients typically were observed overnight in the hospital. Patients with persistent postprocedural pain were administered oral opioid analgesics at the time of discharge.

Pain Assessment and Follow-Up

The patient's pain was the primary end point and was measured using the BPI. We interviewed all patients with the BPI just prior to the procedure, the day following the treatment, weekly for 1 month, and then every 2 weeks for the second through the sixth month. Each patient was asked to answer questions with respect to the lesion that was treated.

The type of malignancy, size, and location of the lesions that were treated are summarized in Table 30.1 Colorectal ($n = 10$), renal ($n = 9$), and lung ($n = 4$) were the most common tumor types treated. The most common sites of tumor involvement were the pelvis ($n = 12$), sacrum

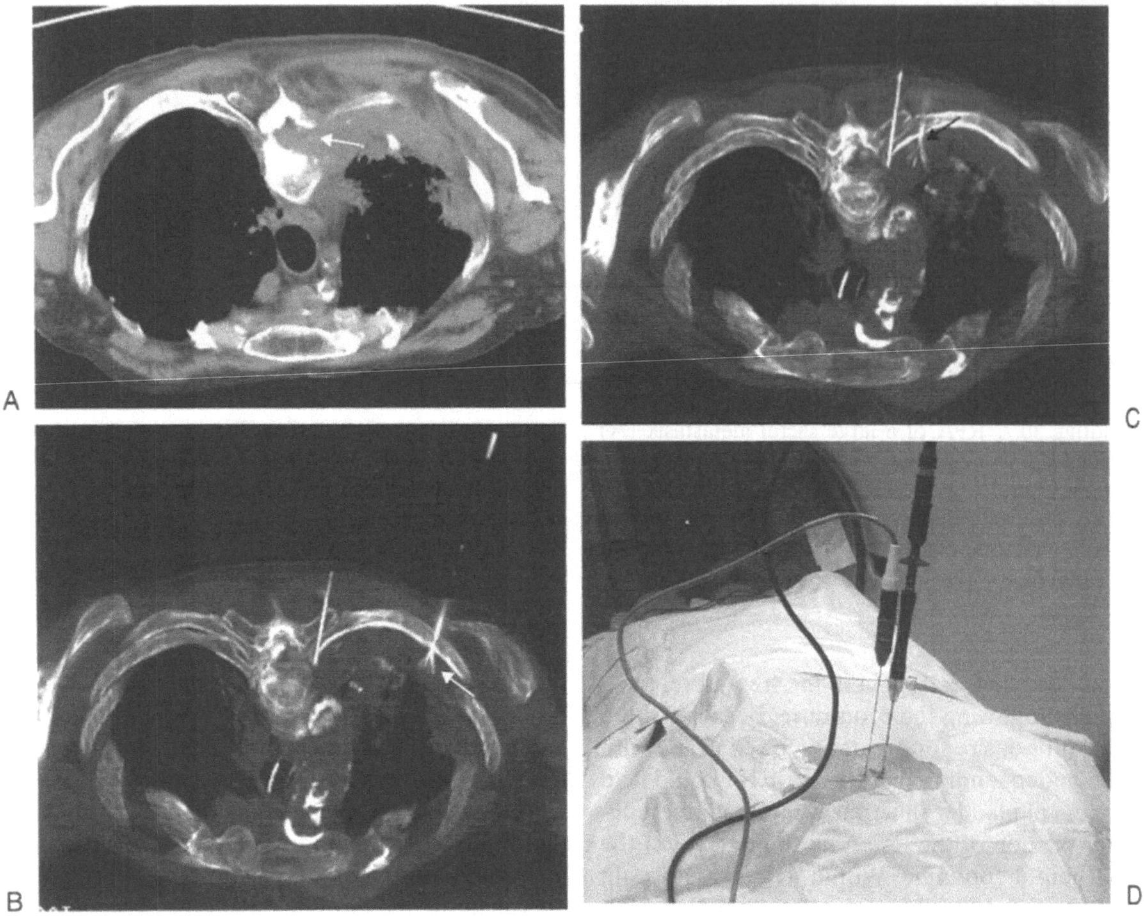

FIGURE 30.8. Metastatic colorectal carcinoma to rib, vertebral body, and pleural surface. (A) Volumetric prone CT demonstrates osteolytic destruction of the lateral portion of the vertebral body (arrow) with associated soft tissue mass anterior to the rib. (B) Prone CT image shows the position of the passive thermocouple probe near the vertebral body pedicle with the RFA electrode deployed laterally (arrow) in the metastatic lesion. (C) Prone CT demonstrates the most medial deployment of the RFA electrode (arrow). Ablation was discontinued when the temperature at the passive thermocouple reached 40°C. (D) Photograph of the RFA electrode in place with adjacent thermocouple located medially. The patient's pain decreased from 10/10 to 3/10 4 weeks following the treatment.

(n = 12), rib (n = 6), and vertebrae (n = 4). Treated lesions were osteolytic, with the exception of two patients who had mixed osteolytic/osteoblastic lesions. The size of the treated lesions ranged from 1 cm (rib) to approximately 18 cm (paraspinal). The median number of ablations per lesion was 3.0 (range 1–14), with an average time per ablation of 11.7 minutes (range 1.1–52.5 minutes). The mean total ablation time was 49.5 minutes (range 8.0–218.9 minutes).

Pain Response to Radiofrequency Ablation

A total of 41/43 patients (95%) experienced a drop in pain that met our a priori definition of a clinically significant benefit (two-point drop). Patients experienced highly significant reductions in worst pain, average pain, pain interference, and improvement in pain relief after RFA of painful metastases involving bone (Fig. 30.9 and Table 30.2). Significant decreases were seen beginning at week 1 and extending to week

TABLE 30.1. Characteristics of patients treated with radiofrequency ablation (RFA).

Number of patients	43	
Women	15	(35%)
Men	28	(65%)
Age (median)	64	(range 28–88)
Tumor type (number)		
Colorectal carcinoma	10	
Renal carcinoma	9	
Lung carcinoma	4	
Sarcoma	3	
Other	17	
Tumor size (longest diameter; cm)*	6.3 cm	(range 1.4–18.0)
Tumor location		
Pelvis	12	
Sacrum	12	
Rib	6	
Vertebrae	4	
Other	9	
Prior radiation to treated site	32	(74%)
Concurrent opioid analgesics	30	(70%)

* Tumor size at presentation. For lesions >5 cm, RFA treatment targeted ablation of the tumor–bone interface, not complete ablation of the tumor.

24 for all pain parameters. Two patients, whose pain responded to initial RFA, required retreatment after a recurrence of pain (≥4/10 worst pain) at 8 and 16 weeks, respectively. Both patients had significant reduction in worst pain (≥4-point drop) following retreatment.

Opioid use was recorded for each patient and converted into morphine equivalents using standardized conversions (30). Following RFA, opioid requirements peaked at week 1 (Table 30.2). At week 4, although opioid requirements were not statistically different from baseline, a trend toward decreasing requirements was seen. By weeks 8 and 12, there were significant reductions in opioid usage. Increases in opioid usage occurred at week 24, although the corresponding pain scores did not increase.

Although the RFA procedure is safe, precautions are necessary to avoid thermal injury to large nerves, vessels, bowel, and bladder. Adverse events following the procedures were noted in three patients. One patient developed

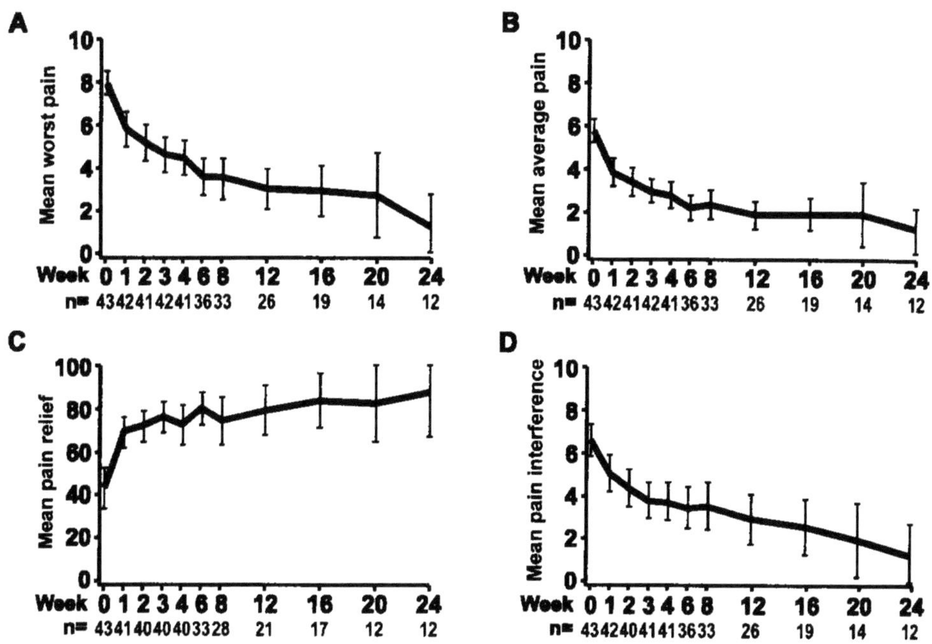

FIGURE 30.9. Mean Brief Pain Inventory (BPI) pain scores over time for patients treated with RFA. (A) Worst pain. (B) Average pain. (C) Pain relief from RFA or medications. (D) Interference of pain in daily activities. Error bars represent the 95% confidence intervals. *n*, the number of patients completing BPI at each time point.

TABLE 30.2. Number of patients, Brief Pain Inventory (BPI) mean pain scores, and opioid requirements at baseline and following RFA.

	Baseline	Day 1	Week 1	Week 4	Week 8	Week 12	Week 24
No. of patients	43	31*	42	41	33	26	12
Worst pain	7.9	7.3	5.8	4.5	3.5	3.0	1.4
(0–10)		$p = .2456$	$p < .0001$	$p < .0001$	$p < .0001$	$p < .0001$	$p = .0005$
Average pain	5.8	4.6	3.9	2.8	2.4	1.9	1.2
(0–10)		$p < .0001$	$p < .0001$	$p < .0001$	$p < .0001$	$p < .0001$	$p = .0005$
Pain interference	6.6	5.6	5.0	3.7	3.5	2.9	1.3
(0–10)		$p = .0825$	$p = .0001$	$p < .0001$	$p < .0001$	$p = .0008$	$p = .0015$
Pain relief	43	64	69	73	74	79	84
(0–100)		$p = .0007$	$p < .0001$	$p < .0001$	$p = .0002$	$p < .0001$	$p = .0029$
Morphine	99.0	97.5	105.7	95.5	40.4	45.4	93.0
equivalent dose					$p = .01$	$p = .01$	$p = .47$

Note: p values are signed rank tests of the null hypothesis that the difference in the current time period minus the baseline value is equal to zero.
* Ultrasound cohort only.

a second-degree skin burn at the grounding pad site. Another patient developed transient bowel and bladder incontinence following RFA of a previously irradiated leiomyosarcoma metastasis that involved the upper sacrum. A third patient developed an acetabular fracture 6 weeks following RFA of a breast cancer metastasis with significant involvement of the ileum, ischium, and acetabulum. This patient required open reduction and fixation of the acetabulum.

Summary

Several case reports and a clinical trial have found a highly significant reduction in pain from metastatic disease with percutaneous ablation. These findings are important, not only because of the magnitude of the benefit, but because it occurred in patients traditionally refractory to most conventional treatments.

These reports and our clinical trial show that RFA of metastatic lesions that involve bone is a safe procedure. Three complications were noted in our trial following treatment with RFA. One patient suffered transient bowel/bladder incontinence following treatment of a sacral metastasis that was previously irradiated. Another patient sustained an acetabular fracture 6 weeks following RFA of a metastatic lesion involving the ileum, ischium, and acetabulum. It was unclear whether RFA contributed to the development of the acetabular fracture. It is possible that injection of polymethylmethacrylate into the ablated tissue, as performed by Groenemeyer and coworkers (21) following ablation of spinal metastases, could result in stabilization of the partially destroyed bone and prevent fracture. One patient suffered a second-degree skin burn at the grounding pad site. Further burns may be prevented through careful monitoring of skin temperature deep to the grounding pads.

Radiofrequency ablation provides an effective, rapid, and durable method for palliation of localized painful metastases that involve bone. This procedure is safe and the relief of pain is significant; the procedure should provide an alternative for the palliation of painful bone metastases when standard treatments fail.

References

1. Nielsen OS, Munro AJ, Tannock IF. Bone metastases: pathophysiology and management policy. J Clin Oncol 1991;9:509–524.

2. Mercadante S. Malignant bone pain: pathophysiology and treatment. Pain 1997;69:1–18.
3. Mantyh PW, Clohisy DR, Koltzenburg M, Hunt SP. Molecular mechanisms of cancer pain. Nat Rev Cancer 2002;2:201–209.
4. Mannion RJ, Woolf CJ. Pain mechanisms and management: a central perspective. Clin J Pain 2000;16:S144–S156.
5. Watkins LR, Goehler LE, Relton J, Brewer MT, Maier SF. Mechanisms of tumor necrosis factor-alpha (TNF-alpha) hyperalgesia. Brain Res 1995; 692:244–250.
6. Sorkin LS, Xiao WH, Wagner R, Myers RR. Tumour necrosis factor-alpha induces ectopic activity in nociceptive primary afferent fibres. Neuroscience 1997;81:255–262.
7. Woolf CJ, Allchorne A, Safieh-Garabedian B, Poole S. Cytokines, nerve growth factor and inflammatory hyperalgesia: the contribution of tumour necrosis factor alpha. Br J Pharmacol 1997;121:417–424.
8. Opree A, Kress M. Involvement of the proinflammatory cytokines tumor necrosis factor-alpha, IL-1 beta, and IL-6 but not IL-8 in the development of heat hyperalgesia: effects on heat-evoked calcitonin gene-related peptide release from rat skin. J Neurosci 2000;20: 6289–6293.
9. Davar G, Hans G, Fareed MU, Sinnott C, Strichartz G. Behavioral signs of acute pain produced by application of endothelin-1 to rat sciatic nerve. Neuroreport 1998;9:2279–2283.
10. Gokin AP, Fareed MU, Pan HL, Hans G, Strichartz GR, Davar G. Local injection of endothelin-1 produces pain-like behavior and excitation of nociceptors in rats. J Neurosci 2001;21:5358–5366.
11. Zhou Z, Davar G, Strichartz G. Endothelin-1 (ET-1) selectively enhances the activation gating of slowly inactivating tetrodotoxin-resistant sodium currents in rat sensory neurons: a mechanism for the pain-inducing actions of ET-1. J Neurosci 2002;22:6325–6330.
12. Massie MJ, Holland JC. The cancer patient with pain: psychiatric complications and their management. J Pain Symptom Manag 1992;7:99–109.
13. Spiegel D, Sands S, Koopman C. Pain and depression in patients with cancer. Cancer 1994; 74:2570–2578.
14. Jeremic B, Shibamoto Y, Acimovic L, et al. A randomized trial of three single-dose radiation therapy regimens in the treatment of metastatic bone pain. Int J Radiat Oncol Biol Phys 1998; 42:161–167.
15. Price P, Hoskin PJ, Easton D. Prospective randomised trial of single and multifraction radiotherapy schedules in the treatment of painful bony metastases. Radiother Oncol 1986;6:247–255.
16. Cole DJ. A randomized trial of a single treatment versus conventional fractionation in the palliative radiotherapy of painful bone metastases. Clin Oncol (R Coll Radiol) 1989;1:59–62.
17. Gaze MN, Kelly CG, Kerr GR, et al. Pain relief and quality of life following radiotherapy for bone metastases: a randomised trial of two fractionation schedules. Radiother Oncol 1997: 109–116.
18. Gangi A, Kastler B, Klinkert A, Dietemann JL. Injection of alcohol into bone metastases under CT guidance. J Comput Assist Tomogr 1999;18: 932–935.
19. Groenemeyer DH, Schirp S, Gevargez A. Image-guided percutaneous thermal ablation of bone tumors. Acad Radiol 2002:467–477.
20. Dupuy DE, Hong R, Oliver B, Goldberg SN. Radiofrequency ablation of spinal tumors: temperature distribution in the spinal canal. AJR 2000;175:1263–1266.
21. Groenemeyer DHW, Schirp S, Gevargez A. Image-guided radiofrequency ablation of spinal tumors: preliminary experience with an expandable array electrode. Cancer J 2002;8:33–39.
22. Patti JW, Neeman Z, Wood BJ. Radiofrequency ablation for cancer-associated pain. J Pain 2002; 3:471–473.
23. Ohhigashi S, Nishio T, Watanabe F, Matsusako M. Experience with radiofrequency ablation in the treatment of pelvic recurrence in rectal cancer; report of two cases. Dis Colon Rectum 2001;44:741–745.
24. Ogunbiyi OA, McKenna K, Birnbaum EH, Fleshman JW, Kodner IJ. Aggressive surgical management of recurrent rectal cancer—is it worthwhile? Dis Colon Rectum 1997;40:150–155.
25. Wong CS, Cummings BJ, Brierley JD, et al. Treatment of locally recurrent rectal carcinoma—results and prognostic factors. Int J Radiat Oncol Biol Phys 1998;40:427–435.
26. Callstrom MR, Charboneau JW, Goetz MP, et al. Painful metastases involving bone: feasibility of percutaneous CT- and US-guided radiofrequency ablation. Radiology 2002;224:87–97.
27. Goetz M, Rubin J, Callstrom M, et al. Percutaneous US and CT-guided radiofrequency ablation of painful metastases involving bone. ASCO 2002; May 24–30:1544.

28. Daut RL, Cleeland CS, Flanery RC. Development of the Wisconsin Brief Pain Questionnaire to assess pain in cancer and other diseases. Pain 1983;17:197–210.
29. Cleeland CS, Gonin R, Hatfield AK, et al. Pain and its treatment in outpatients with metastatic cancer. N Engl J Med 1994;330:592–596.
30. Farrar JT, Young JP Jr, LaMoreaux L, Werth JL, Poole RM. Clinical importance of changes in chronic pain intensity measured on an 11-point numerical pain rating scale. Pain 2001;94:149–158.

31 Radiofrequency Ablation of Osteoid Osteoma

Daniel I. Rosenthal and Hugue Ouellette

Percutaneous radiofrequency treatment of osteoid osteoma has been performed for more than 10 years. It is the preferred method of treatment for most patients in those centers that offer it, and has been shown to be a safe, effective, and cost-effective alternative to operative treatment (1–5). However, many patients continue to be subjected to the increased risks and lengthy recovery of open surgery or to the prolonged discomfort and risks associated with medical therapy. This is presumably because of lack of awareness of the technique or benefits of percutaneous treatment. This chapter provides a detailed description of proper patient selection, technique, and follow-up for those wishing to perform this therapy.

Definition

Osteoid osteoma is a small, benign, but painful bone-forming tumor, which may cause considerable peritumoral inflammation. It is composed of osteoblasts that give rise to variable amounts of woven bone and a loose fibrovascular stroma (6). Unlike osteoblastoma, which may have identical histologic features, osteoid osteoma has little or no growth potential. The nonprogressive nature of the disease is a key aspect of the definition (7). However, since many, or even most, lesions are not observed over time to determine growth, in practice, osteoid osteoma is often differentiated from osteoblastoma on the basis of size (osteoid osteoma being smaller than 1.5 cm). Malignant transformation of an osteoid osteoma has not been described.

Osteoid osteomas comprise approximately 10% of benign bone tumors (8). They are thus rare enough so that the physician who initially sees the patient may fail to consider the diagnosis, but common enough to be encountered in many practices.

Patient Identification

Clinical

The tumors are usually found in the extremities of children and young adults. The typical patient is a late teenage boy. The average age in our series is 17, with a male predominance of 3:1. Patients less than 5 years of age or over 30 are uncommon, although a scattering of very young and very old patients have been reported (9,10).

Osteoid osteomas are painful. They appear to cause pain by two mechanisms. The lesions produce a large quantity of prostaglandin, leading to a variable but often marked inflammation of surrounding tissues (11,12). In this respect, they are similar to chondroblastomas, which also produce prostaglandin (12). In addition, however, osteoid osteomas contain sensory nerves (11,13). The combination of these two features is, we believe, unique among bone tumors (14).

The pain often begins insidiously as a dull ache in the affected part. Because of its characteristic occurrence in young males, it is often ascribed to an athletic injury or to "growing pains". With time, the pain may become sharper and more severe. Although pain may be exacerbated by activity, the tumors are usually painful at rest, and are often most painful at night. This is a useful distinguishing feature from stress fracture, which may have similar imaging features, but does not hurt when the extremity is rested. Superficial lesions are quite sensitive to palpation.

Pain usually responds to nonsteroidal anti-inflammatory medications. Response to medication is often (but not always) rapid and complete. Aspirin and ibuprofen appear to provide symptomatic relief in the greatest number of individuals. Naproxen, if effective, offers the greatest duration of relief. Acetaminophen is less effective. Severe pain may be accompanied by marked muscle wasting, sometimes simulating the presentation of a neuropathy (15).

Imaging

For therapy to be appropriately directed, the tumor must be definitively identified by pre-procedure imaging studies. This can be challenging since the tumor frequently is much smaller than the reactive zone that surrounds it. Typically, osteoid osteoma is an oval or spherical lucency, measuring between 1 and 15 mm in diameter (average 7–8 mm) (Figs. 31.1 to 31.3). Occasionally, tumors may be markedly elongated, measuring several centimeters in longitudinal dimension, but less than 1 cm in transverse diameter (16) (Fig. 31.4). This variation is most often seen in young children. Rarely, a small cluster of tumors may be seen (Fig. 31.5). Such "multicentric" tumors are almost always confined to a small anatomic area within a single bone (17). Failure to recognize that multiple lesions are present may be an uncommon cause of recurrence (18). Involvement of two anatomically remote sites has been reported (19–21), but is exceedingly rare.

The tumor may contain a variable amount of internal ossification, but is rarely completely ossified (Figs. 31.1 and 31.2). The term *nidus* often is used to describe the appearance of osteoid osteoma; however, it is sometimes used to mean the lucent tumor within the zone of reactive sclerosis, and at other times is used to refer to the focal ossification within the tumor. The word *nidus* comes from the Latin term for

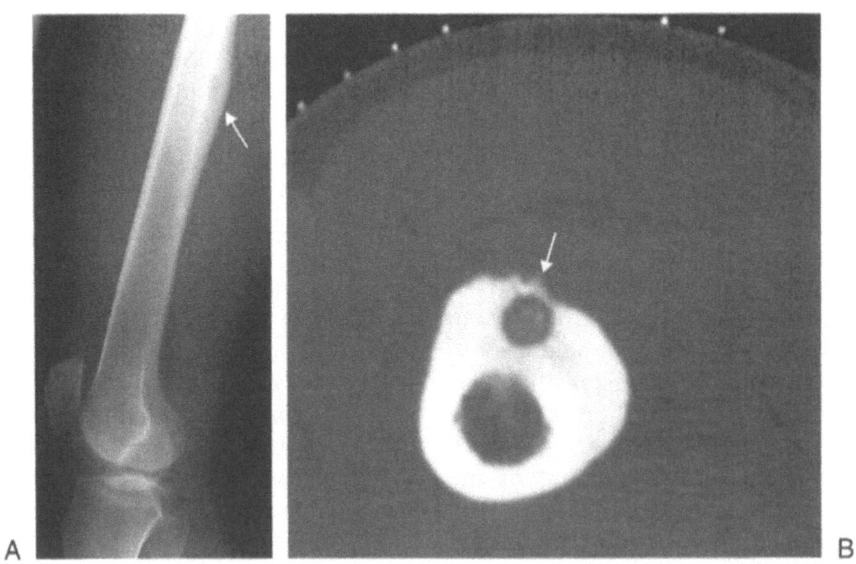

FIGURE 31.1. (A) Plain film of the femur demonstrates a lucency within the posterior cortex of the femur, surrounded by dense periosteal new bone formation (arrow). This is the typical appearance of an intracortical osteoid osteoma, the most common form. (B) Computed tomography (CT) scan through the lesion demonstrates that the tumor is 8 mm in diameter and contains faint internal ossification (arrow).

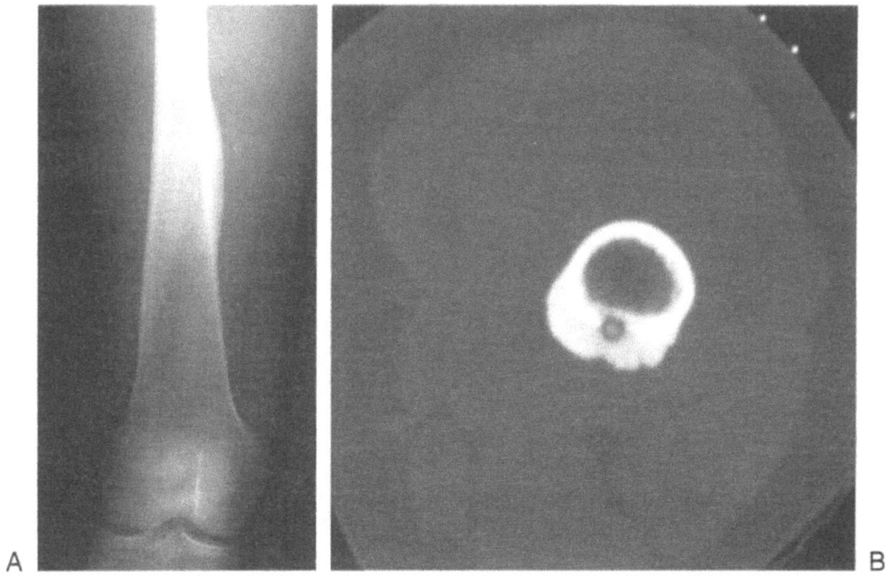

FIGURE 31.2. (A) Plain film demonstrates a lesion with a very similar appearance to that in Fig. 31.1A. (B) CT scan shows that the lesion originated on the periosteal surface of the bone, another common site of origin.

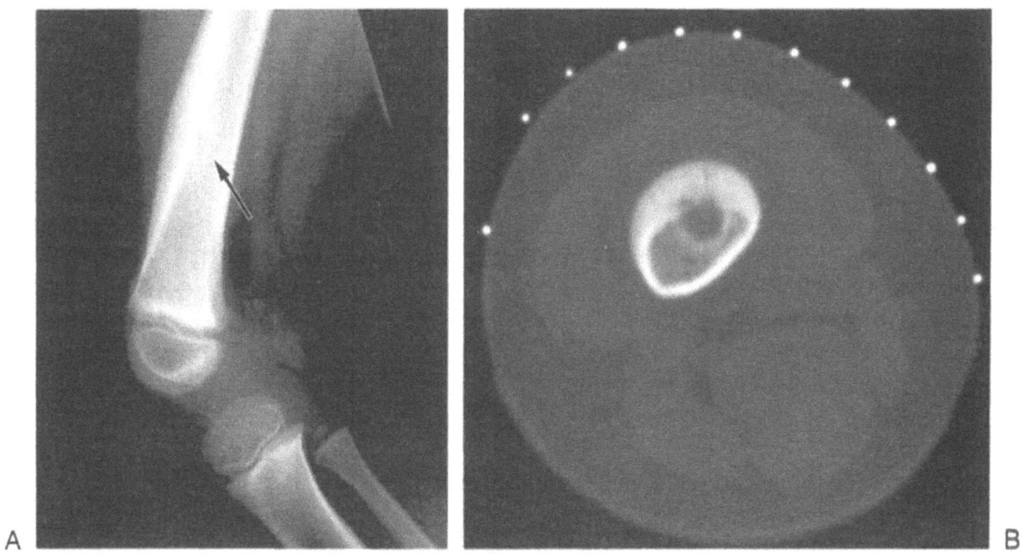

FIGURE 31.3. (A) The lesion (arrow) is difficult to see on this plain radiograph. (B) CT scan shows that the tumor has an intramedullary location, the least common presentation.

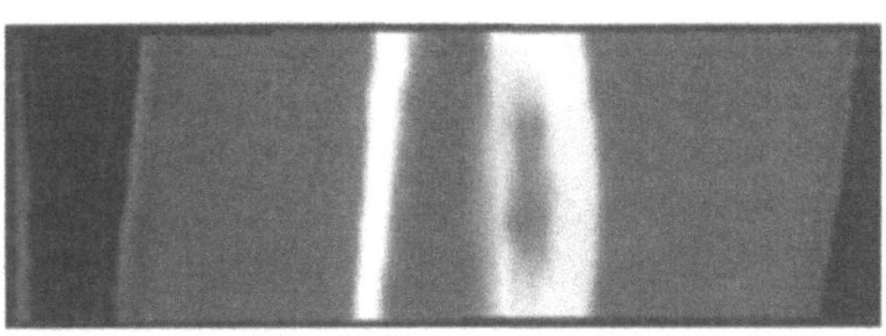

FIGURE 31.4. Reformatted CT scans demonstrate an elongated osteoid osteoma in the cortex of the femur. The tumor measured almost 3 cm in longitudinal dimension, but only 8 mm in axial diameter.

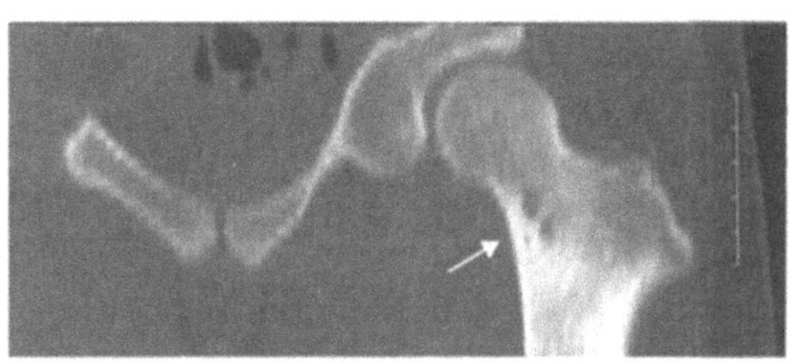

FIGURE 31.5. Reformatted CT scans demonstrate a multicentric osteoid osteoma of the femur, showing two distinct tumors separated by intervening bone (arrow).

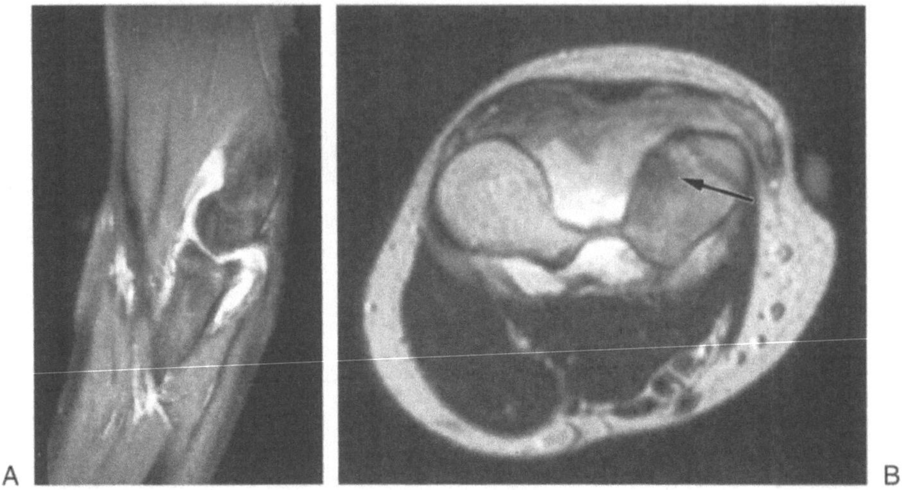

FIGURE 31.6. Sagittal (A) and axial (B) magnetic resonance images of the elbow demonstrate a large joint effusion in response to an intraarticular osteoid osteoma. The tumor itself is difficult to see, but appears as a rounded low-signal area in the humeral condyle (B, arrow).

"nest," and perhaps would be most suitable to describe the lucent tumor, with the tumoral ossification corresponding to the "egg" in the nest. However, in our opinion, the term is ambiguous. Throughout this chapter we refer to "tumor" and "tumor ossification," avoiding the word *nidus*.

Osteoid osteomas arise in cortex and periosteum with equal frequency. Medullary tumors are much less common (Fig. 31.3).

Although any bone may be affected, tumors are most common in the lower extremities. Local pain usually directs imaging studies to the appropriate location. However, referred pain is not rare, especially in younger patients. The most common pattern of referred pain is a tumor of the hip resulting in knee symptoms. Radioisotope scans are reliably abnormal in patients with osteoid osteoma. The tumor produces a small focus of intense uptake that is apparent even in the presence of surrounding tissue reaction. This feature can be useful to identify the location of the abnormality and sometimes may even be diagnostic.

Osteoid osteomas are characteristically (although not universally) surrounded by extensive peritumoral inflammatory changes. Bone marrow, periosteal, and soft tissue edema may be present. Lesions arising within joints may produce a massive joint effusion, simulating an arthropathy (Fig. 31.6) (22). Solid or sometimes layered periosteal ossification and medullary sclerosis are common. The sclerotic bone that surrounds the tumor can be extensive, and can obscure the tumor on plain films. Computed tomography (CT) scan reveals the diagnostic characteristics of osteoid osteoma most reliably. Magnetic resonance imaging (MRI) is highly sensitive to the reactive tissues, including the bone marrow and soft tissue edema that often surround the tumor. However, the tumor itself may be more difficult to identify on MRI (Fig. 31.6) (23). If the characteristic round or oval tumor cannot be identified with imaging studies, radiofrequency treatment should not be attempted.

Other Lesions that May Appear Similar

Several other lesions may cause confusion. Other symptomatic benign bone tumors also may also result in small oval lucencies surrounded by reactive bone. Painful *chondromas* are usually periosteal, but rarely may be intracortical (24,25). Periosteal chondromas usually sit on the bone surface like an egg in a cup, surrounded by a base of periosteal bone, but not by the extensive sclerosis seen with osteoid osteoma (26). *Chondroblastoma* usually is found in the epiphyseal centers of growing bones (as osteoid osteoma also may be). It is usually larger than an osteoid osteoma, and may have a lobulated contour. The surrounding tissue reaction may be very similar to osteoid osteoma. Similarly, *eosinophilic granuloma* (EG) may cause marked marrow edema and periosteal reaction. The lucent center of EG is often larger and more irregular in shape than osteoid osteoma (Fig. 31.7).

In each of these cases, the typical lesion differs in appearance from the typical osteoid osteoma, but atypical lesions may be indistinguishable. However, treatment of a small lesion of any of them by radiofrequency is appropriate and may be curative (27,28).

The very rare *intracortical variant of osteosarcoma* also may appear identical to an osteoid osteoma (29). Small metastases also could have a similar appearance, but fortunately are extremely rare in the age group affected by osteoid osteoma. Radiofrequency treatment of one of these malignant lesions has not been reported, but would almost certainly not be adequate therapy. If the correct diagnosis is revealed by the biopsy performed at the time of treatment, adjuvant therapy could be performed with no adverse consequences for the patient.

There are two entities for which radiofrequency treatment should be regarded as contraindicated. A *stress fracture* would probably be devitalized by radiofrequency treatment, perhaps resulting in delayed healing. Stress fractures can be distinguished on imaging by the absence of the typical oval or spherical lucency. A stress fracture may demonstrate a central lytic area particularly in the tibia, but the lucency is usually less well defined, and more linear. More importantly, the pain due to a stress fracture improves with rest, and seldom disturbs the patient's sleep, while osteoid osteoma generally causes pain that is not activity-dependent.

Treatment of an intracortical *abscess* by radiofrequency could result in formation of an area of devitalized bone. Such an iatrogenic sequestrum could complicate efforts to treat the infection. Most abscesses cause larger and less regular lytic areas, often resulting in lobular, elongated lucencies through the sclerotic bone, resembling an animal's burrow.

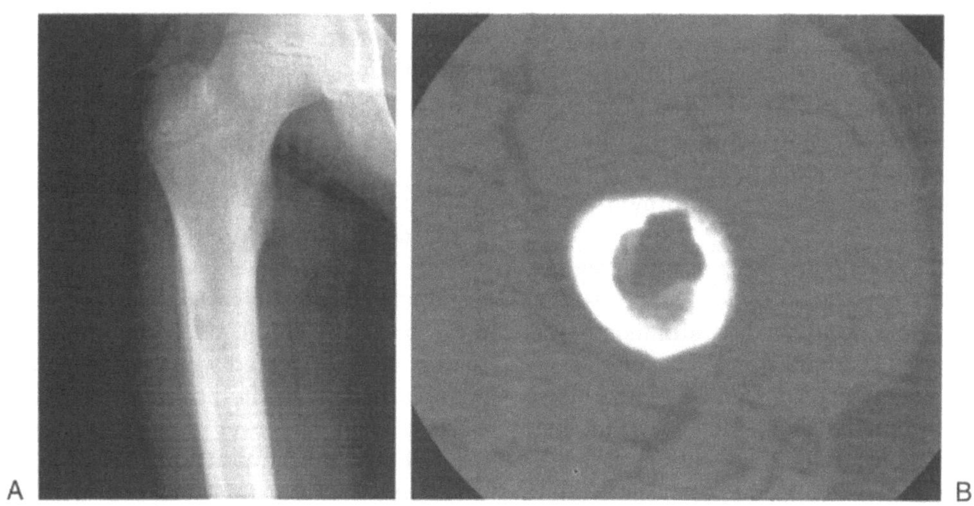

FIGURE 31.7. (A) Plain film showing a 1-cm lytic lesion of the femur, with marked periosteal reaction on the lateral cortex. This lesion was originally thought to represent an osteoid osteoma. (B) A CT scan of the lesion shows that the lesion has an irregular lobulated contour, which would be very unusual for an osteoid osteoma. Biopsy confirmed the diagnosis of eosiophilic granuloma.

Although potentially an abscess may simulate an osteoid osteoma exactly (30), this must be quite uncommon, as we have not yet encountered such a case.

Rationale for Intervention in Osteoid Osteoma

Since growth potential is limited, and since malignant degeneration has not been reported, the primary goal of treatment is elimination of symptoms. There is much anecdotal evidence, and at least small series that suggests that these lesions undergo spontaneous resolution, even if untreated (31–33). The average time to resolution of symptoms is said to be from 3 (32) to 6 years (31). These observations have given rise to the belief that osteoid osteoma may be treated appropriately by nonsteroidal antiinflammatory drugs without surgical or percutaneous intervention (32,34).

However, there is also anecdotal evidence of symptoms persisting for much longer periods without resolution (35–37). Since the majority of patients appear to undergo intervention of some sort, it is difficult to be certain of whether the majority of lesions would regress over time. When surgical treatment was the only alternative, chronic medical therapy was a reasonable alternative. However, percutaneous treatment has significantly lessened the morbidity of treatment, making it less clear why one would elect to have long-term medical therapy. Nonetheless, in considering the pros and cons of percutaneous radiofrequency treatment, all patients should be informed of this option.

There are several instances in which medical treatment is not a good option. Some patients do not tolerate nonsteroidal antiinflammatory medications. Gastrointestinal side effects are relatively common; ulcer formation and bleeding are uncommon. For a few patients, pain relief with nonsteroidal medications is inadequate. If a patient is forced to alter his lifestyle, or is unable to sleep or requires narcotics for pain relief, intervention seems preferable to conservative treatment.

If the untreated tumor is likely to result in structural damage, intervention should be strongly considered. If the lesion is close to an open growth plate, inflammatory hypervascularity may cause overgrowth or premature fusion leading to curvature of the limb or limb-length inequality (38). Similarly, inflammatory effects of intraarticular tumors may cause joint damage that leads to late arthritis (39,40). Spinal lesions often cause scoliosis due to muscle spasm. If left untreated for long periods of time, this may become permanent (41).

Choice of Intervention

Although several effective percutaneous techniques exist, we favor radiofrequency treatment because of its effectiveness, low cost, and favorable complication rate. Laser treatment is also a form of ablative therapy. It can be performed with very small-caliber needles (42,43). However, in our experience this confers no advantage, as sturdy needles often are required to gain access to the lesions and to obtain adequate biopsy material. Laser equipment is also more costly. Percutaneous excision also can be effective (44–46), especially for smaller tumors. Larger lesions are more difficult to remove, and complications due to the extent of bone removal may occur (47). Although success has been reported for alcohol injection (48,49), anatomic localization is more difficult to control and ablative effects are less reliable.

Contraindications to Radiofrequency Ablation

Complete diagnostic certainty is not required prior to intervention, as other benign bone tumors may be treated without harm and with possible benefit to the patient, if they are the cause of pain. However, radiofrequency treatment should not be performed if an infection or a stress fracture is a strong consideration.

If the tumor cannot be identified within the sclerotic bone and reactive edema, percutaneous treatment is not feasible.

If there is no safe access for a needle, treatment is not possible.

Most importantly, vital structures within 1 cm of the tumor could be injured by heat. This is especially true of nerves, making treatment of spinal tumors problematic. A thin shell of bone separating the lesion from the nerve may serve as a relative barrier to thermal transmission (50); however, each spinal case must be considered on its own merits, and we regard spinal location as a relative contraindication.

Proximity to a joint (Fig. 31.8) or a growth plate (Fig. 31.9) does not appear to represent an important problem, as the radiofrequency method is probably less destructive than either the surgical alternative or the continued presence of the tumor in such a location. We are unaware of any clinical consequences of treating a tumor adjacent to a joint or a growth plate.

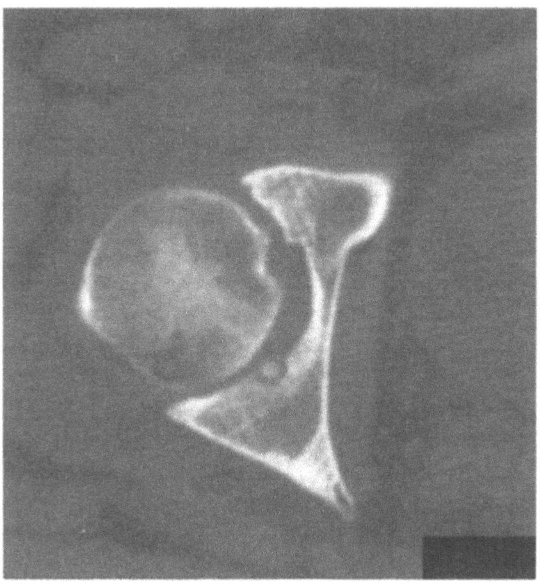

FIGURE 31.8. CT scan demonstrates an osteoid osteoma arising in the subchondral bone of the acetabulum. Although treatment of a lesion in such a location will probably produce some damage to articular cartilage, radiofrequency ablation is less destructive than any other intervention and probably less damaging to the joint than prolonged presence of an untreated tumor.

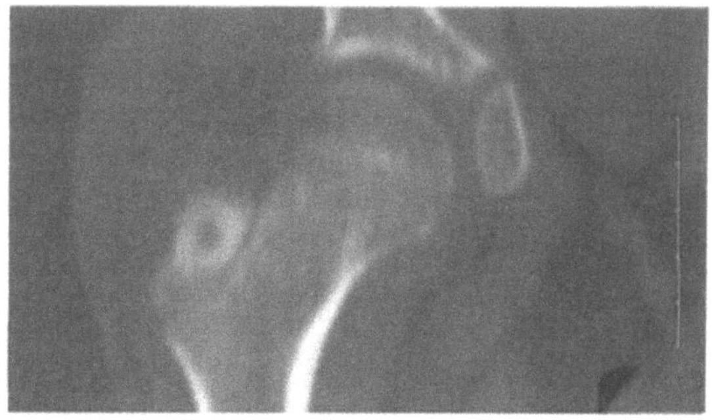

FIGURE 31.9. Reformatted CT images show a tumor arising within the epiphyseal center of the greater trochanter adjacent to the open growth plate.

Preparation for Radiofrequency Treatment

Most patients with osteoid osteoma are healthy children or young adults, and a brief interview will determine suitability for general anesthesia. Preprocedure laboratory testing does not seem necessary. Patients taking pain medication are told to continue until the night before the procedure, despite the known prolongation of bleeding time caused by these agents. Bleeding has not been a problem, perhaps because the radiofrequency treatment acts as a form of cautery.

General anesthesia is desirable for most cases. Osteoid osteomas are very sensitive to touch, and pain caused by needle entry into the tumor is much more intense than pain due to a typical bone biopsy. It cannot be adequately blocked by local anesthesia of the periosteal tissue (27). Furthermore, the small size of the tumors, the frequent presence of dense surrounding bone, and the requirement that no portion of the tumor be more than 5 mm from the electrode make proper positioning of the electrode both important and difficult. Any patient movement can significantly lengthen the procedure. Although spinal anesthesia can often produce adequate analgesia, it is not suitable for children, and often requires a longer interval of recovery before the patient can be discharged.

Once anesthesia is established, a localizing scan using collimation of 3 mm or less is performed. This preliminary scan is used to map the dimensions of the tumor and to establish the best access. Several points should be borne in mind in planning the procedure:

1. No part of the tumor must be more than 5 mm from the exposed tip of the electrode. For lesions that measure more than 1 cm in length, at least two electrode placements are required. Similarly, smaller lesions may require multiple placements if the electrode is not centrally located on the first placement.
2. If it is necessary to penetrate dense cortical or periosteal bone, it is preferable to approach the surface with the drill or needle perpendicular to the surface to minimize the risk of skidding along the cortex.
3. In most cases, the shortest path through the bone is preferred. However, in some instances it may be necessary or advisable to select an approach that requires more extensive drilling. It is perfectly feasible to access a lesion from the opposite side of the bone (Fig. 31.10); however, such an approach requires very careful attention (in all three dimensions). An error made during the early stages of drilling is not easily corrected once the needle is embedded in bone.
4. Thermal diffusion will kill tissue around the tip of the electrode for a distance of 5 to 6 mm. For superficial lesions, there is a risk of skin burn. Although cortical bone appears to confer a margin of safety (41,50), anatomic boundaries are not necessarily thermal boundaries and therefore treatment may not be advisable even though needle placement may be accomplished safely. We generally decline to perform RFA if adequate treatment of a lesion requires electrode placement less than 1 cm away from the spinal cord or an important nerve.

For all imaging after the initial localizing scans, tube current often can be reduced to half or even less than that used for routine imaging to minimize radiation exposure (Fig. 31.11). Sterile skin preparation is followed by placement of a marker needle (usually a 22-gauge spinal needle) and scans are performed to confirm the level prior to making an incision.

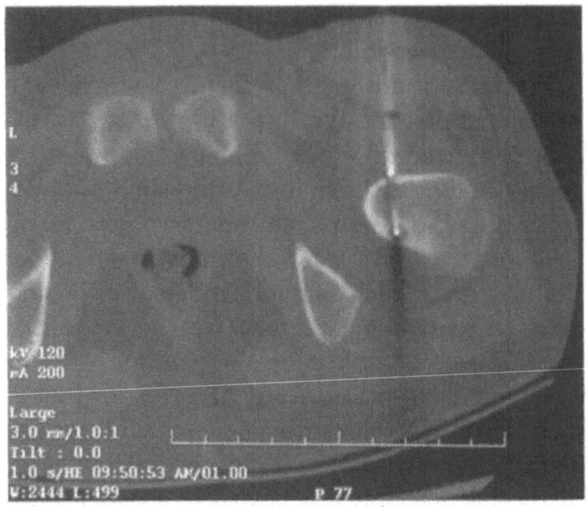

FIGURE 31.10. Direct access to this lesion on the posterior surface of the femoral neck was deemed inadvisable because of the proximity to the sciatic nerve, and the increased difficulty of anesthesia in the prone position. An anterior approach was used, which required drilling through the entire femoral neck.

Equipment

We have found the following combination of equipment to work well under a great variety of circumstances. Access to the bone is obtained using a Bonopty penetration set (Bonopty Bard, Radi Medical Systems, Uppsala, Sweden). This is a disposable hand-operated drill that is placed with a protective cannula. It comes in one size only. It readily penetrates periosteal bone, trabecular bone, and thin cortices. It also can be advanced through solid cortical bone (such as might be found in the midfemur of a young adult) with considerable effort and frequent interruptions to clear the drill channels. When the drill reaches to within 1 mm or less of the tumor, it is exchanged for a 16-gauge, 15-cm Osty-Cut bone biopsy needle (Bard/Angiomed, GmbH & Company Medizintechnik KG) (Fig. 31.12).

When the biopsy device enters the tumor, the patient often exhibits sudden increases in res-

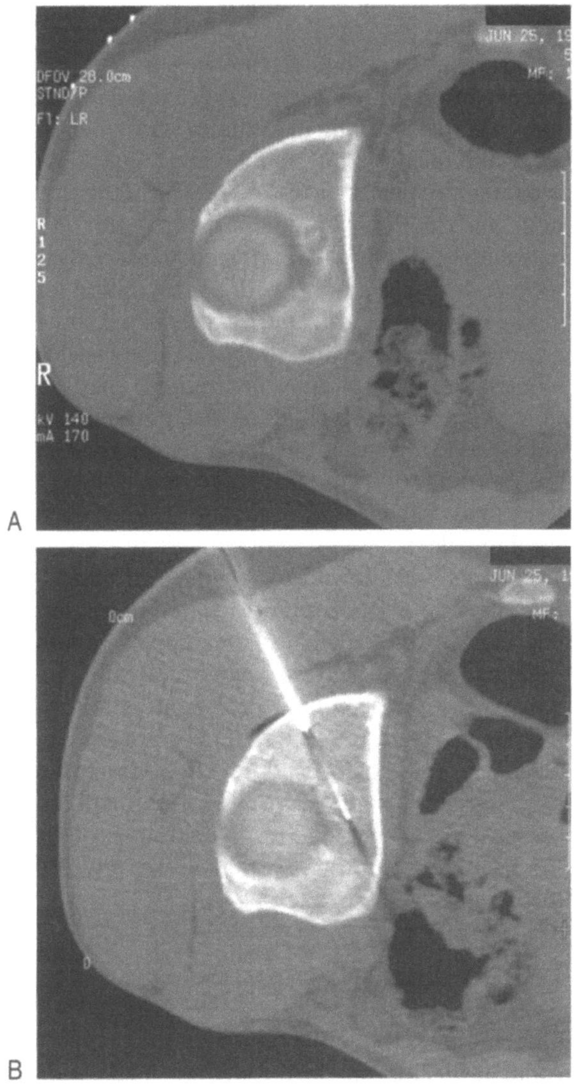

FIGURE 31.11. (A) An image from the initial localizing series performed using conventional exposure factors (140kVp, 170mA). (B) Repeated scans used for needle positioning are done with lower technical factors (120kVp, 70mA in this case) to reduce radiation exposure. Although there is increased mottle on the images, the quality is adequate to perform the procedure.

piratory rate and heart rate (27). This response helps to identify needle placement within the tumor, but placement also should be confirmed by check scans. The biopsy needle is passed through the entire lesion. Plugging the needle with bone on the far side of the lesion helps to retain the specimen upon needle withdrawal.

The biopsy needle is withdrawn, leaving the coaxial drill cannula in place, and the biopsy specimen is sent for routine processing. We have not found frozen section analysis to be advantageous because frozen preparation is suboptimal. The radiofrequency electrode is introduced through the cannula into the hole created by the biopsy needle.

Various electrodes are available on the market. Most of these have been designed for treatment of much larger soft tissue lesions and are not optimal for osteoid osteoma. For the greatest safety, the active tip of the electrode should not exceed the dimensions of the tumor. An electrode that results in a sphere of tissue necrosis approximately 1 to 1.5cm in diameter is ideal.

The dimensions of the electrode must be appropriate to the type of needle that was used for access. The electrode must be of small enough caliber and great enough length to fit through the device used to gain access to the bone, and into the hole made by the biopsy needle. We use a monopolar electrode with an outer diameter (OD) of 1.1mm and an exposed tip of either 5- or 8-mm length (Radionics, Burlington, MA). The smaller electrode is used for average lesions up to approximately 7 or 8mm. The larger electrode is used for bigger tumors.

Check scans are performed following electrode placement. It is important to confirm that

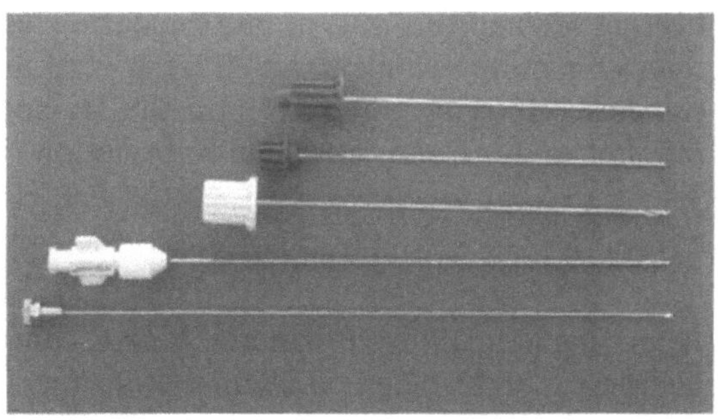

FIGURE 31.12. The top three devices are components of a Bonopty penetration set, consisting of a cannula, stylette, and drill. The lower two are the Osty-Cut bone biopsy needle and its stylette. Notice that the Osty-Cut device is long enough to obtain a biopsy through the Bonopty cannula.

no portion of the tumor is more than 5 or 6 mm away from the exposed portion of the electrode. This is easy to confirm for in-plane distances; however, longitudinal extent may require review of several images. If a part of the tumor is farther away, an additional drill hole, biopsy, and treatment should be performed to encompass the portion of the tumor not covered by the initial thermal lesion. Curiously, the performance of a radiofrequency treatment has no short-term effect upon the interpretability of the biopsy, and the pathologist will not be able to identify the fact that the second specimen has been heated.

Using manual or automatic output controls on the generator, the temperature at the tip of the electrode is gradually (approximately 1 degree/second) increased until it reaches 90°C. Downward adjustment of the generator output is required to maintain this temperature as progressive coagulation of the lesion occurs. The exact time and temperature for treatment is difficult to rationalize on purely scientific grounds. The ultimate size of the thermal lesion depends on the opposing effects of thermal diffusion, and tissue cooling, largely due to blood flow. In the steady state, temperature falls as the fourth power of the distance from the electrode (38), leading to a rather abrupt margin between viable and destroyed tissue. Since the steady state is reached shortly after the target temperature is achieved, sustained application of energy would appear to have little purpose. However, our experience with 4 minutes of heating seemed to result in more recurrences than a 6-minute treatment, which is our current standard. Imaging after treatment is not required and provides no useful information.

Care After the Procedure

Approximately 10 to 20 minutes before completion, a nonsteroidal antiinflammatory medication (Ketorolac, Allergan Pharmaceuticals, 30 mg IV adult dose) is administered intravenously to help with postprocedure pain. If the lesion is superficially located on the bone, injection of local long-acting anesthetic also may be helpful. However, in many instances it does not appear to be effective. A simple bandage or Steri-Strip is adequate. No suture, cast, or brace is required.

Upon awakening from anesthesia, the patient often, but not invariably, complains of pain. The pain is similar to tumor pain in character and location, but may be more intense. It is characteristically most severe within the first hour, and once brought under control with narcotics it steadily improves. It may be necessary to send the patient home with a prescription for a narcotic medication. One or two doses should be adequate, after which the patient may switch to nonsteroidals, or may not require medication. Approximately half of the patients are able to recognize that the tumor pain is gone by the morning following the procedure, although there may be residual procedure-related pain for a few days.

Patients are allowed to resume daily activities immediately. For tumors located in weight-bearing cortex, such as the upper femur, patients are advised to avoid activities involving distance running for 3 months following the procedure, even though we have not observed any postprocedure stress fractures. Leg muscle atrophy and abnormal gait (if present) are expected to resolve spontaneously. We have not required assistance from physical therapists.

Follow-Up

Our routine is to see the patient in the recovery room to decide on postprocedure medication needs, and to speak by telephone the next morning to answer questions. One week later we again telephone to report the results of the biopsy, and to assess the short-term outcome. All subsequent follow-up is performed by the referring clinician.

We do not believe that postprocedure imaging is essential in asymptomatic patents. However, if performed, at approximately 6 weeks after the procedure, it frequently reveals a spherical radiolucent "halo" approximately 1 to 1.5 cm from the electrode site, presumably representing the margins of the necrotic area. Subsequently the periosteal bone produced by the lesion becomes incorporated into the normal cortex and the tumor becomes increasingly and uniformly ossified. Young children may have completely normal imaging studies 6 months after the procedure. Older individuals may still demonstrate focal sclerotic areas even after several years. If the patient has no symptoms, the appearance is irrelevant.

Success Rates

Success of treatment is judged by freedom from pain and tumor recurrence. These are not necessarily identical, as patients may have persistent pain for various reasons other than recurrence.

In our experience it is extremely infrequent for a patient to obtain no relief at all from treatment. However, if there is residual tumor, recurrence of symptoms usually follows after a relatively brief interval. On average, recurrence is apparent between 3 and 6 months after treatment. We have seen occasional cases as late as 18 months. Although the literature documents rare instances after many years (51,52), most authorities agree that a 2-year pain-free interval is sufficient to document cure.

Using this criterion, in our experience approximately 90% of patients have complete and permanent relief of symptoms following a single treatment, 5% have recurrences, and 5% have some form of persistent symptoms but do not desire any further evaluation or therapy (16). Other series document somewhat higher rates of recurrence (53). Recurrence rates following operative intervention appear to be similar (51).

Recurrences are almost invariably in the same location as the initial tumor, or immediately contiguous, and present with the same symptoms. The treatment options for a recurrent lesion are identical to that for the initial lesion (medical, surgical, or percutaneous), although the success rates are lower.

References

1. Barei DP, Moreau G, Scarborough MT, Neel MD. Percutaneous radiofrequency ablation of osteoid osteoma. Clin Orthop 2000;373:115–124.
2. de Berg JC, Pattynama PM, Obermann WR, Bode PJ, Vielvoye GJ, Taminiau AH. Percutaneous computed-tomography-guided thermocoagulation for osteoid osteoma. Lancet 1995; 346(8971):350–351. (Notes: 18 patients with no complications using the ablation method. Patient hospitalized overnight and discharged next morning. Resumed normal activities immediately. All remained pain free except one; f/u 3–15 months. Second treatment eliminated symptoms in the unsuccessful case.)
3. Lindner NJ, Ozaki T, Roedl R, Gosheger G, Winkelmann W, Wortler K. Percutaneous radiofrequency ablation in osteoid osteoma. 2001; 83B(3):391–396. (Notes: Westfalishe Wilhelms Universität, Münster, Germany.)
4. Pinto CH, Taminiau AHM, Vanderschueren GM, Hogendoorn PCW, Bloem JL, Obermann WR. Technical considerations in CT-guided radiofrequency thermal ablation of osteoid osteoma: tricks of the trade. AJR Roentgenol 2002; 179(12):1633–1642.
5. Rosenthal DI, Hornicek FJ, Wolfe MW, Jennings CL, Gebhardt MC, Mankin HJ. Percutaneous radiofrequency coagulation of osteoid osteoma compared with operative treatment. J Bone Joint Surg 1998;80A(6):815–821.
6. Mirra J. Bone Tumors. Philadelphia: JB Lippincott, 1980:97.
7. Gitelis S, Schajowicz F. Osteoid osteoma and osteoblastoma. Orthop Clin North Am 1989; 20(3):313–325.
8. Greenspan A. Benign bone-forming lesions: osteoma, osteoid osteoma, and osteoblastoma. Skel Radiol 1993;22(7):485–500.
9. Habermann ET, Stern RE. Osteoid-osteoma of the tibia in an eight-month-old boy. J Bone Joint Surg Am 1974;56:633–636.
10. Szabo RM, Smith B. Possible congenital-osteoid osteoma of a phalanx. J Bone Joint Surg Am 1985;67:815–816.
11. Greco F, Tamburrelli F, Laudati A, La Cara A, Trapani G. Nerve fibres in osteoid osteoma. Ital J Orthop Traumatol 1988;14(1):91–94.
12. Wold LE, Pritchard DJ, Bergert J, Wilson DM. Prostaglandin synthesis by osteoid osteoma and osteoblastom. Mod Pathol 1988;1(2):129–130.
13. Esquerdo J, Fernandez CF, Gomar F. Pain in osteoid osteoma: histological facts. Acta Orthop Scand 1976;47(5):520–524.
14. O'Connell JX, Nanthakumar SS, Nielson GP, Rosenberg AE. Osteoid osteoma: the uniquely

innervated bone tumor. Mod Pathol 1998;11(2): 175–180.
15. Kiers L, Shield LK, Cole WG. Neurological manifestations of osteoid osteoma. Arch Dis Child 1990;65(8):851–855.
16. Chiou Y-Y, Rosenthal DI, Rosenberg AE. "Beaded" osteoid osteoma: a possible intermediate between solitary and multicentric tumor. Skel Radiol 2003;32(7):412–415.
17. Kenan S, Abdelwahab IF, Klein MJ, Hermann G, Lewis MM. Case report 864. Elliptical, multicentric periosteal osteoid osteoma. Skel Radiology 1994;23(7):565–568.
18. Keret D, Harcke HT, MacEwen GD, Bowen JR. Multiple osteoid osteomas of the fifth lumbar vertebra. Clin Orthop Rel Res 1989;248:163–168.
19. O'Dell CW Jr, Resnick D, Niwayama G, George TG, Linovitz RJ. Osteoid osteoma arising in adjacent bones. Report of a case. J Canad Assoc Radiol 1976;27:298–300.
20. Rand JA, Sim FH, Unni KK. Two osteoid osteomas in one patient: a case report. J Bone Joint Surg 1982;64A(8):1243.
21. Schai F, Friederich N, Kruger A, Jundt G, Herbe E, Buess P. Discrete synchronous multifocal osteoid osteoma of the humerus. Skel Radiol 1996;25(7):667–670.
22. Alani WO, Bartal E. Osteoid osteoma of the femoral neck stimulating an inflammatory synovitis. Clin Orthop Rel Res 1987;223:308–312.
23. Davies M, Cassar-Pullicino VN, Davies AM, McCall IW, Tyrrell PN. The diagnostic accuracy of MR imaging in osteoid osteoma. Skeletal Radiol 2002;31(10):559–569.
24. Abdelwahab IF, Hermann G, Lewis MM, Klein MJ. Case report 588: intracortical chondroma of the left femur. Skel Radiol 1990;19:59–61.
25. Rudman DP, Damron TA, Vermont A, Mathur S. Intracortical chondroma. Skel Radiol 1998; 27(10):581–583.
26. Bauer TW, Dorfman HD, Latham JT. Periosteal chondroma: a clinicopathologic study of 23 cases. Am J Surg Pathol 1982;6(7):631–637.
27. Ramnath RR, Rosenthal DI, Cates J, Gebhardt M, Quinn RH. Intracortical chondroma simulating osteoid osteoma treated by radiofrequency. Skeletal Radiol 2002;31:597–602.
28. Erickson JK, Rosenthal DI, Zaleske DJ, Gebhardt MC, Cates JM. Primary treatment of chondroblastoma with percutaneous radio-frequency heat ablation: report of three cases. Radiology 2001;221(2):463–468.
29. Hasegawa T, et al. Intracortical osteoblastic osteosarcoma with oncogenic rickets. Skel Radiol 1999;28:41–45.
30. Abril JC, Castillo F, Diaz A. Brodie's abscess of the hip simulating osteoid osteoma. Orthopedics 2000;23(3):285–287.
31. Golding JSR. The natural history of osteoid osteoma. J Bone Joint Surg 1954;36B(2):218–229.
32. Kneisl JS, Simon MA. Medical management compared with operative treatment for osteoid osteoma. J Bone Joint Surg 1992;74A(2):179–183.
33. Leicester AW, Trantalis JN. Osteoid osteoma in a young child: successful non-operative management. ANZ J Surg 2001;71:491–493.
34. Saville PD. A medical option for the treatment of osteoid osteoma. Arthritis Rheum 1980;23: 1409–1411.
35. Jackson RP, Reckling FW, Mantz FA. Osteoid osteoma and osteoblastoma. Clin Orthop Rel Res 1977;128:303–313.
36. Kayser M, Muhr G. Eighteen-year anamnesis of osteoid osteoma—a diagnostic problem? Arch Orthop Trauma Surg 1988;107(1):27–30.
37. Vickers CW, Pugh DC, Ivins JC. Osteoid osteoma: a fifteen-year follow-up of an untreated patient. J Bone Joint Surg Am 1959; 41A(2):357–358.
38. Antich PP, Pak CYC, Gonzales J, Anderson J, Sakhaee K, Rubin C. Measurement of intrinsic bone quality in vivo by reflection ultrasound: correction of impaired quality with slow-release sodium fluoride and calcium citrate. J Bone Miner Res 1993;8(3):301–311.
39. Foeldvari I, Schmitz MC. Rapid development of severe osteoarthritis associated with osteoid osteoma in a young girl. Clin Rheumatol 1998; 17(6):534–537.
40. Weber KL, Morrey BF. Osteoid osteoma of the elbow: a diagnostic challenge. J Bone Joint Surg Am 1999;81A(8):1111–1119.
41. Cove JA, Taminiau AH, Obermann WR, Vanderschueren GM. Osteoid osteoma of the spine treated with percutaneous computed tomography-guided thermocoagulation. Spine 2000;25(10):1283–1286.
42. Gangi A, Dietemann JL, Gasser B, et al. Interventional radiology with laser in bone and joint. Radiol Clin North Am 1998;36(3):547–557.
43. Witt JD, Hall-Craggs MA, Ripley P, Cobb JP, Bown SG. Interstitial laser photocoagulation for the treatment of osteoid osteoma. J Bone Joint Surg 2000;82B(8):1125–1128.

44. Amendola A, Vellet D, Willits K. Osteoid osteoma of the neck of the talus: percutaneous, computed tomography-guided technique for complete excision. Foot Ankle Int 1994;15(8): 429–431.
45. Assoun J, Railhac J-J, Bonnevialle P, et al. Osteoid osteoma: percutaneous resection with CT guidance. Radiology1993;188(2):541–547.
46. Atar D, Lehman WB, Grant AD. Tips of the trade. Computerized tomography-guided excision of osteoid osteoma. Orthop Rev 1992; 21(12):1457–1458.
47. Sans N, Galy-Fourcade D, Assoun J, et al. Osteoid osteoma: CT-guided percutaneous resection and follow-up in 38 patients. Radiology 1999;212(3): 687–692.
48. Duda SH, Schnatterbeck P, Harer T, Giehl J, Bohm P, Claussen CD. Treatment of osteoid osteoma with CT-guided drilling and ethanol instillation. Dtsch Med Wochenschr 1997; 122(16):507–510.
49. Sanhaji L, Gharbaoul IS, Hassani RE, Chakir N, Jiddane M, Boukhrissi N. A new treatment of osteoid osteoma: percutaneous sclerosis with ethanol under scanner guidance. J Radiol 1996; 77(1):37–40. (Original in French.)
50. Dupuy DE, Hong R, Oliver B, Goldberg SN. Radiofrequency ablation of spinal tumors: temperature distribution in the spinal canal. AJR 2000;175(5):1263–1266.
51. Norman A. Persistence or recurrence of pain: a sign of surgical failure in osteoid osteoma. Clin Orthop Rel Res 1978;130:263–266.
52. Regan MW, Galey JP, Oakeshott RD. Recurrent osteoid osteoma. Clin Orthop Rel Res 1990;253: 221–224.
53. Vanderschueren GM, Taminiau AHM, Obermann WR, Bloem JL. Osteoid osteoma: clinical results with thermocoagulation. Radiology 2002; 224(1):82–86.

32 Image-Guided Prostate Cryotherapy

Gary Onik

Background of Cryotherapy

The treatment of prostate cancer remains a significant dilemma. The prevalence of prostate cancer is quite high, documented by pathologic studies. It is well accepted that a major proportion of prostate cancers will not be clinically significant (1). Even those cancers with a volume of 0.5 cc or greater have a variable biologic behavior. On the other hand, the treatments for prostate cancer are not without substantial chance for lifestyle-limiting morbidity. Recent information showing minimal survival benefit between no treatment and radical prostatectomy has emphasized the concept of "watchful waiting"; that is, not treating the primary tumor at all has gained acceptance as a viable management alternative in certain patient populations (2). The decision to treat an individual's prostate cancer with a particular therapy or at all, requires a careful assessment of the risk versus benefit for that patient. As the complications and lifestyle limiting side effects of treatments are reduced, these decisions become easier. The reintroduction of ultrasound-guided prostate cryotherapy is founded on the goal of decreasing the morbidity of prostate cancer treatment.

Gondor et al (3) in 1966 first reported the concept of a cryotherapy procedure for the treatment of prostate disease. Subsequently, an open transperineal cryosurgery procedure was developed in which the freezing was carried out on the surface of the prostate with visual monitoring. Using this same approach, Bonney et al (4) reported results of this procedure in 229 patients followed for up to 10 years. Comparison with radical prostatectomy and radiation therapy patients showed equal survival among the various treatment modalities. Although cryosurgery showed some advantages, such as being able to treat patients with large bulky tumors, poor monitoring of the freezing process resulted in complications such as urethrocutaneous and urethrorectal fistulas that limited acceptance of the procedure.

In 1993 Onik et al (5) reported the first series of percutaneous ultrasound-guided and -monitored prostate cryotherapy (Figs. 32.1 and 32.2). This report resulted in a resurgence of interest. As with any new procedure, ultrasound-guided prostate cryotherapy went through a learning curve. Reported results about the control of the cancer as well as complications were variable. A negative perception of the procedure was compounded in that most early series predominantly treated patients who had failed radiation therapy and who had much higher complication rates, particularly that of incontinence (73%) (6,7). The situation was also exacerbated by a high urethral complication rate, caused by use of a rigged urethral warming catheter, when the original catheter was placed back into investigational use by the Food and Drug Administration (FDA) (14% vs. 42%) (8). Despite these early problems, the long-term results from multiple institutions were examined, and finally the Health Care Financing Administration (HCFA) in 1999 removed cryosurgery from the investigational category, placing it alongside radiation and

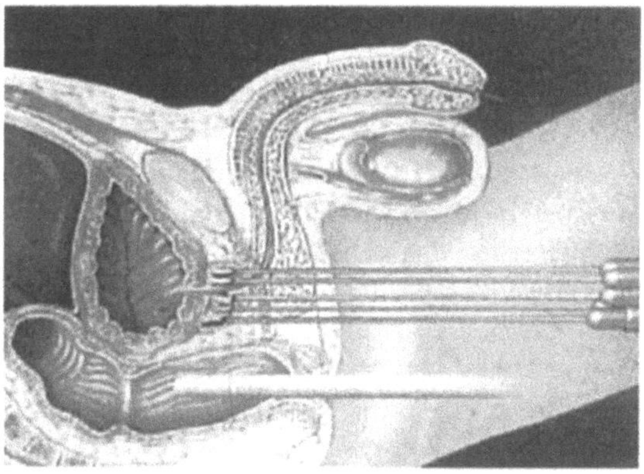

FIGURE 32.1. The transperineal placement of cryoprobes into the prostate using transrectal ultrasound (US) guidance. This is the same approach used for brachytherapy.

radical prostatectomy as a treatment for primary prostate cancer.

The quality of these results, taking into account the early technical variability of the procedure, as well as the urethral warmer problems, is best reflected in the multiinstitutional study recently published by Long et al (9). When they compared cryotherapy to radiotherapy using the same patient risk stratification and success criteria, the results were comparable to both external-beam radiation therapy and brachytherapy. The 5-year biochemical disease-free survival rate with cryotherapy for the low-risk group was 76%, and for comparable brachytherapy the reported series was 75% to 87% and for conformal radiotherapy 67% to 81%. The results were similarly comparable for medium- and high-risk groups. In terms of complications, the incidence of rectal complications was greater for radiation therapy, while the rate of impotence was greater for cryotherapy. Long et al noted that it was remarkable that the results were so similar, despite the substantial disparity in resources and experience between the two therapies. As we will examine, when the latest advances in cryotechniques are considered, the results and complication rates for cryosurgery reported by Long et al can be markedly improved.

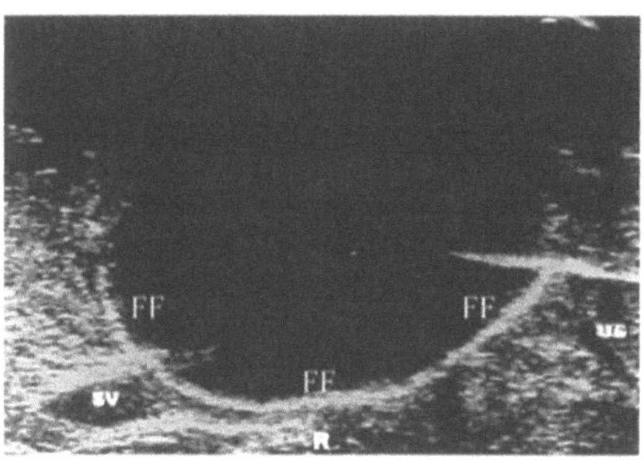

FIGURE 32.2. Transrectal ultrasound showing excellent visualization of the freezing front (FF) as a hyperechoic rim with posterior acoustic shadowing. R, rectal wall; SV, seminal vesicle; UG, urogenital diaphragm.

Patient Selection

When dealing with prostate cancer therapy, the extent and pathologic character of the patient's disease are essential in choosing the proper therapy. Treatments such as radical prostatectomy and radiation have higher recurrence rates as the extent and aggressiveness (Gleason score) of the patient's cancer increase. An advantage of cryotherapy is the flexibility of the procedure to be tailored to treat both high- and low-risk patients, as well as patients who have failed radiation therapy.

The Patient at High Risk for Local Recurrence

The use of cryotherapy for the treatment of solid organ cancers made a resurgence with the advent of ultrasound monitoring of hepatic cryosurgery in 1984 (10). Hepatic cryotherapy filled a unique place in the armamentarium of liver cancer treatment, in that it successfully treated patients with multiple tumors or tumors that were unresectable due to proximity to major vasculature that could not be sacrificed (11,12). Due to its target patient population of previously untreatable patients, with an expected mortality of virtually 100%, imaging-guided hepatic cryotherapy was readily embraced by the surgical oncologic community (13).

In at least one way, prostate cancer is akin to liver cancer in that many patients with prostate cancer are unresectable, based on the likelihood of capsular penetration at the time of definitive treatment. Unfortunately, efforts at preoperative staging have been inadequate to identify this patient population. The difficulty of the situation is further compounded because at the time of radical prostatectomy the surgeon's ability to appreciate capsular penetration and involvement of the neurovascular bundles is inadequate. In a recent study by Vaidya et al (14), there was virtually no correlation between the surgeon's determination of tumor penetration into the periprostatic tissue with involvement of the neurovascular bundle and actual pathologic confirmation. Thus, positive margin rates of 30% to 40% associated with nerve sparing radical prostatectomy are the usual situation.

Using various clinical parameters such as Gleason score, clinical stage, and prostate-specific antigen (PSA) level, preoperative prediction of the statistical chance for capsular penetration can be reasonably assessed (15,16). This approach can lower the positive margin rate when rigorously applied, as demonstrated by Eggleston and Walsh (17). In clinical practice, however, most urologists believe that radical prostatectomy still is the gold standard of treatment. This leads to a natural reluctance to deny a patient the treatment they feel is unproven for cure. Based on the success of cryotherapy in treating unresectable liver cancer, it was hoped that with the ability to freeze into the periprostatic tissue, thereby encompassing tumor capsular penetration, that prostate cryotherapy could improve the outcome in those patients at high risk of positive surgical margins.

Numerous studies on ultrasound-guided prostate cryotherapy have demonstrated successful treatment of patients with stage T3 prostate cancer with demonstrated gross extracapsular disease (18,19). Demonstration of this concept in patients with a "high likelihood" of capsular penetration, based only on statistical analysis, is more problematic, since the exact margin status of the tumor is not known preoperatively or postoperatively following cryotherapy.

One study, in which aggressive periprostatic freezing was facilitated by separating the rectum from the prostate at the time of the operation by a saline injection into Denonvilliers' fascia, showed no local recurrences demonstrated in 61 patients followed for up to 4 years (20). These good results occurred despite the fact that 68% of the patients were considered at high risk of capsular penetration and local failure, based on a Gleason score of 7 or greater, PSA more than 10 ng/mL, having failed radiation therapy, or extensive bilateral disease based on preoperative biopsies.

When cryoablation is carried out aggressively with the aim of a negligible PSA post-treatment, comparison with radical prostatectomy should be possible. In the only published study comparing the outcomes between the two (21), cryotherapy had a 23% greater chance of resulting in a PSA of less than 0.2 ng/mL than did radical prostatectomy (96% vs. 73%). When a 0 PSA was used as the success criterion, cryotherapy maintained an approximately 20% advantage over radical prostatectomy (66.9% vs. 48.2%). As risk for positive margins increased, based on a PSA of 20 or greater, cryotherapy maintained these results, while those of radical prostatectomy deteriorated further (86% vs. 36%). While this study was retrospective and with only a relatively small number of patients, the results are consistent with the original rationale of destroying extracapsular cancer by treating the periprostatic tissues. In addition, these findings are consistent with other studies that show success in treating T3 disease and other high-risk patients.

In two recent cryotherapy reports with 5- and 7-year follow-up in medium- and high-risk patients, the results were superior to other treatment modalities, including conformal radiation therapy, brachytherapy, and radical prostatectomy (22,23). Kaplan-Meyer curves showed virtually no difference among low-, medium-, and high-risk patients. These results are remarkable, and have major implications for overall survival in patients who previously had a poor prognosis. These results, coupled with the low morbidity of the procedure, the ability to be performed in older patients and the ability to be repeated when needed, we believe make cryotherapy the procedure of choice in this subset of patients.

Organ-Confined, Low-Volume, Low Gleason Score Disease (Nerve-Sparing Cryotherapy)

When treating patients with prostate cancer that is organ confined, low morbidity and limited effect on lifestyle become major factors in selection of the treatment option. Cryotherapy has low morbidity, and the procedure can be done on an outpatient basis. Also, there is no need for blood transfusions and no reported incidence of periprocedural cardiovascular or pulmonary complications. The most dreaded local complication of prostate cryoablation, urethrorectal fistula, which occurs due to rectal freezing, has virtually been eliminated by the technique of injecting saline into Denonvilliers' fascia at the time of the procedure, thus creating a large buffer zone between the rectum and the prostate capsule. When failed radiation cases and those patients treated without the original urethral warmer are excluded, cryotherapy has an excellent record in relation to urinary complications, with low incontinence rates of 2% or less (20,24,25). A study published by Robinson et al (26), looking at the quality of life of patients undergoing cryoablation, showed return of urinary function to baseline status in virtually all patients by 1 year postprocedure.

In an effort to prove itself as a viable cancer treatment, cryotherapy has been aggressively aimed at total prostate gland ablation. It is clear, however, that total gland ablation with freezing of both neurovascular bundles has a significant negative impact on sexual function (26). Cryotherapy's high rate of impotence is a major disadvantage compared to nerve-sparing radical prostatectomy and brachytherapy in garnering patients who are interested in maintaining sexual function. In our experience, total cryotherapy has the same impotency rate as non–nerve-sparing radical prostatectomy: virtually 100% in the short and intermediate terms. The same reason that cryotherapy has demonstrated an advantage in treating high-risk patients, however, contributes to this rate of impotence. When cryoablation is properly carried into the periprostatic tissue to encompass any extracapsular tumor that preferentially invades the neurovascular bundles, both bundles are necessarily destroyed. Therefore, in patients at high risk of bilateral extracapsular disease, impotence is an expected side effect, and actually a welcome sign that proper treatment has been carried out. The original thought that sexual dysfunction secondary to cryotherapy would only be temporary, based on the well-known ability of peripheral nerves to regenerate after cryoablation, was erroneous. The parasympathetic system, critical to erection, has its secondary cell bodies in proximity to the prostatic capsule; the destruction of these by cryotherapy is irreversible.

However, nothing limits cryotherapy from being carried out as a nerve-sparing procedure, similar to the approach with radical prostatectomy. The ability of cryotherapy to be repeated is an advantage. Temperature monitoring to prevent freezing of the contralateral neurovascular bundle from the tumor can be used to preserve this structure, and therefore maintain potency.

We have followed a group of nine patients, for as long as 6 years, who underwent unilateral nerve-sparing cryotherapy. The indication for nerve-sparing cryotherapy was the small volume of cancer demonstrated on biopsy, along with the demonstration of unilateral disease by staging procedures. The potency rate (defined as erection sufficient to carry out intercourse to the satisfaction of the patient) was 78% (seven of nine patients), with no patient having evidence for a local recurrence on PSA monitoring or biopsy. The group included high-risk patients, with five of nine having some risk factor for extracapsular disease (three of nine patients had a Gleason score of 7 or above). The potency results were surprising in that only one nerve bundle was spared, but this lack of manipulation spares injury to the blood supply. These results rival bilateral nerve sparing of radical prostatectomy (27). The high potency rate with sparing of only one neurovascular bundle is better than that expected with radical prostatectomy, which has been reported as 13% to 41% (28,29). Brachytherapy has a reported potency rate of 49% 2 years postprocedure (30).

Nerve-sparing cryotherapy is a blend of an aggressive, yet minimally invasive procedure, which accounts for the combination of excellent cancer control and lack of complications. Extensive freezing of the periprostatic tissue is still carried out on the side of the demonstrated tumor. In patients with a high Gleason score, or with cancer demonstrated at the base of the gland, prophylactic freezing of the confluence of the seminal vesicles also can be carried out. The expected incidence of urinary and rectal complications is lower than that for total cryoablation, radical prostatectomy, or brachytherapy. No patient in our series demonstrated persistent incontinence. Importantly, any errors in patient selection are correctable by re-treatment without added morbidity. We believe this treatment approach has major implications, and, if confirmed, could become the treatment of choice for patients with low-risk disease.

Patients with Local Recurrence After Radiation Therapy

Patients who have received a maximal dose of radiation but suffer local recurrence of tumor without evidence of metastatic disease, theoretically are still curable. Unfortunately, radiation destroys the tissue planes needed for a safe and effective attempt at salvage radical prostatectomy. Radical prostatectomy in a salvage situation has reported positive margins in 40% of patients (31) with prohibitive morbidity, demonstrating a 58% incontinence rate and an incidence of rectal injury as high as 15% (32). Consequently, salvage radical prostatectomy rarely is performed in this setting; most patients are placed on palliative hormonal ablation therapy.

The treatment of patients for salvage after radiation therapy was not without difficulties however. Early findings showed poor cancer control results with fewer than 25% of patients reaching PSA levels of 0.2 ng/mL (8) or less, and with positive biopsy rates as high as 35%. Complications in this patient population also were significant. While the incontinence rate for non-salvage cryotherapy patients is less than 2%, significant incontinence for radiation salvage patients can be as high as 46% (33). Advances in cryotherapy technique have improved these results; a study by Ghafar et al (34) demonstrated a 60% success rate at providing an undetectable PSA; the associated incontinence rate was 9%.

Our results are consistent with this aforementioned report. Twenty-four patients who had locally recurrent prostate cancer after radiation therapy were treated with cryotherapy with a mean follow-up of 3 years. The group had a high risk of recurrence—15 of 24 patients had a Gleason score of 7 or above, and four patients had already failed hormone therapy. The median preoperative PSA was 4.7 ng/mL, standard deviation (SD) 3.4 ng/mL, and the postcryotherapy median PSA was 0.01 ng/mL with a SD of 1.4. Of the 24 patients, 19 (79%) have a stable PSA that is undetectable. Of the five unstable patients, all have had negative biopsies. Thus, in these 24 high-risk patients, there is no evidence of local recurrence. In addition, three of the four patients who had failed hormonal therapy have no evidence of recurrent disease. The incontinence rate in these patients was 33%, but does not reflect the recent changes in freezing protocols and urethral warmer changes that have lowered this rate to 10% (34). In addition, patients with severe incontinence that limited lifestyle were treated successfully with artificial sphincter placement.

Based on these results, cryotherapy recently has been approved by Medicare as the only treatment specifically for the indication of recurrent cancer after radiation failure. Based on the potentially curative nature of the procedure, cryotherapy has become the procedure of choice in this difficult group of patients.

Technical Advances in Cryotherapy

Saline Injection into Denonvilliers' Fascia

A major theoretical criticism of prostate cryoablation has been based on the anatomy of the pelvis, in particular the proximity of the prostate capsule to the rectal mucosa. Limited space between the prostate and rectum can result in freezing of the rectal mucosa with resultant urethrorectal fistula. Conversely, fear of urethrorectal fistula can lead to premature cessation of the freezing process. This can lead to a high incidence of tumor recurrence. Even for the experienced operator, it can be said that the procedure at times is a nerve-wracking balancing act between adequate treatment and rectal injury.

Probably the most important advance in the technique of prostate cryoablation that leads to favorable reproducible results relates to the injection of saline into Denonvilliers' fascia at the time of freezing to temporarily increase the space between the rectum and prostate (Fig. 32.3). In over 200 cases, this maneuver has virtually eliminated the risk of rectal freezing and the complication of urethrorectal fistula without adding any additional morbidity in our experience.

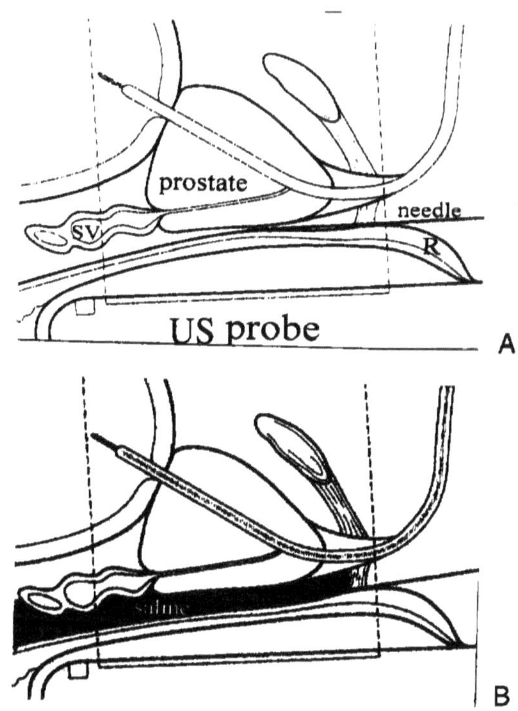

FIGURE 32.3. (A) The placement of a needle into Denonvilliers' fascia between the rectum (R) and the prostate capsule. There is a urethral warming catheter in place. (B) This diagram shows an increase in the space between the rectum and the prostate after saline has been injected.

The elimination of the fear of rectal freezing has numerous consequences that improve the results of cryotherapy. First, with the rectum out of the way, freezing can be extended outside the prostate sufficiently to bring the –35°C isotherm to the capsule of the prostate; this ensures adequate temperatures for cancer destruction throughout the prostate. Second, freezing can be extended far enough outside the prostate to include extracapsular extension of cancer; this improves local control of cancer in high-risk patients. In addition, with more freezing room, cryoprobes can be placed farther into the peripheral zone of the gland, where 80% of cancers reside. This exposes these cancers to faster freezing and colder temperatures, both of which improve cancer destruction. The arrangement of the cryoprobes also can change with a probe being placed into the posterior urethral region to encompass the confluence of the seminal vesicles, thereby preventing recurrence in this region. Last, with this move of cryoprobes into the peripheral zone, the freezing of the periurethral tissue, while still adequate, is less intense, thereby decreasing the possibility of urethral sloughing. With adoption of this technique, the learning curve is shortened, and the future reproducibility of cryotherapy results is assured.

Temperature Monitoring in Critical Areas and Improved Cryoablation Protocols

For reliable destruction of cancer by freezing, temperatures must reach certain critical limits. Recent in vitro and in vivo studies have shown that reaching –35°C with at least two freeze—thaw cycles is needed to destroy prostate cancer cells reliably (35). Marked improvement in clinical results occurs when temperature is monitored by thermocouples placed in critical areas in the prostate and when two full freeze–thaw cycles are performed. Wong et al (7) had 10 failed cases in the first 12 with only ultrasound monitoring; six failures occurred in the next 66 cases after thermocouple monitoring was instituted. A major advantage of cryotherapy, however, is the ability to re-treat local failures. Using thermocouple monitoring and re-treating, the previous failed cases had a negative biopsy rate of 94% (72 of 77 patients) at 30 months.

Salikan et al (24) reported an almost identical experience in which 10 of 69 patients initially had positive biopsies after treatment, with the majority of the 10 occurring early in their cryotherapy experience. Ultimately, after retreatment, 68 of 69 patients (99%) had negative biopsies.

Clearly, temperature monitoring in critical areas of the prostate gland is essential to good cancer control using cryoablation. Temperature monitoring also may help limit complications from overfreezing. Once the target temperature is reached, further freezing becomes a greater liability.

Improved Equipment with Increase from Five to Eight Probes

The original LN2-based freezing equipment now has been replaced by Joule-Thompson argon gas systems. These systems allow faster freezing rates that improve cancer destruction. The more precise control of the freezing process by gas systems also adds to the safety of the procedure.

Increasing the number of probes from five to eight has allowed a more uniform freezing temperature throughout the gland, which also improves results. Lee et al (36) showed that there was a statistically significant difference in total gland ablation (measured by PSA level and absence of glands on subsequent biopsy) between using five liquid nitrogen probes and six to eight argon gas probes (67% vs. 89%). Ultimately, Lee et al achieved a negative biopsy rate of 96% (157 of 163 patients).

Increasing the number of probes beyond eight could have a potentially negative effect. Recent data generated by a "cryoseed system" from Galil Medical Inc. (Haifa, Israel) that utilizes 17-gauge needle probes to create a 1-cm-diameter iceball has shown a decreased ability to totally ablate the prostate gland. These degraded results probably are the result of the short freezing length of these probes and difficulty in accurately overlapping the freezing zones along the length of the gland. All the data currently used to gain acceptance of cryoablation were developed with probes that freeze the length of the gland in one freeze. Departing from this concept jeopardizes much of what has been learned about how to obtain consistent results.

Future Technical Improvements

With recent approval for reimbursement by HCFA, there finally is an incentive for commercial interests to make the investment to technically improve the procedure. At the present time the greatest efforts are being made in improvements already well-established in brachytherapy. Since the freezing capabilities of cryoprobes are highly predictable, planning software to direct proper cryoprobe placement based on gland size and shape is already being developed. Planning software shortly will be coupled to guidance software and hardware that will greatly simplify what now is a totally freehand approach to cryoprobe placement.

While ultrasound is inexpensive and readily available, it still is highly operator dependent and difficult to use by novices. Other cross-sectional imaging techniques such as MRI have the potential to simplify and standardize cryotherapeutic procedures. As opposed to ultrasound (US), in which ice causes shadowing and shows only the leading edge of the iceball, both MRI and CT demonstrate the full extent of the freezing (Fig. 32.4). Using thermodynamic equations, these images can be used to noninvasively calculate temperatures within the iceball and automatically control the cryoprobes to create a specific freezing shape and profile.

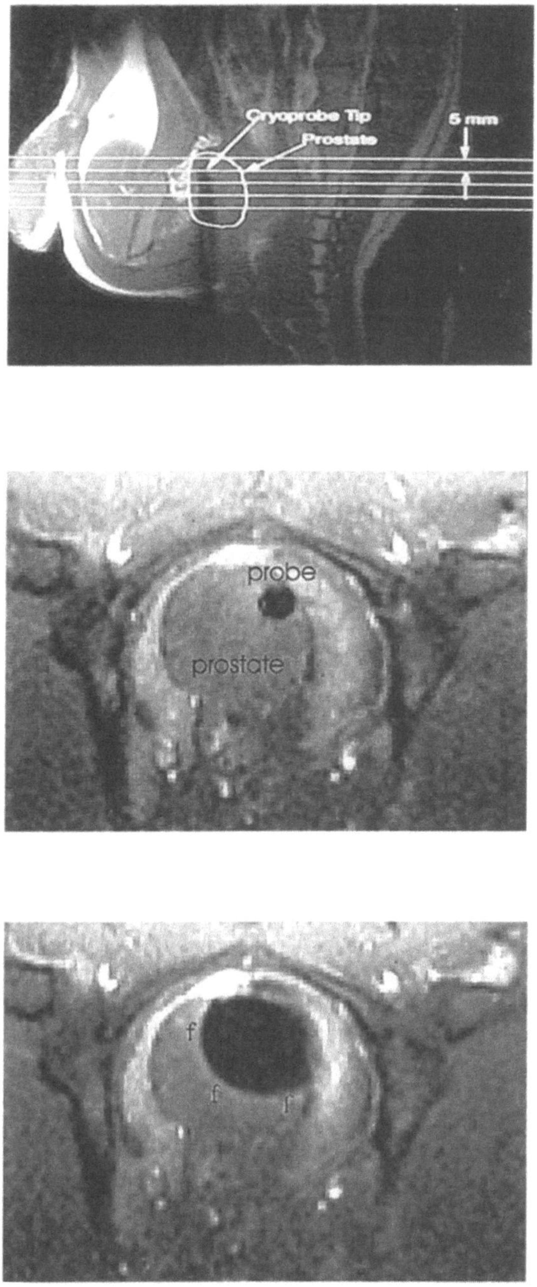

FIGURE 32.4. (A) Sagittal T1-weighted magnetic resonance imaging (MRI) showing a cryoprobe placed transperineally into the prostate of a dog. (B) Axial T1-weighted image of the same dog's prostate gland shows the cryoprobe in place in the anterior portion of the prostate. (C) Axial T1-weighted image shows freezing front (f) extending from the probe into the prostate. Note the asymmetric growth of the iceball, with minimal freezing occurring anteriorly due to the anterior venous complex.

We believe, as the inherent advantages of freezing as with brachytherapy radiation are appreciated, further technical development will continue to occur. Clearly, at the present time we are seeing only the tip of the "iceberg" of the technical potential of cryotherapy.

Conclusions

Ultimately, the choice of treatments also may involve outcomes and economic considerations. This will require us to examine closely what the overall costs are of providing the various treatment options for prostate cancer. For instance, how superior do the results of proton beam therapy have to be over other treatment options to justify building an $80 million facility? Can the expense of providing brachytherapy and external beam radiation in combination be justified if the same patient population can be treated with equally good results by cryotherapy or radical prostatectomy? If clinicians do not consider these factors, the agencies paying the bills likely will. In this regard, cryotherapy likely will be considered a highly cost-effective treatment.

There is the potential for cryotherapy (or some other direct image-guided ablative technology) to become the predominant method of prostate cancer treatment, based on its advantages. The major criticism of the procedure in the near future will be the relatively short follow-up of data compared to more established treatments. Numerous reports validate the ability of cryotherapy to re-treat patients, with no added morbidity, and superior results in treating extracapsular disease.

References

1. Villers A, McNeal JE, Freiha FS, et al. Multiple cancers in the prostate. Morphologic features of clinically recognized vs. incidental tumors. Cancer 1992;70(9):2312–2318.
2. George N. Therapeutic dilemmas in prostate cancer: justification for watchful waiting. Eur Urol 1998;34(suppl 3):33–36.
3. Gondor MJ, Soanes WA, Shulman S. Cryosurgical treatment of the prostate. Invest Urol 1966;3: 372–375.

4. Bonney WW, Fallon B, Gerber WL, et al. Cryosurgery in prostatic cancer survival. Urology 1982;14:37–42.
5. Onik GM, Cohen K, Reyes GD, et al. Transrectal ultrasound-guided percutaneous radical cryosurgical ablation of the prostate. Cancer 1993;72:1291–1299.
6. Pisters LL, von Eschenbach AC, Scott SM, et al. The efficacy and complications of salvage cryotherapy of the prostate. J Urol 1997;921–925.
7. Wong WS, Chinn DO, Chin M, et al. Cryosurgery as a treatment for prostate carcinoma: results and complications. Cancer 1997;79:963–974.
8. Cespedes RD, Pisters LL, von Eschenbach AC, et al. Long-term follow-up of incontinence and obstruction after salvage cryosurgical ablation of the prostate: results in 143 patients. J Urol 1997; 157:237–240.
9. Long JP, Bahn D, Lee F, et al. 5 year retrospective multi-institutional pooled analysis of cancer-related outcomes after cryosurgical ablation of the prostate. Urology 2001;57(3):518–523.
10. Onik GM, Cooper C, Goldberg HI, Moss AA, Rubinsky B, Christianson M. Ultrasonic characteristics of frozen liver. Cryobiology 1984;21: 321–328.
11. Onik G, Rubinsky B, Zemel R, et al. Ultrasound guided hepatic cryosurgery in the treatment of metastatic colon carcinoma: preliminary results. Cancer 1991;67:901–907.
12. Ravikumar TS, Kane R, Cady B, et al. A five year study of cryosurgery in the therapy of liver tumors. Arch Surg 1991;126:1520–1524.
13. Steele G. Cryoablation in hepatic surgry. Semin Liver Dis 1991;14(2):120–122.
14. Vaidya A, Hawke C, Tiguert R, et al. Intraoperative T staging in radical retropubic prostatectomy: Is it reliable? Urology 2001; 57(5):949–954.
15. Partin AW, Yoo JK, Carter HB, et al. The use of prostate specific antigen, clinical stage and Gleason score to predict pathological stage in men with localized prostate cancer. J Urol 1993; 150:110–115.
16. Tawari A, Narayan P. Novel staging tool for localized prostate cancer: a pilot study using genetic adaptive neural networks. J Urol 1998; 160(2):430–436.
17. Eggleston JC, Walsh PC. Radical prostatectomy with preservation of sexual function: pathologic findings in the first one hundred cases. J Urol 1985;134(6):1146–1148.
18. Connolly JA, Shinohara K, Carroll P. Cryosurgery for locally advanced prostate cancer. Semin Urol Oncol 1997;15(4):244–249.
19. Miller RJ, Williams MJ, Sinner M, et al. Percutaneous transperineal cryosurgical ablation of the prostate for the primary treatment of clinical stage C adenocarcinoma of the prostate. Urology 1995;44:676–679.
20. Onik G, Narayan P, Brunelle R, et al. Saline injection into Denonvilliers' fascia during prostate cryosurgery. Jnl Min Invas Therapy 2000; 9(6):423–427.
21. Gould RS. Total cryosurgery of the prostate versus standard cryosurgery versus radical prostatectomy: comparison of early results and the role of transurethral resection in cryosurgery. J Urol 1999;162:1653–1657.
22. Bahn DK, Lee F, Bandalament R, et al. 7-year outcomes in the primary treatment of prostate cancer. Urology 2002;60(2 suppl 1):3–11.
23. Donnelly BJ, Salikan JC, Ernst DS, et al. Prospective trial of cryosurgical ablation of the prostate: five year results. Urology 2002;60(4): 645–649.
24. Salikan JC, Donnely B, Brasher P, et al. Outcome and safety of transrectal US guided percutaneous cryotherapy for localized prostate cancer. J Vasc Intervent Radiol 1999;10(2 pt 1):199–208.
25. De La Taille A, Benson MC, Bagiella E, et al. Cryoablation for clinically localized prostate cancer using an argon based system: complication rates and biochemical recurrence. BJU Int 2000;85:281–286.
26. Robinson JW, Saliken JC, Donnelly BJ, et al. Quality of life outcomes for men treated with cryosurgery for localized prostate cancer. Cancer 86(9):1793–1800.
27. Onik G, Narayan P, Vaughan D, et al. Focal nerve-sparing cryosurgery for the treatment of primary prostate cancer: a new approach to preserving potency. Urology 2002;60(1):109–114.
28. Catalona WJ, Basler JW. Return of erections and urinary continence following nerve sparing radical retropubic prostatectomy. J Urol 1993; 150(3):905–907.
29. Geary ES, Dendinger TE, Freiha FS, et al. Nerve sparing radical prostatectomy: a different view. J Urol 1995;154(1):145–149.
30. Sanchez-Ortiz RF, Broderick GA, Rovner ES, et al. Erectile function and quality of life after interstitial radiation therapy for prostate cancer. Int J Impot Res 12(suppl 3):S18–24.

31. Neerhut GJ, Wheeler T, Cantini M, et al. Salvage radical prostatectomy for radiorecurrent adenocarcinoma of the prostate. J Urol 1988;140(3):544–549.
32. Rainwater LM, Zincke H. Radical prostatectomy after radiation therapy for cancer of the prostate: feasibility and prognosis. J Urol 1988;140(6):1455–1459.
33. Bales GT, Williams MJ, Sinner M, et al. Short-term outcomes after cryosurgical ablation of the prostate in men with recurrent prostate cancer following radiation therapy. Urology 1995;46:676–680.
34. Ghafar MA, Johnson CW, De La Taille, et al. Salvage cryotherapy using an argon based system for locally recurrent prostate cancer after radiation therapy: the Columbia experience. J Urol 2000;166(4):1333–1337.
35. Tatsutani K, Rubinsky B, Onik GM, Dahiya R, Narayan P. The effect of thermal variables on frozen human primary prostatic adenocarcinoma cells. Urology 1996;48(3):441–447.
36. Lee F, Bahn DK, Badalament RA, et al. Cryosurgery for prostate cancer: improved glandular ablation by use of 6 to 8 cryoprobes. Urology 1999;54(1):135–140.

33
Uterine Artery Embolization for Fibroid Disease

Robert L. Worthington-Kirsch

Historical Background

Embolization of the uterine arteries has been the standard of care for management of acute bleeding after childbirth or after gynecologic surgery since the late 1970s (1,2). Through the 1980s, apparently no one in either the interventional radiology or gynecologic communities had thought of treating uterine fibroids by embolization. This may have been due to the minimal interaction between interventional radiology and gynecology practices.

In the late 1980s, Jacques Ravina, a French gynecologist, became interested in the possible utility of embolization as a preemptive measure before gynecologic surgery, such as myomectomy. He was familiar with the utility of embolization for postoperative bleeding and decided to investigate preoperative embolization; he hoped this would decrease intraoperative bleeding, as well as decrease the risk of postoperative hemorrhage. Preoperative embolization of the uterine arteries did indeed prove to be useful to decrease perioperative bleeding complications (3).

In some cases, there was a delay between the embolization and the planned surgery of at least a few days, and in some cases a few weeks. Many of these patients experienced relief of their fibroid-related symptoms from the embolization alone and refused to proceed with the planned gynecologic surgery. Ravina and his group first published their experience with a small series of patients in 1995 (4), and went on to continue their studies of uterine artery embolization (UAE) as a primary treatment for fibroids (5,6).

Uterine artery embolization was introduced in the United States by Bruce McLucas (a gynecologist) and Scott Goodwin (an interventional radiologist), both from UCLA Medical Center in 1996 (7). Francis Hutchins (gynecologist) and Robert Worthington-Kirsch (interventional radiologist) introduced UAE to the eastern U.S. late in 1996 (8). Since then there has been rapid spread of the procedure across the U.S., Europe, and worldwide.

Indications for Uterine Artery Embolization

The first indication for UAE is the presence of symptomatic fibroids. Fibroids (myomas of the uterus) are benign tumors of the uterus. They are extremely common, occurring in as many as 70% or more of women of childbearing age in some racial groups, such as African Americans (9,10).

Fibroids cause symptoms in only a portion of women who have them, probably about 50% (11). In general, fibroids that are not causing any symptoms do not need to be treated. When they do cause symptoms, these fall into one of three symptom groups.

The first and most common symptom is abnormal vaginal bleeding. Fibroids typically cause both an increase in menstrual flow and prolongation of the menses. This abnormal bleeding frequently is accompanied by worsening of dysmenorrhea. The increase in bleeding can be relatively mild or severe. In some patients the menorrhagia can be severe enough that they are unable to leave their homes for several days of each menstrual cycle, or it can cause life-threatening anemia. Fibroids do not have to be in a submucosal position to cause menorrhagia.

The second symptom complex is that of bulk-related symptoms. As the fibroids grow, they enlarge the uterus and cause pressure on adjacent organs. The most common of these symptoms is from pressure on the bladder. While urinary frequency, urgency, and nocturia are most common, occasionally a fibroid in the lower uterine segment can cause pressure on the bladder base and lead to episodes of bladder outlet obstruction. Less commonly, the fibroid uterus can put pressure on the sigmoid and rectum, causing a sensation of rectal pressure and/or constipation, or on the sacrum causing low back pain. The fibroid uterus can also cause dyspareunia.

The third symptom complex concerns problems with fertility. The relationship of fibroids and subfertility is complex and only partially understood (12,13). Most women with fibroid disease have normal fertility. It is clear that a submucosal fibroid may distort the endometrial cavity and interfere with implantation or progression of a pregnancy. However, fibroids elsewhere in the uterus also may have an untoward impact on pregnancy.

It is clear that UAE is an appropriate therapy for women who have abnormal bleeding and/or bulk/pressure symptoms from their fibroid disease (8,14–17). In women who want to maintain future fertility, the utility of UAE is not so clear. The literature suggests that UAE for other indications does not interfere with future fertility (18). There are women who have become pregnant after UAE (19–21), and most have had normal pregnancy outcomes. There are not yet enough data available to predict a fertility rate after UAE with any confidence. At the same time, the data regarding fertility after myomectomy are not of particularly high quality (22). Fertility rates reported for women having myomectomy without selection for size, number, and distribution of fibroids are not particularly high, ranging from 8% to 46% (23,24). While we clearly need more information, the data currently available suggest that fertility after UAE may be similar to fertility after myomectomy. This may be especially true in those women who have multiple fibroids, and are generally regarded as poor candidates for myomectomy.

In the author's opinion, the desire to preserve future fertility is not necessarily a contraindication to UAE in patients who have fibroid symptoms that would otherwise warrant treatment. Given the currently available data, UAE should not be considered for women whose primary fibroid-related issue is subfertility, unless an experienced fertility surgeon feels that the patient is not a candidate for myomectomy.

Patient Selection

Patient selection for UAE is a cooperative process between the interventional radiologist and the referring gynecologist. The first issue is to ensure that fibroids are indeed present and to exclude other significant pelvic pathology. This is done by a combination of the gynecologic examination and imaging studies. The gynecologist should exclude other processes such as endometriosis, pelvic inflammatory disease, and endometrial carcinoma. The author specifically requests endometrial evaluation [by hysteroscopy, endometrial biopsy, or dilatation and curettage (D&C)] in all women with excessive bleeding over age 40, and in all women with abnormal bleeding patterns regardless of age.

Imaging studies confirm the presence of fibroids and exclude other pathology such as undiagnosed adnexal masses or adenomyosis. Adenomyosis commonly can mimic the presentation of fibroid disease, and has been reported as a cause of clinical failure of UAE (25). There has been work to investigate the possibility of treating adenomyosis by UAE (26–28), but the results have not been particularly encouraging.

There are few absolute exclusion criteria for UAE. These include pregnancy, evidence of active pelvic infection, and the presence of an undiagnosed pelvic mass. Needless to say, a history of life-threatening contrast allergy or other major contraindications to arteriography also may be exclusion criteria. When fibroids coexist with adenomyosis, UAE may be successful, so long as the predominant process is fibroid disease, but it may not be the best choice in patients with both fibroids and endometriosis, since UAE will not relieve symptoms caused by endometriosis.

Uterine artery embolization provides symptomatic relief of either abnormal bleeding or bulk/pressure symptoms in the majority of patients, regardless of initial uterine size (16). In the author's opinion, there is no threshold or limit for UAE in terms of uterine or fibroid size. However, patients with large uteri do need to be aware that their uterus may still be palpably enlarged, even after significant volume reduction. Patients with large uteri who desire a "flat belly" are unlikely to be satisfied with the volume reduction afforded by UAE.

Although not formally reported in the literature, there are two known cases in which an exophytic pedunculated fibroid was liberated into the peritoneal cavity after UAE, presumably because of necrosis of the stalk. In these cases, the patients became symptomatic from the infarcted intraperitoneal myoma, and laparotomy was required in both cases. A similar occurrence after surgery for fibroids has been reported (29). This should only be a concern if the peduncle is quite narrow, and the vast majority of exophytic fibroids, even those with a distinct peduncle, are not at risk for this occurrence. The author gives patients who are found to have fibroids on such narrow stalks choices of: (a) deferring UAE for surgical therapy such as hysterectomy or myomectomy; (b) planning limited myomectomy to remove the pedunculated fibroid combined with UAE to manage the remainder of the patient's fibroid disease; or (c) doing a UAE with the knowledge that there is a risk of the fibroid being liberated into the abdomen, which can be managed surgically if the need arises (although the likelihood of that risk is not known).

There is a risk that fibroids may slough into the endometrial cavity and need to pass through the vagina (30–32). The risk appears to be 5% or less in the overall UAE population (15,17). However, it may be as high as 25% in women who have a dominant submucosal myoma (33). Sloughing of a fibroid usually is easily diagnosed and managed by the interventional radiology/gynecology team. The presence of a dominant submucosal myoma, therefore, is not a contraindication to UAE, although the management team should be aware of the situation and potential effects.

Technique

The technique for UAE is well described in the literature (4,8,14,15,17). The uterine artery is typically the first branch of the anterior division of the internal iliac artery, although some anatomic variation has been described (34). When catheterizing the uterine arteries, one should be careful to avoid the cystic artery, which often shares a common trunk with the uterine artery.

The catheter should be positioned in the main segment of the uterine artery. If possible, the catheter tip should be distal to the origin of the cervicovaginal branch of the uterine artery. However, this is not practical in most cases, as the cervicovaginal branch origin is often quite distal.

Once the catheter tip is in position, the uterine artery is embolized (Fig. 33.1). There are several options available to use for embolic material. When UAE was first introduced as a therapy for fibroids, the protocol was simple. The uterine artery was selectively embolized with polyvinyl alcohol (PVA) particles, followed by "capping" with a plug of gelatin sponge. The end point for embolization was to have a static column of contrast in the uterine artery, with only a stump filling when the internal iliac artery was injected. The gelatin sponge cap was thought to both complete the occlusion of the uterine artery and prevent PVA particles from being drawn out of the uterine artery by the Venturi effect, with resulting nontarget embolization.

Razavi and colleagues (35) have shown that UAE with PVA alone is effective without

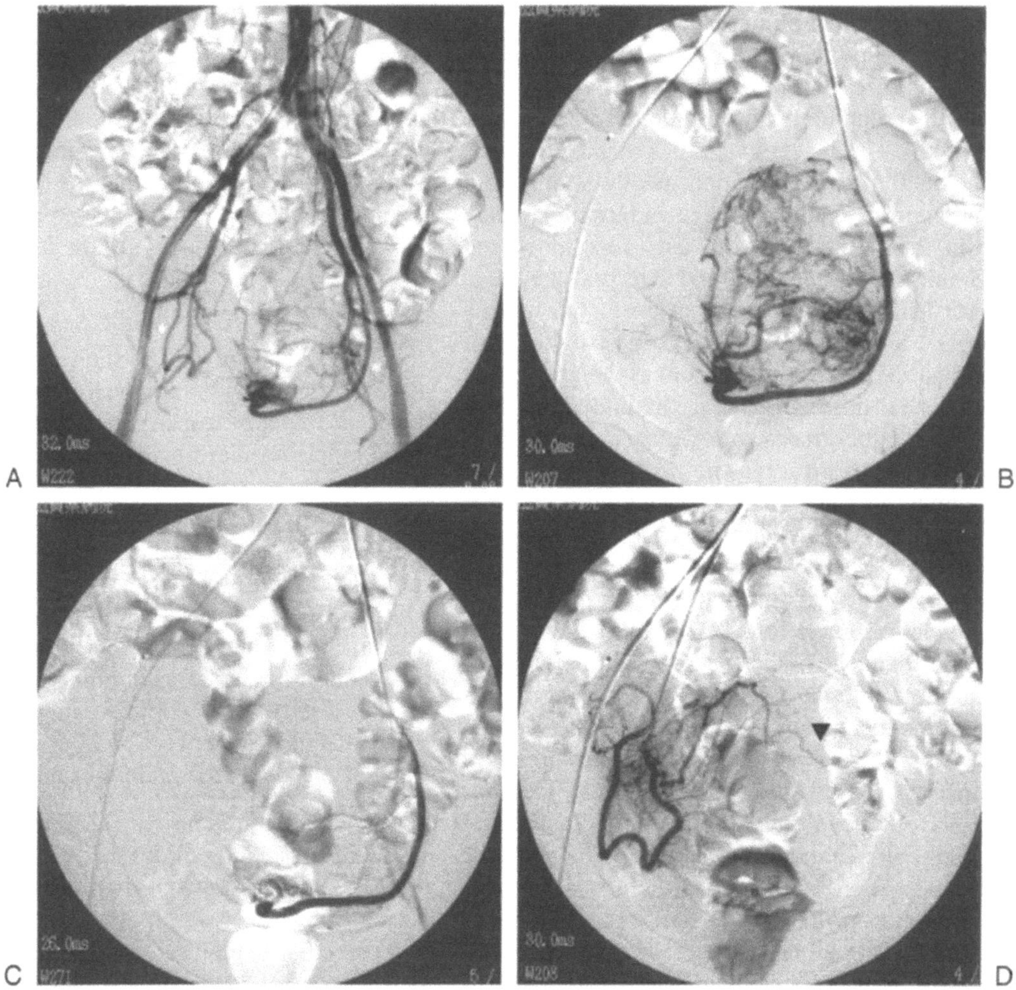

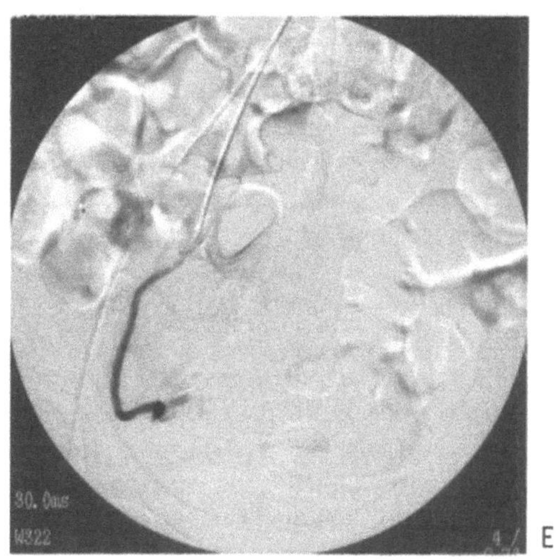

FIGURE 33.1. (A) Mapping pelvic arteriogram in a woman with symptomatic fibroids in a 16-week-sized uterus. Note the enlarged and tortuous uterine arteries (white asterisks). (B) Selective injection of the left uterine artery before embolization. Note how the vessels surround the dominant fibroid forming a perifibroid plexus. (C) After embolization of the left uterine artery with PVA, there is no further flow beyond the main uterine artery segment. (D) Selective injection of the right uterine artery before embolization. Note the collateral vessel filling across the midline into the distribution of the just embolized left uterine artery (black arrowhead). (E) After embolization of the right uterine artery with PVA, there is no further flow beyond the main uterine artery segment. (Images courtesy of Tetsuya Katsumori, MD, Saiseikai Shiga Hospital, Shiga Prefecture, Japan.)

evidence of nontarget embolization. The author's experience has been that uterine arteries embolized with PVA and gelatin sponge are usually completely obliterated at repeat arteriography. This is seemingly in contradiction with the standard teaching that gelatin sponge is a "temporary agent". There must be a tissue reaction that stimulates the body to remove the gelatin sponge, and thus it seems that this reaction leads to durable occlusion of the uterine artery. Since UAE appears to destroy most (if not all) of the fibroids present at the time of the UAE, but does not change the underlying tendency of the uterus to form new fibroids, it is important to preserve the main uterine artery segments after UAE, especially in younger women, if only to preserve access for a second UAE at some point in the future. Given these observations, this author has abandoned the use of gelatin sponge for UAE in all patients.

With the introduction of calibrated microsphere embolic agents, embolization has become technically easier. The chief advantage of calibrated microspheres is that they are more uniformly sized than standard PVA preparations. This results in a more predictable level of embolization and minimizes the clogging of both standard and microcatheters, which is a continuous problem with standard PVA preparations. This difference is so significant that a simple dose equivalence between standard PVA and microspheres cannot be determined (36). The two different preparations behave in markedly different ways. It has quickly become apparent that UAE with calibrated microspheres does not have to be performed to the end point of complete occlusion of the uterine artery. This end point is difficult, if not impossible, to achieve with calibrated microspheres. Comparison of embolization with PVA and microspheres in an animal model shows that PVA forms aggregates that often occlude vessels much more proximally than would be expected from the particle size used. This is apparently what leads to cessation of flow in the main uterine arteries during UAE with standard PVA preparations.

It must be remembered that the aim of embolization is not to occlude the main uterine artery, but to occlude the vessels that supply the fibroid, while sparing the vessels that supply normal uterine tissue as much as possible. Given these observations, what should the arteriographic end point be? One should look for evidence that the flow dynamics of the uterus have significantly changed, and that the blood flow to the perifibroid plexus has been interrupted. The angiographic signs of this are the following:

1. The appearance of new collaterals that were not present on initial injection of the uterine artery. This may be the sudden appearance of filling across the utero-ovarian anastomosis, or the appearance of vessels cross-filling to the opposite uterine artery.
2. An increase in resistance of the uterine body vessels to further injection of contrast. This can be manifested by the beginning of reflux in the uterine artery proximal to the catheter tip, dilation of the uterine artery when pressure is exerted on the injection syringe, or cessation of flow in the ascending ramus of the uterine artery with contrast staining of the lower uterine segment.
3. Occlusion of the main uterine artery.

It appears that one can achieve the more subtle of these end points more easily with calibrated microspheres than with standard PVA preparations. However, it also should be noted that there has been little or no observed difference in the safety or clinical efficacy of UAE using standard PVA compared to calibrated microspheres.

One of the most important technical considerations when performing UAE is the possibility of flow across the utero-ovarian anastomosis. If embolic material is allowed to reflux across this anastomosis into the ovary, there is risk of damage to the ovary (37,38). The severity of the risk to ovarian function is unclear (39,40). Usually one can see flow across the anastomosis, either on the initial injection of the uterine artery or developing as the embolization proceeds. In these cases, careful monitoring of the injection pressure during embolization can minimize or eliminate reflux of embolic material into the ovarian artery. It is important to recognize that the ovary itself is several centimeters cephalad from the utero-ovarian anastomosis, so reflux of material a very short way across this anastomosis should be harmless. On the other hand, there are times when there is significant flow into the uterus from the ovarian artery. This may occur as collateral flow that is recruited by the demands of the fibroids (41,42), or in cases of anatomic variation in the uterine artery in which part of all of the uterine artery branches are "replaced" by the ovarian artery (43). When there is significant flow to the uterus from the ovarian artery that persists after embolization of the uterine arteries, there is a good chance that the clinical results of UAE will be less than optimal. This is especially true when the ovarian artery supplies a portion of the uterus independent of the uterine artery. In these cases, supplemental embolization of the ovarian artery should be considered, either at the same sitting (if the informed consent for the UAE has included the possibility of ovarian artery embolization) or at a later date.

The ovarian arteries usually both arise directly from the aorta, although either (more commonly the right) may originate from the renal artery. Once catheterized, there are several choices of technique to embolize the ovarian artery:

1. Embolize the ovarian artery from its midportion, just as one would embolize the uterine artery. This carries the highest risk of damaging the ovary.
2. Embolize the proximal ovarian artery with a larger particle such as a gelatin sponge "torpedo" or a coil; this preserves the ovary, but would not get embolic material into the perifibroid vessels—rather relying on decreasing the pressure head into the uterus as a supplement to the embolization of the uterine arteries to infarct the fibroids.
3. Advance a microcatheter down the ovarian artery and into the anastomotic branch, so that the embolization is into the uterus beyond the origin of the branches into the ovary. This option requires not only superb microcatheter skills, but also a large amount of procedure and fluoroscopy time (44).
4. Embolize the ovarian artery with larger particles, which should then bypass the smaller branches into the ovary itself and be washed down into the uterus. Pelage et al (45) have presented evidence suggesting that the branch vessels into the ovary proper are typically 500 to 600 μm in diameter, so embolization with particles larger than 650 to 700 μm should largely preclude any particles getting into the ovary itself.

Almost all patients develop significant cramping after the procedure is completed, similar to that seen with spontaneous degeneration of a myoma. This usually requires IV narcotics for pain control, as well as loading doses of nonsteroidal antiinflammatory drugs (NSAIDs) such as ibuprofen. The acute postprocedure pain lasts 4 to 8 hours, after which patients begin to feel better (46). By the morning after UAE, all patients are discharged from the hospital on oral medications.

Outcomes

All the published series of significant size report similar outcomes with UAE (6,15,17). Technical success is reported at greater than 95%. Recovery is typically rapid, with the majority of patients returning to full activities within 21 days of the procedure. Length of hospitalization, return to work, and return to normal activity levels all appear to be shorter with UAE than for patients who undergo surgical treatment for fibroids (47). The paradigm for postprocedure management is the same as for management of acute spontaneous fibroid infarction, that is, NSAIDs (such as ibuprofen), supplemented by narcotics (such as oxycodone) as needed (48).

There are two management issues that have to be watched for during the recovery phase. About 10% of patients develop a fever and malaise, sometimes accompanied by nausea and vomiting (15). This is similar to the postembolization syndrome seen after embolization of other solid organs (49) or the post ablation syndrome. In most cases, this resolves in 3 to 5 days, but can persist for a week or longer. Postembolization syndrome can be differentiated from infection by the absence of worsening pelvic pain or purulent vaginal discharge.

As has been mentioned above, a small number of patients slough fibroids vaginally after UAE (30–32). This may occur as early as several days after UAE, or as long as several months after the procedure. Fibroid slough presents as the relatively abrupt onset of crampy abdominal pain and odorous vaginal discharge. These patients should be treated with oral antibiotics to prevent ascending infection. In most cases, the sloughed fibroid will pass spontaneously within 24 to 36 hours, with resolution of symptoms. Although the fibroid may pass spontaneously beyond this period, a longer delay increases the risk for ascending infection. The author routinely requests that the referring gynecologist perform a dilation and evacuation (D&E) to remove the sloughed fibroid if it has not passed within 48 hours of the onset of symptoms.

The majority of women experience no interruption in their menstrual cycle after UAE. There is risk for amenorrhea after UAE, particularly for women over 45 years of age (50–52). Approximately 90% of women have improvement or normalization of menstrual flow after UAE (6,8,15,17).

Uterine and fibroid volumes decrease after UAE, although the degree of volume reduction is variable. At 3 months after UAE, 35% to 50% reduction in overall uterine volume is typical (6,15,17). Volume reduction continues in many women for at least 12 months after UAE; 80% to 85% of women who have pressure symptoms caused by fibroid bulk report improvement in those symptoms within 3 months of UAE (6,15,17). This is independent of the presence of, or change in, abnormal bleeding (16). Symptomatic relief (both from menorrhagia and bulk-related symptoms) after UAE appears to be lasting.

Complications

Complications of UAE have proven to be rare. Infection can develop, particularly in the setting of a sloughing fibroid that is not managed aggressively; this may lead to urgent or emergent hysterectomy. The incidence of this occurrence is less than 1 in 200 cases (17). In one patient, an infection has led to overwhelming sepsis and death (53). There is one report of patient mortality from pulmonary embolus the day after UAE (54). Overall, the mortality risk associated with UAE is nearly an order of magnitude lower than the mortality risk associated with hysterectomy for fibroids (54). The overall risk of complication seems to be lower for UAE than for hysterectomy (47,55).

Future Directions

Much about UAE is currently unknown. Projects are ongoing to formally compare UAE to surgical therapies such as hysterectomy and myomectomy, and to gather long-term outcome data. New embolization materials are being developed, and refinements to both the technique of embolization and patient management are evolving rapidly. Many questions about the place of UAE for younger women, particularly those who want to preserve fertility, remain and are a ripe field for further research.

Conclusion

Uterine artery embolization has been established as a valuable ablative therapy for the management of fibroid disease. It affords durable therapy for fibroid symptoms by a procedure that is less invasive than traditional surgical therapies. The advantages of UAE over surgical treatment include shorter hospitalization, lower complication risk, and faster recovery.

References

1. Heaston DK, Mineau DE, Brown BJ, Miller FJ. Transcatheter arterial embolization for the control of persistent massive puerperal hemorrhage after bilateral surgical hypogastric artery ligation. AJR 1979;133:152–154.
2. Oliver JA, Lance JS. Selective embolization to control massive hemorrhage following pelvic surgery. Am J Obstet Gynecol 1979;135:431–432.
3. Ravina JH, Merland JJ, Herbreteau D, Houdart E, Bouret JM, Madelenat P. Embolisation pre-

operatoires des fibromes uterins. Presse Med 1994;23:1540.
4. Ravina JH, Herbreteau D, Ciraru-Vigneron N, et al. Arterial embolisation to treat uterine myomata. Lancet 1995;346:671–672.
5. Ravina JH, Aymard A, Ciraru-Vigneron N, et al. Embolisation artérielle particulaire: un nouveau traitement des hémorragies des léiomyomes utérins. Presse Med 1998;27:299–303.
6. Ravina JH, Ciraru-Vigneron N, Aymard A, Ferrand J, Merland JJ. Uterine artery embolisation for fibroid disease: results of a 6 year study. Min Invas Ther Allied Technol 1999;8:441–447.
7. McLucas B, Goodwin SC. A fibroid treatment with promise—and a catch. Obstet Gynecol Manag 1996;8:53–57.
8. Worthington-Kirsch RL, Hutchins FL, Popky GL. Uterine artery embolization for the management of leiomyomas: quality of life assessment and clinical response. Radiology 1998;208: 625–629.
9. Cramer SF, Patel D. The frequency of uterine leiomyomas. Am J Clin Pathol 1990;94:435–438.
10. Schwartz SM. Epidemiology of uterine leiomyomata. Clin Obstet Gynecol 2001;44:316–326.
11. Greenberg MD, Kazamel TIG. Medical and socioeconomic impact of uterine fibroids. Obstet Gynecol Clin North Am 1995;22:625–636.
12. Forman RG, Reidy J, Nott V, Braude P. Fibroids and fertility. Min Invas Ther Allied Technol 1999; 8:415–419.
13. Rice JP, Kay HH, Mahony BS. The clinical significance of uterine leiomyomas in pregnancy. Am J Obstet Gynecol 1989;160:1212–1215.
14. Goodwin SC, Vedantham S, McLucas B, Forno AE, Perella R. Uterine artery embolization for uterine fibroids: results of a pilot study. J Vasc Intervent Radiol 1997;8:517–526.
15. Hutchins FL, Worthington-Kirsch RL, Berkowitz RP. Selective uterine artery embolization as primary treatment for symptomatic leiomyomata uteri: a review of 305 consecutive cases. J Am Assoc Gynecol Laparosc 1999;6:279–284.
16. Delaney ML, Worthington-Kirsch RL, Hutchins FL, Berkowitz RP. Uterine artery embolisation for the management of myomata in patients without complaints of menorrhagia. Min Invas Ther Allied Technol 1999;8:455–458.
17. Spies JB, Ascher SA, Roth AR, Kim J, Levy EB, Gomez-Jorge J. Uterine artery embolization for leiomyomata. Obstet Gynecol 2001;98:29–34.
18. Stancato-Pasik A, Mitty HA, Richard HM III, Eshkkar NS. Obstetric embolotherapy: effect on menses and pregnancy. Radiology 1996;201: 179.
19. Ravina JH, Ciraru-Vigneron N, Aymard A, LeDref O, Merland JJ. Pregnancy after embolization of uterine myoma: report of 12 cases. Fertil Steril 2000;73:1241–1243.
20. McLucas B, Goodwin S, Adler L, Rappaport A, Reed R, Perella R. Pregnancy following uterine artery embolization. Int J Gynecol Obstet 2001; 74:1–7.
21. Pelage JP, Walker WJ. Uterine artery embolisation for symptomatic fibroids and pregnancy. J Vasc Intervent Radiol 2002;13:S65.
22. Myers ER, Barber MD, Couchman GM, et al. Evidence report: management of uterine fibroids. US Agency for Healthcare Research and Quality (AHRQ), Contract No. 290-97-0024, Task Order 4, 2000.
23. Bernard G, Darai E, Poncelet C, Benifla JL, Madelenat P. Fertility after hysteroscopic myomectomy: effect of intramural myomas associated. Eur J Obstet Gynecol Reprod Biol 2000; 88:85–90.
24. Sudik R, Harsch K, Steller J, Daume E. Fertility and pregnancy outcome after myomectomy in sterility patients. Eur J Obstet Gynecol Reprod Biol 1996;65:209–214.
25. Smith SJ, Sewall LE, Handelsman A. A clinical failure of uterine artery embolization due to adenomyosis. J Vasc Intervent Radiol 1999;10: 1171–1174.
26. Siskin GP, Tublin ME, Stainken BF, Dowling K, Dolen EG. Uterine artery embolization for the treatment of adenomyosis. AJR 2001;177:297–302.
27. Kim MS, Wan JW, Lee DY, Ahn CS. Uterine artery embolization for adenomyosis without fibroids. Clin Radiol 2004;59:520–526.
28. Katsumori TK, Ueda M, Nishino T, Bamba M, Katsumori T, Kushima R. Cellular changes following uterine artery embolization for the treatment of adenomyosis. Cytopathology 2001;12: 270–272.
29. Worthington-Kirsch RL, Hutchins FL. Retained myoma fragment after LASH procedure—case report and imaging findings (letter). Clin Radiol 2001;56:777–778.
30. Berkowitz RP, Hutchins FL, Worthington-Kirsch RL. Vaginal expulsion of submucosal fibroids following uterine artery embolization: a report of three cases. J Reprod Med 1999;44:373–376.
31. Abhara S, Spies JB, Scialli AR, Jha RC, Lage JM, Nikolic B. Transcervical expulsion of a fibroid

as a result of uterine artery embolization for leiomyomata. J Vasc Intervent Radiol 1999;10: 409–411.
32. Jones K, Walker WJ, Sutton C. Sequestration and extrusion of intramural fibroids following arterial embolization: a case series. Gynaecol Endosc 2000;9:300–313.
33. McLucas B. Management of the post-embolization patient. Presented at New Trends in Myoma Management Including Uterine Fibroid Embolization, St. Thomas' Hospital, London, England, 1 June 2001.
34. Gomez-Jorge J, Kyoung A, Spies JB. Uterine artery anatomy relevant to uterine leiomyomata embolization. Presented at SCVIR Uterine Artery Embolization (UAE) Conference, Washington, DC, 14 October 2000.
35. Razavi MK, Rhee J, Sze DY, Kee ST, Semba CP, Dake MD. Recanalization of uterine arteries after embolization for symptomatic leiomyomas: evidence on MRA. J Vasc Intervent Radiol 2000; 11:S286.
36. Levine A, Kim D, Termin P, Worthington-Kirsch RL. Comparison of embosphere and PVA embolization agents in a porcine renal model. Presented at Cardiovascular and Interventional Radiological Society of Europe (CIRSE) 2001 Annual Meeting and Postgraduate Course, Gothenburg, Sweden, 22–26 September 2001, (manuscript in preparation).
37. Ryu RK, Chrisman HB, Omary RA, et al. The vascular impact of uterine artery embolization: prospective sonographic assessment of ovarian arterial circulation. J Vasc Intervent Radiol 2001;12:1071–1074.
38. Stringer NH, Grant T, Park J, Oldham L. Ovarian failure after uterine artery embolization for treatment of myomas. J Am Assoc Gynecol Laparosc 2000;7:395–400.
39. Chrisman HB, Saker MB, Ryu RK, et al. The impact of uterine fibroid embolization on resumption of menses and ovarian function. J Vasc Intervent Radiol 2000;11:699–703.
40. Spies JB, Roth AR, Gonsalves SM, Murphy-Skrzniarz KM. Ovarian function after uterine artery embolization for leiomyomata: assessment with use of serum follicle stimulating hormone assay. J Vasc Intervent Radiol 2001;12: 437–442.
41. Nikolic B, Spies JB, Abhara S, Goodwin SC. Ovarian artery supply of uterine fibroids as a cause of treatment failure after uterine artery embolization: a case report. J Vasc Intervent Radiol 1999;10:1167–1170.
42. Matson M, Nicholson A, Belli AM. Anastamoses of the ovarian and uterine arteries: a potential pitfall and cause of failure of uterine embolization. Cardiovasc Intervent Radiol 2000;23:393–396.
43. Worthington-Kirsch RL, Walker WJ, Adler L, Hutchins FL. Anatomic variation in the uterine arteries: a cause of failure of uterine artery embolisation for the management of symptomatic fibroids. Min Invas Ther Allied Technol 1999;8:397–402.
44. Andrews RT, Bromley PJ, Pfister ME. Successful embolization of collaterals from the ovarian artery during uterine artery embolization for fibroids: a case report. J Vasc Intervent Radiol 2000;11:607–610.
45. Pelage JP, Laurent A, Wassef M, et al. Uterine artery embolization in sheep: comparison of acute effects with polyvinyl alcohol and calibrated microspheres. Radiology 2002;224:436–445.
46. Worthington-Kirsch RL, Koller NE. Time course of pain after uterine artery embolization for fibroid disease. Medscape Women's Health Journal 2002;7:http://www.medscape.com/viewarticle/430765.
47. Worthington-Kirsch RL. Uterine artery embolization for leiomyomata using embosphere microspheres: interim results of a phase II comparative study. Presented at New Trends in Embolotherapy Symposium sponsored by Biosphere Medical associated with CIRSE 2002, 5–9 October 2002, Luzerne, Switzerland.
48. Rapkin AJ. Pelvic pain and dysmenorrhea In: Berek JS, ed. Novak's Gynecology. 12th ed. Baltimore: Williams & Wilkins, 1996: 405.
49. Hemingway AP. Complications of embolotherapy. In: Kadir S, ed. Current Practice of Interventional Radiology. Philadelphia: B.C. Decker, 1991: 104–109.
50. Chrisman HB, Saker MB, Ryu RK, et al. The impact of uterine fibroid embolization on resumption of menses and ovarian function. J Vasc Intervent Radiol 2000;11:699–703.
51. Spies JB, Roth AR, Gonsalves SM, Murphy-Skrzniarz KM. Ovarian function after uterine artery embolization for leiomyomata: assessment with use of serum follicle stimulating hormone assay. J Vasc Intervent Radiol 2001;12: 437–442.
52. Tulandi T, Sammour A, Valenti D, Child TJ, Seti L, Tan SL. Ovarian reserve after uterine artery embolization for leiomyomata. Fertil Steril 2002; 78:197–198.

53. Vashisht A, Studd JWW, Carey AH, et al. Fibroid embolisation: a technique not without significant complications. Br J Obstet Gynaecol 2000;107: 1166–1170.
54. Lanocita R, Frigerio LF, Patelli G, et al. A fatal complication of percutaneous transcatheter embolization for the treatment of fibroids. Presented at the 2nd International Symposium on Embolization of Uterine Myomata, the Society for Minimally Invasive Therapy, 11th International Conference, Boston, 16–18 September 1999.
55. Walker WJ, Worthington-Kirsch, RL. Fatal septicemia after uterine fibroid embolisation (letter). Lancet 1999;354(9191):1730.
56. Spies JB, Cooper JM, Worthington-Kirsch RL, Lipman JC, Benenati JF, McLucas B. Uterine artery embolization (UAE) using embospheres: initial results of a phase II comparative study. Presented at SCVIR 2002, 27th Annual Scientific Meeting, 6–11 April 2002, Baltimore.

34
Applications of Cryoablation in the Breast

John C. Rewcastle

The use of cryoablation in the breast has been anecdotally investigated since the mid-1800s (1). Recently, however, more concerted and structured research has been conducted that builds upon the modern understanding of cryobiology and several advances in technology.

Freezing and thawing of tissue result in necrosis. It is important to note that cryotherapy injures not only individual cells at the time of therapy (*direct damage*), but also the tissue as a whole by impairing the microvasculature (*indirect damage*) (2). Unlike radiation, the ability of cryotherapy to ablate tissue is dependent not on the nuclear characteristics of individual cells, but rather on the exposure of the entire tumor volume to a lethal freezing process. Cellular survival during cryoablation depends not only on the freezing and thawing rates, but, most importantly, on the lowest temperature reached and the hold time at subzero temperatures (3). During cryoablation, ice, which is essentially pure water, initially forms outside the cell, increasing the extracellular concentration. It does not form initially inside the cells as the lipid membrane blocks ice crystal growth, resulting in an osmotic imbalance. Direct cellular injury can result and is due to two damage mechanisms: intracellular ice formation (IIF) and solution effects.

Freezing rates are high enough within only a few millimeters of the cryoprobe to induce IIF (4,5). Although IIF is usually a lethal event associated with irreversible membrane damage, it is not known if cell death is a cause or a result of IIF, and several mechanistic theories exist (6).

The majority of the iceball experiences lower freezing rates that lead to cellular dehydration that result from the osmotic imbalance [5, 6]. This mechanism has been termed "solution effects" and there exist several hypotheses, but no consensus, as to its physical basis. Resulting solute concentration alone has been held responsible for the damage, as has attainment of a critical minimum volume shrinking, beyond which the membrane is damaged (6).

Direct injury does not completely destroy all cells. In the hours and days following cryoablation, indirect damage occurs. Microvasculature endothelial cells also are damaged by the direct injury mechanisms, resulting in ischemia that greatly enhances cell kill within the iceball. This may be the dominant killing mechanism during cryosurgery (6). In vitro studies have shown that induced apoptosis also may play a role (7). Enhancing apoptosis with adjuvant chemotherapy may indeed lead to a significant increase in in vivo cryoinjury, and investigations are ongoing (8).

Several reports have noted that the integrity of some structures is not compromised by exposure to cryogenic temperatures. For example, the renal collecting system is not damaged during cryotherapy even when exposed to very low temperatures unless it is physically punctured with a probe, and transmural lesions are created routinely during cardiac cryoablation without impairing the integrity of the heart wall (9,10). There also exists some evidence of an immunologic response to cryoablation, but experimental results have been inconsistent and its existence, let alone significance, remains controversial (2).

The other significant advance in cryoablation has been the recent introduction of high-pressure gas cryoablation systems that exploit the Joule-Thompson (J-T) effect. The J-T effect, a behavior characteristic of high-pressure gas, predicts that gas changes temperature as it expands through a narrow port into a lower pressure zone. This is a constant enthalpy expansion that, in the case of argon gas, results in rapid cooling to the boiling point of argon gas (–186°C). To accomplish this, high-pressure (3000 psi) ambient temperature argon gas is circulated to the cryoprobe tip where it expands rapidly as it drops to room pressure (15 psi). The expanded gases are circulated back to the cryogenic unit through the larger outer lumen of the cryoprobe and the supply hose. The venting of used gas, usually into the room, occurs at the cryogenic machine. Freezing is controlled by a computer-modulated gas regulator that opens and closes the gas flow supply to the cryoprobe.

Under the J-T effect, some gases, such as helium, warm rather than cool when expanded. Accordingly, helium can be incorporated into the cryogenic system to act as a rapidly responsive cryoprobe heater as it expands to ambient pressure. It is noteworthy that both argon and helium are inert and therefore, safe gases.

The gas systems provide finely adjustable and rapid system responses (seconds) to user input. This is in comparison to liquid nitrogen systems that had a lag time of up to 2 minutes. They also support rapid conversion from cooling to heating, effected through computer-automated switching of argon to helium. The gas cryoprobes, which can modulate between –186°C and +40°C in about 30 seconds, do not demonstrate any clinically perceptible promotion of freezing during the interval switch.

It is the understanding of cryobiology as well as the introduction of advanced argon gas–based cryomachines operated under ultrasound guidance that allow for the accurate removal of heat from a target tissue. This has led to investigations of cryoablation for the treatment of biopsy-proven fibroadenomas, the use of a cryoprobe as a localization tool to assist in lumpectomy, and the use of cryoablation as a primary breast cancer therapy.

Cryoablation for the Treatment of Biopsy-Proven Fibroadenomas

Approximately 10% of women experience a fibroadenoma in their lifetime (11). Fibroadenomas are considered aberrations of normal breast tissue rather than benign tumors (12), and consist of combined proliferation of epithelial and connective tissue elements, usually developing in the lobular region (11). Most fibroadenomas stop growing after becoming 2 to 3 cm in size, with 15% spontaneously regressing and 5% to 10% progressing (11,13).

Historically, surgical resection has been the treatment of choice for breast fibroadenoma. The advantages include providing a definitive diagnosis while eliminating the source of patient anxiety, and alleviating the need for follow-up monitoring, which relies on long-term patient compliance. Drawbacks to excision include the cost and morbidity (cosmetic or ductal damage), which may be unnecessary in a benign lesion that may resolve spontaneously remit (11,14). There is also the awareness that resection of every fibroadenoma would place a huge burden on the health care system (14).

In the past decade there has been a growing acceptance of conservative management (i.e., observation and monitoring) with a corresponding push to reserve resection for limited circumstances. Unfortunately, definitive diagnosis is seldom certain with conservative management (15). Some physicians have expressed great reluctance about letting a lump remain in a breast in a patient who will most likely be lost to follow-up, so that regular monitoring cannot take place (16). Further, there remain abundant indications in the literature for resection. Some of these indications include an increase in lesion size, lack of regression by age 35 (11), a higher risk of phylloides tumor in masses >3 cm (17), multiple fibroadenomas (14), and a mass that is psychologically disturbing to the patient

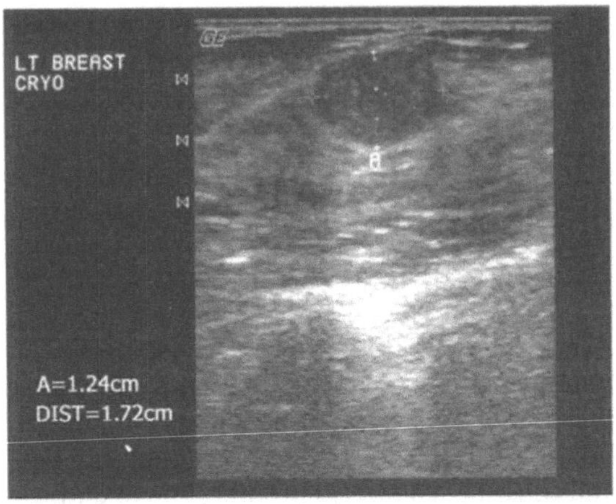

FIGURE 34.1. Ultrasound visualization of a breast lesion.

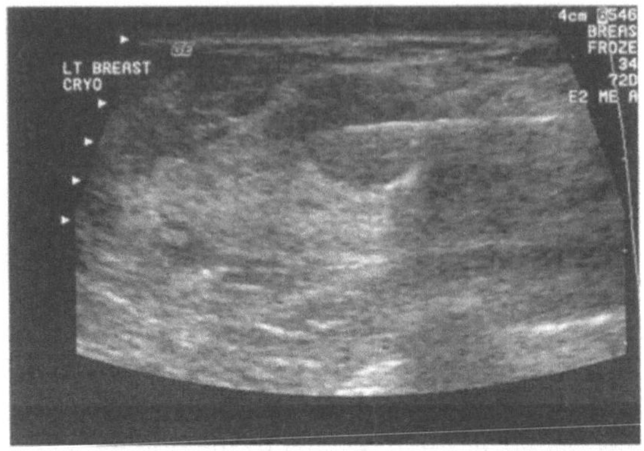

FIGURE 34.2. Ultrasound visualization of a cryoprobe placed in the center of the breast lesion.

(18). Further, with epidemiologic evidence that the mean age of fibroadenoma diagnosis is the mid-20s and the mean age of diagnosis of fibroadenoma containing a carcinoma is 43 years, Deschenes et al (19) recommend that all fibroadenomas diagnosed in women older than 30 years be excised.

Cryoablation presents as a minimally invasive treatment option for women with biopsy-proven fibroadenomas. In fact, cryoablation seems to be ideally suited for this application as it has a proven ability to target and ablate tissue in situ, does not require physical removal of the fibroadenoma or treatment of large amounts of surrounding normal tissue, and requires only a 3- to 4-mm incision for the insertion of a cryoprobe. The combination of these factors has led to several clinical trials assessing the ability of cryoablation to effectively treat fibroadenomas.

Kaufman et al (20) reported a series of 50 patients with 57 biopsy proven fibroadenomas. Cryoablation was performed in the operating room only for the first seven patients who underwent intravenous sedation, after which all patients were treated comfortably in the office with local anesthesia. The size of the treated lesions varied from 7 to 42 mm.

The procedure consists of locating the lesion on ultrasound (Fig. 34.1), then advancing a cryoprobe into the center of the lesion (Fig. 34.2). Using a treatment algorithm based on lesion size, an iceball forms and engulfs each lesion and exposes it to temperatures of –40°C or less. A double freeze–thaw cycle is used routinely.

Numerous studies have shown that tissues exposed to –40°C or less during two subsequent freeze–thaw cycles will, without question, be ablated (21). Figure 34.3 shows the hyperechoic rim of an iceball as observed on ultrasound. Note that only the proximal edge of the iceball is visible as near 100% sonographic reflection occurs at the interface between frozen and unfrozen tissue. Figure 34.4 demonstrates the relation between the ultrasound probe and the iceball. In the situation shown one would observe an ultrasound image akin to that in Figure 34.3. If the lesion is near the skin surface, saline can be injected between the lesion and skin to increase their physical separation. There are no instances in which the skin was damaged by an approaching iceball. Discomfort is transient in all patients and rarely requires medica-

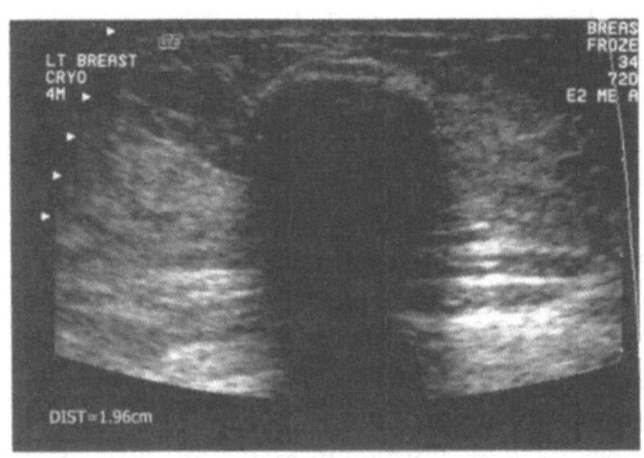

FIGURE 34.3. Ultrasound visualization of an iceball. The hyperechoic rim is the proximal iceball edge.

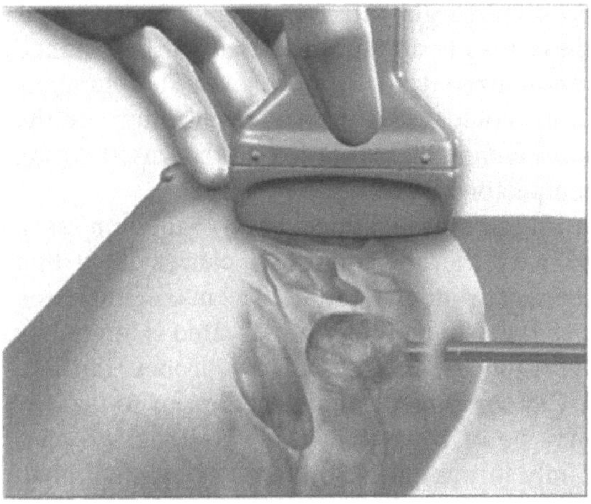

FIGURE 34.4. Drawing of the breast surface, ultrasound probe, and iceball. This situation would produce an ultrasound image like that in Figure 34.3.

tions other than acetaminophen or ibuprofen. As expected, localized swelling and skin ecchymosis are observed, but typically resolve within 3 weeks. Breast appearance returns to baseline universally within 6 weeks.

Following initial swelling progressive absorption of the fibroadenoma is observed on ultrasound. At 6 months the average volume decrease is 65% and 92% at 12 months. Patient satisfaction is excellent.

In a similar study Littrup et al (22) treated 42 biopsy-proven fibroadenomas in 27 patients. Minimal discomfort was reported with the use of local anesthesia. No significant complications occurred. Again, patient satisfaction was excellent. Fibroadenoma volume reduction at 12 months was observed under ultrasound to be 73%.

Cryoprobe-Assisted Lumpectomy

Over the past 30 years various techniques have been utilized for the preoperative localization of nonpalpable or barely palpable breast lesions, the most common of which is guidewire localization using mammographic or ultrasonographic guidance. The purpose of needle-localized procedures was always twofold: (1) diagnosis, and (2) excision of a malignancy with an adequate tumor-free margin of normal tissue. Needle-wire localization procedures almost always accomplish diagnosis, but are very poor at ensuring a tumor-free margin in the specimen. Although the definition of a "clear margin" remains controversial, surgical margin involvement with breast cancer almost always results in obligatory reexcision or mastectomy. For wire-localized procedures, the reexcision rate (requiring return of the patient to the operating room for a second procedure) often is reported to be between 40% and 60% (23–30).

The essence of a cryoprobe-assisted lumpectomy is that the tumor and a margin are enclosed by an iceball localized prior to surgical excision. Under ultrasound guidance a cryoprobe is inserted into the center of the tumor. The cryoprobe is then engaged until an iceball is created that encloses not only the entire tumor, but also a margin. Once large enough, the operation of the cryoprobe can be modified such that the iceball no longer grows, but maintains a static size. The iceball enclosing the tumor is then surgically excised, which may prove to be a superior localization methodology than needle wire localization.

Tafra et al (31) report a pilot study of 24 patients who underwent a cryoprobe-assisted lumpectomy for their ultrasound visible breast cancers. All lesions were localized successfully and the negative margin rate for patients with a margin greater than 6mm was 5.6%. Although this study is neither large nor comparative the results are compelling compared to the reported positive margin rate in the literature. As a follow-up, a multicenter randomized trial is planned that compares cryoprobe-assisted localization to needle wire localization.

Cryoablation as a Primary Therapy for Breast Cancer

There is very little in the literature regarding the use of cryoablation as a primary therapy for breast cancer. A single case study of in situ cryoablation of breast cancer was published by Staren et al (32). There are, however, two similar studies in which patients underwent cryoablation prior to surgical excision. Pfleiderer et al (33) used a 3-mm cryoprobe to ablate 16 lesions in 15 patients. There were no complications associated with the cryoablation procedure and all patients underwent resection within 5 days. The authors concluded that the invasive components of small tumors can be treated effectively with cryoablation, but remnant ductal carcinoma in situ (DCIS) components not observed prior to treatment may be problematic. Further, they recommend that multiple cryoprobes be used if the lesion is greater than 15 mm.

In a similar study, Sabel et al (34) reported on 29 patients with ultrasound-visible breast cancer <2.0 cm who underwent a double freeze–thaw cycle cryoablation utilizing a single cryoprobe. The cryoprobe design changed mid-study from a diameter of 2.4 mm to 2.7 mm. Subsequent standard surgical resection was performed on all patients 1 to 4 weeks post-cryoablation. The procedure was very well tolerated with no complications and no need for narcotic pain medications. Pathologic examination found that all tumors <1.0 cm were 100% ablated; 100% ablation also was achieved in invasive ductal carcinoma without a significant DCIS component (<25% on biopsy) when the carcinoma size was between 1.0 and 1.5 cm. These results have formed the basis of a planned multicenter trial. It is expected that additional independent trials regarding cryoablation as a primary therapy for breast cancer also will begin shortly.

Both these studies clearly demonstrate the ability of cryoablation to effectively treat a target volume. The size and number of probes will dictate the maximum size of lesion that can be treated.

Conclusion

Cryoablation is being used in several different ways in the management of benign and malignant breast tumors. Results from the treatment of fibroadenomas are encouraging and cryo now represents a safe and effective alternative with minimal cosmetic impact for women who choose to have definitive action taken. The negative margin rates from the cryoprobe-assisted lumpectomy pilot study are significant as they represent almost a tenfold reduction in the positive margin rate following lumpectomy. If these results are substantiated in the planned randomized trial, cryoprobe-assisted lumpectomy could replace wire localization as the most common localization method used during lumpectomy.

Initial investigations of cryoablation as a primary therapy for breast cancer show that there are potential pitfalls. The maximum lesion size that can be effectively treated is limited by the number and size of cryoprobes. Further, DCIS components undetected prior to therapy may be of concern. These two issues are certainly surmountable by careful treatment planning and diagnosis.

Cryoablation has the ability to ablate in a uniform and confluent manner without removing a breast mass or leaving an unsightly scar. This results in a therapy that is effective, safe, and attractive to the patient due to minimal quality-of-life impact. The use of cryoablation for the treatment of both benign and malignant breast conditions is sure to increase in the future.

Acknowledgments. The author would like to acknowledge the assistance of Trena Depel and Mark Rose in the preparation of this manuscript.

References

1. Arnott J. Practical illustrations of the remedial efficacy of a very low or anesthetic temperature. Lancet 1850;2:257–259.
2. Hoffmann NE, Bischof JC. The cryobiology of cryosurgical injury. Urology 2002;60(2 suppl1): 40–49.
3. Smith DJ, Fahssi WM, Swanlund DJ, Bischof JC. A parametric study of freezing injury in AT-1 rat prostate tumor cells. Cryobiology 1999;39(1):13–28.
4. Bischof JC, Smith D, Pazhayannur PV, Manivel C, Hulbert J, Roberts KP. Cryosurgery of dunning AT-1 rat prostate tumor: thermal, biophysical, and viability response at the cellular and tissue level. Cryobiology 1997;34(1):42–69.
5. Rewcastle JC, Muldrew K, Sandison GA. In vitro injury mapping for single cryoprobe cryosurgery. Cryobiology 2001;43:322.

6. Gage AA, Baust J. Mechanisms of tissue injury in cryosurgery. Cryobiology 1998;37(3):171–186.
7. Baust JM, Van B, Baust JG. Cell viability improves following inhibition of cryopreservation-induced apoptosis. In Vitro Cell Dev Biol Anim 2000;36(4):262–270.
8. Clarke DM, Baust JM, Van Buskirk RG, Baust JG. Chemo-cryo combination therapy: an adjunctive model for the treatment of prostate cancer. Cryobiology 2001;42(4):274–285.
9. Lustgarten DL, Keane D, Ruskin J. Cryothermal ablation: mechanism of tissue injury and current experience in the treatment of tachyarrhythmias. Prog Cardiovasc Dis 1999;41(6):481–498.
10. Sung GT, Gill IS, Meraney AM. Effect of interventional cryoinjury to the renal collecting system (abstract). J Urol 2000;163:113.
11. Sperber F, Blank A, Metser U, et al. Diagnosis and treatment of breast fibroadenomas by ultrasound-guided vacuum-assisted biopsy. Arch Surg 2003;138:796–800.
12. Houssami N, Cheung MNK, Dixon M. Fibroadenoma of the breast. Med J Aust 2001;174:185–188.
13. Pick PW, Iossifide IA. Occurrence of breast carcinomas within a fibroadenoma: a review. Arch Pathol Lab Med 1984;108:590–593.
14. Greenberg R, Skornick Y, Kaplan O. Management of breast fibroadenoma. J Gen Intern Med 1998;13:640–645.
15. Takei H, Lino Y, Horiguchi J, et al. Natural history of fibroadenomas based on the correlation between size and patient age. Jpn J Clin Oncol 1999;29:8–10.
16. Alle K. Conservative management of fibroadenoma of the breast: author's reply. Br J Surg 1996;83:1799.
17. Gordon PB, Gagnon FA, Lanzkowsky L. Solid breast masses diagnosed as fibroadenoma at fine-needle aspiration biopsy: acceptable rates of growth at long-term follow-up. Radiology 2003; 229:233–238.
18. Drukker BH. Breast disease: a primer on diagnosis and management. Int J Fertil 1997;42:278–287.
19. Deschenes L, Jacob S, Fabia J, Christen A. Beware of breast fibroadenomas in middle-aged women. Can J Surg 1985;28:372–374.
20. Kauffman CS, Bachman B, Littrup PJ, et al. Office-based ultrasound-guided cryoablation of breast fibroadenomas. Am J Surg 2002;184: 394–400.
21. Larson TR, Robertson DW, Corica A, Bostwick DG. In vivo interstitial temperature mapping of the human prostate during cryosurgery with correlation to histopathologic outcomes. Urology 2000;55:547–552.
22. Littrup PJ, Freeman-Gibb L, Andea A, et al. Cryotheapy for breast fibroadenomas. Radiology 2005;234:63–72.
23. Pittinger TP, Maronian NC, Poulter CA, Peacock JL. Importance of margin status in outcome of breast-conserving surgery for carcinoma. Surgery 1994;116:605–608.
24. Blair SL, O'Shea KE, Orr RK. Surgeon variability in treating nonpalpable breast cancer: surgical oncology as a value-added specialty. Ann Surg Oncol 1998;5:28–32.
25. Velanovich V, Lewis FR Jr, Nathanson SD, et al. Comparison of mammographically guided breast biopsy techniques. Ann Surg 1999;229: 625–630.
26. Tartter PI, Kaplan J, Bleiweiss I, et al. Lumpectomy margins, reexcision, and local recurrence of breast cancer. Am J Surg 2000;179:81–85.
27. Luu HH, Otis CN, Reed WP Jr, Garb JL, Frank JL. The unsatisfactory margin in breast cancer surgery. Am J Surg 1999;178:362–366.
28. Jardines L, Fowble B, Schultz D, et al. Factors associated with a positive reexcision after excisional biopsy for invasive breast cancer. Surgery 1995;118:803–809.
29. Chinyama CN, Davies JD, Rayter Z, et al. Factors affecting surgical margin clearance in screen detected breast cancer and the effect of cavity biopsies on residual disease. Eur J Surg Oncol 1997;23:123–127.
30. Rahusen FD, Taets van Amerongen AHM, Van Diest PJ, Borgstein PJ, Bleichrodt RP, Meijer S. Ultrasound-guided lumpectomy of nonpalpable breast cancers: a feasibility study looking at the accuracy of obtained margins. J Surg Oncol 1999; 72:72–76.
31. Tafra L, Smith SJ, Woodward JE, et al. Pilot trial of cryoprobe assisted breast-conserving surgery for small ultrasound visible cancers. Ann Surg Oncol 2003;10(9):1018–1024.
32. Staren ED, Sabel MS, Gianakakis LM, et al. Cryosurgery of breast cancer. Arch Surg 1997; 132:28–33.
33. Pfleiderer SO, Freesmeyer MG, Marx C, et al. Cryotherapy of breast cancer under ultrasound guidance: initial results and limitations. Eur Radiol 2002;12:3009–3014.
34. Sabel MS, Kaufman CS, Whitworth P, et al. Cryoablation of early stage breast cancer: work in progress report of a multi-institutional trial. Ann Surg Oncol 2004;11(5):542–549.

35
Percutaneous Ablation of Breast Tumors

Bruno D. Fornage and Beth S. Edeiken

The surgical management of breast cancer has evolved gradually over the past century from the exclusive use of radical mastectomy to the current practice of segmental mastectomy and radiation therapy. This less aggressive surgical approach in the management of breast cancer extended to treatment of the axilla. The latter led to the recent introduction and subsequent acceptance of lymphatic mapping and sentinel node biopsy as an alternative strategy to the routine use of formal levels I and II axillary dissection in clinically node-negative patients.

In light of this trend toward less invasive local therapy approaches for small tumors, interest has emerged in evaluating nonsurgical ablative modalities for treating primary tumors. However, whereas previous applications of radiofrequency ablation (RFA) or cryotherapy—such as RFA of bone metastases, RFA or cryotherapy of liver tumors, and cryotherapy of prostate cancer—often are performed for palliation and improvement of quality of life, not cure, for patients with an otherwise poor prognosis and for whom the therapeutic alternatives incur more risk or simply are not available, the challenge of minimally invasive therapy of small breast cancer is that patients already have an excellent prognosis. Therefore, if the percutaneous ablation fails, these patients may have lost their best chance for cure of a clearly treatable cancer. Besides this ethical issue, the main technical obstacle to the development of these therapeutic modalities is the inability to validate the clear pathologic margins of the ablated tissue. Currently, surgical excision with pathologic examination of the margins is the only procedure that provides this crucial information. Obviously, these ethical and technical limitations are of lesser concern in the treatment of benign breast masses.

Nonsurgical image-guided ablative techniques are available. Some of these techniques use devices that are inserted percutaneously into the breast to either heat or cool the tumor sufficiently to cause complete cell death. Others, which involve the injection of chemical agents such as pure ethanol, have been used in the treatment of liver tumors, but these are increasingly losing popularity because they are difficult to control. Thus, the various modalities that are currently available to ablate breast lesions fall into two general categories: thermotherapy—hyperthermia induced by application of radiofrequency current (i.e., RFA), laser irradiation, microwave irradiation, or insonation with high-intensity focused ultrasound (HIFU) waves—and cryoablation therapy.

Thermotherapy

Radiofrequency Ablation

With RFA, heat is produced through the application of a high-frequency alternating current that flows from the tip of an uninsulated electrode into the surrounding tissue. The electrode itself is not the source of heat; rather, frictional heating is caused when the ions in the tissue attempt to follow the rapidly changing direction of the alternating current. The tissue heats resistively in the area that is in contact with the electrode tip, and heat is then transferred conductively to more distant tissue.

The promising clinical experience with this modality in tumor sites other than the breast, at the cost of minimal morbidity, provided ample motivation to investigate its effectiveness in treating primary breast cancer. In addition, the breast provides a favorable environment because there are no major vessels that could cause convectional heat loss (i.e., "heat sink") during the treatment, and injuries to the skin or chest wall can be avoided by excluding lesions that are too close to these structures. On the negative side, primary breast cancers are usually ill-defined, with irregular or spiculated margins that are difficult to delineate with sufficient accuracy by imaging. Only those small invasive carcinomas that have clear-cut margins and no or little associated ductal carcinoma in situ (DCIS), determined by core biopsy specimens, are good candidates for percutaneous ablation.

The goal of RFA of primary breast cancer is to achieve a lethally thermal lesion that encompasses not only the tumor, but also a margin of surrounding normal tissue to destroy possible peripheral microscopic disease. The initial report exploring the feasibility of RFA for the treatment of breast tumors was published by Jeffrey et al (1) on five women with locally advanced invasive breast cancer, four of whom had received preoperative chemotherapy with or without radiation therapy. The authors concluded that RFA was effective in causing invasive breast cancer cell death, but that its use would be applicable mostly to tumors smaller than 3 cm.

Radiofrequency ablation of the breast is done under sonographic guidance and occasionally under stereotactic guidance (2). In a pilot "ablate and resect" study at the University of Texas M. D. Anderson Cancer Center, we investigated the feasibility of using sonographically guided RFA for the local treatment of small (T1) invasive breast tumors (3,4). A meticulous pre-RFA sonographic study was performed to ensure that the tumor was small, solitary, and well visualized on sonography, and that its margins were well-demarcated from the adjacent tissues. We required the presence of a 1-cm distance between the tumor and both the skin and underlying chest wall for the lesion to be eligible (Fig. 35.1). Before we performed the RFA procedure, we took care to collect satisfactory core biopsy specimens to establish a definitive pathologic diagnosis, and to test the tumor tissue for hormonal receptors and other factors such as Her-2-Neu, because after RFA no other tumor tissue was available.

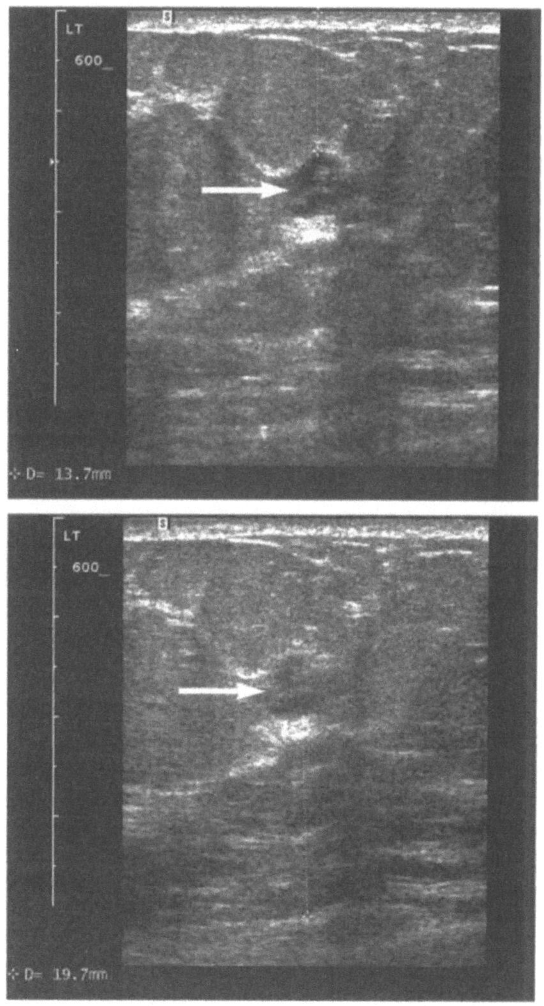

A
B

FIGURE 35.1. Sonograms of a small mucinous carcinoma of the breast. The tumor is well circumscribed (arrow) and lies at a safe distance from both (A) the skin surface (1.4 cm) and (B) the chest wall (2.0 cm).

A

B

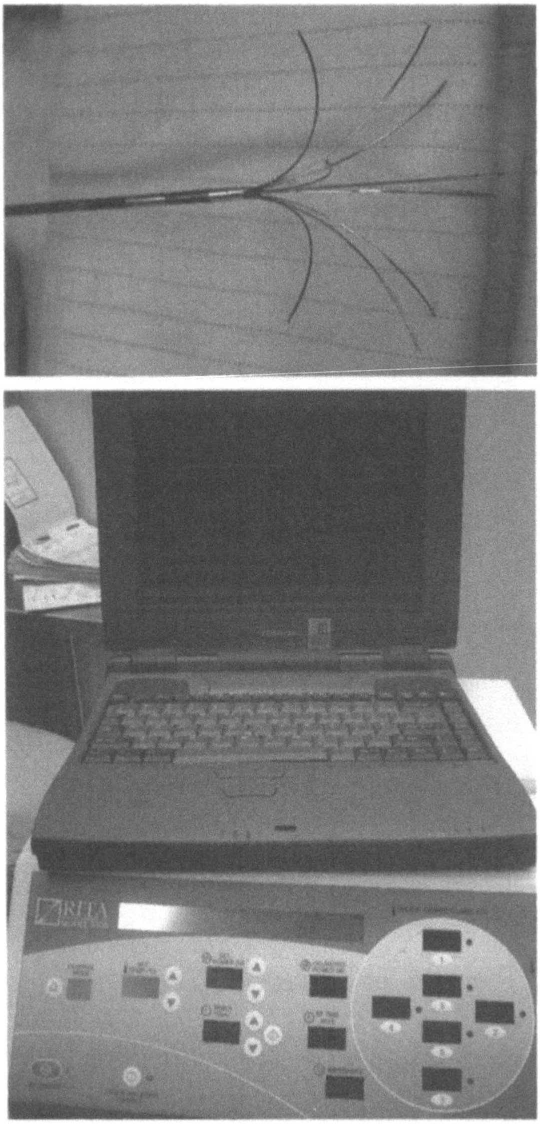

FIGURE 35.2. Radiofrequency ablation instrumentation (RITA Medical Systems, Mountain View, CA). (A) Photograph shows the multiarray needle-electrode with its nine secondary prongs fully deployed. (B) Photograph shows the radiofrequency generator and the laptop computer, whose screen graphically displays the temperatures recorded in real time at the tips of five of the prongs.

For our study, we used a RITA RFA device (RITA Medical Systems, Mountain View, CA), which consists of a multiple-array needle-electrode with several curved, flexible stainless steel secondary electrodes (prongs) that can be deployed over a distance of 3 cm, and a radiofrequency generator (Fig. 35.2). After we had three-dimensionally located the target lesion, the needle-electrode was inserted percutaneously through the tissues until its tip abutted the lesion (Fig. 35.3). The prongs were then deployed through the mass under full real-time sonographic monitoring (Fig. 35.4). Then the needle-electrode was connected to the generator, and the target temperature was set at 95°C. Thermocouples at the tips of some of the prongs of the device provided continuous real-time monitoring of the actual temperatures at those sites. A laptop computer, using proprietary software developed by RITA Medical Systems, displayed the curves of the temperatures at these sites in real time, the power output of the generator, and the impedance of the tissues over time (Fig. 35.5). The target temperature, once reached, was maintained for 15 minutes. No saline injections were used.

We noted no specific sonographic change during the procedure that would reliably reflect the pathologic changes induced by the RFA and therefore help to determine the extent of the thermal lesion. Instead, as the procedure progressed, the sonographic visibility of the lesion decreased, and sometimes the lesion was obscured completely at the end of the proce-

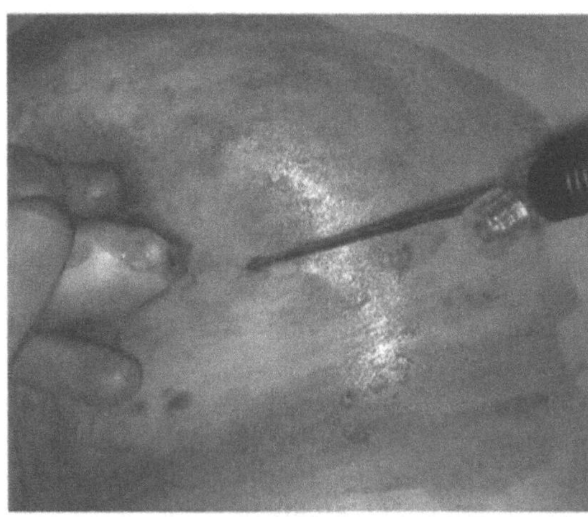

FIGURE 35.3. Sonographically guided insertion of the radiofrequency ablation needle-electrode. Photograph shows that the cannula is aligned with the scan plane of the high-frequency linear-array transducer.

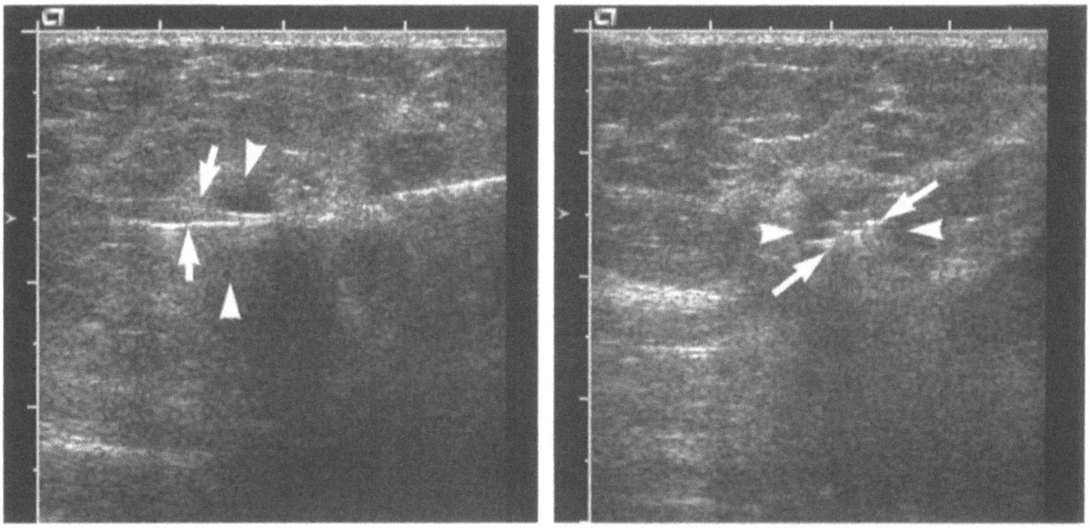

A B

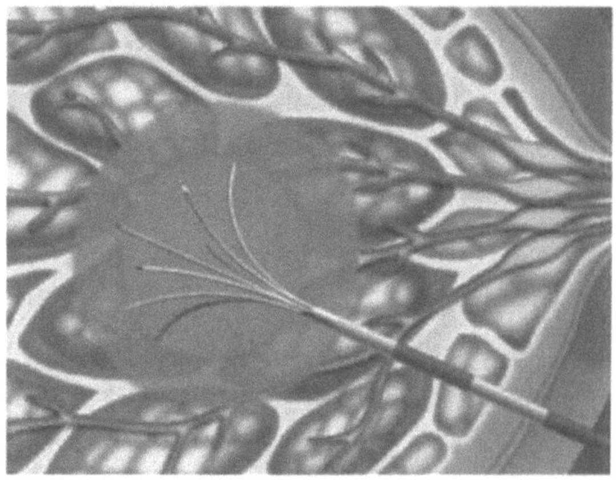

C

FIGURE 35.4. Deployment of the prongs of the radiofrequency ablation device. (A) Longitudinal sonogram shows two prongs (arrows) traversing the small carcinoma (arrowheads). (B) Transverse sonogram shows the cross sections of multiple prongs (arrows) in the central portion of the rounded tumor (arrowheads). (C) Diagram illustrates the expected ablation volume achieved around the deployed prongs of the multiarray device.

dure by an ill-defined area of increased echogenicity (Fig. 35.6). As we had expected, color Doppler imaging performed after the procedure was complete showed the complete extinction of any preexisting vascularity in and around the tumor within the ablated volume.

On gross pathologic examination, a hyperemic ring, measuring about 3 to 4 cm in diameter, was seen around the tumor, representing the outer limit of the ablated lesion (Fig. 35.7). On hematoxylin and eosin staining, a thermal effect was evident in the target lesions, including the presence of disrupted cell outlines, preserved nuclear staining, and increased cytoplasmic eosinophilia. Viability staining with reduced nicotinamide adenine dinucleotide (NADH)-diaphorase confirmed the nonviability of the cells in the ablated volume.

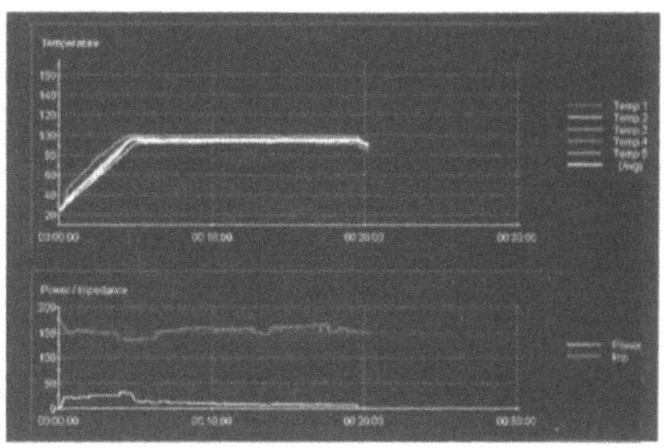

FIGURE 35.5. Screenshot of the laptop computer displays the temperatures recorded at the tips of five of the prongs, which have reached the target temperature of 95°C and have been maintained at that level for 15 minutes (top). The graph also displays the power output and the tissue impedance (bottom).

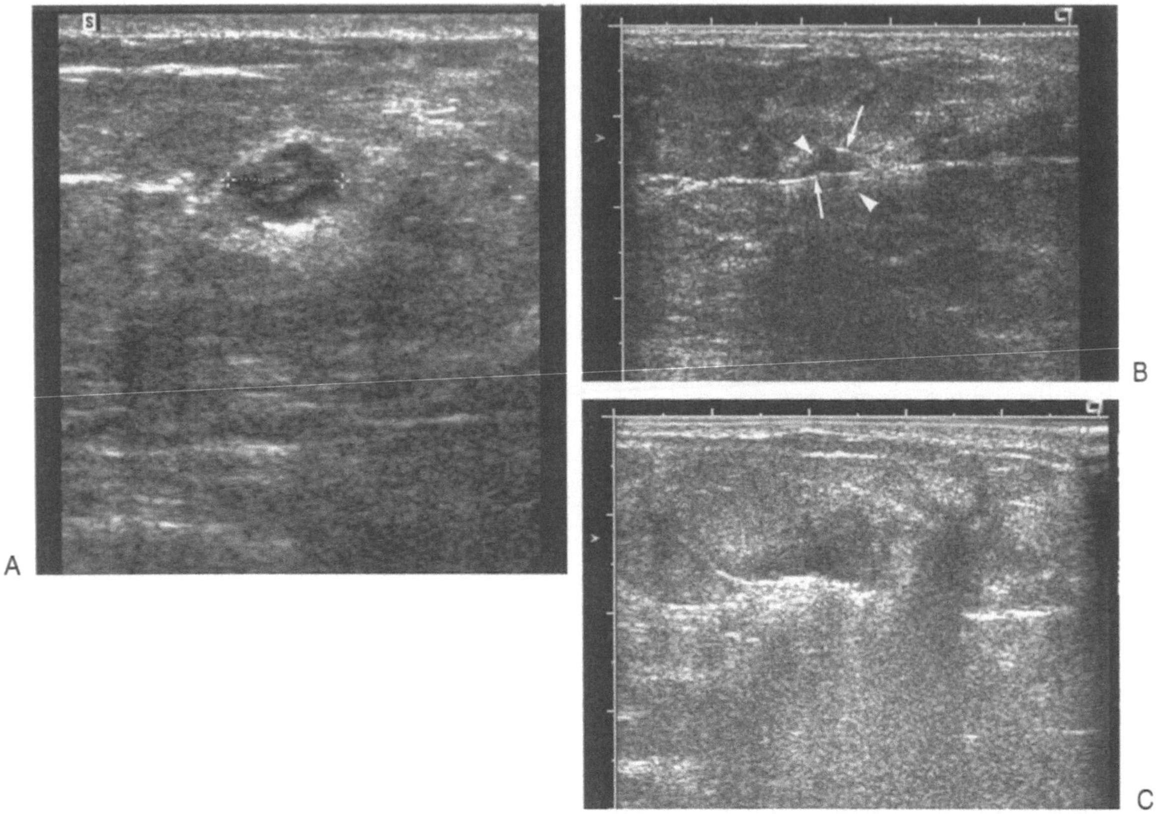

FIGURE 35.6. Changes in the sonographic appearance of a small carcinoma during radiofrequency ablation (RFA). (A) Pre-RFA sonogram shows the small (0.9 cm), well-defined tumor (calipers). (B) Sonogram obtained at the beginning of the RFA procedure shows the prongs (arrows) inserted through the lesion (arrowheads). (C) Sonogram obtained at the end of the RFA session shows that the tumor is no longer identifiable owing to the substantial increase in echogenicity of the adjacent tissues, which obscures the lesion.

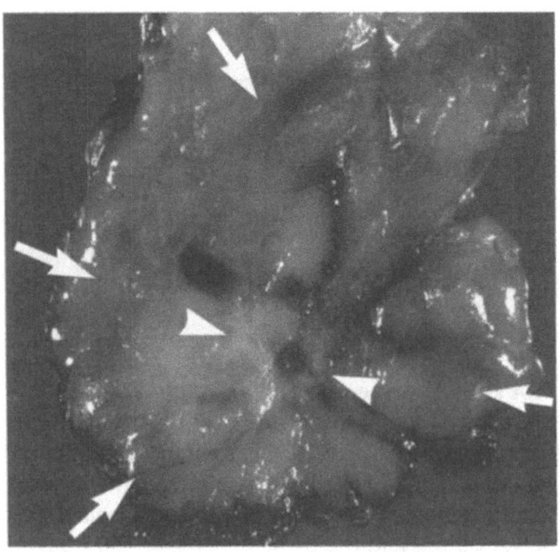

FIGURE 35.7. Photograph of the breast tissue specimen excised after completion of radiofrequency ablation (RFA) shows a reddish hyperemic ring (arrows) defining the extent of the ablation zone. Note the small tumor (arrowheads) in the center of the ring and the tract of the RFA device through the small tumor.

No complications, such as burn of the overlying skin or underlying chest wall, occurred, probably as a result of our stringent patient selection criteria. A case of full skin burn during breast RFA has been reported in another study (5).

In our study, the target lesion delineated by sonography was ablated completely in 100% of the cases (Fig. 35.7). In one case of a tumor that had been downstaged by preoperative chemotherapy from a 4-cm palpable mass to a sonographically and mammographically determined residua of about 1 cm in diameter, RFA ablated the small residua; however, pathologic examination revealed extensive invasive and in situ carcinoma around it. Therefore, we believe that patients who have been treated with preoperative chemotherapy should not be offered RFA as a therapeutic option. Our study has been expanded to include two other centers with less favorable results, raising the issues of both appropriate selection of cases and operator dependence. Thus, before RFA can be used as a replacement for the standard-of-care therapy of small breast cancer, that is, lumpectomy followed by radiation therapy, important questions and serious concerns need to be addressed.

The optimal RFA treatment parameters, that is, those that ensure ablation of the tumor with sufficient margin and the least damage to the surrounding tissues, are not yet fully established. They will likely vary, according to the histopathologic type of the tumor and the composition of the surrounding breast tissue. It is conceivable that our RFA protocol overtreats the lesions that might be destroyed equally well with a shorter RF session, lower target temperature, or both. The use of animal models should provide information about this possible dose-effect relationship.

The true microscopic extent of the tumor, which may be very large and at times extremely asymmetric, cannot be determined accurately either sonographically or by any other currently available imaging technique. In the absence of surgical resection with pathologic evaluation of the specimen, any residual disease in or at the periphery of the ablated volume would go undetected and could lead to a higher risk of local recurrence, even if RFA is followed by radiation therapy. For this reason, ill-defined tumors that are not well demarcated from surrounding tissues on imaging, including invasive lobular carcinomas, should not be considered targets for curative RFA. Tumors with a substantial DCIS component on diagnostic core biopsy specimens also should be excluded.

The use of real-time sonography during RFA has been ineffective in both monitoring the formation and assessing the extent of the thermal lesions. By sonography, the margins of the tumor are obscured by a diffuse area of hyperechogenicity and sometimes disappear completely as the RFA progresses. Therefore, the only—but critical—role of sonographic guidance is to ensure that the device is placed in the exact geometric center of the target, and that the prongs are deployed in such a manner as to generate an ablation volume that will concentrically encompass the tumor. For the time being, until an imaging modality is developed that can accurately ascertain the margins of the ablation volume during the procedure, the use of RFA as a curative option for early breast cancer requires a certain amount of overtreatment.

Will all ablated tumors proceed to complete necrosis? To date, we have information on the effectiveness of the ablation derived only from immediate evaluation of the target tissue through special viability staining. Whether this type of assessment is predictive of eventual complete necrosis of the treated tumor if left in situ after RFA will need to be confirmed.

How difficult will it be after RFA to follow patients with only standard imaging modalities (mammography and sonography) and physical examination? Whether extensive fat necrosis and its associated early calcifications will interfere with the early detection of recurrence remains to be determined. Imaging with magnetic resonance imaging (MRI), positron emission tomography (PET), or both is expected to play a crucial role in the follow-up of these patients. However, even the use of sophisticated imaging modalities may not prevent the need for extensive sampling of the periphery of the ablated lesion with core needle biopsies to detect microscopic recurrent or residual disease.

What will the long-term cosmetic results of RFA be? Although it may be predicted that the cosmetic results would be excellent, the extent of tissue retraction and fibrosis, and the ultimate effect of radiation therapy on a thermally treated area not only are unknown, but may vary from patient to patient.

The most important end point for future trials designed to use RFA as an alternative curative procedure to lumpectomy followed by radiation therapy, is long-term local control. Will RFA, which causes a coagulative necrosis of the tumor and a surrounding rim of tissue, adequately mimic a surgical procedure and yield similar results in long-term local control? Since the expected 5-year recurrence rate is only a few percent with surgery, experience with large numbers of patients will be needed to determine whether any statistically significant difference exists between the two treatments.

After our pilot RFA study at the University of Texas M. D. Anderson Cancer Center was successful, we designed a protocol for the use of RFA as a replacement for lumpectomy of cancers up to 1.5 cm (Fig. 35.8) (6). Patients will undergo core biopsy at the periphery of the ablated zone 4 weeks after the RFA procedure to assess local tumor control, and will undergo imaging procedures and quality-of-life evaluations at 6-month intervals for the first 2 years and annually thereafter through year 5. The results of this study will indicate whether RFA is oncologically and cosmetically appropriate for the local treatment of primary breast cancer.

The best results in all sonographically guided interventional procedures are achieved by radiologists highly skilled in sonography, and the RFA procedure is no exception. RFA requires the highest level of eye–hand coordination and three-dimensional (3D) sonographic "vision." A major issue regarding the skills required for the procedure will be the degree of operator dependence. Although the sonographically guided percutaneous insertion of the RFA probe appears similar to that of a core biopsy needle, there is a notable difference between the two procedures. For a sonographically guided core biopsy to be successful, the operator needs to hit any part of the target lesion (including its edge) only once in four to six attempts. However, to ensure successful RFA, the device must be placed in the geometric center of the tumor, which requires accurate 3D mental images of the location of the tips of the deployed prongs and the anticipated shape and size of the ablation volume, with no room for guesswork. Thus, the placement of the RFA device inside the target lesion requires a greater level of skill than does merely hitting the target with an automated biopsy gun. It is doubtful that the expertise required to perform curative RFA of breast cancer in terms of the accuracy of the 3D placement of the device and prediction of an acceptable size thermal lesion is exportable to the general surgical

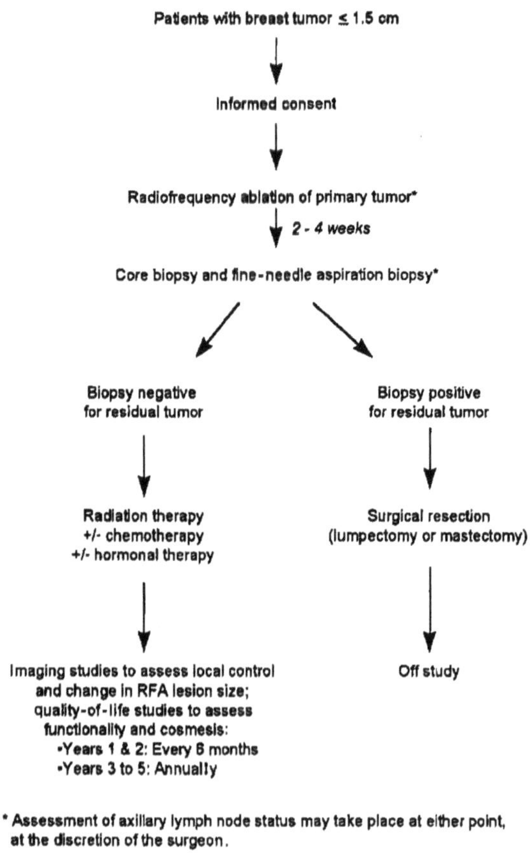

FIGURE 35.8. Protocol of a future study, designed to test radiofrequency ablation as an alternative to breast conservation surgery and radiation therapy for the local treatment of small (≤1.5 cm) breast carcinomas.

community. We therefore believe that a team approach involving an expert interventional sonologist is a prerequisite.

Which patients should be offered this alternative therapy for breast cancer? Until RFA proves equivalent to breast conservation surgery and applicable to a wider range of patients, patients who are not candidates for surgery (or are poor candidates) would benefit from curative RFA, as would elderly patients with slow-growing tumors and a lower risk of recurrence. Selected patients with local recurrences also could be considered for RFA. Finally, some consideration should be given to the concept of performing RFA (or any other percutaneous ablation technique) on a tumor prior to its surgical excision in an attempt to minimize dissemination of tumor cells during tumor manipulation.

Laser Irradiation

Laser-irradiation thermotherapy is another ablation technique based on interstitial hyperthermia (7). Various lasers have been used for this purpose. Recently, diode lasers have largely replaced neodymium:yttrium-aluminum-garnet (Nd:YAG) lasers because of their small size, portability, and lower cost.

An advantage of laser fibers is their small size: a bare fiber can be inserted through a needle as small as 22 gauge. A treatment zone of about 1 cm can be expected to result from a precharred laser tip when tissue is exposed to 2 to 3 W of continuous laser power for about 10 minutes. The laser energy may be split into as many as four fibers for simultaneous treatment through multiple needles. Recently developed diffuser tips have extended the treatment zone to 3 cm. Laser-irradiation thermotherapy has been performed under sonographic (8), stereotactic (9,10), or MRI (11,12) guidance.

In a recent study of stereotactically guided laser ablation of breast cancer, 54 tumors (50 invasive and four in situ; 51 masses and three areas of microcalcification) with a mean diameter of 1.2 cm were treated on a stereotactic table, using a 16- to 18-gauge 805-nm laser probe, with an optic fiber transmitting a predetermined amount of laser energy (9). First, four metallic markers were placed in the tumor, and one thermocouple was inserted at a distance of 1 cm from the laser fiber tip. Then 50 mL of local anesthetic were infused. The target temperature, as measured by the thermocouple, was 60°C. The average treatment time was 30 minutes. The ablated lesions were surgically removed for pathologic evaluation 1 to 8 weeks later, and a 2.5- to 3.5-cm hemorrhagic ring was seen surrounding the necrotic tumors. Complete tumor ablation was achieved in only 70% of cases, but this figure includes both the results obtained during the authors' learning curve and technical failures. In two patients who refused to undergo subsequent surgical excision, the unresected tumors first showed shrinkage, followed by the development of a 2- to 3-cm oil cyst and fibrosis, proven by needle core biopsies (9). This group of investigators also reported earlier that they observed total tumor ablation with negative margins whenever 2500 J/mL of tumor were administered or when the thermal sensors recorded 60°C. In that study, microscopic examination 1 week after the ablation showed disintegration of malignant cells, with a peripheral acute inflammatory response and extensive fibrosis, noted 4 to 8 weeks after the ablation (10).

Laser ablation also can be performed under MRI guidance. An important advantage of MRI guidance is the availability of accurate phase-sensitive temperature mapping that can monitor the extent of the thermal lesion during the procedure (13).

Insonation with High-Intensity Focused Ultrasound (HIFU) Waves

Another approach to local tissue destruction has been through the use of HIFU waves, delivered by a series of transducers that focus the waves onto a predetermined area within the breast that rapidly heats to the point of tissue destruction. Unlike other ablation techniques, insonation with HIFU waves does not involve percutaneous insertion of a device inside the lesion. A disadvantage of this technique, however, is the substantial risk that the target lesion will move during the procedure and therefore be missed. Another limitation is the relatively small amount of tissue that can be treated at a time.

Magnetic resonance imaging has been the imaging modality of choice for guidance with the HIFU ablation technique. A few clinical research studies have been undertaken with HIFU of breast tumors, mostly concentrating on the treatment of fibroadenomas (14,15). In one series of 11 fibroadenomas in nine patients, HIFU waves were used under MRI guidance with temperature-sensitive phase difference–based imaging during each sonication to monitor both the location of the focus and the increase in temperature, which ranged from 13° to 50°C (15). Three of the 11 lesions were not treated adequately because of insufficient acoustic power, patient movement, or both. One case of transient edema of the pectoralis muscle was noted 2 days after the procedure (15).

Cryoablation Therapy

Cryoablation, once a popular technique for treating liver metastases, is regaining the favor of some investigators, especially for treating fibroadenomas. This is due in part to the advent of new, compact, easy-to-use cryoablation systems that use argon gas, which reaches freezing temperatures faster than liquid nitrogen. Because the very cold temperatures achieved in cryoablation are anesthetic, this procedure can be performed safely under local anesthesia with little or no sedation of the patient.

During cryoablation of both normal and malignant breast tissue, ice initially forms in the connective tissue, then propagates and surrounds fat cells in normal adipose tissue and clumps of tightly packed malignant cells in cancer (16).

The thermal variables involved in cryoablation include cooling rate, temperature gradient, freezing interface velocity, final freezing temperature, holding time at the final temperature, warming (thaw) rate, and number of freeze–thaw cycles (17). Cellular damage increases with faster cooling because of the higher probability of intracellular ice formation. A double freeze–thaw cycle increases cell damage, which is sufficient for complete cell destruction at a final temperature of –40°C if a 25°C/minute cooling rate is used and at –20°C if a 50°C/minute cooling rate is used (17).

In a study in rats, mice, dogs, and sheep that used a 3-mm cryoprobe and liquid nitrogen for cryoablation of mammary adenocarcinomas, a single short (<7 minutes) freeze killed only tumors smaller than 1.5 cm in diameter, despite an apparent temperature decrease to –40°C at the periphery of the tumors (18). If the iceball fully encompassed the tumor and was maintained for at least 15 minutes, 100% tumor kill was achieved, independent of tumor size. In this study, two freeze–thaw cycles, each consisting of a 15-minute freeze and a 10-minute thaw, were most effective. No procedure-related complications were noted (18). This same group of investigators also treated one human patient who had two invasive lobular carcinomas: the specimens obtained during core needle biopsies performed 4 and 12 weeks after the well-tolerated cryoablation procedure were negative for residual disease (18).

A more recent study involved 16 breast cancers with a mean (± standard deviation) size of 2.1 ± 0.8 cm that were treated with a 3-mm cryoprobe inserted under sonographic guidance for two freeze–thaw cycles of a 7- to 10-minute freeze and a 5-minute thaw (19). The mean diameter of the iceball after the second freeze cycle was 2.8 ± 0.3 cm. Five tumors smaller than 1.6 cm showed no residual invasive cancer after treatment, but two of them had DCIS in the surrounding tissues, whereas tumors of 2.3 cm or larger showed incomplete necrosis.

Cryoablation is well suited for use under sonographic guidance because the hyperechoic front edge of the iceball that is created appears sharp sonographically (Fig. 35.9). This allows accurate real-time visibility and control of the extent of the thermal lesion, which is not possible with RFA. As a result, the procedure is easily tailored to the size of the lesion. If needed to protect the skin, sterile saline can be injected under sonographic guidance at the periphery of the iceball.

At our institution, we have used an argon-based device (Visica System; Sanarus Medical,

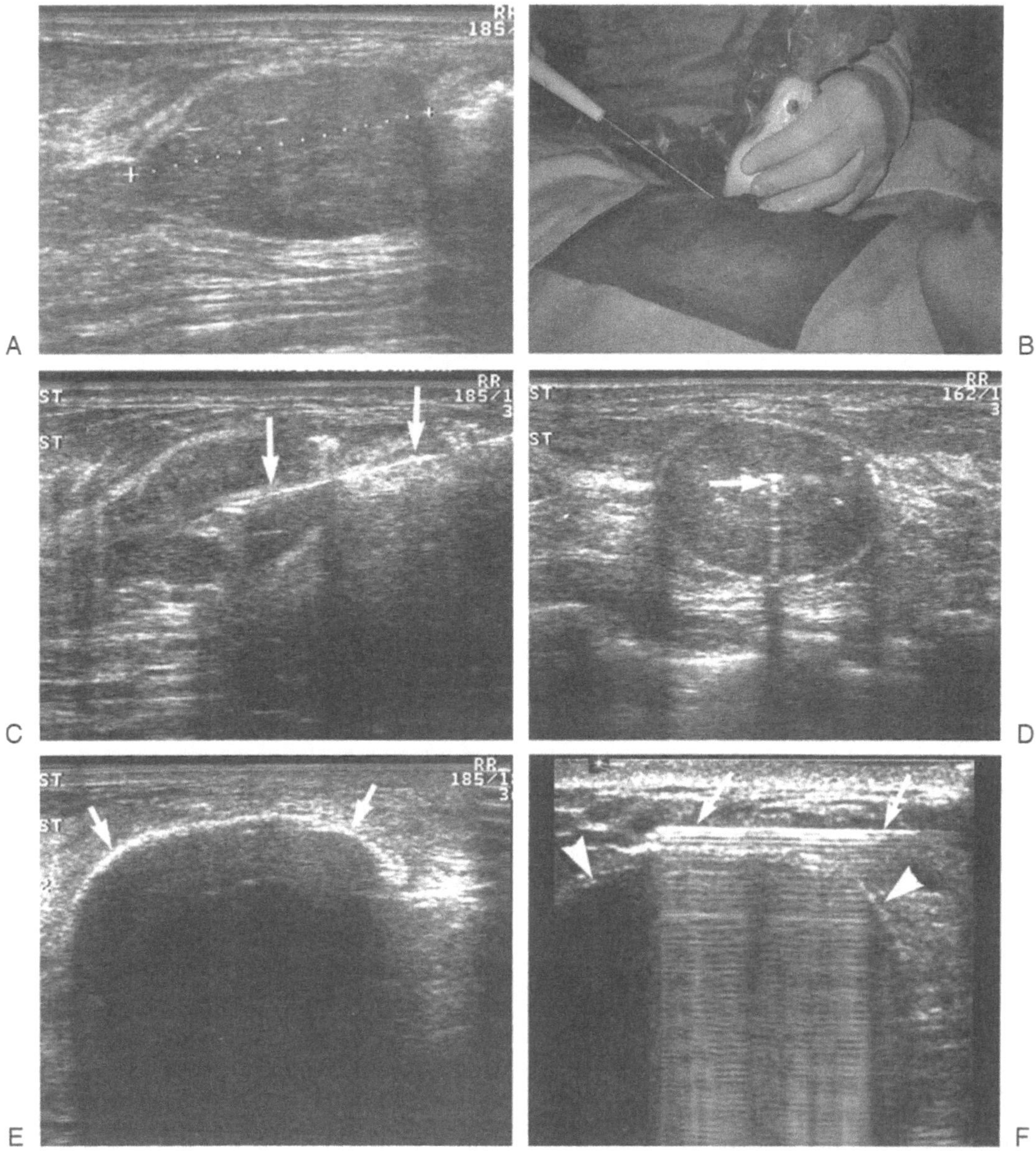

FIGURE 35.9. Cryoablation of a large fibroadenoma in a 25-year-old woman who had undergone five previous excisional biopsies for fibroadenomas. (A) Sonogram shows a large fibroadenoma (calipers). (B) Photograph shows insertion of the cryoprobe through the breast under sonographic guidance. (C) Longitudinal sonogram shows the cryoprobe (arrows) advancing through the center of the oval lesion. (D) Transverse sonogram confirms the correct position of the cryoprobe (arrow) through the central portion of the target lesion. Note the typical comet-tail artifact associated with the metallic probe. (E) Longitudinal sonogram obtained during the cryoablation shows the iceball (arrows) encompassing the fibroadenoma. (F) Sonogram shows that saline is injected between the iceball (arrowheads) and the skin under sonographic guidance to avoid the development of skin lesions. Arrows point to the needle. Note the marked reverberations behind the probe. (G) Photograph of the breast 24 hours later shows no evidence of hematoma. (H) Sonogram obtained 8 months later shows a 75% reduction in the volume of the lesion.

(*continued*)

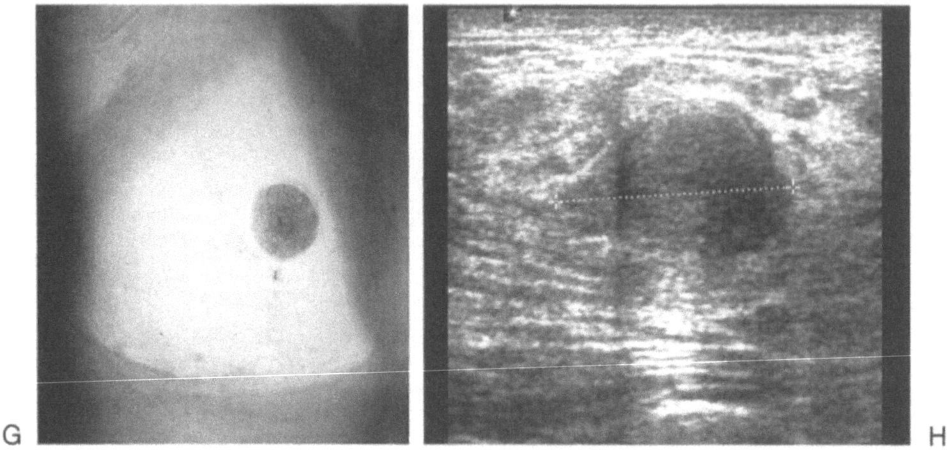

FIGURE 35.9. (*continued*)

Inc., Pleasanton, CA) with a cryoprobe that is 2.4 mm in diameter and is placed under sonographic guidance. Two 8- to 10-minute cycles of freezing separated by a thaw of the same duration usually have been applied to 2- to 3-cm fibroadenomas. An improved algorithm that allows more rapid treatment combines a cycle of active "high freeze" (to reach the target temperature) and one of "low freeze" (to maintain the low target temperature). The respective durations of the two cycles are tailored to the size of the lesion, and the total freeze time does not exceed 10 minutes; the relative duration of high freeze increases from 2 minutes for a fibroadenoma of less than 1.0 cm, to 10 minutes for a fibroadenoma of 3.6 to 4.0 cm (Table 35.1).

TABLE 35.1. Relative durations of high and low freeze cycles* for percutaneous cryoablation of fibroadenomas according to lesion size.

Fibroadenoma size (cm)	Freeze cycle duration (minutes) High	Low
<1.0	2	0
1.0–1.5	2	4
1.6–2.0	3	5
2.1–2.5	5	5
2.6–3.0	6	4
3.1–3.5	8	2
3.6–4.0	10	0

* Freeze cycles are categorized as "high", for reaching the target temperature, and "low", for maintaining the low target temperature.

Common transient postprocedure side effects of cryoablation of breast masses are local swelling and ecchymosis, which resolve within 2 to 3 weeks. Treated fibroadenomas shrink over 6 to 12 months. In one multicenter study, 57 core biopsy-proven fibroadenomas ranging from 0.8 to 4.2 cm, with a mean size of 2.1 cm, were cryoablated using two freeze cycles for a total duration of 6 to 30 minutes (20). The procedures were performed under local anesthesia, most of them in an office setting. The median tumor volume decreased by 65% at 6 months and 92% at 12 months. No skin injury and little or no pain during and after the procedure were noted, and the cosmetic results and degree of patient satisfaction were excellent. The authors recommended the use of cryoablation as an alternative to surgical excision of fibroadenomas (20).

Conclusion

As more small, nonpalpable solid masses are detected by screening mammography, the natural desire in the medical community is for the development of systems capable of completely destroying these masses in the least invasive manner (i.e., with the least trauma, pain, and inconvenience to the patient), with optimal cosmetic results, yet without sacrificing the chance for cure. Although several modalities already appear capable of achieving this goal, important issues remain to be resolved before they can become the standard of care for breast diseases, particularly breast cancer. From a technical standpoint, a substantial amount of information on treatment methods remains to be collected for each percutaneous ablation technique ("How would you like your tumor—cooked or frozen?"). Eventually, in addition to being compared with current standards of care, all these different techniques will need to be compared with one another ("Does frying kill better than freezing?"). Further studies, especially ones evaluating long-term outcome, are mandatory before the current standard-of-care treatment of small breast cancer can be altered. Progress should be made only with caution and without being driven by technology. Nonetheless, these new treatment options are attractive alternatives, especially for benign breast diseases such as fibroadenomas, provided they prove to be both safe and efficacious.

References

1. Jeffrey SS, Birdwell RL, Ikeda DM, et al. Radiofrequency ablation of breast cancer: first report of an emerging technology. Arch Surg 1999;134:1064–1068.
2. Elliott RL, Rice PB, Suits JA, Ostrowe AJ, Head JF. Radiofrequency ablation of a stereotactically localized nonpalpable breast carcinoma. Am Surg 2002;68:1–5.
3. Mirza AN, Fornage BD, Sneige N, et al. Radiofrequency ablation of solid tumors. Cancer J 2001;7:95–102.
4. Fornage BD, Sneige N, Ross M, Singletary SE, Mirza AN, Edeiken BS. US-guided percutaneous radiofrequency ablation in the local treatment of small invasive breast carcinoma. Radiology 2002;225(P):459.
5. Izzo F, Thomas R, Delrio P, et al. Radiofrequency ablation in patients with primary breast carcinoma: a pilot study in 26 patients. Cancer 2001;92:2036–2044.
6. Singletary SE, Fornage BD, Sneige N, et al. Radiofrequency ablation of early-stage invasive breast tumors: an overview. Cancer J 2002;8:177–180.
7. Steger AC, Lees WR, Walmsley K, Brown SG. Interstitial laser hyperthermia: a new approach to local destruction of tumours. BMJ 1989;299:362–365.
8. Basu S, Ravi B, Kant R. Interstitial laser hyperthermia, a new method in the management of fibroadenoma of the breast: a pilot study. Lasers Surg Med 1999;25:148–152.
9. Dowlatshahi K, Francescatti DS, Bloom KJ. Laser therapy for small breast cancers. Am J Surg 2002;184:359–363.
10. Dowlatshahi K, Fan M, Gould VE, Bloom KJ, Ali A. Stereotactically guided laser therapy of occult breast tumors: work-in-progress report. Arch Surg 2000;135:1345–1352.
11. Harms SE. MR-guided minimally invasive procedures. Magn Reson Imaging Clin N Am 2001;9:381–392.
12. Vogl TJ, Mack MG, Straub R, et al. MR-guided laser-induced thermotherapy with a cooled power laser system: a case report of a patient with a recurrent carcinoid metastasis in the breast. Eur Radiol 2002;12(suppl 4):S101–S104.
13. Huber PE, Jenne JW, Rastert R, et al. A new noninvasive approach in breast cancer therapy using magnetic resonance imaging-guided focused ultrasound surgery. Cancer Res 2001;61:8441–8447.
14. Hynynen K, Pomeroy O, Smith DN, et al. MR imaging-guided focused ultrasound surgery of fibroadenomas in the breast: a feasibility study. Radiology 2001;219:176–185.
15. Hong JS, Rubinsky B. Patterns of ice formation in normal and malignant breast tissue. Cryobiology 1994;31:109–120.
16. Rui J, Tatsutani KN, Dahiya R, Rubinsky B. Effect of thermal variables on human breast cancer in cryosurgery. Breast Cancer Res Treat 1999;53:185–192.
17. Staren ED, Sabel MS, Gianakakis LM, et al. Cryosurgery of breast cancer. Arch Surg 1997;132:28–34.
18. Pfleiderer SO, Freesmeyer MG, Marx C, Kuhne-Heid R, Schneider A, Kaiser WA. Cryotherapy of breast cancer under ultrasound guidance: initial results and limitations. Eur Radiol 2002;12:3009–3014.
19. Kaufman CS, Bachman B, Littrup PJ, et al. Office-based ultrasound-guided cryoablation of breast fibroadenomas. Am J Surg 2002;184:394–400.
20. Kaufman CS, Bachman B, Littrup PJ, et al. Office based ultrasound-quided cryoablation of breast fibroadenomas. Am J Surg 2002;184:394–400.

36
Complications of Tumor Ablation

Lawrence Cheung, Tito Livraghi, Luigi Solbiati, Gerald D. Dodd III, and Eric vanSonnenberg

Percutaneous and surgical ablation procedures are flourishing, in large part because of the relative paucity and the acceptability of complications. However, serious and fatal complications have occurred, albeit rarely, with ablation. This chapter identifies those complications, describes their underlying cause, and, when possible, discusses strategies to avoid them.

When initially considering a patient for tumor ablation, awareness of both the frequency and scope of complications that can occur with the various procedures is necessary to accurately weigh the potential benefits of the intervention against its attendant risks. These risks also should be evaluated relative to those of the alternatives under consideration, such as surgical resection, aggressive chemotherapy, or a course of radiation therapy.

Although each local ablation technique possesses its own characteristic dangers, there are general guidelines that can be followed to minimize the severity and rate of complications. Preprocedure, patients should be evaluated carefully with regard to lesion size and location, feasibility of access routes, and degree of underlying clinical comorbidities. Bleeding and infection are potentially common to all interventional procedures; thus, coagulation tests should be performed on all patients and normalized whenever possible, and prophylactic antibiotics ought to be considered for those at increased risk of infection. The procedure itself should be performed meticulously, with attentive monitoring of vital signs, and care given to maintaining the sterility of the field and equipment. Postprocedure follow-up with appropriate clinical, laboratory, and imaging studies is critical to detect and remedy any complications as early as possible.

Complications of ablation should not be confused with those of the associated procedures that may precede or follow the ablation, such as biopsy, fluid infusion techniques, or possibly surgery. Even fine-needle biopsy that may immediately precede the ablation has its associated complications that may be serious and major (1).

In classifying complications as major or minor, a major complication is one that, if left untreated, might threaten the patient's life, lead to substantial morbidity and disability, or result in a lengthened hospital stay. All other complications are considered minor. They will be categorized in this chapter primarily according to the mechanism of ablation, and by the organ in which they occur. We include the reported literature, as well as our own personal experience.

Percutaneous Ethanol Injection (PEI)

Hepatic

Percutaneous ethanol injection most frequently is used for liver tumors, primarily hepatocellular carcinoma (HCC). In numerous large studies of PEI in the liver, it has consistently been shown to be a safe procedure, with mortality rates ranging from 0.09% to 0.97%, and major complication rates of 1.7% to 4.6% (2–4). Some of these studies include data for both conventional and single-session PEI. Conventional PEI generally is used to treat lesions less than 5 cm in greatest dimension, and involves injecting small amounts of ethanol, ranging from 1 to 15 mL depending on lesion size. It does not require general anesthesia and often is performed in multiple sessions. In contrast, single-session PEI is used to treat large lesions (>5 cm) by performing multiple passes and injecting significantly more ethanol during a single session. The procedure is performed under general anesthesia, and the volume of ethanol injected can exceed 100 mL. If the results of conventional and single-session PEI are analyzed separately, single-session PEI has increased complication rates, with one study reporting mortality and major complication rates of 1.71% and 6.29%, respectively, for single-session PEI, compared with 0.27% and 0.54% for conventional PEI (4).

Mortality

Reported causes of death from PEI in the liver include bleeding gastroesophageal varices, hemoperitoneum, and acute liver failure (2–5). Bleeding varices are the result of worsening portal hypertension from the procedure. When ethanol is injected into a lesion, it causes thrombosis of tumor vessels; however, it also can induce thrombosis of small vessels in regions of the liver adjacent to the lesion. This leads to a sudden increase in venous portal pressure, and if superimposed upon chronic portal hypertension from advanced cirrhosis, can result in massive variceal bleeding.

Most instances of fatal intraperitoneal hemorrhage are caused by the rupture of highly vascular HCCs that are located superficially, that is, either against or protruding into the liver capsule (2,4). Death from acute liver failure after PEI occurs primarily in patients with Child-Pugh class B or C cirrhosis, as their limited residual liver function renders the patient vulnerable to acute decompensation, even from mild to moderate insults (4).

Other causes of death from PEI that have been reported include hemothorax and massive hepatic necrosis (4,6). A case complicated by hemothorax was performed using an intercostal approach and was thought to be due to accidental rupture of the intercostal artery (4). A case of hepatic necrosis was attributed to an intratumoral arterioportal shunt that allowed the injected ethanol to spread diffusely throughout the liver (6).

Major Complications

Major complications that can occur with PEI in the liver include variceal bleeding, intraperitoneal bleeding, and hemothorax as discussed above, as well as hemobilia, subcapsular hematoma, portal vein thrombosis, biloma, sepsis, liver abscess, septic cholangitis, hepatic infarct of segments adjacent to the lesion, acute liver failure, and worsening of hepatic function with Child-Pugh class progression. The presence of a biloenteric anastomosis is a major risk factor for septic complications either during or soon after PEI (7), and postprocedure fevers in these patients should be evaluated carefully. Prophylactic antibiotics are mandatory for ablation in these patients.

Another major complication of PEI is neoplastic seeding along the needle tract, with a reported incidence ranging from 0.01% to 1.4%. Tumor seeding may be seen intraperitoneally in the liver and abdominal cavity, subcutaneously in the chest wall or abdominal wall, along the diaphragm, and cutaneously (8–10). Metastatic tumor spread to the lung also has occurred following PEI in the liver (11), leading to the concern that partial tumor necrosis following ethanol injection may increase embolization of tumor cells; however, there have been no other descriptions of this phenomenon.

Other rare complications of PEI include syncope, hypotension, hypoventilation, pneumothorax, gastric ulcer formation, splenic abscess, intestinal perforation, and acute renal failure from acute tubular necrosis (2–5,12–14).

Minor Complications

The most common minor complications following PEI are pain, fever, nausea, and vomiting, all of which are self-limited. Transient intoxication also is seen, especially with single-session PEI, during which the large volume of injected ethanol can lead to blood alcohol levels greater than 100 mg/dL (5). Asymptomatic right pleural effusions occasionally are detected on routine follow-up imaging, and generally resolve spontaneously.

Thyroid

There has been limited usage of PEI to treat benign thyroid nodules. Pain and fever are the most commonly reported side effects after the procedure. Other complications include transient dysphonia and Horner's syndrome (15,16), which relate to the proximity of the thyroid nodule to the recurrent laryngeal nerve and cervical sympathetic chain, respectively. Common jugular vein thrombosis also has been reported as a minor complication that resolves without treatment (16).

Radiofrequency Ablation (RFA)

Hepatic

Mortality rates for hepatic RFA have ranged from 0.3% to 1.6%, and major complication rates, from 2.4% to 5.7% (17,18). The risk of major complications increases with the number of ablation sessions, although not with tumor size (17). The choice of single versus cluster electrodes has not been found to affect complication rates significantly (17). In one study that compared percutaneous and intraoperative RFA, the mortality rate was 0.9% (2/216) for percutaneous RFA, compared with 2.4% (3/123) for intraoperative RFA (18). Similar types of complications, both major and minor, were seen in the two groups.

Mortality

Causes of death following RFA in the liver include intestinal perforation with subsequent peritonitis and multiorgan failure, acute liver failure, and massive hemoperitoneum following rupture of a superficial HCC nodule (17,18).

The colon has the highest risk of perforation from thermal damage, likely due to its thin wall and relative immobility when compared with the small bowel. Characteristic of thermally induced perforation is having the target lesion located within 1 cm of the liver capsule and adjacent to a gastrointestinal lumen. A second risk factor for intestinal perforation appears to be prior abdominal surgery with the formation of fibrotic adhesions that affix parts of the gastrointestinal tract to the liver (17). These adhesions probably impair normal peristalsis and preclude movement of the bowel away from the liver, thereby resulting in intraprocedural heating.

Acute liver failure following RFA can be secondary to various causes. There have been several cases of total portal vein thrombosis, from both intraoperative RFA with application of the Pringle maneuver, and from percutaneous RFA without balloon occlusion of the portal vein (18). One patient developed liver failure secondary to right hepatic duct stenosis following ablation of a lesion near the hepatic hilum (17). Apparently, the large bile ducts are susceptible to thermal damage; thus, lesions near the hepatic hilum or large bile ducts should be approached with care. Another case of fatal acute liver failure occurred in a patient who underwent right hepatectomy that was extended to segment IV along with RFA of a lesion in segment III (18). A large area of radiofrequency destruction was found in the remaining liver, and the patient lacked sufficient residual function to compensate.

Other deaths following hepatic RFA include a case of bile pulmonary embolism (19), one patient with pancreatic cancer who died suddenly 3 days postprocedure of unknown cause, and a patient with obesity and diabetes mellitus who developed peritonitis from *Staphylococcus aureus* that was attributed to an unknown break in sterile technique (17).

Major Complications

In addition to the complications discussed above, other major complications following hepatic RFA include liver abscess formation, tumor seeding, hypoxemia, and hemothorax. Patients with biloenteric anastomoses are at significantly higher risk for developing liver abscesses, similar to PEI (17,18). Patients with diabetes mellitus also appear to be at higher risk for septic complications (17). Patients with either of these conditions should receive prophylactic antibiotics prior to RFA.

The incidence of tumor seeding following RFA in the liver is around 0.5% in most large studies (17,18,20), although rates as high as 12.5% (4/32) have been reported in one study with a limited number of patients (21). The risk of tumor seeding is increased with subcapsular lesions, highly undifferentiated HCC, and high baseline serum α-fetoprotein level with HCC lesions (17,21). To decrease the risk of tumor seeding, the initial probe placement should be performed as carefully as possible to minimize the number of passes through the liver. Furthermore, after the ablation is complete, RF energy can be delivered to the probe during its withdrawal, thus cauterizing the probe tract.

Hypoxemia has been seen in a small number of patients following RFA. The cause remains to be elucidated, although there is speculation that it is caused by acute lung inflammation from the overexpression of cytokines that has been demonstrated with experimental cryoablation in animals, but has yet to be seen with RFA (22,23). Although the hypoxemia is transient and self-resolving after several days, it may prolong hospital stay due to the need to rule out pulmonary embolism.

Major complications that have been reported rarely include segmental hepatic infarction, common bile duct stenosis, biloma, blood in the gallbladder from hemobilia, acute cholecystitis, sepsis, hyperkalemia, diaphragmatic paresis, pulmonary embolism, pleural effusion requiring thoracentesis, pneumothorax requiring drainage, and cardiac arrest (17,18,24,25).

There also has been a report of two cases of severe intraprocedural hypertension requiring temporary cessation of the procedure and the administration of intravenous labetalol or hydralazine (26). Both of these patients had lesions in the posterior aspect of the right lobe of the liver, in proximity to the right adrenal gland. In one patient, measurement of catecholamines during the hypertensive crisis revealed massive elevations above normal levels. This has prompted speculation that intraprocedural heating of the adrenal gland may stimulate the release of catecholamines. Therefore, the possibility of a hypertensive crisis should be considered when ablating liver lesions near the right adrenal gland.

Minor Complications

The most common minor complication following RFA in the liver is postprocedure low-grade fever and general malaise, which has been described as the "postablation syndrome" (27). Symptom severity and duration correlate roughly with the volume of tumor ablated, and more aggressive procedures tend to result in more severe and prolonged symptoms. Although the symptoms generally resolve within 2 to 7 days, the syndrome can persist for up to 3 weeks with very large areas of necrosis.

Other minor complications include periprocedural and postprocedural pain, self-limiting intraperitoneal and subcapsular bleeding, asymptomatic arterioportal shunts, small pleural effusions, and pneumothoraces that do not require treatment. Skin burns were seen much more frequently before comprehensive guidelines for grounding pad safety were developed (28).

Pulmonary

The use of RFA to treat pulmonary lesions, either primary or metastatic, is relatively new, and data on the complications of this procedure are limited. Nevertheless, the initial reports on pulmonary RFA, all of which have employed a percutaneous approach, indicate that it is a safe procedure, with mortality rates ranging from 0% to 3.7% and major complication rates of 11% to 30% (29–34).

Mortality

Reported deaths following pulmonary RFA include one case of acute respiratory distress syndrome (30) and two pulmonary hemorrhages (31,35). The case of acute respiratory distress syndrome occurred 4 days after the RFA procedure in a patient who had recently been diagnosed with pneumonia. This has led to speculation that inflamed, consolidated lung parenchyma is more susceptible to thermal damage from RF energy due to a difference in its conductivity relative to normal, aerated lung. Until more data are available regarding this complication, it is recommended that patients with pneumonia should wait until the consolidation has resolved completely before undergoing RFA.

Concerning the two pulmonary hemorrhages, one was detected within 2 hours of the procedure in a patient who was taking clopidogrel, an inhibitor of platelet aggregation, at the time of the procedure (35). Based on this report, the authors advise that patients taking clopidogrel should discontinue the medication 1 week prior to RFA, similar to elective surgery when bleeding is a risk. The other reported case of pulmonary hemorrhage occurred 2 days after treatment and also was attributed to platelet dysfunction (31).

Major Complications

The primary major complication of pulmonary RFA is pneumothorax requiring thoracostomy tube placement for drainage. The incidence of pneumothorax that warrants drainage ranges from 6.6% to 30% in the largest studies (29–31). The risk of pneumothorax is significantly increased when the RF probe traverses normal lung parenchyma, and pneumothorax occurs more frequently in centrally located tumors than in those that are peripheral (30). Whenever possible, a transparenchymal route to the lesion should be avoided.

Other reported major complications include a cerebral infarction thought to be secondary to an air embolism (34), obstructive pneumonia (30), and a large pleural effusion complicating a pneumothorax (29).

Minor Complications

Two intraprocedural complications that have been reported are persistent cough that requires a reduction in RF energy from >100 W to 80 W (30), and pain that necessitates a conversion from local anesthesia to intravenous sedation (29). There is also a high incidence of intraprocedural pneumothorax that does not require drainage, as high as 67% (four of six) in one small series (32).

Common postprocedure complications include fever and malaise, consistent with the postablation syndrome, as well as pain and dyspnea. Other minor complications that have been reported are asymptomatic pleural effusion, mild intrapulmonary hemorrhage with transient hemoptysis, expectoration of small amounts of desiccated tissue (29), subcutaneous emphysema, and severe myalgia. From our own experience, we had one patient who developed a skin burn on the back, and another with transient dysphonia following RFA of a lesion in proximity to the aortic arch, near the origin of the left recurrent laryngeal nerve.

Renal

Various centers currently perform RFA to treat renal lesions; early experience indicates that there is minimal morbidity and mortality associated with the procedure (36–40). With over 100 patients reported, there has been only one death following renal RFA—a patient with a history of severe pulmonary disease who died from aspiration pneumonia 3 days after an uneventful procedure (39). There was no evidence of renal hemorrhage or direct injury to the lungs from the ablation itself.

Major Complications

The few major complications reported are representative of problems that have been seen with RFA in the liver, such as bleeding, injury to adjacent structures, and tumor seeding. One patient with a central lesion developed a large perirenal hematoma and blood in the renal pelvis. A clot formed in the collecting system causing anuria, and the patient required cystoscopic ureteral stent placement and a blood transfusion (36).

Another patient suffered a small burn injury to the liver immediately adjacent to a right-sided, anterior renal lesion during RFA (39). Injuries to adjacent structures are thought to be relatively rare, because of the surrounding perirenal fat. This provides a buffer that may help dissipate heat and protect nearby organs.

A single instance of tumor seeding has been reported following renal RFA. The patient developed a 5-mm, cutaneous metastasis at the electrode insertion site, which was immediately resected and has not recurred during the 16 months since the procedure (40). This complication illustrates the importance of careful clinical follow-up. As in the liver, cauterization of the probe tract may help prevent tumor seeding if the probe has traversed normal renal parenchyma.

Another important question that has been raised is whether the renal collecting system is susceptible to thermal injury during ablation of centrally located lesions. Although a number of deep, medial lesions have been ablated without complications (36,37), there are two recent reports of injuries to the collecting system (40,41). One patient was incidentally found to have a dilated upper pole calyx on routine follow-up computed tomography (CT) scan obtained 2 months after the procedure; this was believed to be secondary to heat-induced stricture of the collecting system (40). A more serious case has been reported in a patient who developed flank pain, mild hydronephrosis, and mildly delayed contrast excretion 2 weeks after treatment. Six months after ablation, the patient had persistent, severe hydronephrosis and delayed contrast excretion; anatomic and functional imaging revealed complete ureteropelvic junction obstruction and that the affected kidney was contributing only 8% to overall renal function. Open nephrectomy was performed and confirmed the presence of a fibrotic lesion in the collecting system at the site of RFA (41). These studies suggest that fibrosis and stricturing of the renal collecting system with subsequent obstruction are potential complications of renal RFA, and that care should be taken to avoid including the renal pelvis or ureteropelvic junction within the treatment zone whenever possible.

Minor Complications

The most common minor complications following renal RFA are periprocedural pain and nausea, asymptomatic perirenal hematomas, and transient microscopic or macroscopic hematuria. Other reported minor complications include transient intraprocedural hypertension (mean blood pressure, 215/100 mm Hg) that resolved spontaneously after the procedure (40), subcapsular hematoma (38), pain with hip flexion, and paresthesia in the periumbilical region or the skin of the ipsilateral flank (37,40). The cases of pain during hip flexion resolved without treatment within 2 weeks, and may reflect temporary injury to the psoas muscle. The instances of paresthesia are likely due to injuries to the intercostal, lumbar, ilioinguinal, or iliohypogastric nerves that are located close to the kidney. In some cases, the paresthesia persisted for months, and may indicate permanent nerve damage.

Bone

In a multicenter study of percutaneous RFA of bony metastases, 43 patients were treated, and one (2.3%) major complication was seen (42). The patient suffered an acetabular fracture 6 weeks after RFA of a lesion that involved the acetabulum, ileum, and ischium. Although the presence of tumor alone predisposes to pathologic fracture, it is possible that tumor necrosis in the acetabulum from the ablation also contributed. Two minor complications also were reported in the study: one second-degree skin burn at the grounding pad site and one case of transient bowel and bladder incontinence following RFA of a previously irradiated sacral metastasis.

In one of the only reported cases of intrauterine RFA during pregnancy, the ablation of a sacrococcygeal teratoma resulted in the birth of a newborn with an open posterior hip dislocation and loss of sciatic nerve function (43).

Adrenal

In a series of 15 adrenal lesions in eight patients treated with RFA, the only complication was a delayed polymicrobial abscess in a 9-cm lesion that was discovered 11 weeks after the procedure (44). The abscess was treated successfully with prolonged catheter drainage and antibiotics. Another series of 13 adrenal masses in 12 patients had no major complications (45). The only minor complication reported was a small hematoma in a patient with preexisting thrombocytopenia from chemotherapy. No patients in either study developed hypertension during the procedure, despite a recent report of catecholamine release and life-threatening hypertension during the ablation of liver lesions near the right adrenal gland (26).

Breast

Several pilot studies have examined RFA of breast lesions followed by surgical resection (46–49). The only major complication occurred in a study of 26 patients, one of whom developed a full-thickness skin burn following RFA of a lesion immediately beneath the skin (46). The minor complications reported were small breast ecchymoses in some patients, and there was one 5-mm skin burn that did not require treatment (47,48). In one study of 20 patients, there were no complications reported (49).

Cryoablation

Hepatic

Cryoablation of hepatic tumors has been used since the 1980s, traditionally via laparotomy. Currently, laparoscopic and percutaneous approaches are gaining popularity (50–52). Mortality rates following open cryoablation range from 1.2% to 7.5%, and major complication rates vary from 5.9% to as high as 45.0% (53–56). Numerous studies have observed a correlation between the volume of liver being ablated and the risk of major complications, such as parenchymal fracture, coagulopathy, and acute renal failure from myoglobinuria (55,57,58). The specific liver volume at which complications begin to increase significantly has been estimated at >30% to 35% liver volume, lesions >5 to 10cm diameter, and a total estimated area of lesions >30 cm^2 (53–55,57). Currently, there is no evidence regarding the relative safety of open, surgical cryoablation versus the laparoscopic or percutaneous routes.

Two retrospective studies have attempted to compare the complication rates of cryoablation and RFA for hepatic tumors using either an open or percutaneous approach (50,59). In the study that performed either cryoablation or RFA intraoperatively, the rate of major complications for cryoablation was 40.7% (22/54) versus 3.3% (3/92) for RFA (59). However, the other study that used a percutaneous approach for both procedures failed to show significant differences in the major complication rates: 29% (9/31) for cryoablation and 26% (8/31) for RFA (50). The choice of treatment modality was based on the preference and training of the individual surgeons in the first study, and on the random availability of probes in the second. A third study that used the laparoscopic approach treated lesions smaller than 5 cm with RFA and those from 5 to 8 cm with cryoablation. The authors found major complication rates of 24% (4/17) for cryoablation, and 3.4% (1/29) for RFA (51).

Mortality

One of the most common causes of death following hepatic cryoablation is a syndrome consisting of thrombocytopenia, disseminated intravascular coagulation, acute respiratory distress syndrome, hypotension, and multiorgan failure. This constellation of symptoms has been termed the "cryoshock phenomenon", due to its similarities to septic shock, although without evidence of systemic infection (60). Although some patients have the full syndrome, many have various combinations of the primary symptoms. The exact mechanism of cryoshock remains to be elucidated; however, there is evidence that large-volume freezing and multiple freeze–thaw cycles stimulate release of cytokines similar to those seen in septic shock, including tumor necrosis factor-α and interleukin-6 (23,61). The cryoshock phenomenon is highly specific, both to cryoablation and to the liver as the target organ. However, it is seen following cryoablation of both primary liver tumors and metastatic lesions, which suggests it may be the surrounding, normal liver tissue that is releasing the mediators of cryoshock in response to cryotrauma, rather than the tumor. It is known that the Kupffer cells of the liver have a propensity to release cytokines following injury, including tumor necrosis factor-α and interleukin-6. Another explanation for the specificity of cryoshock to the liver could be that the volume of tissue frozen with hepatic cryoablation typically is greater than with prostate or renal cryoablation.

Severe hemorrhage is another major cause of mortality associated with cryoablation. Although the coagulopathy of cryoshock may contribute to the high frequency of hemorrhage, the predominant source of significant bleeding comes from fracturing of the liver parenchyma during the rapid freeze–thaw cycles, analogous to the cracks that form in an ice cube when placed in warm water. The cracks in the hepatic parenchyma extend from the center of the iceball to the outer margin of the freeze zone. In most instances, the bleeding comes from the fractured hepatic vessels, although there is one report of a fatal hemorrhage from the iceball cracking into the right hepatic vein (59). The risk of parenchymal fractures can be decreased by minimizing any movement or torque on the cryoprobe during the freezing process, especially when the freeze is near completion and the liver is at its coldest. Furthermore, attempts to retract the probe should not be made until the iceball has thawed completely, thus allowing the probe to be removed with minimal resistance.

Other causes of death following cryoablation include liver failure from insufficient residual function, colonic perforation from freezing injury, sepsis, acute myocardial infarction, and pulmonary embolism. Rare causes of death include variceal hemorrhage, hepatorenal syndrome, portal vein thrombosis, strangulated bowel obstruction, acute pancreatitis, ischemic stroke, and delayed intraabdominal rupture of the cryoablated area that led to multiorgan failure (50,54,55,61,62).

Major Complications

Cryoshock, parenchymal fracture with subsequent hemorrhage, freezing injury to adjacent structures such as the colon, and acute liver failure are all major causes of morbidity, as well as mortality. In addition to these, the most common complications following cryoablation are hypothermia, injury to the biliary system, renal insufficiency secondary to myoglobinuria, hepatic abscess, and symptomatic pleural effusion.

Hypothermia associated with the cryoablation procedure can be severe, with a drop in core temperature below 33.5°C. In addition to the cardiac complications of arrhythmia and myocardial ischemia, hypothermia can induce or worsen coagulopathy. The incidence of hypothermia can be decreased by using Bair Hugger heating blankets (Arizant Healthcare, Prairie, MN) during the procedure and by increasing the patient's core temperature to 38.2°C prior to performing cryoablation (53,63).

Injuries to the biliary system are also potential complications. Although the large blood vessels are protected from thermal injury by the warming effect of flowing blood, the large bile ducts are susceptible to freezing damage. Necrosis of the bile duct epithelium can lead to bile leakage with biloma formation, biliary strictures, or biliary-cutaneous fistulas. If the tumor to be ablated lies near the large bile ducts, one technique for protecting them from thermal damage is to circulate warm saline through a catheter placed in the bile ducts (64). Another technique that has been described involves the placement of metal stents in the large bile ducts approximately 2 days prior to cryoablation (53). The stents help preserve the integrity of the bile ducts during the freezing process, and may aid in their reepithelialization if injured.

Myoglobinuria is seen in many patients following cryoablation. Although usually transient, myoglobinuria occasionally can progress to acute tubular necrosis with renal insufficiency. The incidence of acute tubular necrosis can be reduced, albeit not entirely negated, by ensuring adequate hydration prior to the procedure, initiating mannitol diuresis during the procedure, and alkalinzing the urine postprocedurally (53,65).

Hepatic abscesses can develop in the ablated tumor, generally in the weeks following the procedure. Delayed abscess formation, more than 1 year after the procedure, also has been observed (66). Many patients develop pleural effusions following hepatic cryoablation, and while most are asymptomatic and resolve in less than 2 weeks, those that cause dyspnea or do not resolve spontaneously require thoracentesis or placement of a thoracostomy tube.

Other reported complications include subcapsular hematoma, wound infection, wound dehiscence, injury to the diaphragm, pneumothorax, right lower lobe pneumonia, mental status changes, unexplained fever, severe nausea and vomiting, and acute pancreatitis (51,54,59,61).

Minor Complications

Minor complications following hepatic cryoablation include the postablation syndrome of low-grade fever and malaise, periprocedural and postprocedural pain, nitrogen skin burns (51), transient elevation of liver enzymes, asymptomatic pleural effusions, myoglobinuria, and transient thrombocytopenia or coagulopathy that does not require transfusion of platelets or fresh frozen plasma.

Prostate

Although prostate cryoablation first began to be performed in the late 1960s (67), complication rates were unacceptably high, due to the inability to place cryoprobes precisely or to monitor the freezing process accurately. Technological advances in the past 15 years, which include transrectal ultrasound guidance and monitoring (68), as well as placement of a urethral warming device (69), markedly decreased complications. A recent development is the transition from liquid nitrogen to gas-driven probes that permit the use of cryoprobes with a much smaller diameter; this avoids the need for tract dilatation, and allows the direct placement of more probes into the tumor (70).

Mortality following prostate cryoablation is extremely rare, with most large studies reporting no deaths (71–73). A multicenter survey reported only three deaths out of 5432 patients (0.06%), two from pulmonary embolism, and one from a complicated rectourethral fistula (56). Major complication rates are discussed individually for the most common problems, and although many of these, such as impotence and incontinence, are not life threatening, they do have a significant impact on quality of life. Salvage cryoablation following failed radiotherapy has higher complication rates than primary cryoablation (74), as is discussed further below.

Major Complications

Impotence is the most common complication following prostate cryoablation, with reported rates of 53% to 93% in previously potent individuals (71–73,75). The neurovascular bundles in the prostate that carry the cavernosal nerves responsible for erectile function generally are ablated during the procedure to ensure complete destruction of the tissue at the periphery of the prostate gland. It is hypothesized that since the nerves are not cut, they have the potential to recover their function over time, and that patients may recover potency. One study reported that 19 of 373 patients (5.1%) regained erectile function over an average of 16.4 months (73), while another reported that at 3 years, 18 of 38 (47%) had resumed sexual intercourse, five (13%) spontaneously and 13 (34%) with the aid of sildenafil or prostaglandin (75). Nerve-sparing, unilateral cryoablation currently is being investigated, and in a pilot study, seven of nine patients (78%) retained potency following the procedure (76).

Urinary incontinence is another common complication, although the exact incidence varies both with the method of assessment and whether the patient is undergoing primary or salvage cryoablation. Reported incontinence rates for primary cryoablation have ranged from 7.5% to 15.9% using a broad definition that includes any degree of leakage (71–73). The incidence of severe incontinence that requires the daily use of urinary pads has been reported from 3% to 4.3% (71,73). Early studies that examined salvage cryoablation following failed radiotherapy found postprocedure incontinence rates as high as 73% (74), while in more recent studies only 7.9% to 20% required urinary pads (77,78).

Urethral sloughing occurs when the urethra is injured by the freezing process and allows necrotic prostate tissue to enter the urinary tract. The signs and symptoms of urethral sloughing include dysuria, pyuria, and obstruction. Catheterization sometimes is successful at dislodging the obstructing tissue, as well as facilitating urinary drainage; however, more severe cases may require transurethral resection of necrotic prostate tissue. The incidence of urethral sloughing that necessitates transurethral resection of the prostate ranges from 2.5% to 13% in patients who undergo primary cryoablation (72,73,79), with comparable results for salvage therapy (74,77). It is important to use an approved urethral warming device, as these devices offer better protection against urethral sloughing than those that have not been approved (72).

Rectourethral fistula formation is a severe complication that can occur if the freeze zone extends too far posteriorly. Although formerly a common problem prior to the implementation of transrectal ultrasound monitoring, the incidence of rectourethral fistula formation in recent large studies ranges from 0% to 0.5% for primary cryoablation (71–73). Rates are slightly higher in those undergoing salvage therapy, from 0% to 3.3% in the largest studies (71,74,77,78); however, incidence as high as 11% (2/18) has been reported (80).

Other reported major complications following prostate cryoablation include prostatic abscess, testicular abscess (75), perirectal abscess (80), sepsis, urethritis, epididymitis, urinary tract infection, bladder outlet obstruction, bladder neck contracture, ureteral obstruction, urethral stricture, stone formation in the prostatic urethra (81), prostatocutaneous fistula, rectovesical fistula (56), and vesicourethral fistula (78).

Minor Complications

The most common minor complications of prostate cryoablation include transient hematuria, rectal pain, pelvic pain, osteitis pubis (82), scrotal swelling, and penile tingling or numbness. The rectal and pelvic pain frequently can be managed with nonsteroidal antiinflammatory medications once abscess and urinoma have been ruled out. Osteitis pubis, or inflammation of the pubic symphysis, can be managed similarly. The scrotal swelling and penile paresthesia usually are transient and resolve spontaneously.

Renal

A small but increasing number of centers have begun performing renal cryoablation via an open (83–85), laparoscopic (85–88), or percutaneous (89) approach. Although the total number of patients treated is relatively small, it has proven to be a safe procedure with no reported deaths and relatively few major or minor complications.

Major Complications

An important major complication that has been reported is renal parenchymal or capsular fracture during the thawing cycle that may lead to hemorrhage (83,86). The technique to minimize the risk of renal fractures is similar to that in the liver: cryoprobes should be inserted gently with a minimum of torque, they should not be disturbed during the freezing process, and retraction of the probes should not be attempted until the iceball has thawed, to allow probe removal with a minimum of force or stress on the tissue.

Other major, intraprocedural complications that have occurred include a tear in the splenic capsule with the loss of approximately 1000 mL of blood (83), and cryoinjury to the pancreas, with subsequent pancreatitis from the inadvertent extension of the probe through and beyond a lesion in the left kidney (88). Major, postprocedural complications include chronic renal failure that necessitated hemodialysis (83), superficial wound abscess (89), congestive heart failure (83), dyspnea requiring 24-hour intubation, and paralytic ileus (87).

There has been concern that cryoablation of lesions near the collecting system may result in caliceal injury, leading to urinary extravasation and possible fistula formation. However, there have yet to be any reports of urine leakage or fistula formation, despite the probable freezing of the collecting system in some patients. Recent animal studies have demonstrated that the renal pelvis can be frozen with minimal risk of injury (90,91).

Minor Complications

Reported minor complications following renal cryoablation include small perirenal hematomas (89), elevations of amylase and lipase for 24 to 48 hours, asymptomatic electrocardiogram changes, transient atrial fibrillation (88), small pelvic vein thrombosis, and transient worsening of hemiparesis in a patient with a prior left cerebrovascular accident (85).

Laser-Induced Interstitial Thermotherapy (LITT)

Hepatic

Most of the available data concerning complications following hepatic LITT are from studies using a percutaneous approach for laser fiber placement. There is less experience with LITT than with RFA or cryoablation; however, in the few large studies that have been reported, mortality from LITT is low, ranging from 0.3% to 1.0% (92,93). Major complications have occurred at rates of 3.2% to 4.7%, when based on the number of patients treated (4,92); however, many patients underwent multiple treatment sessions that indicate that the risk per LITT procedure is actually lower. Also, LITT can be performed as an inpatient or outpatient procedure, and one study comparing complications in the two groups found that there was no significant difference in the rates of the two most common complications: pleural effusion and subcapsular hematoma (92).

Mortality

Reported deaths following hepatic LITT include two patients who developed acute liver failure following the procedure, one from a massive hepatic infarction (94) and another with Child-Pugh class C cirrhosis who died 2 months after treatment (93). Another death occurred 4 weeks after treatment from jejunal perforation with subsequent peritonitis and adult respiratory distress syndrome (92). It is unclear whether the perforation was due to thermal damage suffered during the procedure or from stress ulceration. Other cases of intestinal perforation have not been reported. One case of multisystem organ failure (95), and one death from presumed septic shock have been reported (92). One patient with a known history of cirrhosis and severe esophageal varices died 2 weeks after LITT from massive variceal bleeding of the esophagus (92).

Major Complications

The most common major complications following hepatic LITT are pleural effusions that require thoracentesis and hepatic abscess formation. Pleural effusions are a common occurrence postprocedurally, and although most are small, asymptomatic, and resolve spontaneously, a small number that persist or cause dyspnea require drainage. The risk of hepatic abscess is significantly increased in patients who have undergone prior hepatobiliary surgery, especially Whipple procedures for pancreatic adenocarcinoma (92).

Other major complications that have been reported include injury to the major bile ducts, segmental infarction from either coagulation of a major arterial vessel or from extensive laser-induced necrosis, intraperitoneal hemorrhage (92), systemic febrile reaction (96), paralytic ileus, and acute liver failure in patients with advanced cirrhosis (4). Intraprocedural bradycardia (heart rate <30) precluded the completion of one procedure (96). Only two cases of tumor seeding from the needle tract have been reported (94). In a study of 899 patients, there were no skin burns observed, which can be partly attributed to the use of light protection systems (LPS; Dornier Medizintechnik, Germering, Germany) with a fast automatic switch-off function to prevent the fiberoptic bundles from being burned (92).

Minor Complications

The most common minor complications of hepatic LITT are pain, fever, nausea, and asyptomatic pleural effusion. Other reported minor complications include abdominal wall bruising, intrahepatic hematoma, subcapsular hematoma, subcutaneous hematoma, mild intraperitoneal bleeding, transient biloma, local wound infection, and pneumothorax requiring only intraprocedural evacuation (92–96).

Microwave Coagulation Therapy (MCT)

Hepatic

Data on the complications of hepatic MCT are remarkably scarce. In one of the largest reported series involving 234 patients, there were no deaths or major complications (97). Overall, the rate of major complications ranges from 0% to 11% (97–101). In one study that compared percutaneous and intraoperative MCT, complications including hepatic abscess formation were much more common in the intraoperative group (99). This could be due partly to a larger mean lesion size in patients for whom an open or laparoscopic approach was chosen (4.5 cm) versus the percutaneous approach (3.4 cm).

A prospective, randomized trial that compared MCT and RFA for the treatment of HCC found that major complications occurred in 4 of 36 patients (11%) treated with MCT versus 1 of 36 (2.8%) for RFA (102). Although the mean lesion size was found to be similar between the two groups, the number of treatment sessions per nodule was significantly higher in the MCT group than in the RFA group (2.4 vs. 1.1). This led to a prolonged treatment course in those undergoing MCT.

Major Complications

The reported major complications following hepatic MCT include acute liver failure (100), ascites, intraperitoneal hemorrhage (101), subcapsular hematoma, liver abscess, subcutaneous abscess (102), cholangitis, persistent fever (100), and needle-tract seeding. Although the incidence of needle-tract seeding generally is low following MCT, one study found three cases out of 63 patients (4.8%)—one on the surface of the liver and two on the abdominal wall (99). Another case report described an instance of generalized intraperitoneal seeding following hepatic MCT, with numerous small nodules found in the omentum, visceral serosa, and in the pouch of Douglas (103).

Minor Complications

The most commonly reported minor complications following hepatic MCT are periprocedural pain and low-grade fever, which occur in a majority of patients. Other minor complications include pleural effusion, small subcapsular hematoma, subcutaneous hematoma, and minor skin burns. Clinically insignificant hepatic infarction, pneumothorax (101), portal vein thrombosis, and arterioportal shunt also have been described (99).

Conclusion

The popularity of tumor ablation has blossomed, due, in part, to its favorable safety profile compared to other treatment options. Although serious complications have occurred with ablation procedures, the risk of such events is acceptably low. Furthermore, the field of tumor ablation is still relatively new, and there is a learning curve associated with it, as with all procedures. Indeed, several long-term studies have indicated that many more complications occurred earlier in the respective authors' experience (17,92). It is expected that as proficiency in tumor ablation increases, potential complications can be anticipated and averted, furthering the safety of ablation and entrenching its role in therapeutic oncology.

References

1. Bret PM, Sente JM, Bretagnolle M, et al. Ultrasonically guided fine-needle biopsy in focal intrahepatic lesions: 6 years experience. Can Assoc Radiol J 1986;37:5–8.
2. Di Stasi M, Buscarini L, Livraghi T, et al. Percutaneous ethanol injection in the treatment of hepatocellular carcinoma. A multicenter survey of evaluation practices and complication rates. Scand J Gastroenterol 1997;32:1168–1173.

3. Livraghi T, Giorgio A, Marin G, et al. Hepatocellular carcinoma and cirrhosis in 746 patients: long-term results of percutaneous ethanol injection. Radiology 1995;197:101–108.
4. Giorgio A, Tarantino L, de Stefano G, et al. Complications after interventional sonography of focal liver lesions. A 22-year single-center experience. J Ultrasound Med 2003;22:193–205.
5. Livraghi T, Vettori C, Torzilli G, et al. Long-term results of single-session percutaneous ethanol injection in patients with large hepatocellular carcinoma. Cancer 1998;83:48–57.
6. Boucher E, Carsin A, Raoul JL, et al. Massive hepatic necrosis secondary to treatment of hepatocellular carcinoma by percutaneous alcoholization. Gastroenterol Clin Biol 199;22: 459–461.
7. de Baère T, Roche A, Amenabar JM, et al. Liver abscess formation after local treatment of liver tumors. Hepatology 1996;23:1436–1440.
8. Miki K, Makuuchi M, Takayama T, et al. Peritoneal seeding of hepatocellular carcinoma after ethanol injection therapy. Hepato-Gastroenterology 2000;47:1428–1430.
9. Ishii H, Okada S, Okusaka T, et al. Needle tract implantation of hepatocellular carcinoma after percutaneous ethanol injection. Cancer 1998; 82:1638–1642.
10. Casella G, Cacopardo E, Rovere G, et al. Cutaneous seeding after ultrasound-guided percutaneous ethanol injection for treatment of hepatocellular carcinoma. J Clin Ultrasound 2001;29:354–358.
11. Matsumata T, Okamoto M, Ishikawa H, et al. Necrosis of the hepatocellular carcinoma nodule can aggravate metastasis. Nippon Geka Gakkai Zasshi 1998;99:197–200.
12. Elgindy N, Lindolm H, Gunven P. High-dose percutaneous ethanol injection therapy of liver tumors. Patient acceptance and complications. Acta Radiologica 2000;41:458–463.
13. Seki S, Kitada T, Otogawa K, et al. Gastric ulcer as a rare complication of percutaneous ethanol injection for hepatocellular carcinoma. Am J Gasteroenterol 2002;97:770–771.
14. Isobe H, Sakamoto S, Nawata H. Splenic abscess as a complication of percutaneous ethanol injection therapy for hepatocellular carcinoma. J Clin Gastroenterol 1992;15:167–179.
15. Komorowski J, Kuzdak K, Pomorski L, et al. Percutaneous ethanol injection in treatment of benign nonfunctional and hyperfunctional thyroid nodules. Cytobios 1998;95:143–150.
16. Angelini F, Nacamulli D, De Vido D, et al. Treatment of hot thyroid nodule with percutaneous ethanol injection: indications, complications, and prognostic factors. Radiologia Medica 1996; 91:774–780.
17. Livraghi T, Solbiati L, Meloni MF, et al. Treatment of focal liver tumors with percutaneous radio-frequency ablation: complications encountered in a multicenter study. Radiology 2003; 226:441–451.
18. de Baère T, Risse O, Kuoch V, et al. Adverse events during radiofrequency treatment of 582 hepatic tumors. AJR. Am J Roentgenol 2003; 181:695–700.
19. Schmidt-Mutter C, Breining T, Gangi A, et al. Fatal bile pulmonary embolism after radiofrequency treatment of a hepatocellular carcinoma. Surg Endosc 2003;17:2028–2031.
20. de Sio I, Castellano L, De Girolarno V, et al. Tumor dissemination after radiofrequency ablation of hepatocellular carcinoma. Hepatology 2001;34:609–610.
21. Llovet JM, Vilana R, Bru C, et al. Increased risk of tumor seeding after percutaneous radiofrequency ablation for single hepatocellular carcinoma. Hepatology 2001;33:1124–1129.
22. Chapman W, Debelak J, Pinson CW, et al. Hepatic cryoablation, but not radiofrequency ablation, results in lung inflammation. Ann Surg 2000;231:752–761.
23. Seifert J, France M, Zhao J, et al. Large volume hepatic freezing: association with significant release of the cytokines interleukin-6 and tumor necrosis factor-alpha in a rat model. World J Surg 2002;26:1333–1341.
24. Yamamoto T, Kubo S, Hirohashi K, et al. Secondary hemocholecyst after radiofrequency ablation therapy for hepatocellular carcinoma. J Gastroenterol 2003;28:399–403.
25. Verhoeven B, Haagsma E, Appeltans B, et al. Hyperkalaemia after radiofrequency ablation of hepatocellular carcinoma. Eur J Gastroenterol Hepatol 2002;14:1023–1024.
26. Onik G, Onik C, Medary I, et al. Life-threatening hypertensive crises in two patients undergoing hepatic radiofrequency ablation. AJR Am J Roentegenol 2003;181:495–497.
27. Napier D, Dodd G, Hubbard L, et al. Post-ablation syndrome following radiofrequency thermal ablation of liver tumors. Presented at SGR 29th Annual Meeting. March 12, 2000. Kauai, Hawaii.
28. Goldberg SN, Solbiati L, Halpern EF, et al. Variables affecting proper system grounding for

radiofrequency ablation in an animal model. J Vasc Interv Radiol 2000;11:1069–1075.
29. King J, Glenn D, Clark W, et al. Percutaneous radiofrequency ablation of pulmonary metastases in patients with colorectal cancer. Br J Surg 2004;91:217–223.
30. vanSonnenberg E, Shanker S, Morrison PR, et al. Radiofrequency ablation of thoracic lesions: part II initial clinical experience—technical and multidisciplinary considerations in 30 patients. AJR 2005;184:381–390.
31. Dupuy D, Mayo-Smith W, DiPetrillo T, et al. Clinical experience of pulmonary radiofrequency ablation in 27 patients. Radiological Society of North America Proceedings, Chicago, November 2001;Abstract 389.
32. Nishida T, Inoue K, Kawata Y, et al. Percutaneous radiofrequency ablation of lung neoplasms: a minimally invasive strategy for inoperable patients. J Am Coll Surg 2002;195: 426–430.
33. Sewell P Jr, Jackson M, Vance R, et al. Assessing radiofrequency ablation of non-small cell lung cancer with positron emission tomography (PET). Radiology 2000;217 (Suppl):334.
34. Lee J, Jin K, Kim C, et al. Percutaneous radiofrequency ablation for inoperable lung malignancies: a preliminary report. Radiological Society of North America Proceedings, Chicago, November 2001;Abstract 390.
35. Vaughn C, Mychaskiw G II, Sewell P. Massive hemorrhage during radiofrequency ablation of a pulmonary neoplasm. Anesth Analg 2002;94: 1149–1151.
36. Gervais D, McGovern F, Wood B, et al. Radiofrequency ablation of renal cell carcinoma: early clinical experience. Radiology 2000;217: 665–672.
37. Pavlovich C, McClellan W, Choyke P, et al. Percutaneous radio frequency ablation of small renal tumors: initial results. J Urol 2002;167: 10–15.
38. de Baere T, Kuoch V, Smayra T, et al. Radio frequency ablation of renal cell carcinoma: preliminary clinical experience. J Urol 2002;167: 1961–1964.
39. Su L, Jarrett T, Chan D, et al. Percutaneous computed tomography-guided radiofrequency ablation of renal masses in high surgical risk patients: preliminary results. Urology 2003; 61(Suppl 4A):26–33.
40. Mayo-Smith W, Dupuy D, Parikh P, et al. Imaging-guided percutaneous radiofrequency ablation of solid renal masses: techniques and outcomes of 38 treatment sessions in 32 consecutive patients. AJR Am J Roentgenol 2003; 180:1503–1508.
41. Johnson D, Saboorian M, Duchene D, et al. Nephrectomy after radiofrequency ablation-induced ureteropelvic junction obstruction: potential complication and long-term assessment of ablation adequacy. Urology 2003;62: 351–352.
42. Goetz M, Callstrom M, Charboneau J, et al. Percutaneous image-guided radiofrequency ablation of painful metastases involving bone: a multicenter study. J Clin Oncol 2004;22: 300–306.
43. Ibrahim D, Ho E, Scherl SA, et al. Newborn with an open posterior hip dislocation and sciatic nerve injury after intrauterine radiofrequency ablation of a sacrococcygeal teratoma. J Pediatr Surg 2003;38:248–250.
44. Wood B, Abraham J, Hvizda J, et al. Radiofrequency ablation of adrenal tumors and adrenocortical carcinoma metastases. Cancer 2003;97: 554–560.
45. Mayo-Smith W, Dupuy D. Adrenal neoplasms: CT-guided radiofrequency ablation—preliminary results. Radiology 2004;231:225–230.
46. Izzo F, Thomas R, Delrio P, et al. Radiofrequency ablation in patients with primary breast carcinoma: a pilot study in 26 patients. Cancer 2001;92:2036–2044.
47. Burak W, Agnese D, Povoski S, et al. Radiofrequency ablation of invasive breast carcinoma followed by delayed surgical excision. Cancer 2003;98:1369–1375.
48. Hayashi A, Silver S, van der Westhuizen N, et al. Treatment of invasive breast carcinoma with ultrasound-guided radiofrequency ablation. Am J Surg 2003;185:429–435.
49. Fornage B, Sneige N, Ross M, et al. Small (≤2-cm) breast cancer treated with US-guided radiofrequency ablation: feasibility study. Radiology 2004;231:215–224.
50. Adam R, Hagopian E, Linhares M, et al. A comparison of percutaneous cryosurgery and percutaneous radiofrequency for unresectable hepatic malignancies. Arch Surg 2002;137: 1332–1339.
51. Tait LS, Yong SM, Cuschieri A. Laparoscopic in situ ablation of liver cancer with cryotherapy and radiofrequency ablation. Br J Surg 2002; 89:1613–1619.
52. Lezoche E, Paganini A, Feliciotti F, et al. Ultrasound-guided laparoscopic cryoablation

of hepatic tumors: preliminary report. World J Surg 1998;22:829–836.
53. Sarantou T, Bilchik A, Ramming K. Complications of hepatic cryosurgery. Semin Surg Oncol 1998;14:156–162.
54. Sohn R, Carlin A, Steffes C, et al. The extent of cryosurgery increases the complication rate after hepatic cryoablation. Am Surg 2003;69: 317–322.
55. Crews K, Kuhn J, McCarty T, et al. Cryosurgical ablation of hepatic tumors. Am J Surg 1997;174:614–617.
56. Seifert J, Morris D. World survey on the complications of hepatic and prostate cryotherapy. World J Surg 1999;23:109–114.
57. Cha C, Lee F, Rikkers L, et al. Rationale for the combination of cryoablation with surgical resection of hepatic tumors. J Gastrointest Surg 2001;5:206–213.
58. Onik G, Atkinson D, Zemel R, et al. Cryosurgery of liver cancer. Semin Surg Oncol 1993;9:309–317.
59. Pearson AS, Izzo F, Fleming RY, et al. Intraoperative radiofrequency ablation or cryoablation for hepatic malignancies. Am J Surg 1999; 178:592–599.
60. Morris D, Ross W, Iqbal J, et al. Cryoablation of hepatic malignancy: an evaluation of tumor marker data and survival in 110 patients. Gastrointest Cancer 1996;1:247–251.
61. Seifert J, Stewart G, Hewitt P, et al. Interleukin-6 and tumor necrosis factor-alpha levels following hepatic cryotherapy: association with volume and duration of freezing. World J Surg 1999;23:1019–1026.
62. Yeh K, Fortunato L, Hoffman J, et al. Cryosurgical ablation of hepatic metastases from colorectal carcinomas. Am Surg 1997;63:63–68.
63. Weaver ML, Ashton J, Zemel R. Treatment of colorectal liver metastases by cryotherapy. Semin Surg Oncol 1998;14:163–170.
64. Silverstein JC, Staren E, Velasco J. Thermal bile duct protection during liver cryoablation. J Surg Oncol 1997;64:163–164.
65. Weaver ML, Atkinson D, Zemel R. Hepatic cryosurgery in treating colorectal metastases. Cancer 1995;76:210–214.
66. Cozzi P, Stewart G, Morris D. Thrombocytopenia after hepatic cryotherapy for colorectal metastases: correlates with hepatocellular injury. World J Surg 1994;18:774–777.
67. Gonder M, Soanes W, Shulman S. Cryosurgical treatment of the prostate. Invest Urol 1966;3: 372–378.
68. Onik G, Cobb C, Cohen J, et al. US characteristics of frozen prostate. Radiology 1988;168: 629–631.
69. Cohen J, Miller R. Thermal protection of urethra during cryosurgery of prostate. Cryobiology 1994;31:313–316.
70. Zisman A, Pantuck A, Cohen J. Prostate cryoablation using direct transperineal placement of ultrathin probes through a 17-gauge brachytherapy template: technique and preliminary results. Urology 2001;58:988–993.
71. Han K, Cohen J, Miller R, et al. Treatment of organ-confined prostate cancer with 3rd generation cryosurgery: preliminary multi-center experience. J Urol 2003;170:1126–1130.
72. Long J, Bahn D, Lee F, et al. Five-year retrospective, multi-institutional pooled analysis of cancer-related outcomes after cryosurgical ablation of the prostate. Urology 2001;57:518–523.
73. Bahn D, Lee F, Badalament R, et al. Targeted cryoablation of the prostate: 7-year outcomes in the primary treatment of prostate cancer. Urology 2002;60(2 Suppl 1):3–11.
74. Pisters L, von Eschenbach A, Scott S, et al. The efficacy and complications of salvage cryotherapy of the prostate. J Urol 1997;157:921–925.
75. Donnelly B, Saliken J, Ernst D, et al. Prospective trial of cryosurgical ablation of the prostate: five-year results. Urology 2002;60: 645–649.
76. Onik G, Narayan P, Vaughan D, et al. Focal "nerve-sparing" cryosurgery for treatment of primary prostate cancer: a new approach to preserving potency. Urology 2002;60:109–114.
77. Ghafar M, Johnson C, De La Taille A, et al. Salvage cryotherapy using an argon based system for locally recurrent prostate cancer after radiation therapy: the Columbia experience. J Urol 2001;166:1333–1338.
78. Chin J, Pautler S, Mouraviev V, et al. Results of salvage cryoablation of the prostate after radiation: identifying predictors of treatment failure and complications. J Urol 2001;165: 1937–1942.
79. Wieder J, Schmidt JD, Casola G, et al. Transrectal ultrasound-guided transperineal cryoablation in the treatment of prostate carcinoma: preliminary results. J Urol 1995;154:435–441.
80. Long J, Fallick M, LaRock D, et al. Preliminary outcomes following cryosurgical ablation of the prostate in patients with clinically localized prostate carcinoma. J Urol 1998;159:477–484.

81. Aus G, Bergdahl S, Hugosson J, et al. Stone formation in the prostatic urethra after cryotherapy for prostate cancer. Urology 1997; 50:615–617.
82. Seigne J, Pisters L, von Eschenbach AC. Osteitis pubis as a complication of prostate cryotherapy. J Urol 1996;156:182.
83. Rukstalis D, Khorsandi M, Garcia F, et al. Clinical experience with open renal cryoablation. Urology 2001;57:34–39.
84. Delworth M, Pisters L, Fornage B, et al. Cryotherapy for renal cell carcinoma and angiomyolipoma. J Urol 1996;155:252–255.
85. Rodriguez R, Chan D, Bishoff J, et al. Renal ablative cryosurgery in selected patients with peripheral renal masses. Urology 2000;55:25–30.
86. Gill I, Novick A, Meraney A, et al. Laparoscopic renal cryoablation in 32 patients. Urology 2000;56:748–753.
87. Nadler R, Kim S, Rubenstein J, et al. Laparoscopic renal cryosurgery: the Northwestern experience. J Urol 2003;170:1121–1125.
88. Lee D, McGinnis D, Feld R, et al. Retroperitoneal laparoscopic cryoablation of small renal tumors: intermediate results. Urology 2003;61: 83–88.
89. Shingleton W, Sewell P. Percutaneous renal tumor cryoablation with magnetic resonance image guidance. J Urol 2001;165:773–776.
90. Chosy S, Nakada S, Lee F, et al. Monitoring renal cryosurgery: predictors of tissue necrosis in swine. J Urol 1998;159:1370–1374.
91. Sung G, Gill I, Hsu T, et al. Effect of intentional cryoinjury to the renal collecting system. J Endourol 1999;13(S1):A14.
92. Vogl T, Straub R, Eichler K, et al. Malignant liver tumor treated with MR imaging-guided laser-induced thermotherapy: experience with complications in 899 patients (2520 lesions). Radiology 2002;225:367–377.
93. Giorgio A, Tarantino L, de Stefano G, et al. Interstitial laser photocoagulation under ultrasound guidance of liver tumors: results in 104 treated patients. Eur J Ultrasound 2000;11:181–188.
94. Gilliams A, Lees W. Survival after percutaneous, image-guided, thermal ablation of hepatic metastases from colorectal cancer. Dis Colon Rectum 2000;43:656–661.
95. Tranberg K, Moller P, Hannesson P, et al. Interstitial laser treatment of malignant tumors: initial experience. Eur J Surg Oncol 1996;22: 47–54.
96. Christophi C, Muralidharan V. Chronic liver diseases: epidemiology, pathophysiology, diagnosis and treatment. J Gastroenterol Hepatol 2001;16:548–552.
97. Dong B, Liang P, Yu X, et al. Percutaneous sonographically guided microwave coagulation therapy for hepatocellular carcinoma: results in 234 patients. AJR Am J Roentgenol 2003;180: 1547–1555.
98. Liang P, Dong B, Yu X, et al. Prognostic factors for percutaneous microwave coagulation therapy of hepatic metastases. AJR Am J Roentgenol 2003;181:1319–1325.
99. Mitsuzaki K, Yamashita Y, Nishiharu T, et al. CT appearance of hepatic tumors after microwave coagulation therapy. AJR Am J Roentgenol 1998;171:1397–1403.
100. Yamanaka N, Tanaka T, Oriyama T, et al. Microwave coagulonecrotic therapy for hepatocellular carcinoma. World J Surg 1996;20: 1076–1081.
101. Abe T, Shinzawa H, Wakabayashi H, et al. Value of laparoscopic microwave coagulation therapy for hepatocellular carcinoma in relation to tumor size and location. Endoscopy 2000;32: 598–603.
102. Shibata T, Iimuro Y, Yamamoto Y, et al. Small hepatocellular carcinoma: comparison of radiofrequency ablation and percutaneous microwave coagulation therapy. Radiology 2002;223: 331–337.
103. Sato M, Tokui K, Watanabe Y, et al. Generalized intraperitoneal seeding of hepatocellular carcinoma after microwave coagulation therapy: a case report. Hepato-Gastroenterol 1999;46: 2561–2564.

Section VI
Perspectives

37 Tumor Ablation for Patients with Lung Cancer: The Thoracic Oncologist's Perspective

Bruce E. Johnson and Pasi A. Jänne

Lung cancer is the second most frequent cause of cancer in both men and women in the United States (1). There were an estimated 91,800 lung cancer cases in men and 80,100 cases in women in the United States in 2003. The most effective treatment for patients with localized lung cancer is surgical resection. Radiation therapy and chemotherapy also are established effective treatments in patients with more advanced lung cancer. The role of tumor ablation in the management of patients with lung cancer is evolving. To understand the current and future potential role in the management of patients with lung cancer, it is important to have information about the available therapies for the different stages of lung cancer.

Conventional Treatment for Patients with Lung Cancer

Treatment of lung cancer is effective if the lung cancer is detected when it has not spread locally to the structures in the chest wall, mediastinum, bones, or the lymph nodes in the mediastinum (stages I and II). Patients should be treated with surgical resection by removing the affected lobe or lung if they can physiologically tolerate the removal of one to three of the five lobes of their lungs. Seventy percent to 80% of these patients with the earliest stages of lung cancer are alive and free of lung cancer at 5 years if the lung cancer is less than 3 cm and there is no lymph node or metastatic cancer involvement (2,3). Some patients have inadequate respiratory reserve to tolerate surgical resection of their lung cancer. There is an extensive experience in treating these patients with radiotherapy to the primary lesion in the lung; approximately 20% of these patients are alive 5 years after the start of the radiotherapy (4,5). However, only approximately 26% of patients presenting with lung cancer have their cancer localized to single lobe and without any evidence of spread to the lymph nodes in the mediastinum or bloodstream. Most patients are unable to be treated with these effective local therapies alone (6).

Patients with lung cancer most commonly present when the cancer has spread locally in the chest, into the lymph nodes in the mediastinum (stage III), and systemically through the lymphatic system or bloodstream (stage IV). Patients with cancer spread to the structures in the chest or lymph nodes in the mediastinum are most commonly treated with multiple therapeutic modalities. These represent approximately 33% of patients who develop lung cancer. Fit patients with stage III lung cancer are treated with combination chemotherapy and chest irradiation (7–9). The therapy is much less effective than surgical treatment of patients with stage I and II non–small-cell lung cancer because patients with stage III lung cancer have an expected 5-year survival of 5% to 15%. The therapies currently available to patients with lung cancer that has spread through the bloodstream are relatively ineffective. Approximately 41% of patients present with lung cancer that has spread through the lymphatic system or bloodstream. The use of combination chemotherapy for patients with stage IV lung cancer evokes response rates in 20%, the median survival is 7 to 9 months (1 to 2 months longer than in patients who are not treated with combination chemotherapy), and only 2% of patients are alive 5 years after the start of their chemotherapy (10–13).

Development of Radiofrequency Ablation for Patients with Lung Cancer

There is more than 10 years of experience using radiofrequency to ablate metastatic and primary cancers in the liver; extensive follow-up of these patients after this treatment has documented its efficacy (14–18). Research in this area has led to the development of probes that can ablate tumors greater than 1 cm, which is important for the treatment of lung cancers (18).

The success of this percutaneous approach has prompted developing techniques to use radiofrequency ablation (RFA) in the lung for both primary lung lesions and metastases. There are currently several potential uses for tumor ablation in patients with lung cancer including those with lung cancer whose lung function is not adequate to tolerate a surgical resection or localized radiation therapy. The other common indications are inpatients who have a local problem either in the initial cancer or in a metastatic site that cannot be irradiated or undergo surgical resection. This can be due either to the location of the tumor, or to the growth of the tumor after primary radiation therapy. The local problems can include development of a metachronous lung cancer, lobar obstruction, pain caused by localized tumor masses, obstruction caused by a tumor mass, or isolated metastatic disease.

Animal Model of Lung Cancer Treated with Radiofrequency Ablation

An animal model has been developed to test the safety and efficacy of RFA in rabbits. The VX2 carcinoma cell line is injected into the lungs of New Zealand rabbits. The growth of the lung tumor(s) can be monitored by computed tomography or magnetic resonance imaging. The lung tumors reach a size of 1 cm in a few weeks (19–21). The cancers then grow within the lungs and spread systemically. The rabbits go on to die from their cancer within 3 months in the absence of any treatment. The course of these cancers growing within the lung can be altered by treatment with RFA. Twenty-five rabbits have been treated with a radiofrequency generator capable of producing 150 W of power (Radionics, Burlington, MA). The probe of the generator was passed percutaneously through the chest wall and into the lesion. The size of the lesions and position of the probe were verified by imaging. The tumor was ablated by applying power to the radiofrequency generator for several minutes as determined by size of the lesions and previous experimental results. The treatment caused complications in the rabbits: two rabbits developed significant pneumothoraces requiring surgery or euthanasia, and a third rabbit developed a pyothorax after being treated with RFA.

Twenty-three of the rabbits were sacrificed a few hours to 2 months after treatment with RFA. Histologic examination of the tumors in the lungs showed necrosis in the lesions within a few hours and eventual eradication of the tumor in most rabbits after the treatment. One of the experiments followed the animals for several months after their treatment (19). Rabbits were sacrificed and their tumors examined histologically. More than half of the rabbits had their tumors eradicated. Four rabbits treated with RFA were not sacrificed and lived longer than 3 months, the time when all rabbits inoculated with VX2 and not treated with RFA had died from their cancer. The information generated from this animal model and information from treating patients with primary liver cancer and liver metastases supported going forward into treatments of lung tumors in humans with RFA.

Tumor Ablation of Primary and Metachronous Lung Cancers

The standard treatment of lung cancer localized to the lung without evidence of spread to the lymph nodes or through the bloodstream is surgical resection. However, not all patients can tolerate a pulmonary resection. Approximately 90% of patients with lung cancer are current or former cigarette smokers with some degree of pulmonary impairment. In addition, patients developing lung cancer in the United States usually are elderly with a median age of 69 years and comorbid diseases that preclude surgical resection. Patients with severe pulmonary impairment or comorbid diseases should undergo a careful evaluation by an experienced general thoracic surgeon to determine if they should have an attempt at surgical resection.

The other group of patients who are potential candidates are those who had undergone a successful surgical resection of their non–small-cell lung cancer. These patients may have one to three lobes removed to resect their non–small-cell lung cancer adequately. Patients treated successfully for non–small-cell lung cancer have a 2% risk per year of developing a second lung cancer in their remaining lung (22). These patients have diminished pulmonary reserve and may not be able to undergo further resections. Patients who are unable to undergo an initial or repeat surgical resection should be referred to radiation oncologists. There is substantial literature about patients who were unable or unwilling to undergo a surgical resection and who then are treated with radiation therapy to the primary lesions. Doses of approximately 6000 cGy are administered to the primary tumor mass. Approximately 20% of patients with stage I and II non–small-cell lung cancer treated with chest radiotherapy alone will be alive 5 or more years after this treatment (4,5).

For those patients who are unable or unwilling to undergo surgery and/or radiation therapy, local treatment including RFA may be considered. Intraparenchymal cancers in the lung may well be suited to RFA because the air in the surrounding pulmonary parenchyma provides insulation around the cancer (23). Therefore, the energy generated from the radiofrequency probe may be concentrated in the lesions, while having relatively little effect in the surrounding tissues. However, some tumor masses near major blood vessels or the heart are not appropriate candidates for tumor ablation because of potential damage to the vascular structures that might lead to bleeding complications. Figure 37.1 shows a lesion invading blood vessels and Figure 37.2 shows a lesion near the heart and aorta.

There are examples in the literature of patients whose primary lung cancers, synchronous lung cancers, or metachronous lung cancers have been treated with RFA and have not

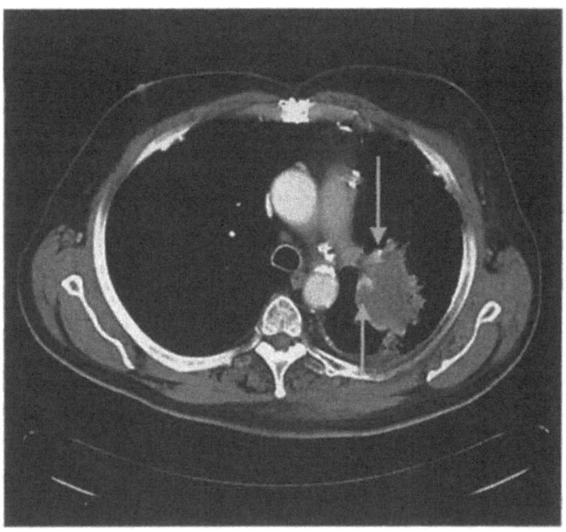

FIGURE 37.1. Non–small-cell lung carcinoma with vascular invasion. The patient presented with a tumor in the left lung that could not be resected due to poor pulmonary reserve. The patient was treated with primary radiation therapy and 12 months later the tumor began to enlarge. Tumor ablation was considered, but not attempted due to vascular invasion (arrows) of the tumor mass near large branches of the pulmonary artery.

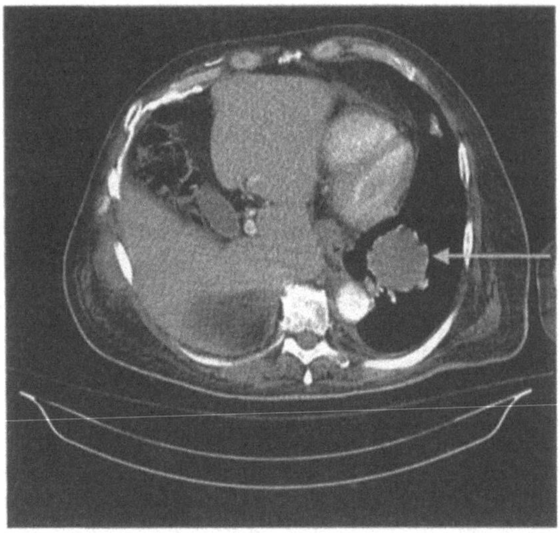

FIGURE 37.2. Metastatic mesothelioma adjacent to the heart. The patient was treated with a right-sided extrapleural pneumonectomy, but developed contralateral pulmonary metastases. Tumor ablation of the mass adjacent to the heart (arrow) was considered, but deferred because of the proximity to the heart.

recurred after follow-up of 1 to 3 years (Table 37.1). The information thus far is anecdotal, with approximately 10 patients reported in the peer-reviewed published literature. Thus, it is yet another local therapy that can be employed if surgical resection and/or radiation therapy are deemed to be inappropriate and the cancer can be controlled for an extended period of time. Further research will be needed to define the role of tumor ablation in these patient populations.

There are potential complications associated with the RFA. Dupuy et al (23) reported pneumothoraces in 20% of patients treated with RFA with most requiring chest tube placement. This is an important potential complication, because patients who undergo RFA because of poor pulmonary reserve and then develop significant pneumonthorax may develop life-threatening pulmonary insufficiency. Therefore, the procedure should be performed in a setting in which patients can be treated with respiratory support and emergent chest tube placement. Other side effects include pleurisy, development of a pleural effusion, and a pro-

TABLE 37.1. Literature review on patients with lung cancer treated with radiofrequency ablation.

Patient (reference)	Age	Stage	Previous treatment	Reason for ablation	Outcome
1. Male (23)	78	III	None	Shrink mass before chest RT	Alive at 27 months
2. Male (23)	75	Metachronous stage I	Pneumonectomy	Eradicate nodule plus brachytherapy	Alive 11 months
3. Female (23)	69	I	None	Eradicate nodule	Alive at 24 months
4. Male (23)		I	None	Eradicate nodule	Alive 1 week later
5. Male (24)	70	IV	Surgery and chemotherapy	Eradicate nodule	Died from complications of bleeding within 1 month
6. Male (28)	59	2 stage I NSCLC (metachronous in RUL and RLL)	None	Eradicate nodules	Alive at 10 months
7. Male (29)	45	IV	Chemotherapy and chest RT	Eradicate nodule	Alive at 3 months
8. Female (29)	66	IB	None	Shrink nodule before external RT	Died at nursing home 2 months after procedure
9. Male (30)	56	Metachronous lung cancers	Surgery	Eradicate nodule	Alive at 2 years
10. Male (30)	72	Metachronous lung cancer	Surgery	Eradicate nodule	Alive at 1 year

Abbreviations: RT, chest radiotherapy; RLL, right lower lobe; RUL, right upper lobe; NSCLC, nonsmall cell lung cancer.

ductive cough. Patients also can develop bleeding following treatment with tumor ablation. A patient was treated with RFA of a lesion in the right lung (patient number 5, Table 37.1). Two hours after the procedure he developed pulmonary hemorrhage and eventually died from complications within the next month (24). The patient was being treated with an antiplatelet agent (clopidogrel) that may have contributed to this bleeding complication. The authors recommend that patients be questioned closely about the use of antiplatelet agents before attempting an ablative procedure.

Tumor Ablation of Locally Recurrent or Metastatic Lung Cancer

Patients with non–small-cell lung cancer treated with radiation can redevelop symptomatic cancer progression in the same area. Patients with stage III non–small-cell lung cancer will relapse within the radiation portal approximately 20% of the time (25). This can rarely be treated with surgical resection or a second course of radiation therapy. These patients are potential candidates for percutaneous or endobronchial RFA if there is adequate distance from the vital structures of the pulmonary artery, aorta, and heart to the lesion.

A common local problem caused by lung cancer is bronchial obstruction. This can occur in approximately 20% of patients with lung cancer at the time of presentation (26) and a greater percentage in patients followed during their disease course. The bronchial obstruction can be treated with external irradiation, endobronchial irradiation, stenting, photodynamic therapy, cryotherapy, laser therapy, or RFA. Radiofrequency ablation has been used commonly to treat patients with bronchial obstruction. There has been a series of 94 patients with lung cancer treated with RFA including 50 with a previous course of chest irradiation or chemotherapy (27). Forty-six of the 50 patients were able to have more than 50% of the luminal obstruction cleared following treatment with RFA. Thus, this is one of many methods to relieve bronchial obstruction. Further research will be needed to determine which of the many modalities of treatment is appropriate for different clinical situations.

Tumor ablation also has been used for patients developing a local problem related to tumor masses. This can be due to contiguous spread to the bone from an underlying lung cancer that can give rise to severe bone pain. One early report documents a patient with lung cancer that spread to the sternum, and the patient underwent external irradiation; the lung cancer had grown in the previously irradiated area and caused bone pain (23). He was treated with RFA with subsequent relief of the pain.

Our multidisciplinary group also has utilized RFA in patients with metastatic lung cancer. One example is a patient who has been treated for osseous pain from a lesion in the pulmonary parenchyma that eroded into both ribs and vertebra (Fig. 37.3). Another patient developed a localized relapse in the left adrenal gland and liver 6 years after treatment of the primary lung cancer (Fig. 37.4). The patient was treated with RFA of the adrenal and liver lesion. These are

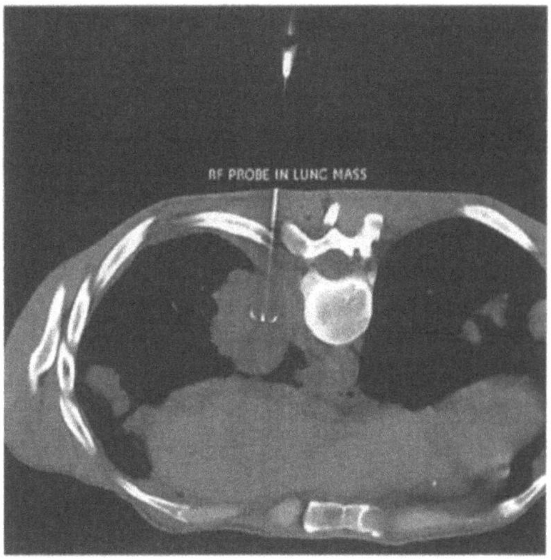

FIGURE 37.3. Patient developed a mass in the periphery of the lower lobe that caused back pain. The probe is shown in place in the middle of the mass. The patient had partial relief of the pain following the procedure.

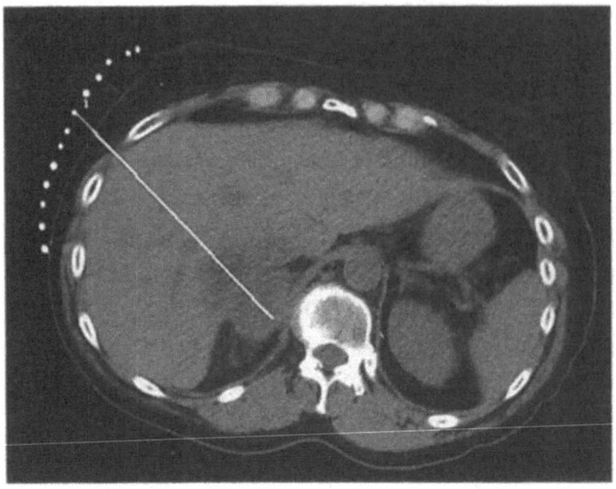

FIGURE 37.4. Patient presented with enlarging right adrenal and liver lesions 6 years after resection of her T3N0M0 non–small-cell lung cancer. The lesions continued to grow during multiple courses of chemotherapy. Metastatic evaluation showed no other evidence of cancer, so she underwent radiofrequency ablation. This view shows planning of the probe into the adrenal and liver lesion. The treatment has controlled the lesion 3 months after the radiofrequency ablation.

anecdotal examples of effective RFA treatment of painful bony lesions and ablative treatment of isolated recurrences.

Thus, tumor ablation using radiofrequency has been applied by percutaneous application as well as by endobronchial administration. Both have been shown to be effective therapies for some localized pulmonary lesions, as well as endobronchial tumors. Radiofrequency ablation also can play a role in metastatic or recurrent lesions in areas not amenable to surgery or radiation therapy (32,33). This can include relief of painful bony lesions or isolated metastases to the liver. The role of this local modality in patients who are unable to undergo surgery and/or irradiation likely will expand. Further clinical research will be needed to define the role of RFA in patients with airway obstruction in relationship to cryotherapy, laser treatment, and photodynamic therapy. Further clinical research also will be needed to define its role for management of metastatic lesions.

References

1. Jemal A, Murray T, Samuels A, Ghafoor A, Ward E, Thun MJ. Cancer statistics, 2003. CA Cancer J Clin 2003;53:5–26.
2. Mountain CF. Revisions in the international system for staging lung cancer. Chest 1997;111: 1710–1717.
3. Naruke T, Tsuchiya R, Kondo H, Asamura H. Prognosis and survival after resection for bronchogenic carcinoma based on the 1997 TNM-staging classification: the Japanese experience. Ann Thorac Surg 2001;71:1759–1764.
4. Gauden S, Ramsay J, Tripcony L. The curative treatment by radiotherapy alone of stage I non-small cell carcinoma of the lung. Chest 1995;108: 1278–1282.
5. Langendijk JA, Aaronson NK, de Jong JM, et al. Quality of life after curative radiotherapy in stage I non–small-cell lung cancer. Int J Radiat Oncol Biol Phys 2002;53:847–853.
6. Fry WA, Phillips JL, Menck HR. Ten-year survey of lung cancer treatment and survival in hospitals in the United States: a national cancer data base report. Cancer 1999;86:1867–1876.
7. Dillman RO, Herndon J, Seagren SL, Eaton WL, Green MR. Improved survival in stage III non–small-cell lung cancer: seven-year follow-up of Cancer and Leukemia Group B (CALGB) 8433 Trial. J Nat Cancer Inst 1996;88:1210–1215.
8. Furuse K, Fukuoka M, Kawahara M, et al. Phase III study of concurrent versus sequential thoracic radiotherapy in combination with mitomycin, vindesine, and cisplatin in unresectable stage III non–small-cell lung cancer. J Clin Oncol 1999;17:2692–2699.
9. Sause WT, Scott C, Taylor S, et al. Radiation Therapy Oncology Group (RTOG) 88-08 and Eastern Cooperative Group (ECOG) 4588: preliminary results of a phase III trial in regionally advanced, unresectable non-small cell lung cancer. J Natl Cancer Inst 1995;87:198–205.
10. Group N-SCLCC. Chemotherapy in non–small cell lung cancer: a meta-analysis using updated data on individual patients from 52 randomized clinical trials. Br Med J 1995;311:899–909.
11. Kelly K, Crowley J, Bunn PA Jr, et al. Randomized phase III trial of paclitaxel plus carboplatin versus vinorelbine plus cisplatin in the treatment of patients with advanced non–small-cell lung cancer: a Southwest Oncology Group trial. J Clin Oncol 2001;19:3210–3218.
12. Schiller JH, Harrington D, Belani CP, et al. Comparison of four chemotherapy regimens for

advanced non–small-cell lung cancer. N Engl J Med 2002;346:92–98.
13. Breathnach OS, Freidlin B, Conley B, et al. Twenty-two years of phase III trials for patients with advanced non-small-cell lung cancer: sobering results. J Clin Oncol 2001;19:1734–1742.
14. Livraghi T, Solbiati L, Meloni MF, Gazelle GS, Halpern EF, Goldberg SN. Treatment of focal liver tumors with percutaneous radio-frequency ablation: complications encountered in a multicenter study. Radiology 2003;226:441–451.
15. Solbiati L, Livraghi T, Goldberg SN, et al. Percutaneous radio-frequency ablation of hepatic metastases from colorectal cancer: long-term results in 117 patients. Radiology 2001;221:159–166.
16. Curley SA, Izzo F, Delrio P, et al. Radiofrequency ablation of unresectable primary and metastatic hepatic malignancies: results in 123 patients. Ann Surg 1999;230:1–8.
17. Curley SA, Izzo F, Ellis LM, Nicolas Vauthey J, Vallone P. Radiofrequency ablation of hepatocellular cancer in 110 patients with cirrhosis. Ann Surg 2000;232:381–391.
18. Gazelle GS, Goldberg SN, Solbiati L, Livraghi T. Tumor ablation with radio-frequency energy. Radiology 2000;217:633–646.
19. Miao Y, Ni Y, Bosmans H, et al. Radiofrequency ablation for eradication of pulmonary tumor in rabbits. J Surg Res 2001;99:265–271.
20. Goldberg SN. Gazelle GS, Compton CC, Mueller PR, McLoud TC. Radio-frequency tissue ablation of VX2 tumor nodules in the rabbit lung. Acad Radiol 1996;3:929–935.
21. Goldberg SN, Gazelle GS, Compton CC, McLoud TC. Radiofrequency tissue ablation in the rabbit lung: efficacy and complications. Acad Radiol 1995;2:776–784.
22. Johnson BE. Second lung cancers in patients after treatment for an initial lung cancer. J Natl Cancer Inst 1998;90:1335–1345.
23. Dupuy DE, Mayo-Smith WW, Abbott GF, DiPetrillo T. Clinical applications of radiofrequency tumor ablation in the thorax. Radiographics 2002;22(Spec No.):S259–S269.
24. Vaughn C, Mychaskiw G 2nd, Sewell P. Massive hemorrhage during radiofrequency ablation of a pulmonary neoplasm. Anesth Analg 2002;94:1149–1151.
25. Andre F, Grunenwald D, Pujol JL, et al. Patterns of relapse of N2 nonsmall-cell lung carcinoma patients treated with preoperative chemotherapy: should prophylactic cranial irradiation be reconsidered? Cancer 2001;91:2394–2400.
26. Vaaler AK, Forrester JM, Lesar M, Edison M, Venzon D, Johnson BE. Obstructive atelectasis in patients with small cell lung cancer. Incidence and response to treatment. Chest 1997;111:115–120.
27. Marasso A, Bernardi V, Gai R, et al. Radiofrequency resection of bronchial tumours in combination with cryotherapy: evaluation of a new technique. Thorax 1998;53:106–109.
28. Rose SC, Fotoohi M, Levin DL, Harrell JH. Cerebral microembolization during radiofrequency ablation of lung malignancies. J Vasc Intervent Radiol 2002;13:1051–1054.
29. Dupuy DE, Zagoria RJ, Akerley W, Mayo-Smith WW, Kavanagh PV, Safran H. Percutaneous radiofrequency ablation of malignancies in the lung. AJR 2000;174:57–59.
30. Nishida T, Inoue K, Kawata Y, et al. Percutaneous radiofrequency ablation of lung neoplasms: a minimally invasive strategy for inoperable patients. J Am Coll Surg 2002;195:426–430.
31. Shankar S, vanSonnenberg E, Silverman SG, Tuncali K, Morrison PR. Management of pneumothorax during percutaneous radiofrequency ablation of a lung tumor: technical note. J Thorac Imaging 2003;18:106–109.
32. Morrison PR, vanSonnenberg E, Shankar S, et al. Radiofrequency ablation in the thorax; part 1—Experiments in the porcine model. AJR 2005;184:375–380.
33. vanSonnenberg E, Shankar S, Morrison PR, et al. Radiofrequency ablation in the chest; part 2—Initial clinical experience with emphasis on adjunctive procedures and multidisciplinary input. AJR 2005;184:381–390.

38
Ablative Therapies for Gastrointestinal Malignancies: The Gastrointestinal Oncologist's Viewpoint

Matthew Kulke

Surgical resection, radiation therapy, and systemic chemotherapy are the primary treatment modalities for patients with gastrointestinal malignancies. Ablative therapies such as radiofrequency ablation (RFA) and cryoablation hold potential as alternative treatment options that, in the appropriate setting, may be both efficacious and well tolerated. However, while ablative therapies are used commonly in the treatment of gastrointestinal malignancies, their precise role in such patients is poorly defined. Initial studies of ablative therapies have focused on malignancies such as colorectal cancer, hepatocellular carcinoma, and neuroendocrine tumors, in which surgical resection, particularly of metastatic lesions, has played an important role. Ablative therapies are less likely to play a significant role in the treatment of gastric and pancreatic cancer, which are more commonly associated with widespread dissemination and peritoneal disease.

Ablative Therapies in Colorectal Carcinoma

Ablative therapies for colorectal cancer usually are considered in patients with relatively limited hepatic metastases. Interest in the ablation of hepatic metastases from colorectal cancer stems from the historical success of hepatic resection in this setting. Several series have firmly established hepatic resection as a potentially curative procedure in patients with limited hepatic disease. In a large, multiinstitutional French study, over 1800 patients undergoing surgical resection for colorectal cancer metastases were found to have a 5-year survival rate of 25% (1). Other large series have reported 5-year survival rates of 25% to 37% for patients undergoing complete resection of liver metastases (2–8).

Patient selection plays a critical role in determining who may benefit from hepatic resection. The presence of extrahepatic sites of disease is a uniformly poor prognostic factor, and is usually a contraindication to hepatic resection (2,5,7,8). Exceptions to this general rule include extrahepatic disease limited to a resectable local recurrence, or potentially resectable pulmonary metastases. The synchronous presentation of hepatic metastases and a primary tumor, as compared to the development of hepatic metastases following resection of the primary, also is an adverse prognostic factor (5,7,8). Some studies have suggested that the presence of four or more hepatic metastases is a contraindication to surgery. However, a recent study from Memorial Sloan-Kettering Cancer Center found that patients undergoing complete resection of four or more metastases experienced a 5-year survival of 24%, suggesting that in properly selected patients, resection of multiple metastases is potentially beneficial (2).

Ablative therapies, such as cryoablation or RFA, generally are reserved for patients whose liver metastases are not considered surgically resectable, but may still be amenable to therapy

TABLE 38.1. Selected studies of radiofrequency ablation in patients with metastatic colorectal cancer.

Study	No. of Patients	No. of Lesions	Median follow-up (months)	Disease-free survival
Rossi, 1996 (32)	11	13	22	1
Rossi, 1998 (33)	14	19	12	2
De Baere, 2000 (9)	68	121	13.7	NA
Solbiati, 2001 (10)	117	179	36	36%

with curative intent. Such scenarios include location of tumors located close to a blood vessel, or the presence of comorbidities that may preclude surgery. Studies of RFA in patients with metastatic colorectal cancer are limited by inconsistent selection criteria and short follow-up (Table 38.1). In an early Italian study, 14 patients with hepatic metastases underwent RFA. Of these patients, only two patients remained disease-free. In a subsequent French study, de Baere and colleagues (9) treated 68 patients, the majority of whom had metastases from colorectal cancer. The initial results of this study were encouraging, with successful ablation of 91 of 100 treated metastases. However, the longer-term benefits of these procedures were not reported. Long-term results from RFA were reported first by Solbiati and colleagues (10), who performed RFA in 117 patients with metastases from colorectal cancer. With a median follow-up time of 3 years, an overall survival rate of 36% was achieved. These results are similar to those achieved with surgical resection, and warrant a direct comparison between these two treatment modalities.

Interpretation of the results of cryoablation in the treatment of hepatic metastases from colorectal cancer similarly is limited by a lack of strict selection criteria and short follow-up. Disease-free survival rates appear similar to those of patients undergoing RFA, and range from 11%–40%, with no studies reporting median follow-up beyond 3 years (Table 38.2).

The potential benefit of ablative therapy as a strictly palliative treatment for patients with hepatic metastases from colorectal cancer has not been studied. Currently, the standard palliative approach to patients with unresectable metastatic colorectal cancer is systemic chemotherapy. First-line treatment, utilizing a combination chemotherapy regimen containing irinotecan, 5-fluorouracil, and leucovorin, has clearly been shown to result in palliation of symptoms and improvement in overall survival (11). Combinations of 5-fluorouracil and oxaliplatin also have activity in patients with metastatic colorectal cancer. Oxaliplatin is used commonly for the treatment of colorectal cancer in Europe, and was recently approved for use as second-line therapy for metastatic colorectal cancer in the United States (12).

The toxicities associated with systemic chemotherapy have led to studies of hepatic-directed therapy in patients with extensive hepatic metastases not amenable to surgical resection. Several studies have evaluated the palliative benefit of chemotherapy infused directly into the hepatic artery. This technique provides higher concentrations of chemotherapy directly to the metastatic sites, while limiting systemic toxicity. Hepatic arterial infusion has been shown to result in higher response rates than systemic chemotherapy, resulting in

TABLE 38.2. Selected studies of cryoablation in patients with metastatic colorectal cancer.

Study	No. of Patients	Median follow-up (months)	Disease-free survival
Onik, 1993 (12)	69	12–15	40%
Ravikumar, 1991 (34)	24	24	28%
Weaver, 1995 (35)	47	30	11%

TABLE 38.3. Selected studies of radiofrequency ablation in patients with hepatocellular carcinoma.

Study	No. of Patients	No. of Lesions	Median follow-up (months)	Disease-free survival
Rossi, 1996 (32)	39	41	22.6	23 (59%)
Ianitti, 2002 (36)	30	NA	36*	3 (60%)*
Kuvshinoff, 2002 (37)	11	NA	9	6 (53%)

* Results from only five patients reported.

shrinkage of liver metastases in approximately 50% of cases (13,14). However, these trials have failed to demonstrate a meaningful survival benefit associated with the hepatic arterial infusion, in large part because of the subsequent development of extrahepatic disease. Based on this experience, it is difficult to recommend RFA or cryoablation as a strictly palliative treatment outside of a clinical trial setting.

Ablative Therapies in Hepatocellular Carcinoma

Currently, the only established cure for hepatocellular carcinoma is partial or total hepatectomy with liver transplantation. Partial hepatectomy is curative in over 30% of selected patients (15,16). The operative mortality associated with partial hepatectomy has decreased to less than 5% in recent years, in large part due to improved operative technique and better patient selection. Baseline hepatic function is one of the most important factors that influence patient outcome. Poor prognostic factors in patients being considered for hepatic resection include the presence of cirrhosis, portal hypertension, thrombocytopenia, and coagulopathy (4). In patients with poor underlying hepatic function, hepatic transplantation may be considered. The limited number of livers available for transplantation, however, has limited the utility of hepatic transplantation as a routine treatment for hepatocellular carcinoma.

In patients who are not candidates for hepatic resection, or for whom transplantation is not feasible, other treatment modalities can be considered, although none has been demonstrated to be beneficial. Chemoembolization, a technique in which the hepatic arterial vessels supplying the tumor are occluded, is associated with tumor response rates in excess of 50%. Two studies in which chemoembolization was performed in patients prior to liver transplantation demonstrated encouraging long-term survival rates (17,18). The long-term benefit of chemoembolization in patients who do not undergo transplantation, however, remains uncertain. Systemic chemotherapy has played little role in the treatment of patients with unresectable hepatocellular carcinoma. Doxorubicin and 5-fluorouracil–based regimens have failed to demonstrate significant activity in this disease, and do not improve patient survival significantly (19,20).

The limited treatment options available to patients with unresectable hepatocellular carcinoma have made newer techniques such as RFA and cryoablation potentially attractive alternatives. Initial small studies of RFA in patients with hepatocellular carcinoma show relatively high rates of disease-free survival, although follow-up times remain short. The successful use of cryoablation also has been reported in patients with hepatocellular carcinoma (21,22) (Table 38.3).

Ablative Therapies in Neuroendocrine Tumors

The clinical course of patients with metastatic carcinoid and pancreatic neuroendocrine tumors is highly variable. Some patients with indolent tumors may remain symptom-free for years, even without treatment, while others more clearly require therapy. Several options are available for the treatment of metastatic neuroendocrine tumors. While cytotoxic therapy has played only a limited role in the management of patients with metastatic neuroendocrine tumors, treatment with somatostatin analogues, surgical resection, hepatic artery embolization, and, more recently, RFA and cryoablation can be considered in appropriate patients.

Patients with metastatic neuroendocrine tumors often become symptomatic from hormonal hypersecretion rather than from tumor bulk. This is especially true for patients with small bowel or appendiceal carcinoid tumors, in whom symptoms are typically absent until hepatic metastases supervene. The secretion of serotonin and other vasoactive substances into the systemic circulation results in the carcinoid syndrome. The carcinoid syndrome is characterized by episodic flushing, wheezing, diarrhea, and the eventual development of carcinoid heart disease. Symptoms of the carcinoid syndrome can be controlled successfully by the administration of somatostatin analogues in approximately 90% of cases (23). Actual radiologic tumor regression following treatment with somatostatin analogues is rare, however (24).

Resection of hepatic metastases also can effectively palliate symptoms of hormonal hypersecretion, and may, in some cases, result in long-term survival. In one series of 74 patients undergoing hepatic resection for metastatic disease, over 90% experienced symptomatic relief, and the 4-year survival rate exceeded 70% (25). In general, resection is undertaken only in patients with a limited number of hepatic metastases, and is most successful when undertaken with curative intent. Hepatic artery occlusion or embolization is an alternative therapy for patients who are not candidates for hepatic resection. The response rates associated with embolization, as measured either by decrease in hormonal secretion or by radiographic regression, generally are greater than 50% (26,27). However, the duration of response can be brief, ranging from 4 to 24 months in uncontrolled series (27). Furthermore, the potential for treatment-associated morbidity, which can include abdominal pain, nausea, elevated liver function tests, and infection, needs to be weighed against the potential benefits of this procedure.

Other approaches to the treatment of hepatic metastases include the use of RFA and cryoablation, either alone or in conjunction with surgical debulking. Most published reports are small case studies of fewer than 40 patients (28). In the series with the longest follow-up, 31 symptomatic patients with metastatic carcinoid, islet cell tumor, or medullary thyroid cancer, underwent resection, cryosurgery, and/or RFA (29). Symptoms were eliminated in 27 (87%), and 16 had progressive or recurrent disease with a median follow-up of 26 months.

Ablative Therapies in Gastric Cancer

Surgical resection is the only potentially curative treatment for patients with gastric cancer. Despite surgical resection, over 50% of patients subsequently develop metastatic disease. In contrast to colorectal cancer, hepatocellular carcinoma, and neuroendocrine tumors, the pattern of metastatic spread in patients with gastric cancer often involves the peritoneum. Because of the high incidence of peritoneal disease, there is rarely an indication for metastatectomy or ablation in such patients.

Ablative Therapies in Pancreatic Cancer

Patients with early-stage pancreatic cancer are candidates for pancreaticoduodenectomy (Whipple resection), which is the only potentially curative option for this disease. Unfortunately, only 15% of patients with pancreatic cancer are candidates for surgical resection. The remaining patients generally present with locally unresectable disease due to involvement of peripancreatic lymph nodes and the celiac vessels, or with distant metastases. Combinations of systemic chemotherapy and external-beam radiation therapy have been shown to palliate symptoms effectively and prolong survival in patients with locally advanced disease (30). As with gastric cancer, pancreatic cancer frequently is associated with peritoneal carcinomatosis. Systemic chemotherapy with gemcitabine has been shown to improve quality of life and overall survival in patients with metastatic pancreatic cancer (31). A role for ablative therapies in either locally advanced or metastatic pancreatic cancer, therefore, is uncertain.

References

1. Nordlinger B, Guiguet M, Vaillant J, et al. Surgical resection of colorectal carcinoma metastases to the liver: a prognostic scoring system to improve case selection based on 1568 patients. Cancer 1996;77:1254–1262.
2. Fong Y, Fortner J, Sun R, Brennan M, Blumgart L. Clinical score for predicting recurrence after hepatic resection for metastatic colorectal cancer: analysis of 1001 consecutive cases. Ann Surg 1999;230:309–321.
3. Hughes K, Rosenstein R, Songerabodi S, et al. Resection of the liver for colorectal carcinoma metastases: a multi-institutional study of long-term survivors. Dis Colon Rectum 1988;31:1–4.
4. Jamison R, Donohue J, Nagorney D, Rosen C, Harmsen W, Ilstrup D. Hepatic resection for metastatic colorectal cancer results in cure for some patients. Arch Surg 1997;132:505–510.
5. Jenkins L, Milikan K, Bines S, Staren E, Doolas A. Hepatic resection for metastatic colorectal cancer. Am Surg 1997;63:605–610.
6. Rees M, Plant G, Bygrave S. Late results justify resection for multiple metastases from colorectal cancer. Br J Surg 1997;84:1136–1140.
7. Scheele J, Stang R, Alterndorf-Hofmann A, Paul M. Resection of colorectal liver metastases. World J Surg 1995;19:59–71.
8. Wanebo H, Chu Q, Vezeridis M, Soderberg C. Patient selection for hepatic resection of colorectal carcinoma metastases. Arch Surg 1996; 131:322–329.
9. de Baere T, Elias D, Dromain C, et al. Radiofrequency ablation of 100 hepatic metastases with mean follow-up of more than 1 year. AJR 2000; 175:1619–1625.
10. Solbiati L, Livraghi T, Goldberg SN, et al. Percutaneous radio-frequency ablation of hepatic metastases from colorectal cancer: long-term results in 117 patients. Radiology 2001;221:159–166.
11. Saltz L, Cox J, Blanke C, et al. Irinotecan plus fluorouracil and leucovorin for metastatic colorectal cancer. N Engl J Med 2000;343:905–914.
12. Onik G, Atkinson D, Zemel R, Weaver M. Cryosurgery of liver cancer. Semin Surg Oncol 1993;9:309–317.
13. Chang A, Schneider P, Sugarbaker P, Simpson C, Culnane M, Steinberg S. A prospective randomized trial of regional versus systemic continuous 5-fluorodeoxyuridine chemotherapy in the treatment of liver metastases. Ann Surg 1987;206: 685–693.
14. Kemeny N, Daly L, Reichman B, Gellar N, Botet J, Oderman P. A randomized study of intrahepatic versus systemic infusion of fluorodeoxyuridine in patients with liver metastases from colorectal cancer. Ann Intern Med 1987;107: 459–465.
15. Hanazaki K, Kajikawa S, Shimozawa N, et al. Survival and recurrence after hepatic resection of 386 consecutive patients with hepatocellular carcinoma. J Am Coll Surg 2000;191:381–388.
16. Shimada M, Rikimaru T, Sugimachi K, et al. The importance of hepatic resection for hepatocellular carcinoma originating from nonfibrotic liver. J Am Coll Surg 2000;191:531–537.
17. Mazzaferro V, Regalia E, Doci R, et al. Liver transplantation for the treatment of small hepatocellular carcinomas in patients with cirrhosis. N Engl J Med 1996;334:693–699.
18. Venook A, Ferrell L, Roberts J, et al. Liver transplantation for hepatocellular carcinoma: results with preoperative chemoembolization. Liver Transplant Surg 1995;1:242–248.
19. Lai C, Wu P, Chan G, Lok A, Lin H. Doxorubicin vs. no antitumor therapy in an inoperable hepatocellular carcinoma: a prospective randomized trial. Cancer 1988;62:479–483.
20. Falkson G, MacIntyre J, Moertel C, Johnson L, Scherman R. Primary liver cancer: an Eastern Cooperative Oncology Group trial. Cancer 1984; 54:970–977.
21. Perglozzi J, Auster M, Conaway G, Sardi A. Cryosurgery for unresectable primary hepatocellular carcinoma: a case report and review of the literature. Am Surg 1999;65:402–405.
22. Sheen A, Poston G, Sherlock D. Cryotherapeutic ablation of liver tumours. Br J Surg 2002;89: 1396–1401.
23. Kvols L, Moertel C, O'Connell M, Schutt A, Rubin J, Hahn R. Treatment of the malignant carcinoid syndrome: evaluation of a long-acting somatostatin analog. N Engl J Med 1986;315: 663–666.
24. Leong W, Pasieka J. Regression of metastatic carcinoid tumors with octreotide therapy: two case reports and a review of the literature. J Surg Oncol 2002;79:180–187.
25. Que F, Nagorney D, Batts K, Linz L, Kvols L. Hepatic resection for metastatic neuroendocrine carcinomas. Am J Surg 1995;169:36–42.

26. Ruszniewski P, Rougier P, Roche A, et al. Hepatic arterial chemoembolization in patients with liver metastases of endocrine tumors. A prospective phase II study in 24 patients. Cancer 1993;71:2624–2630.
27. Moertel C, Johnson C, McKuskic M, et al. The management of patients with advanced carcinoid tumors and islet cell carcinomas. Ann Intern Med 1994;120:302–309.
28. Hellman P, Ladjevardi S, Skogseid B, Akerstrom G, Elvin A. Radiofrequency tumor ablation using cooled tip for liver metastases of neuroendocrine tumors. World J Surg 2002;26:1052–1056.
29. Chung M, Pisegna J, Spirt M. Hepatic cytoreduction followed by a novel long-acting somatostatin analog: a paradigm for intractable neuroendocrine tumors metastatic to the liver. Surgery 2001;130:954–962.
30. GITSG. Treatment of locally unresectable carcinoma of the pancreas: comparison of combined-modality therapy to chemotherapy alone. J Natl Cancer Inst 1988;80:751–755.
31. Burris H, Moore M, Andersen J, et al. Improvements in survival and clinical benefit with gemcitabine as first-line therapy for patients with advanced pancreas cancer: a randomized trial. J Clin Oncol 1997;15:2403–2013.
32. Rossi S, DiStasi M, Buscarini E, et al. Percutaneous RF interstitial thermal ablation in the treatment of hepatic cancer. AJR 1996;167:759–768.
33. Rossi S, Buscarini E, Garbagnati F, et al. Percutaneous treatment of small hepatic tumors by an expandable RF needle electrode. AJR 1998;170:1015–1022.
34. Ravikumar T, Kane R, Cady B, Jenkins R, Clouse M, Jr. A 5-year study of cryosurgery in the treatment of liver tumors. Arch Surg 1991;126:1520–1523.
35. Weaver M, Atkinson D, Zemel R. Hepatic cryosurgery in treating colorectal liver metastases. Cancer 1995;76:210–214.
36. Iannitti D, Dupuy D, Mayo-Smith W, Murphy B. Hepatic radiofrequency ablation. Arch Surg 2002;137:422–427.
37. Kuvshinoff B, Ota D. Radiofrequency ablation of liver tumors: influence of technique and tumor size. Surgery 2002;132:605–612.

39 Treatment of Hepatocellular Carcinoma by Internists

Shuichiro Shiina, Takuma Teratani, and Masao Omata

Hepatocellular carcinoma (HCC) is one of the most common malignancies in the world, especially in Taiwan, Japan, Korea, and China, as well as in sub-Saharan Africa (1). This cancer has been increasing in the United States (2) and other countries (3).

Treatment of HCC is different from that of other solid tumors, in that surgery plays a limited role. The resectability rate of this cancer is notably low, due to multiple lesions or underlying cirrhosis (4). It is estimated that only 20% to 30% of patients with HCC can be candidates for hepatic resection. Still worse, the cancer recurs frequently, even after curative surgical resection (5,6). Approximately 80% of patients who receive curative surgical resection develop recurrence within 5 years after surgery, due to intrahepatic metastases that cannot be detected by imaging modalities before resection, and multicentric carcinogenesis that arises from underlying cirrhosis metachronously. Orthotopic liver transplantation may be an effective treatment in some cases, but shortage of organ donors has led to a restricted indication for HCC. Thus, various nonsurgical therapies have been introduced for HCC.

Transcatheter arterial chemoembolization and image-guided percutaneous tumor ablation are widely performed for HCC. Unlike in the United States, in Japan many transcatheter arterial chemoembolizations and most image-guided percutaneous tumor ablations have been performed not by radiologists, but by internists. This is because internists have access to angiography and to ultrasound. Furthermore, ultrasound examination is chiefly performed by internists.

In most hospitals in Japan, internists (gastroenterologists or hepatologists) perform ultrasound examination of the abdominal organs, although radiologists and surgeons also have access to the examination. Internists perform almost all interventional ultrasound procedures. Image-guided percutaneous tumor ablations, such as percutaneous ethanol injection therapy (PEIT), percutaneous microwave coagulation therapy (PMCT), and radiofrequency ablation (RFA), are performed chiefly by hepatologists and gastroenterologists. In our hospital, we hepatologists perform almost all image-guided percutaneous tumor ablation procedures for liver tumors.

In our department, we have treated 90% of previously untreated patients with HCC by image-guided percutaneous tumor ablation, because of the local curability, minimal effect on residual liver function, and easy repeatability for recurrence. We have performed PEIT since 1985, PMCT since 1995, and percutaneous RFA since 1999 (Fig. 39.1), with satisfactory long-term results. This chapter details our experience.

Percutaneous Ethanol Injection Therapy

Introduction of PEIT (7) brought about a drastic change in the treatment of HCC. It has enabled us to treat HCC effectively by nonsur-

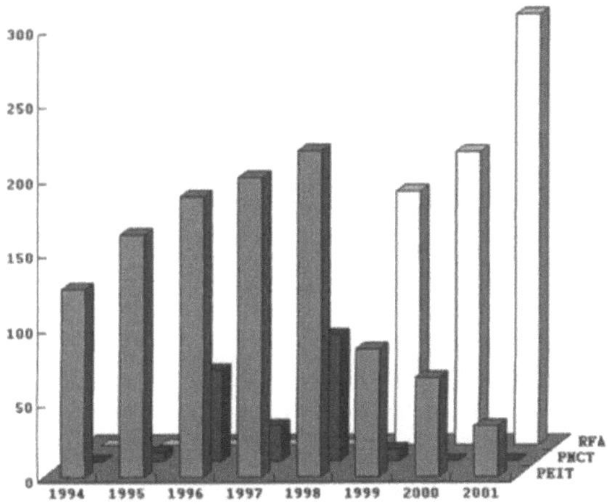

FIGURE 39.1. Transition of image-guided percutaneous tumor ablation for liver tumors at the Department of Gastroenterology, University of Tokyo. There was a drastic shift from percutaneous ethanol injection therapy (PEIT) and percutaneous microwave coagulation therapy (PMCT) to radiofrequency ablation (RFA). Today we perform ethanol injection only on patients who are allocated to ethanol injection because of a randomized controlled trial. All other patients are treated by RFA.

gical measures (8–10). Histopathologic examinations after PEIT have indicated its capacity to destroy the tumor completely in most cases (11), and it has achieved considerably high long-term survival rates (12–14). In Japan, PEIT generally has been accepted as an alternative to surgery for small HCCs (15).

General requirements we currently utilize for PEIT are listed in Table 39.1.

Between 1985 and 1998, 849 new patients with HCC were admitted to our institution. Among them, 756 patients (89%) were treated by PEIT. Ages of the patients ranged from 35 to 87 years (mean 63 years). Eighty-four percent had cirrhosis. There was one lesion in 357 patients (47%), two in 173 (23%), three in 79 (10%), and four or more in 147 (19%). The maximum diameter was 1.0cm or less in 21 patients (3%), 1.1 to 2.0cm in 206 (27%), 2.1 to 3.0cm in 236 (31%), 3.1 to 5.0cm in 222 (29%), and 5.1 cm or more in 71 (9%).

TABLE 39.1. General requirements for percutaneous ethanol injection therapy

Unresectable lesions or refusal of surgery
Absence of apparent vascular or biliary invasion
Absence of uncontrollable ascites
Absence of marked bleeding tendency; prothrombin times ≥35% and platelet count ≥40,000/mm^3
Serum bilirubin level <4.0mg/dL
Informed consent

We have employed the multiple-needle insertion technique to perform PEIT (16) (Fig. 39.1). By inserting multiple needles and changing the depth of the needle tips, we can inject ethanol into several portions in a single treatment session. In some cases, we have also used PEIT with the computed tomography (CT) assistance method. In this method, we first insert needles under ultrasound guidance, and then use CT to confirm that the tip of the needle is in the proper site. By using the multiple-needle insertion technique and the CT assistance method, we can apply PEIT to lesions more than 5cm in diameter, and thus we can treat almost all patients with HCC by PEIT.

We perform PEIT twice a week, until it is assumed that ethanol is injected throughout the lesion. Then, CT is performed to determine whether or not there is any viable cancer. If there remains any undestroyed portions, PEIT is repeated until CT confirms entire tumor necrosis; ethanol is injected into possible viable parts until they are destroyed completely.

In cases of three or fewer lesions, we usually perform PEIT without combining transcatheter arterial embolization (TAE). In cases of four or more lesions, we first perform TAE and then add PEIT for main lesions and/or lesions not treated sufficiently by TAE. Among the 756 patients, PEIT alone was performed in 597 (79%) and TAE was combined in the remaining 159.

With regard to long-term efficacy, the survival rates of all 756 patients treated by PEIT were 89% at 1 year, 64% at 3 years, 39% at 5 years, and 18% at 10 years. In 394 patients who had three or fewer lesions and all patients whose lesions were 3cm or less in diameter, survival was 93% at 1 year, 76% at 3 years, 50% at 5 years, and 27% at 10 years. Furthermore, in 594 patients in whom all lesions detected by imaging modalities underwent PEIT for a potentially curative treatment, survival was 93% at 1 year, 72% at 3 years, 47% at 5 years, and 24% at 10 years. In the remaining 130 patients, whom we classify into the absolutely noncurable group, only main lesions were treated by PEIT; some were left untreated by PEIT because of too many lesions.

Major complications that were encountered included peritoneal bleeding in nine patients, seeding of cancer cells in eight, hemobilia in seven, and massive hepatic infarction in three. There were three procedural deaths.

Percutaneous Microwave Coagulation Therapy

The microwave delivery system (Microtaze; Azwell, Osaka, Japan) consists of a generator (Fig. 39.2) and an electrode (Fig. 39.3). The electrode is connected to the generator by a soft coaxial cable.

In PMCT, heat destroys the cancer tissue generated by microwave energy emitted from the inserted electrode (17,18). The tissue around the electrode is coagulated in a spindle shape at the level of the monopolar electrode, but not beyond; PMCT typically destroys a certain amount of tissue, although the necrotic area it induces is smaller than that with PEIT.

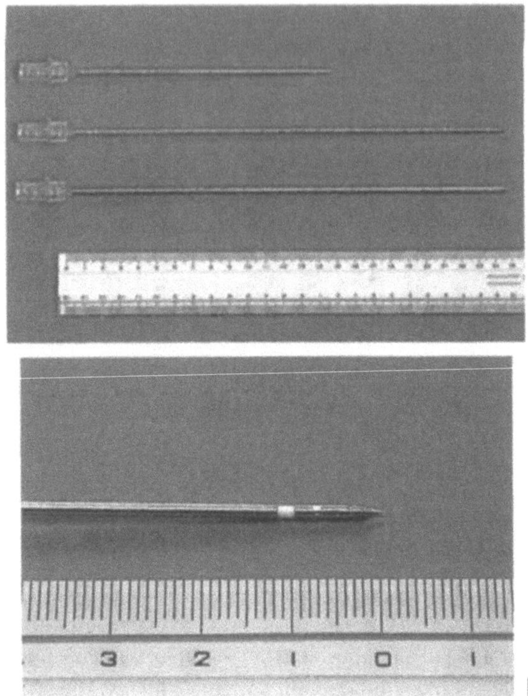

A

B

FIGURE 39.3. Microwave electrodes for percutaneous liver tumor ablation. (A) The electrodes are 1.6 or 2.0mm in diameter and 15 or 25cm in length. The electrodes consist of a stainless steel needle (external electrode) with a 1-cm-long monopolar electrode (internal electrode) at the tip. (B) Tip of the electrode. The distal 2.0cm is the active radiating portion. Microwaves are emitted between the external and internal electrodes, which resemble magnetic dipoles; therefore, microwave coagulation proceeds from the base of the monopolar electrode.

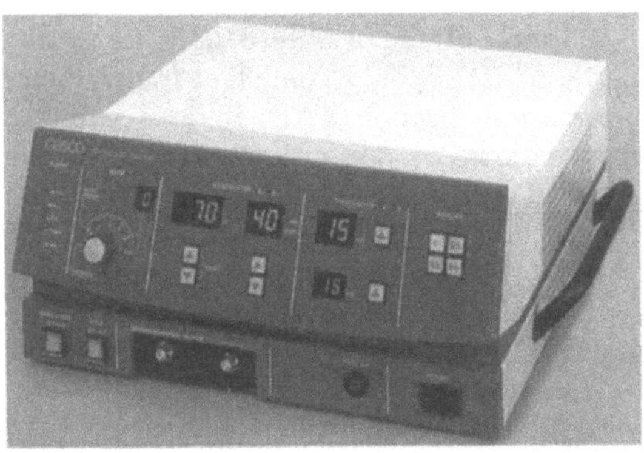

FIGURE 39.2. Microwave generator. Microwave generator is a surgical equipment originally developed in Japan to realize bloodless surgery particularly for fragile parenchymatous organs, like liver. Microwave generator emits a 2450-MHz microwave. In the treatment of liver tumors, not only percutaneous approach but also laparotomic and laparoscopic approaches are applied.

General requirements we currently utilize for PMCT are listed in Table 39.2. They are somewhat different from those of PEIT, because a considerably large introducing needle (14 gauge) is used and one treatment session tends to be more invasive.

We have performed PMCT on 186 patients with HCC, including the primary lesion in 122 patients, and recurrent lesions in the remaining 64. Among the 122 patients with previously untreated HCCs, there was one lesion in 67 (55%), two in 30 (25%), three in 12 (10%), and

TABLE 39.2. General requirements for percutaneous microwave coagulation therapy.

Unresectable lesions or refusal of surgery
Absence of apparent vascular or biliary invasion
Absence of uncontrollable ascites
Absence of marked bleeding tendency; prothrombin times ≥50% and platelet count ≥50,000/mm³
Serum bilirubin level <2.0mg/dL
Lesions in portions where the electrode can be inserted and held safely
Informed consent

four or more in 13 cases (11%). The maximum diameter was 1.0cm or less in 5 patients (4%), 1.1 to 2.0cm in 44 (36%), 2.1 to 3.0cm in 36 (30%), 3.1 to 5.0cm in 26 (21%), and 5.1cm or more in 11 (9%); PMCT alone was performed in 54 patients (44%), combination therapy of PEIT and PMCT was performed in 51 (42%), and the remaining 17 (14%) received all three—PEIT, PMCT, and TAE.

Under ultrasound (US) guidance, introducing needles were inserted first and then the electrode was introduced coaxially through the needles. Radiation for dielectric heating was performed at 65 to 85W for 60 seconds. We created an introducing needle with scales, a stopper for the electrode, and a guide needle with scales, so that the electrode can be inserted into each portion of the lesion systematically (19).

Enhanced CT scan was utilized in all 122 patients to evaluate therapeutic effect of PMCT. In 110 patients for potentially curative treatment, CT demonstrated complete necrosis of the lesion with a safety margin. In the remaining 12 patients in whom PMCT was used only palliatively, CT showed effective mass reduction. With regard to long-term efficacy, the survival rates of all 122 patients treated by PMCT were 90% at 1 year, 87% at 2 years, and 68% at 3 years. Local recurrence of the treated lesions was encountered in four cases.

Major complications occurred in nine (7%) of the 122 patients in whom PMCT was used for the primary lesion: massive pleural effusion requiring drainage in three, liver abscess in three, hemoperitoneum, hemothorax, and subcapsular hematoma that required blood transfusion in one each, and pyothorax in one. Complications were more common when the number of ablations was high in an attempt to destroy all lesions completely in one day.

Radiofrequency Ablation

Radiofrequency ablation recently has been introduced into the treatment of HCC (20–22). In Japan, RFA has been widely used clinically since 1999; more than 700 hospitals perform RFA.

With RFA, an electrode is inserted into the tumor under image guidance. Then radiofrequency energy is emitted from the exposed portion of the electrode, which is converted into heat and causes necrosis of the tumor. Heat may be conducted considerably homogeneously in all directions; the capsule or septa of the hepatic lesion may not prevent heat conduction. Thus, therapeutic efficacy seems more reproducible with RFA.

General requirements for RFA are equal to those for PMCT. RFA can be used in many cases in which PMCT is difficult. This is because a much larger area can be destroyed by a single ablation, and thus fewer electrode insertions are needed to accomplish the treatment by RFA.

We have performed RFA on 636 patients with HCC. There was one lesion in 258 patients (41%), two in 168 (26%), three in 88 (14%), four in 58 (9%), and five or more in 64 (10%). The maximum diameter was 2.0cm or less in 221 patients (35%), 2.1 to 3.0cm in 243 (38%), 3.1 to 4.0cm in 108 (17%), 4.1 to 5.0cm in 31 (5%), and 5.1cm or more in 33 (5%). Radiofrequency ablation was performed with a cooltip electrode (Radionics, Burlington, MA) in 629 patients and with an expandable-type electrode (RITA, Mountain View, CA) in the other seven patients. Two or three days after it was assumed that entire tumor was destroyed by RFA, CT was performed to determine whether or not there remained any viable cancer tissue. If there were any possible undestroyed portions, RFA was repeated until CT confirmed necrosis of the entire tumor.

Lesions were judged to be treated successfully by RFA in 634 (99.7%) of the 636 cases by the final CT (Figs. 39.4 and 39.5). By using the artificial pleural effusion technique and the guide needle method, we could ablate lesions on the surface of the liver, beneath the diaphragm, near large vessels, adjacent to other organs, and those that were detected definitively by CT, but that could not be identified clearly by ultrasound. In the remaining two cases, we gave up RFA because a lesion was not detected by ultrasound and did not seem to be able to be approached safely because of the location of the lesion. All lesions were judged totally necrotic by the final CT. The mean number of treatment sessions was 2.3 ± 1.4, and the duration of hospital stay was 14.3 ± 7.8 days.

With a mean follow-up of 16 months, 12 patients (1.9%) developed local recurrence of the treated lesions. Local recurrences developed in cases in which the border of the lesion was poorly defined before the treatment, or when CT scan slices after the treatment were different from those before the treatment due to differences in inhaling or exhaling, or due to body movement when ablation was limited by advanced liver dysfunction, or when there were too many lesions (greater than 10). The local recurrence rate was much lower than those reported by most other investigators. This is probably because we repeated RFA until CT confirmed complete destruction of the tumors.

Complications occurred in 37 (5.8%) of the 636 cases: liver abscess in eight cases, seeding of malignant cells in six cases, portal vein thrombus in five cases, intraperitoneal bleeding in four cases, skin burn in three cases, transient jaundice in two cases, transient liver failure due to massive hepatic infarction in two cases, massive pleural effusion in two cases, and bile peritonitis, septic shock, gastric ulcer due to antibiotics, transient deterioration of liver function due to hepatic vein injury, and abdominal wall burn with infection in one case each. Only one patient with bile peritonitis underwent emergency surgery. All other patients recov-

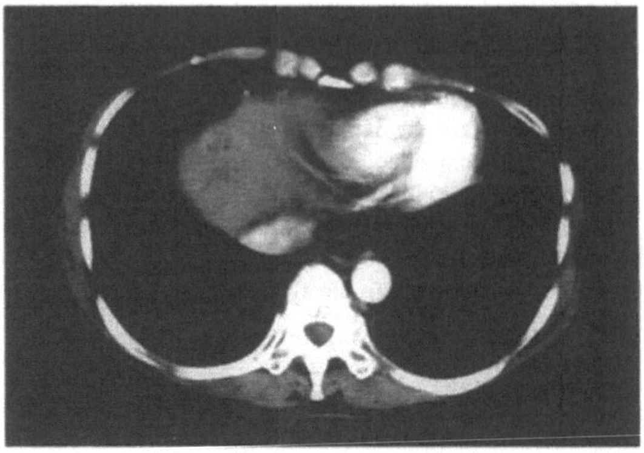
A

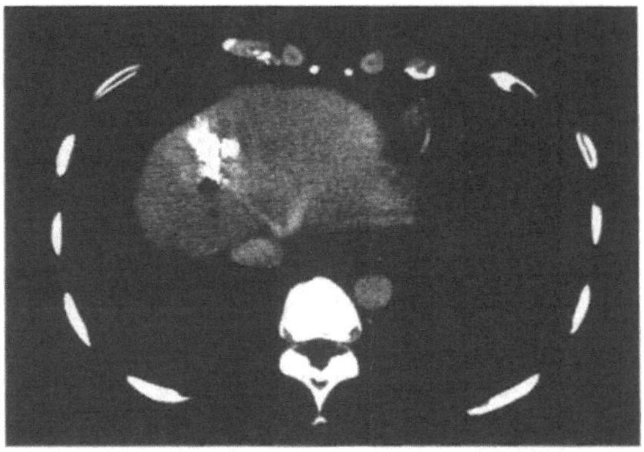
B

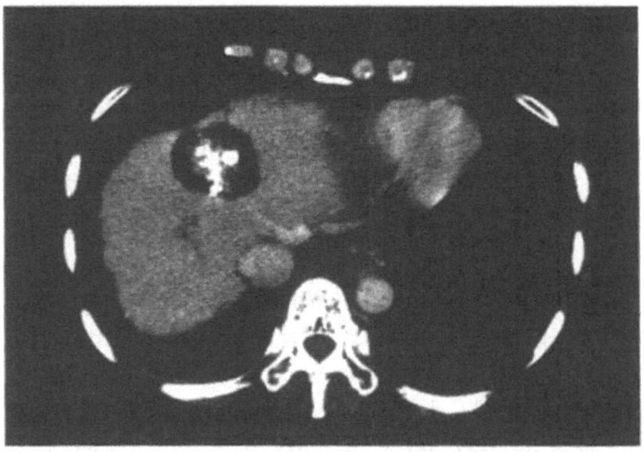
C

FIGURE 39.4. (A) Our first case of RFA. A 61-year-old woman had received microwave ablation under thoracoscopic guidance for a lesion beneath the diaphragm in S4. She was, however, found to have a local recurrence a year later. (B) The patient received chemoembolization for the local recurrence. Then she was referred to our institution for further treatment. There is Lipiodol deposit in the lesion. (C) Computed tomography (CT) scan taken 2 days after RFA. Single insertion of electrode and 12 minutes ablation achieved a nonenhancing area surrounding the Lipiodol deposit.

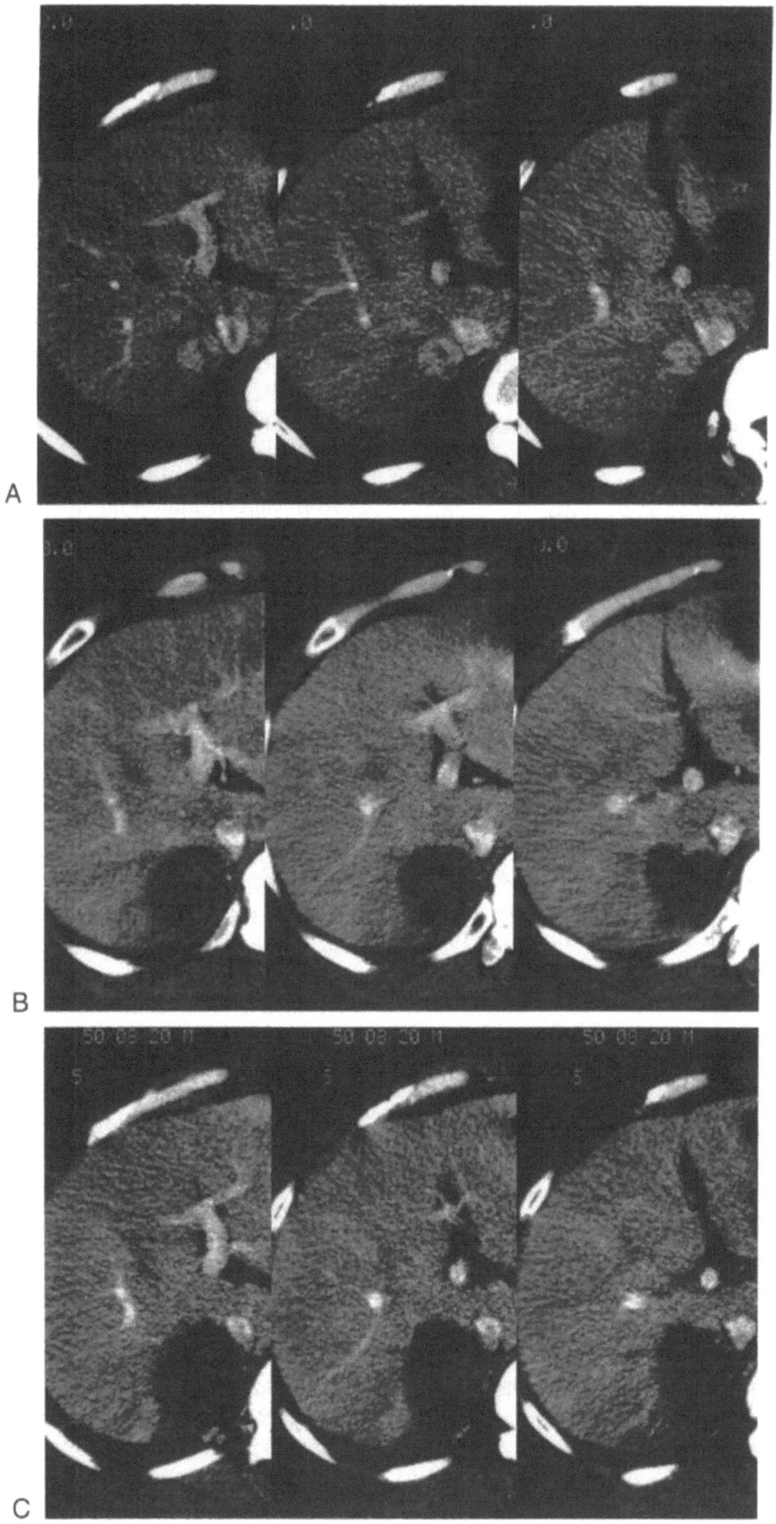

FIGURE 39.5. (A) Our second case of RFA. A 48-year-old man was found to have a lesion 3.6 cm adjacent to the inferior vena cava (IVC). (B) CT scan taken 3 days after the first RFA. There was no apparent undestroyed portion. However, we performed RFA again, because there was no sufficient safety margin near the IVC. (C) CT scan taken after the second RFA. We concluded that safety margin adjacent to the IVC had also been obtained. Thus, we stopped further treatment.

ered with nonsurgical measures. There was no mortality related to RFA.

Discussion

In Japan, primary liver cancer is the fourth most common malignancy and was responsible for 34,311 deaths in 2001. More than 95% of primary liver cancer is HCC. Thus, periodic examination of high-risk subjects, using imaging modalities and tumor markers, are common practice in Japan to detect HCC at an early stage. Patients with hepatic cirrhosis or chronic hepatitis and hepatitis B surface antigen (HBsAg) carriers are regarded as high-risk subjects to develop HCC.

We have treated 90% of new patients with HCC by PEIT, PMCT, and RFA, with considerable success.

Percutaneous ethanol injection therapy can destroy a relatively large area by a single ablation. However, it is difficult to predict an extent of an ablated area in PEIT, because distribution of injected ethanol is affected a great deal by the capsule and septa of the lesion. In PMCT, a certain size of necrosis can be obtained reproducibly, because heat is conducted homogeneously in all directions; the capsule or septa of the lesion may not prevent conduction. However, the size of necrosis induced is considerably small (1.5 cm in diameter and 2 cm in length).

RFA has a similar advantage to PEIT in necrosing a large volume of tumor in one session, and similar to PMCT in destroying a certain size of tissue reproducibly. Radiofrequency energy emitted from the electrode is converted into heat, which reliably causes necrosis up to 3 cm in diameter. Therapeutic efficacy is more reproducible with RFA than with PEIT or PMCT. Thus, RFA requires fewer treatment sessions and shorter hospital stay to achieve complete necrosis of lesions. Because of local curability, minimal effect on residual liver function, and repeat therapy for recurrence, image-guided percutaneous tumor ablation, especially RFA, plays an important role in the treatment of HCC; RFA also will be useful in the treatment of metastatic liver tumors.

References

1. Okuda K, Okuda H. Primary liver cell carcinoma. In: McIntyre N, Benhamou J-P, Bircher J, Rizzetto M, Rodes J, eds. Oxford Textbook of Clinical Hepatology. Vol 2. Oxford, England: Oxford University Press, 1991:1019–1052.
2. El-Serag HB, Mason AC. Rising incidence of hepatocellular carcinoma in the United States. N Engl J Med 1999;340:745–750.
3. Saracci R, Repetto F. Time trends of primary liver cancer: indication of increased incidence in selected cancer registry populations. J Natl Cancer Inst 1980;65:241–247.
4. Liver Cancer Study Group of Japan. Survey and Follow-Up Study of Primary Liver Cancer in Japan: Report 14. Kyoto: Shinko-insatsu, 2000.
5. Balsells J, Charco R, Lazaro JL, et al. Resection of hepatocellular carcinoma in patients with cirrhosis. Br J Surg 1996;83:758–761.
6. Gouillat C, Manganas D, Saguier G, Duque-Campos R, Berard P. Resection of hepatocellular carcinoma in cirrhotic patients: long-term results of a prospective study. J Am Coll Surg 1999;189:282–290.
7. Sugiura N, Takara K, Ohto M, Okuda K, Hirooka N. Percutaneous intratumoral injection of ethanol under ultrasound imaging for treatment of small hepatocellular carcinoma. Acta Hepatol Jpn 1983;24:920.
8. Livraghi T, Festi D, Monti F, Salmi A, Vettori C. US-guided percutaneous alcohol injection of small hepatic and abdominal tumors. Radiology 1986;161:309–312.
9. Shiina S, Yasuda H, Muto H, et al. Percutaneous ethanol injection in the treatment of liver neoplasms. AJR 1987;149:949–952.
10. Sheu JC, Sung JL, Huang GT, et al. Intratumoral injection of absolute ethanol under ultrasound guidance for the treatment of small hepatocellular carcinoma. Hepatogastroenterology 1987;34:255–261.
11. Shiina S, Tagawa K, Unuma T, et al. Percutaneous ethanol injection therapy for hepatocellular carcinoma. A histopathologic study. Cancer 1991;68: 1524–1530.
12. Shiina S, Tagawa K, Unuma T, et al. Percutaneous ethanol injection therapy of hepatocellular carcinoma: analysis of 77 patients. AJR 1990;155: 1221–1226.

13. Ebara M, Ohto M, Sugiura N, et al. Percutaneous ethanol injection for the treatment of small hepatocellular carcinoma. Study of 95 patients. J Gastroenterol Hepatol 1990;5:616–626.
14. Livraghi T. Percutaneous ethanol injection of hepatocellular carcinoma: survival after 3 years in 70 patients. Ital J Gastroenterol 1992;24:72–74.
15. Shiina S, Imamura M, Omata M. Percutaneous ethanol injection therapy (PEIT) for malignant liver neoplasms. Semin Intervent Radiol 1997;14:295–303.
16. Shiina S, Hata Y, Niwa Y, et al. Multiple-needle insertion method in percutaneous ethanol injection therapy for liver neoplasms. Gastroenterol Jpn 1991;26:47–50.
17. Seki T, Wakabayashi M, Nakagawa T, et al. Ultrasonically guided percutaneous microwave coagulation therapy for small hepatocellular carcinoma. Cancer 1994;74:817–825.
18. Murakami R, Yoshimatsu S, Yamashita Y, Matsukawa T, Takahashi M, Sagara K. Treatment of hepatocellular carcinoma: value of percutaneous microwave coagulation. AJR 1995;164:1159–1164.
19. Shiina S, Imamura M, Obi S, et al. Percutaneous microwave coagulation therapy for liver tumors. J Microwave Surg 1997;15:65–69.
20. Buscarini L, Fornari F, Rossi S. Interstitial radiofrequency hyperthermia in the treatment of small hepatocellular carcinoma: percutaneous US-guidance of electrode needle. In: Anderegg A, Despland PA, Otto R, Henner H, eds. Ultraschall-diagnostik 91. Berlin: Springer-Verlag, 1992, pp. 218–222.
21. Rossi S, Di Stasi M, Buscarini E, et al. Percutaneous ultrasound-guided radiofrequency electrocautery for the treatment of small hepatocellular carcinoma. J Intervent Radiol 1993;8:97–103.
22. Livraghi T, Goldberg SN, Lazzaroni S, Meloni F, Solbiati L, Gazelle GS. Small hepatocellular carcinoma: treatment with radio-frequency ablation versus ethanol injection. Radiology 1999;210:655–661.

40
The Surgeon's Perspective on Hepatic Radiofrequency Ablation

David A. Iannitti

Surgeons continue to have an important role in the management of patients with hepatic malignancies. Throughout the decades, modern surgical techniques have improved outcomes in patients undergoing hepatic surgery. However, the majority of hepatic malignancies continue to be unamenable to surgical resection. These patients continue to be challenging for clinicians. Surgeons have carried out hepatic tumor ablation since the 1970s; therefore, a vast experience has been gained in terms of techniques, outcomes, and patient selection for tumor ablation. Cryosurgical ablation has been performed for the past several decades, and long-term patient outcome data currently are available. The experience and outcome with cryoablation can be extrapolated to more modern modalities of tumor ablation, such as with radiofrequency energy. In the early 1990s, developments in laparoscopic surgery influenced hepatic surgery. Laparoscopic hepatic tumor ablation with cryosurgical and radiofrequency probes is available to selected patients today. Therefore, the experience surgeons have gained in managing patients with hepatic malignancies should help to select appropriate patients for hepatic radiofrequency ablation (RFA).

A number of hepatic malignancies can be treated with RFA, the most common being metastatic colorectal carcinoma and hepatocellular carcinoma. If one is to consider RFA of these malignancies, it is important to understand the natural history of these diseases, as well as responses to traditional treatment such as systemic and regional chemotherapy, and the outcomes of hepatic resection.

Colorectal Carcinoma

There are approximately 140,000 new cases of colorectal carcinoma diagnosed in the United States annually (1). At the time of initial diagnosis, 25% of patients have hepatic metastases. Additionally, 20% to 25% of patients develop metastatic disease within 5 years of diagnosis. Therefore, 70,000 patients per year are at risk of developing metastatic disease from colorectal carcinoma. Approximately 60% of patients with metastatic disease have liver involvement, whereas 20% of patients have liver metastases only. Unfortunately, only 25% of patients with metastatic colorectal carcinoma to the liver are amenable to surgical resection. Survival is dependent on the extent of hepatic disease. Patients with a solitary hepatic metastasis have a median survival of 25 months, patients with unilobar multicentric disease have a median survival of 17 months, and patients with diffuse bilobar metastatic disease have a median survival of 3 to 6 months. Few, if any, patients with metastatic colorectal carcinoma to the liver untreated will survive 5 years (2–4).

Standard chemotherapy agents for colorectal carcinoma are 5-fluorouracil (5-FU) and folinic acid (leucovorin). These chemotherapy agents usually are well tolerated by patients; however, in the presence of metastatic disease, there is a low response rate and no significant improvement in median or long-term survival (5,6). New chemotherapy agents approved by the Food and Drug Administration (FDA) include irinotecan (CPT-11) and oxaliplatin. These agents can be used alone, in combination with each other, or in combination with 5-FU and/or leucovorin (7–10). Oxaliplatin, 5-FU, and leucovorin currently appear to be the most effective systemic therapy regime for metastatic colorectal cancer (11–13). However, long-term studies still are pending at this time. Investigational agents such as epidermal growth factor receptor inhibitors and signal transduction pathway inhibitors, including tyrosine kinase inhibitors, currently are being studied in patients with advanced colorectal metastatic disease (14).

Hepatic artery infusion for regional chemotherapy of the liver for metastatic colon cancer was popularized in the 1980s. The standard chemotherapy agent for hepatic artery infusion is 5-fluorodeoxyuridine (FUDR) (15). There have been mixed reviews in the literature evaluating hepatic artery infusion. There does appear to be some short-term survival improvement over systemic chemotherapy (16,17). Hepatic artery infusion in combination with current systemic agents continues to be evaluated by clinical trials; long-term data still are pending (18).

Hepatic resection continues to be the most effective treatment for metastatic colon cancer to the liver (19). Hepatic surgery has undergone significant improvement, particularly over the past 10 years; operative mortality associated with hepatic resections in major centers is less than 3%. Overall morbidity from these procedures is in the 10% to 15% range (20,21). A number of factors affect long-term survival in patients who undergo hepatic resection for metastatic colon cancer to the liver. These include the number and distribution of lesions, resection margins, size of metastases, synchronous versus metachronous development of metastases, the presence of extrahepatic disease, the type of resection (wedge versus anatomic resection), age, gender, blood loss, blood transfusion requirement, primary tumor characteristics, as well as carcinoembryonic antigen (CEA) level all have been shown to affect long-term outcomes (22–24). However, if the patient does undergo hepatic resection for liver-only metastatic disease with clear surgical margins, overall survival at 3, 5, and 10 years is approximately 40%, 30%, and 20%, respectively (25,26). The role of adjuvant therapy following hepatic resection generally is indicated; however, sufficient long-term data with current chemotherapeutic agents are inadequate.

Following hepatic resection, approximately 60% of patients develop recurrent disease within 5 years. The liver is involved in 45% to 75% of cases, and the liver only is affected in 40% of patients with recurrent disease. Only one third of patients with liver-only recurrent metastatic colorectal cancer are candidates for reresection (27,28). The data for repeat hepatic resections for recurrent metastatic colon cancer exist; however, there is a small number of patients per study. However, reresection has been associated with a median survival of greater than 30 months, with a 5-year survival of 16% to 32% (29,30). This suggests that this may be a population of patients who would benefit from operative therapy. Since 75% of patients with metastatic colorectal cancer to the liver are not candidates for surgery, treatment options, such as hepatic tumor ablation, may be preferable in these patients. There are many reasons for patients not to be surgical candidates, such as multicentric disease, bilobar disease, local anatomic invasion, juxtaposition to the major vascular pedicles or structures, and the presence of advanced cirrhosis or other comorbid medical conditions (31). Therefore, the indications for patients to undergo hepatic tumor ablation of colorectal metastases include unresectable tumors, recurrent hepatic tumors, and the inability to tolerate surgery.

Hepatocellular Carcinoma

Hepatocellular carcinoma is a prevalent worldwide disease with approximately 250,000 to one million new cases diagnosed per year (32,33). The incidence in the United States is approximately 1.8 per 100,000, and in some countries it is as high as 30 per 100,000 (32,34). Hepatocellular carcinoma is associated with cirrhosis in approximately 80% of patients. In many patients, viral hepatitis B or C infections also are associated (35–37). Hepatocellular carcinoma demonstrates a variable growth rate, with a median doubling time of approximately 4 months. The median survival of all patients diagnosed with hepatocellular carcinoma in North America who did not receive treatment was approximately 9 months (38). Systemic chemotherapy for hepatocellular carcinoma is ineffective. The standard agent is doxorubicin (Adriamycin), which is associated with cardiac toxicity and a less than 20% response rate (39). Other agents, such as liposomal doxorubicin, thalidomide, and octreotide have been used; however, these alternative agents are associated with low response rates and no proven survival benefit (40–42). Investigational research for treatment of hepatocellular carcinoma includes vascular endothelial growth factor receptor inhibitors, cell surface antibody therapy, and gene therapy; however, the results of systemic chemotherapy for hepatocellular carcinoma are poor.

Regional chemotherapy with hepatic artery chemoembolization or infusion does appear to have higher response rates than systemic therapy. Typical agents used for chemoembolization or infusion are doxorubicin, cisplatinum, mitomycin C, and ethiodized oil (Lipiodol). These agents can be used in diffuse infiltrative disease to regionally perfuse the liver and can be repeated on a regular basis. Hypervascular nodular tumors can be infused initially, and then followed by selective embolization of the feeding artery to the lesion. This treatment can be used in preparation for surgery, for ablation, or as the primary therapy for these tumors (43). Past data have demonstrated that there have been highly variable responses to regional chemotherapy; however, current prospective randomized trials suggest there can be significant tumor response with some improvement in survival with regional chemotherapy for hepatocellular carcinoma. Two- and 4-year survivals with treatment average 45% and 13%, respectively (44,45).

Surgical resection continues to be the treatment of choice for hepatocellular carcinoma; however, the majority of patients have extensive disease or impaired liver function that precludes hepatic resection. The operative mortality for patients undergoing hepatic resection for hepatocellular carcinoma is higher than in other diseases, approximately 11%, with a range of 0% to 25%. Hepatic resection for hepatocellular carcinoma is associated with 1-, 3-, and 5-year survival rates of 82%, 44%, and 31%, respectively (46,47). Recurrence of the disease is high following hepatic resection, with a cumulative recurrence rate at 5 years of 75% (47,48). Since the majority of patients with hepatocellular carcinoma are not candidates for hepatic resection because of the advanced stage of the tumor and underlying liver disease, patients with isolated disease may be good candidates for hepatic RFA.

Historical Development of Tumor Ablation

The concept of tumor ablation certainly is not new, as ablation techniques have been described for more than a century. In 1845 Arnott described using iced saline to treat dermal malignancies. Throughout the mid-1900s, various cryogens were developed, including Freon-12, by Paul in 1942, and liquid nitrogen by Arlington in 1950. An insulated cryotherapy probe was used for treatment of hepatic malignancies by Cooper in 1963. Cryoablation was a fairly popular technique in the 1980s and early 1990s. Cryogens such as argon gas can be used for cryosurgical therapy of liver tumors. Later developments in cryoablation systems and probes have allowed cryotherapy to be carried out percutaneously (49).

Radiofrequency ablation also has been present since the early 1900s. In 1912, Cushing used radiofrequency energy for destruction of central nervous system tumors. This technology recently has been improved and modified for treatment of numerous soft tissue tumors. Animal studies that evaluated tissue temperature tolerance have concluded that normally perfused tissue can tolerate maximal temperatures of approximately 45°C. Temperatures above 50°C are cytotoxic to tumors. As tissue temperatures rise, proteins denature, membranes rupture, and cells dehydrate. Radiofrequency energy can raise tissue temperatures to 100°C, which results in effective coagulative necrosis of tumors. In the 1990s, other thermal sources were developed, such as laser and microwave energy for tumor ablation. In 1998 the FDA approved RFA for therapy of hepatic tumors (50,51).

Radiofrequency Ablation Materials and Operative Techniques

Radiofrequency generators have been used extensively for the treatment of hepatic tumors. There are essentially two types of radiofrequency generators that are applicable for hepatic tumor ablation. These are the impedance-based systems (RITA, Radiotherapeutics, Mountain View, CA) and the output-based systems (Radionics; Burlington, MA). The tumor ablation concept is as follows: a radiofrequency needle probe is passed into the tumor, and then radiofrequency waves from 460 to 480 kHz are emitted through the tumor. Local ion agitation from the current raises the tissue temperature above the cytotoxic threshold (51).

In the impedance-based systems, the current is begun at a low level, and as the tissue impedance increases, the wattage increases for higher current until the volume of tissue within the deployable array reaches up to 100°C. In the output-based system, the local tissue temperature is cooled to approximately 20°C. The generator is run at maximal output. The local cooling effect maintains low tissue impedance and therefore maximal current is used at the outset of the ablation through completion.

These RFA systems can be used in open OR laparoscopic surgery, as well as percutaneously under real-time radiographic guidance. The basic technique for ablation is relatively similar. When performing an operative ablation, the abdomen is explored thoroughly, either with open surgical or laparoscopic techniques. The presence of extrahepatic disease is associated with poor outcomes and precludes a patient's undergoing local tumor ablation (28,31,52). Once the presence of extrahepatic disease has been ruled out, then the liver is examined thoroughly with intraoperative ultrasound. Ultrasound is the most sensitive and accurate means of assessing the extent, location, size, and characteristics of hepatic tumors (53). When all tumors have been located and characterized, the ablations are planned and executed. Under real-time radiographic guidance, the RF probe is inserted to the deep margin of the tumor without traversing a major vascular portal pedicle. The ablation is performed according to the standards of the particular system that is being used. The overall goal is to achieve at least a 1-cm margin of coagulative necrosis circumferentially beyond the periphery of the tumor margin.

Radiofrequency ablation can be supplemented by vascular inflow occlusion to the liver, known as the Pringle maneuver. This maneuver can be carried out by open surgical techniques, as well as laparoscopically. Inflow occlusion clearly has demonstrated a decrease in the time required for ablation, as well as increase in the zone of thermocoagulation (54,55). The temperature of the margins of the tumor should be evaluated during the time of ablation and should be greater than 50°C. With larger tumors, greater than 3 cm in diameter, the practitioner should perform overlapping zones of ablation, often with multiple passes of the radiofrequency probe to various margins of the tumor to achieve complete tumor ablation.

As with any invasive procedure, there are risks associated with hepatic RFA. The overall morbidity averages 0.5%, major complications approximately 2%, and minor complications up to 6%. Various complications have been described from hepatic RFA; these include skin burns, thrombocytopenia, renal failure, colonic perforation, bleeding, bile leak and strictures, hepatic abscess, fever, liver dysfunction, segmental infarct, portal venous thrombosis, diaphragmatic paralysis, systemic hemolysis, pneumothorax, and pacemaker dysfunction (56–58).

Outcomes of Hepatic Tumor Ablation

As mentioned previously, hepatic cryoablation has been performed since the 1970s. Considerable experience and knowledge have been gained from cryoablation. These lessons can and should be applied to RFA. It is clear from surgical resection and open surgical cryoablation that if the patient has extrahepatic metastatic disease, survival does not differ significantly whether ablation is carried out or not. Therefore, extrahepatic peritoneal metastatic disease is a contraindication to ablation.

There has been considerable experience with cryosurgical ablation for metastatic colorectal carcinoma to the liver. The majority of treated patients generally have been considered to have unresectable metastatic disease for a variety of reasons; however, it has been demonstrated that median survival of patients undergoing "complete" cryoablation live approximately 36 months, while patients undergoing "incomplete" cryoablation have a median survival of 24 months (59). Outcomes for cryoablation for metastatic colorectal carcinoma also correlate with the patient's preablation CEA level. Patients with CEA levels greater than 100 ng/mL have significantly worse survival than patients with CEA levels less than 100 ng/mL (60). Five-year survival following surgical cryoablation for metastatic colorectal carcinoma is approximately 25% (60–62); this survival outcome is higher than with systemic or regional chemotherapy.

The largest experience of cryosurgical ablation for hepatocellular carcinoma (167 patients) is reported by Zhou et al (63,64) from China. Eighty-six percent of patients were noted to have cirrhosis. Overall survival reported at 1, 3, and 5 years was 73.5%, 47.7%, and 31.7%, respectively. Survival was improved in patients who had tumors smaller than 5 cm. The survival for patients undergoing cryoablation appears to rival that of patients undergoing hepatic resection.

Radiofrequency ablation outcomes for hepatic malignancies have been reported in a number of published studies; however, most studies have short-term follow-up and are performed in an uncontrolled fashion for a variety of pathologies (58,65–68). Curley et al (55) reported their experience in 123 patients with 169 tumors. Thirty-nine percent were primary liver cancers, and 61% had metastatic disease. There were no deaths in the series, and a 2.4% complication rate. With a 15-month follow-up, there was noted to be a 1.8% local recurrence rate, and a 27.6% distant recurrence rate. Jiao et al (69) reported a series of 35 patients, including eight patients with hepatocellular carcinoma. Four patients were noted to have a 90% reduction in α-fetoprotein (AFP) level. One patient died at 2 months; however, the remainder of the patients had no evidence of disease at a 10-month follow-up. Four of 17 patients expired, while at 7.6 months the remainder of the patients had no evidence of disease. Solbiati et al (70) reported 50% disease-free survival at 16.6 months with 2-year survival of 61.5% in patients with gastrointestinal malignancies. Rossi et al's (68) series of patients with small hepatocellular carcinomas had a median survival of 44 months, and a 10% local recurrence rate. Francica and Marone (71) evaluated 15 patients with cirrhosis who had 20 hepatocellular carcinomas; there was a 64% disease-free survival for treated patients at 1 year. Solbiati et al (72) in a follow-up report in 2001, demonstrated overall survival of patients undergoing hepatic RFA at 1, 2, and 3 years of 93%, 62%, and 41%, respectively. In our experience of 123 patients (20-month median follow-up), 52 patients were treated for colorectal metastases. One-, 2-, and 3-year survival rates were 87%, 77%, and 50%, respectively. In 30 patients with hepatocellular carcinoma with a 21-month median follow-up, 1-, 2-, and 3 year survival rates were 92%, 75%, and 60%, respectively (58).

Surgical vs. Percutaneous Ablation

Since there are currently a number of delivery mechanisms for RFA, one should consider whether a patient would benefit from an open surgical, laparoscopic, or percutaneous approach. Currently the majority of patients undergoing RFA of hepatic malignancies undergo the percutaneous approach. However, several considerations should be given prior to treatment of patients. First is the accuracy of diagnostic imaging for detection of hepatic and extrahepatic tumors. Bilchik et al (73) reported 308 patients with unresectable hepatic tumors. All patients underwent laparoscopy with laparoscopic and intraoperative ultrasound. There was a 12% incidence of occult metastatic extrahepatic peritoneal disease that was not appreciated by preoperative diagnostic imaging studies. Additionally, 33% of patients had additional lesions not recognized by preoperative diagnostic imaging. Jarnagin et al (74) reported a trial of 416 patients with "resectable" hepatic metastatic colorectal carcinomas. Twenty-one of these patients were deemed to be unresectable since 11% had unrecognized occult extrahepatic metastatic disease, and 10% were noted to have disease greater than predicted by preoperative diagnostic imaging. Despite the most current diagnostic imaging techniques available, approximately 10% to 20% of patients will have unrecognized extrahepatic peritoneal metastatic disease. These patients clearly have been shown not to benefit from hepatic tumor ablation. Intraoperative ultrasound, performed either open or laparoscopically, demonstrates additional lesions not recognized by preoperative diagnostic imaging in up to 40% of patients. Therefore, laparoscopic or surgical exploration with intraoperative ultrasound currently is the most accurate method to assess patients with hepatic malignancy. This approach should be carefully considered when a patient is to undergo a planned ablation procedure (75,76).

For practical reasons, the operative approaches may be more feasible than a percutaneous approach. Patients with more than three lesions, may benefit from vascular inflow occlusion. Also, lesions high on the dome of the liver can be difficult to access percutaneously. Transthoracic approaches have been reported; however, there can be associated with pneumothoraces and/or diaphragm injury, such as perforation or paralysis (77). Finally, hepatic tumors that are juxtaposed to other structures, such as the stomach, colon, or gallbladder, also may benefit from an operative approach, particularly a laparoscopic approach when either the gallbladder can be removed or the adjacent structures can be retracted, while the tumor can be more safely ablated with decreased risk of visceral injury.

Summary

Practitioners carrying out hepatic tumor RFA should apply the lessons learned from hepatic surgery. Traditional systemic as well as regional treatments generally are ineffective, are associated with significant toxicity, and usually do not alter patient survival. However, continued research into newer agents may affect survival. Systemic chemotherapy for metastatic colorectal cancer should be considered strongly in patients as an adjuvant following tumor ablation to decrease the risk of recurrence or prolong the time to recurrence. Patients with larger hepatocellular carcinomas (>4 cm) may benefit from preablation hepatic artery chemoembolization to produce a more efficacious tumor ablation. Surgical resection continues to be the gold standard for survival; however, in patients with metastatic colorectal carcinoma and hepatocellular carcinoma, the majority are not candidates for hepatic resection for a variety of reasons. Therefore, tumor ablation appears to be the most effective treatment for patients with unresectable disease that is confined to the liver. Open surgical, laparoscopic, and percutaneous techniques can be carried out; however, careful patient selection for the approach should be made between the surgeon and the interventional radiologist.

References

1. Wingo P, Tong T, Bolden S. Cancer Statistics, 1995. CA Cancer J, Clin 1995;45:8.
2. Wagner JS, Adson MA, van Heerdon JA, et al. The natural history of hepatic metastases from colorectal cancer. A comparison with resective treatment. Ann Surg 1984;199:502–508.

3. Fong Y, Blumgart LH. Hepatic colorectal metastases: current status of surgical therapy. Oncology 1998;12:1489–1498.
4. Stangl R, Altendof-Hoffman A, Charnley RM, et al. Factors influencing the natural history of colorectal liver metastases. Lancet 1994;343: 1404–1410.
5. Scheithauer W, Rosen H, Kornkek GV, et al. Randomised comparison of combination chemotherapy plus supportive care in patients with metastatic colorectal cancer. BMJ 1993;306: 752–755.
6. Moertel CG, Fleming TR, MacDonald JS, et al. Levamisole and fluorouracil for adjuvant chemotherapy of resected colon carcinoma. N Engl J Med 1990;322:352–358.
7. Douillard JY, Cunningham D, Roth AD, et al. Irinotecan combined with fluorouracil compared with fluorouracil alone as first-line treatment for metastatic colorectal cancer: a multicentre randomized trial. Lancet 2000;355:1041–1047.
8. Rougier P, Van Cutsem E, Bajetta E, et al. Randomized trial of irinotecan versus fluorouracil by continuous infusion after fluorouracil failure in patients with metastatic colorectal cancer. Lancet 1998;352:1407–1412.
9. Saltz LB, Cox JV, Blanke C, et al. Irinotecan plus fluorouracil and leucovorin for metastatic colorectal cancer. Irinotecan Study Group. N Engl J Med 2000;343:905–915.
10. Cunningham D, Pyrhonen S, James RD, et al. Randomized trial of irinotecan plus supportive care versus supportive care alone after fluorouracil failure for patients with metastatic colorectal cancer. Lancet 1998;352:1413–1418.
11. de Gramont R, Figer A, Seymore M, et al. Leucovorin and fluorouracil with or without oxaliplatin as first line treatment for advanced colorectal cancer. J Clin Oncol 2000;18:2938–2947.
12. Levi F, Zidani R, Vannetzel JM, et al. Randomised multicentre trial of chronotherapy with oxaliplatin, fluorouracil, and folinic acid in metastatic colorectal cancer. Lancet 1997;350: 681–686.
13. Giachetti S, Itzhaki M, Gruia G, et al. Long-term survival of patients with unresectable colorectal cancer liver metastases following infusional chemotherapy with 5-fluorouracil, leucovorin, oxaliplatin, and surgery. Ann Oncol 1999;10: 663–669.
14. Shaheen RM, Ahmed SA, Liu W, et al. Inhibited growth of colon cancer carcinomatosis by antibodies to vascular endothelial and epidermal growth factor receptors. Br J Cancer 2001;85: 584–589.
15. Chang AE, Schneider PD, Sugerbaker PH, et al. A prospective randomized trial of regional versus systemic continuous 5-fluorodeoxyuridine chemotherapy in the treatment of colorectal liver metastases. Ann Surg 1987;206:685–693.
16. Rougier P, Laplanche A, Huguier M, et al. Hepatic arterial infusion of floxuridine in patients with liver metastases from colorectal carcinoma: long-term results of a prospective randomized trial. J Clin Oncol 1992;10:1112–1118.
17. Lorenz M, Muller HH. Randomized, multicenter trial of fluorouracil plus leucovorin administered either via hepatic arterial or intravenous infusion versus fluorodeoxyuridine administered via hepatic arterial infusion in patients with nonresectable liver metastases from colorectal carcinoma. J Clin Oncol 2000;18:243–254.
18. Kemeny N, Gonen M, Sullivan D, et al. Phase I study of hepatic arterial infusion of floxuridine and dexamethasone with systemic irinotecan for unresectable hepatic metastases from metastatic colon cancer. J Clin Oncol 2001;19:2687–2695.
19. Scheele J, Stangl R, Altendorf-Hofman A. Hepatic metastases from colorectal cancer: impact of surgical resection on the natural history. Br J Surg 1990;77:1241–1246.
20. Bradley AL, Chapman WC, Wright JK, et al. Surgical experience with hepatic colorectal metastasis. Am Surg 1999;65:560–566.
21. Harmon KE, Ryan JAJ, Beihl TR, et al. Benefits and safety of hepatic resection for colorectal metastases. Am J Surg 1999;177:402–404.
22. Nagashima I, Oka T, Hamada C, et al. Histopathological prognostic factors influencing long-term prognosis after surgical resection for hepatic metastases from colorectal cancer. Am J Gastroenterol 1999;94:739–743.
23. Taylor M, Forster J, Langer B, et al. A study of prognostic factors for hepatic resection for colorectal metastases. Am J Surg 1997;173:467–471.
24. Altendorf-Hofmann A, Scheele J. A critical review of the major indicators of prognosis after resection of hepatic metastases from colorectal carcinoma. Surg Oncol Clin North Am 2003; 162–192.
25. Jamison RL, Donohue JH, Nagorney DM, et al. Hepatic resection for metastatic colorectal cancer results in cure for some patients. Arch Surg 1997;132:505–510.

26. Ohlsson B, Stenram U, Tranberg KG, et al. Resection of colorectal metastases: 25-year experience. World J Surg 1998;22:268–276.
27. Holm A, Bradley E, Aldrete JS. Hepatic resection of metastases from colorectal carcinoma. Morbidity, mortality, and pattern of recurrence. Ann Surg 1989;209:428–434.
28. Fong Y, Fortner J, Sun RL, et al. Clinical score for predicting recurrence after hepatic resection for metastatic colorectal cancer: analysis of 1001 consecutive cases. Ann Surg 1999;230:309–318.
29. Bismuth H, Adam R, Navarro F, et al. Re-resection for colorectal liver metastases. Surg Oncol Clin North Am 1996;5:353–364.
30. Nakamura S, Sakaguchi S, Nishiyama R, et al. Aggressive repeat liver resection for hepatic metastases of colorectal carcinoma. Surg Today 1992;22:260–264.
31. Ekberg H, Tranberg KG, Andersson R, et al. Determinants of survival in liver resection for colorectal secondaries. Br J Surg 1986;73:727–731.
32. El-Serag HB. Epidemiology of hepatocellular carcinoma. Clin Liver Dis 2001;5:87–107.
33. Bosch FX, Ribes J, Borras J. Epidemiology of primary liver cancer. Semin Liver Dis 1999;19:271–285.
34. El-Serag HB, Mason AC. Risk factors for the rising rates of primary liver cancer in the United States. Arch Intern Med 2000;160:3227–3230.
35. Chu CM. Natural history of chronic hepatitis B virus in adults with emphasis on the occurrence of cirrhosis and hepatocellular carcinoma. J Gastroenterol Hepatol 2000;15(suppl):E25–E30.
36. Colombo M. Hepatitis C virus and hepatocellular carcinoma. Semin Liver Dis 1999;19:263–269.
37. Ikeda K, Saitoh S, Suzuki Y, et al. Disease progression and hepatocellular carcinogenesis in patients with chronic viral hepatitis: a prospective observation of 2215 patients. J Hepatol 1998;28:930–938.
38. El-Serag HB, Mason AC, Key C. Trends in survival of patients with hepatocellular carcinoma between 1977 and 1996 in the United States. Hepatology 2001;33:62–65.
39. Nerenstone SR, Ihde DC, Freidman MA. Clinical trials in primary hepatocellular carcinoma: current status and future directions. Cancer Treat Rev 1988;15:1–31.
40. Heneghan MA, O'Grady JG. Liver transplantation of malignant liver disease. Ballieres Clin Gastroenterol 1999;13:575–591.
41. Patt YZ, Hassan NM, Lozano RD, et al. Durable clinical response of refractory hepatocellular carcinoma to orally administered thalidomide. Am J Clin Oncol 2000;23:319–321.
42. Kouroumalis E, Skordilis P, Thermos K, et al. Treatment of hepatocellular carcinoma with octreotide: a randomized controlled trial. Gut 1998;42:442–447.
43. Ahrar K, Gupta S. Hepatic artery embolization for hepatocellular carcinoma: technique, patient selection, and outcomes. Surg Oncol Clin North Am 2003;12:105–126.
44. Group d'Etude et de Traitement du Carcinome Hepatocellulaire. A comparison of ethiodized oil chemoembolization and conservative treatment for unresectable hepatocellular carcinoma. N Engl J Med 1995;332:1256–1261.
45. Bruix J, Llovet JM, Castells A, et al. Transarterial chemoembolization versus symptomatic treatment in patients with advanced hepatocellular carcinoma: results of a randomized controlled trial in a single institution. Hepatology 1998;27:1578–1583.
46. Nagorney DM, Gigot JF. Primary epithelial hepatic malignancies: etiology, epidemiology, and outcome after subtotal and total hepatic resection. Surg Oncol Clin North Am 1996;5:283–300.
47. Fong Y, Sun RL, Jarnigin W, Blumgart LH. An analysis of 412 cases of hepatocellular carcinoma at a Western center. Ann Surg 1999;229:790–799.
48. Belghiti J, Panis Y, Farges O, et al. Intrahepatic recurrence after resection of hepatocellular carcinoma complicating cirrhosis. Ann Surg 1991;214:114–117.
49. Ravikumar TS. Interstitial therapies for liver tumors. Surg Oncol Clin North Am 1996;5:365–377.
50. LeVeen RF. Laser hyperthermia and radiofrequency ablation of hepatic lesions. Semin Intervent Radiol 1997;14:313–324.
51. Siperstein A, Gitomirsky A. History and technological aspects of radiofrequency thermoablation. Cancer J 2000;6(suppl):S293–303.
52. Adson MA, van Heerden JA. Adson MH, et al. Resection of hepatic metastases from colorectal cancer. Arch Surg 1984;119:647–651.
53. Kane RA, Hughes LA, Cua EJ, et al. The impact of intraoperative ultrasonography on surgery for liver neoplasms. J Ultrasound Med 1994;13:1–6.
54. de Baere T, Bessoud B, Dromaine C. Percutaneous radiofrequency ablation of hepatic tumors during temporary hepatic venous occlusion. AJR 2002;178:53–59.
55. Curley SA, Izzo F, Delrio P, et al. Radiofrequency ablation of unresectable primary and

metastatic hepatic malignancies; results of 123 patients. Ann Surg 1999;230:1–11.
56. Scaife CL, Curley SA. Complication, local recurrence, and survival rates after radiofrequency ablation for hepatic malignancies. Surg Oncol Clin North Am 2003;12:243–255.
57. Livraghi T, Goldberg SN, Lazzaroni S, et al. Hepatocellular carcinoma: radiofrequency ablation of medium and large lesions. Radiology 2000;214:761–768.
58. Iannitti DA, Dupuy DE, Mayo-Smith WW, et al. Hepatic radiofrequency ablation. Arch Surg 2002;137:422–427.
59. Shafir M, Shapiro R, Sung M, et al. Cryoablation of unresectable malignant liver tumors. Am J Surg 1996;171:27–31.
60. Weaver ML, Ashton JG, Zemel R. Treatment of colorectal liver metastases by cryotherapy. Semin Surg Oncol 1998;14:163–170.
61. Tanden VR, Harmantas A, Gallinger S. Long-term survival after hepatic cryotherapy versus surgical resection for metastatic colorectal carcinoma: a critical review of the literature. Can J Surg 1997;40:175–181.
62. Ravikumar TS, Cady B, Jenkins R, et al. A 5-year study of cryosurgery in the treatment of liver tumors. Arch Surg 1991;126:1520–1524.
63. Zhou XD, Tang ZY, Yu YQ, et al. The role of cryosurgery in the treatment of hepatic cancer: a report of 113 cases. J Cancer Res Clin Oncol 1993;102:100–102.
64. Zhou XD, Tang ZY, Yu YQ. Ablative approach for primary liver cancer. Surg Oncol Clin North Am 1996;5:370–390.
65. Dupuy DE, Zagoria RJ, Akerley W, Mayo-Smith WW, Kavanaugh PV, Safran H. Percutaneous RF ablation of malignancies in the lung. AJR 2000; 174:57–60.
66. Jeffrey SS, Birdwell RL, Ikeda DM, et al. Radiofrequency ablation of breast cancer: first report of an emerging technology. Arch Surg 1999;134:1064–1068.
67. Gervais DA, McGovern FJ, Wood BJ, et al. Radio-frequency ablation of renal cell carcinoma: early clinical experience. Radiology 2000; 217:665–672.
68. Rossi S, Buscarini E, Garbagnati F, et al. Percutaneous treatment of small hepatic tumors by an expandable RF needle electrode. AJR 1998; 170(4):1015–1022.
69. Jiao LR, Hansen PD, Havlik R, et al. Clinical short-term results of radiofrequency ablation in primary and secondary liver tumors. Am J Surg 1999;177(4):303–306.
70. Solbiati L, Ierace T, Goldberg SN, et al. Percutaneous US-guided radiofrequency ablation of liver metastases: treatment and follow-up in 16 patients. Radiology 1997;202:195–203.
71. Francica G, Marone G. Ultrasound-guided percutaneous treatment of hepatocellular carcinoma by radiofrequency hyperthermia with a "cooled-tip needle." A preliminary clinical experience. Eur J Ultrasound 1999;9(2):145–153.
72. Solbiati L, Livraghi T, Goldberg, et al. Percutaneous radiofrequency ablation of hepatic metastases from colorectal cancer: long-term results in 117 patients. Radiology 2001;221:159–166.
73. Bilchik AJ, Wood TF, Allegra D, et al. Cryosurgical ablation and radiofrequency ablation for unresectable hepatic malignant neoplasms. Arch Surg 2000;135(6):657–662.
74. Jarnagin WR, Fong Y, Ky A, et al. Liver resection for metastatic colon cancer: assessing the risk of occult irresectable disease. J Am Coll Surg 1999; 188(1):33–42.
75. Kokudo N, Bandai Y, Imanishi H, et al. Management of new hepatic nodules detected by intraoperative ultrasonography during hepatic resection for hepatocellular carcinoma. Surgery 1996;119:634–640.
76. Lo CM, Lai ECS, Liu CL, et al. Laparoscopy and laparoscopic ultrasound avoid exploratory laparotomy in patients with hepatocellular carcinoma. Ann Surg 1998;227:527–532.
77. Shibata T, Iimuro Y, Ikai I, et al. Percutaneous radiofrequency ablation therapy after intrathoracic saline solution infusion for liver tumor in the hepatic dome. J Vasc Intervent Radiol 2002; 13(3):313–315.

41 Radiofrequency Tumor Ablation in Children

William E. Shiels II and Stephen D. Brown

Historical Perspective

Percutaneous image-guided radiofrequency (RF) tumor ablation continues to gain momentum in adult patients as a viable and effective therapeutic option in the treatment of solid tumors in a variety of locations including the skeleton, liver, spleen, kidney, adrenal gland, and lung (1–6). In all these areas, the basic concept of RF tumor ablation is similar: localized and contained heat generation systematically induces focal coagulative necrosis and cell death. Cytotoxicity is best induced when regional temperatures reach and maintain 50° to 100°C. In children, RF tumor ablation has been used most widely in the treatment of osteoid osteoma. Percutaneous RF ablation (RFA) has fewer indications in the pediatric population, and hence, has been slower to evolve in the treatment of diseases of the liver, kidney, lung, and soft tissues.

Application of RF energy in children has been most widely applied in the form of surgical Bovie electrocautery. It is generally considered that the nature and character of the coagulative necrotic reaction of the tissues to heating with RFA in infants and children is similar to that in adults. Historically, RFA of tissue has been performed in children for a variety of conditions. In pediatric cardiac electrophysiology laboratories, atrial and ventricular ablations using RF have been performed safely and effectively for many years (7–10). Reports in the otolaryngology literature have described using RFA to treat lingual lymphatic malformations and tonsillar hypertrophy in children (11,12). Recently, RF has been applied in utero to treat fetal sacrococcygeal teratomas as well as to occlude vessels in the umbilical cord and placenta in complications related to monochorionic pregnancies (13–16). Reports of RF tumor ablations in children have been limited predominantly to the musculoskeletal system and osteoid osteomas (2–4). Treatment of hepatoblastoma in children as young as 1 year old has been mentioned briefly in the literature (17). This chapter reviews details of unique care issues in percutaneous RFA in children with respect to general patient care concerns and organ-specific RFA applications. The general aspects of RF physics, tissue reaction, cellular dynamics, and instrumentation have been discussed in earlier chapters and are not addressed here.

Clinical Applications

General Procedural Issues

Although many adult percutaneous RFA procedures in organs such as the liver, lung, and kidney may be successfully performed in adults with conscious sedation, children are not tolerant of similar pain experiences. Thus, general anesthesia is required for most, if not all, RFA procedures. Even with liberal use of periosteal local anesthesia, patients still react to the pain of RF bone ablation if anesthesia is limited to deep sedation. Rosenthal et al (18) recently described the pain reaction in patients undergoing treatment of osteoid osteoma using general anesthesia; the pain caused elevations in cardiac and respiratory rates as biopsy needles entered the tumor. In our clinical experience, pain also can be significant enough to cause elevation in blood pressure and heart rate when the RFA heat reaches sensitive structures such as the pleura during RFA of the lung.

The use of prophylactic antibiotics is variable among authors and in specific tissue applications. Our experience, and that of other authors (2–4), demonstrates that RFA of osteoid osteomas is successfully performed without infectious complications in the absence of prophylactic antibiotics. Authors vary in the use of prophylactic antibiotics when treating focal hepatic and renal malignancies (2,5,6,19–21). In the liver, prophylactic antibiotics may be most appropriate in clinical situations such as severe cirrhosis, immunosuppression, concomitant infection, and biliary pathology that entail bile stasis, duct dilation, or earlier biliary bypass surgery. In a large multicenter experience, hepatic abscess was a complication in 0.3% of 2320 patients in whom 3554 liver lesions were treated with RFA (6). In our limited pediatric experience, we administer a single dose of preprocedural antibiotics when treating focal liver lesions, and, to date, none of our cases has been complicated by abscess formation or sepsis.

The potential for thermal skin burns exists with RFA due to heat distribution at the skin site of grounding pads used with monopolar RF systems. Thermal burns are best avoided with the use of large surface area foil grounding pads, placed with the longest surface edge facing the RF electrode, at a distance of 25 to 50 cm from the electrode (22). In adults, the thigh is often recommended as a good location for placement of four large (100 cm^2 each) foil pads. In young children, the thighs may be too small for placement of the large foil pads. As an alternative, the buttocks serve well as a large surface area placement site for the foil pads when RFA is performed in the upper body and trunk.

Young children present with smaller body surface areas than their adult counterparts. Given the relatively greater ratio of tumor volume to body surface area, the potential exists for greater total body heating effect when large surface areas are treated with RFA in children. In our experience, total body temperature elevation has not been encountered in the treatment of focal lesions such as osteoid osteoma or focal liver tumors. On the other hand, body core temperature elevation to as high as 40°C has been documented when treating large metastatic lung lesions, and has responded well to the use of a hypothermic blanket. When treating large-volume tumors (5- to 8-cm diameter), we routinely place the patient on a hypothermic blanket (Medi-Therm II; Gaymar, Orchard Park, NY) prior to beginning the RFA procedure. The use of a hypothermic blanket as cool as 20°C maintains body temperature at or below 38°C during prolonged RFA treatment of large volume tumors in the chest.

Pain control after treatment is a critical issue and Benign Bone Lesions in children that requires a plan for each specific organ system and lesion being treated with RFA. In the treatment of osteoid osteoma, intraprocedural local anesthesia is coupled with oral analgesics for effective pain control. In the liver and lung, pain from liver capsular and pleural distention usually requires the administration of intravenous narcotic analgesics for effective pain management. We have found that pain following RFA is greatest 12 to 24 hours following treatment in the liver and lung, due to accumulation of edema and subsequent increased ablation volume. The pain of postablation syndrome usually subsides after a few days, and is well managed with narcotic analgesia.

Osteoid Osteoma and Benign Bone Lesions

Osteoid osteoma treatment is the most common application for RFA in children. Lesions occur in both the axial and appendicular skeleton. Osteoid osteoma is a nonneoplastic localized inflammatory focus of eosinophils and histiocytes that causes intense recurrent bone pain. Prior to RFA of osteoid osteoma, treatment regimens included long-term use of nonsteroidal antiinflammatory drugs and surgical or percutaneous resection (2–4). Radiofrequency ablation therapy of osteoid osteoma can be curative in 90% to 94% of patients with a single treatment, and 100% of patients with two treatments (3,4).

In treating children with osteoid osteoma, general anesthesia is routinely used for RFA. Computed tomography is the imaging guidance modality of choice. Prior to RFA, biopsy specimens are obtained for histologic confirmation of the correct diagnosis, or to clarify an alternative diagnosis such as intracortical chondroma (23).

The biopsy needle serves as the guide for the RF electrode. In our experience, a 14-gauge coaxial bone biopsy needle (Ackerman; Cook, Bloomington, IN) may function well for the majority of the cases (Fig. 41.1). We have, on occasion, experienced difficulty passing a 17-gauge RF electrode through the coaxial 14-gauge needle lumen. As an alternative to the relatively tight fit of a 14/17-gauge coaxial needle/electrode system, an 11-gauge bone biopsy needle (M-1 or M-2; Cook, Bloomington, IN) provides excellent torque control for penetrating dense sclerotic bone, delivers a generous biopsy specimen for pathologic analysis, and avoids the potential of tight coupling friction of the guiding needle and electrode. Bupivacaine local anesthesia can be administered into the periosteum prior to biopsy and into the treatment site at the completion of RF treatment to best provide protracted local anesthesia and begin the pain management regimen.

Our current practice utilizes a 200-W RF generator (Radionics, Burlington, MA) with a single needle 17-gauge RF electrode, using either the 0.5- or 1.0-cm exposed tip, depending on the size of the treated lesion. After the biopsy is obtained, the outer cannula of the biopsy needle, then subsequently the RF electrode are placed into the center of the nidus and the biopsy cannula is retracted away from the electrode tip. Depending on the size of the lesion, one to two RFA applications are used, with each application providing heat to 90°C for 4 to 5 minutes. Following RFA, patients are discharged under an oral analgesic regimen for pain control. Pain typically subsides in 2 to 3 days. Relief of the osteoid osteoma pain usually occurs within 12 to 24 hours. The postprocedural pain is notably different from the original pain of the osteoid osteoma. Our experience with osteoid osteomas parallels that of other authors who have used RFA to provide an effective cure without complications, and to avoid surgical incisions and long-term convalescence (2–4). The authors have treated benign bone tumors such as chondroblastoma

A

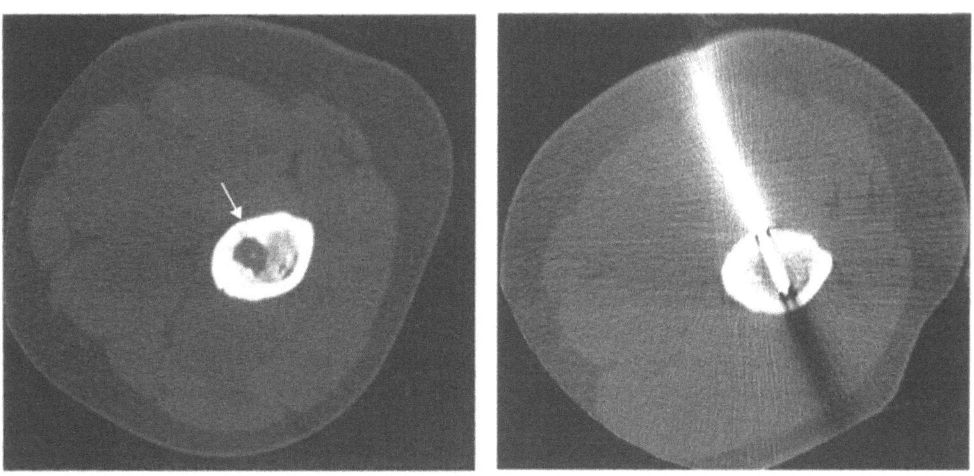

B

Figure 41.1. A 17-year-old boy with osteoid osteoma, treated with radiofrequency ablation, and then asymptomatic, with 18 months follow-up. (A) Computed tomography (CT) image of the right femoral osteoid osteoma nidus (arrow). (B) CT image during radiofrequency ablation (RFA) with the coaxial biopsy needle retracted and the RF electrode in the nidus.

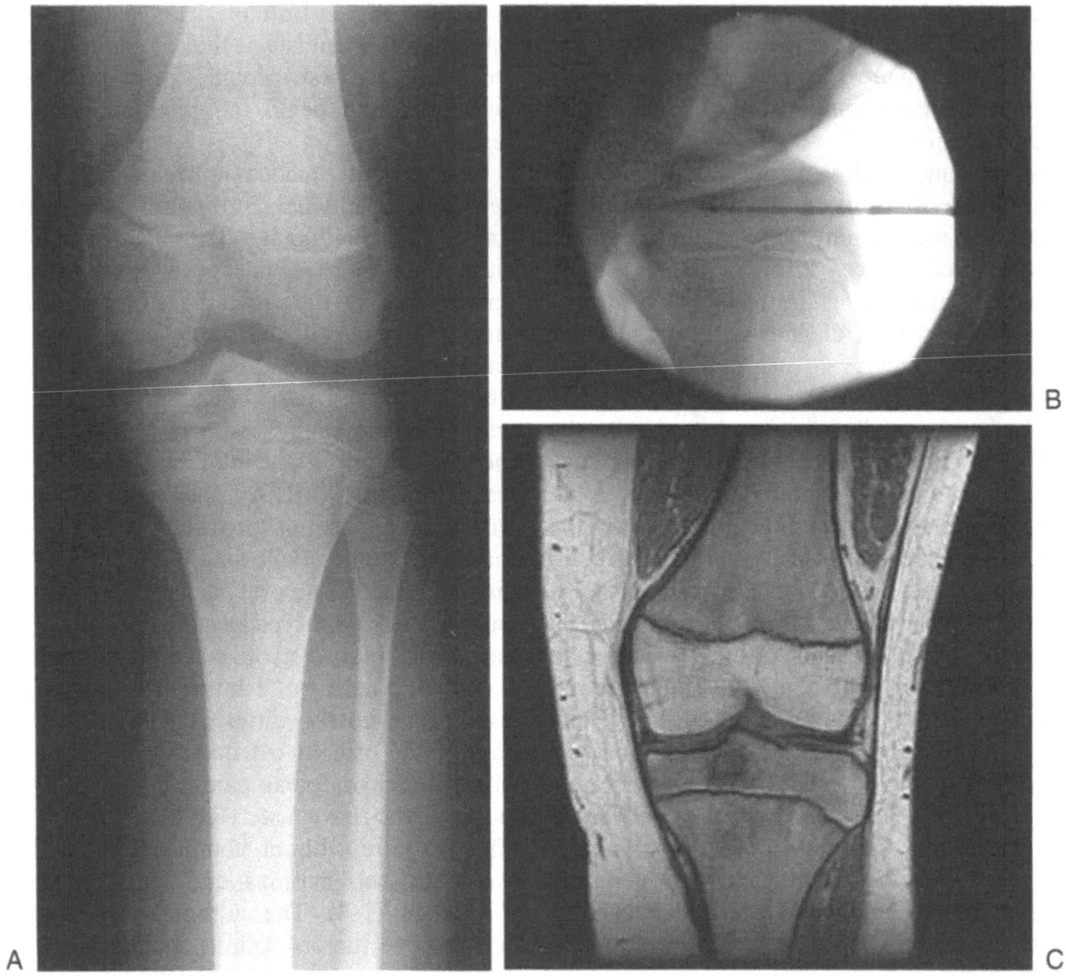

FIGURE 41.2. Eleven-year-old male with tibial chondroblastoma treated successfully with RF ablation. (A) Plain radiograph of the left knee showing the focal lytic chondroblastoma in the proximal tibial epiphysis. (B) Fluoroscopic spot film image during RF ablation procedure. (C) Follow-up MR image with no residual tumor and lack of injury to the articular cartilage.

(Fig. 41.2) with success, avoiding operative damage to articular cartilage and physis.

Hepatic Tumor Ablation

The majority of experience documented in adult hepatic tumor RFA is in the treatment of hepatocellular carcinoma or metastatic disease from organs such as the colon, lung, and breast (1,2,5,6). Treatment of hepatic tumors (hepatoblastoma) in children has been reported sporadically (17). In our clinical practice, focal liver tumors that have been treated with RFA include hepatoblastoma, hepatic adenoma, and metastatic leiomyosarcoma. Patients with hepatoblastoma who present the greatest clinical challenge are those with Beckwith-Wiedemann syndrome who develop multiple hepatoblastomas over time. Indeed, these are ideal candidates for RFA, given the risks of repeated surgeries for resection (Fig. 41.3). Hepatocellular carcinoma in our pediatric patients has presented with multiple lesions

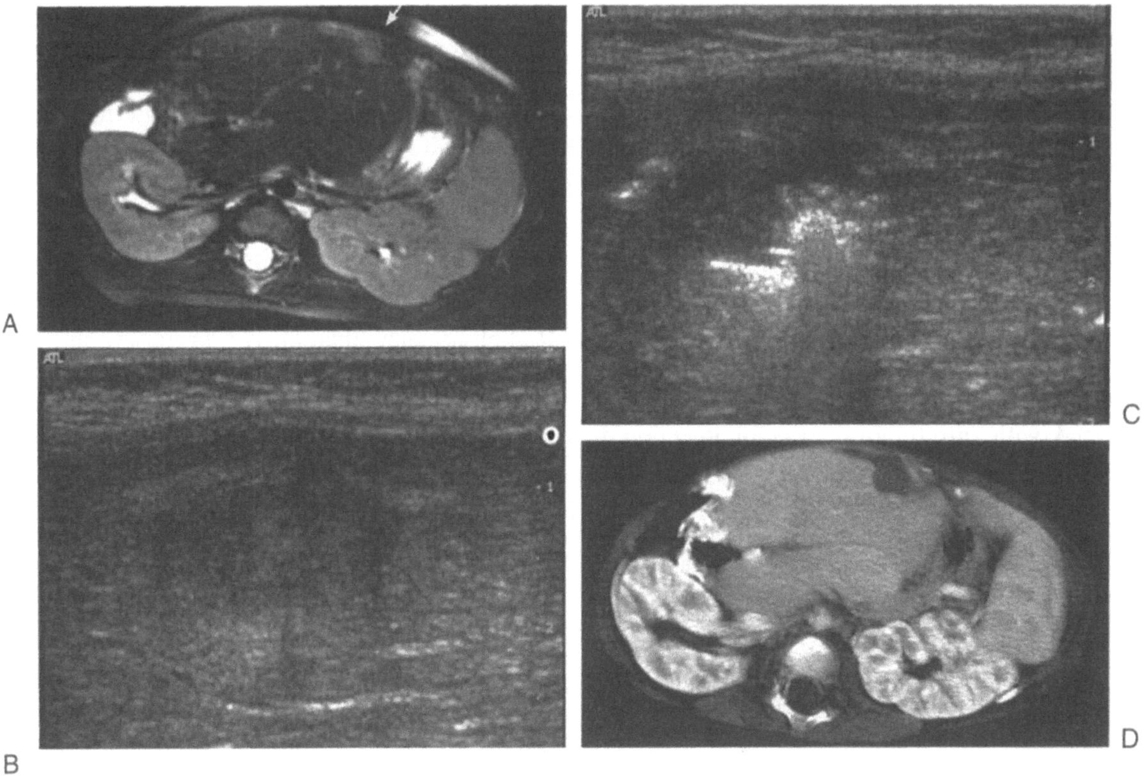

FIGURE 41.3. A 2-year-old boy with Beckwith-Wiedemann syndrome and focal hepatoblastoma, treated with RFA. Pretreatment magnetic resonance imaging (MRI) (A) and ultrasound (B) of the focal hepatoblastoma. (C) Sonogram during RFA with water-cooled electrode demonstrates echogenic RF coagulation necrosis in the tumor. (D) CT image at 1-month follow-up demonstrating complete ablation of the focal hepatoblastoma.

(more than four), precluding effective curative options with RFA. In these patients with large, multifocal tumor burden, either systemic chemotherapy or chemoembolization is considered to be a more appropriate treatment option.

General anesthesia is used for RFA of hepatic tumors in our patients. Single-dose prophylactic antibiotics are administered prior to the onset of RFA treatment. A percutaneous approach is used in the majority of hepatic tumor RFAs. Certain situations are performed more appropriately in an open surgical environment, particularly to avoid the potential for thermal damage and subsequent perforation in lesions next to the stomach, colon, gallbladder, or other hollow viscus (2). Recent experience has shown that in a small series of patients, RFA of hepatic tumors adjacent to the gallbladder may be performed successfully without major complications (24). In RFA treatment of pediatric liver tumors, we use a 200-W RF generator with internally cooled electrodes (Radionics; Burlington, MA), either as a single electrode or as a cluster of electrodes for larger lesions. Overlapping RFAs are performed, with each site reaching a target temperature of at least 60°C over 12 minutes.

In the treatment of focal liver tumors, the experience in children is currently small, as pediatric-unique guidelines are being developed. At the current time, the authors would apply guidelines similar to those in the adult literature, such that we can expect complete tumor ablation in 90% of patients with tumors smaller than 2.5 cm in diameter (2,5,25). Tumors that are 2.5 to 3.5 cm in diameter can be expected to be ablated in 70% to 90% of cases;

ablation of tumors that are >3.5 to 5.0cm in diameter will be seen in only 50% to 70% of cases. In large tumors (>3.5cm) and in conditions such as the Beckwith-Wiedemann syndrome with recurrent hepatoblastoma, palliation using RFA is a reasonable goal if treatment can prolong life expectancy with limited systemic symptoms and few minor complications. The volume of effective tumor ablation can be enlarged using hypertonic saline tumor pretreatment or combined chemoembolization (26,27). Most recently, a promising combination therapy technique has been developed with intratumoral ethanol injection in conjunction with RFA (28). In this technique, tumors that were injected with alcohol immediately prior to RFA resulted in consistently larger areas of ablation than tumors treated solely with RFA, with no increase in complications. Furthermore, RFA appears to potentiate the uniform distribution of alcohol in the tumors, which is a challenge in tumors treated with only ethanol injection. Benign hepatic lesions treated with RFA offer an alternative to partial hepatectomy (Fig. 41.4).

Lung and Renal Tumor Ablation

Radiofrequency ablation is a promising minimally invasive option for treatment of solid lung malignancies in children and adults (2,29). Unlike adults, children rarely present with primary solid malignancies of the lung. Furthermore, relative contraindications to surgery for lung tumors such as chronic obstructive pulmonary disease (COPD) are much less frequent in children than in adults. In our clinical

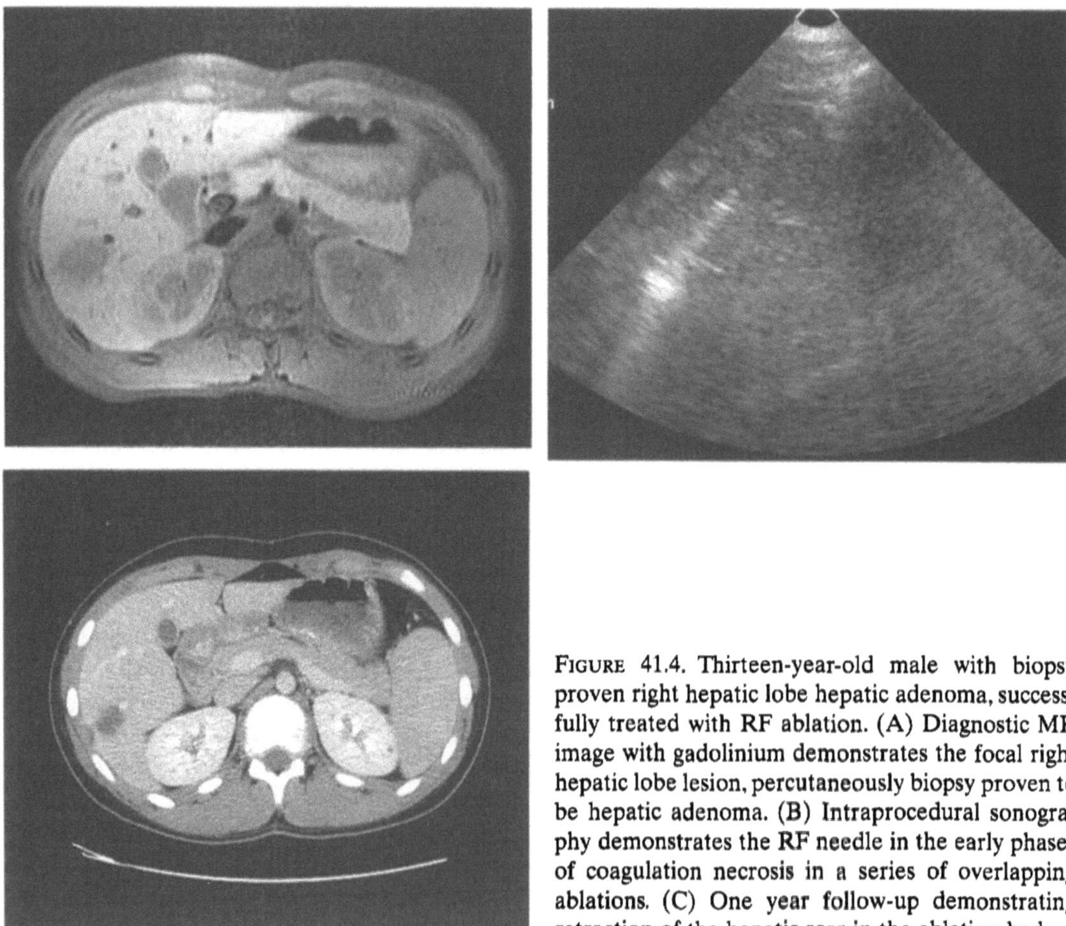
A B C

FIGURE 41.4. Thirteen-year-old male with biopsy proven right hepatic lobe hepatic adenoma, successfully treated with RF ablation. (A) Diagnostic MR image with gadolinium demonstrates the focal right hepatic lobe lesion, percutaneously biopsy proven to be hepatic adenoma. (B) Intraprocedural sonography demonstrates the RF needle in the early phases of coagulation necrosis in a series of overlapping ablations. (C) One year follow-up demonstrating retraction of the hepatic scar in the ablation bed.

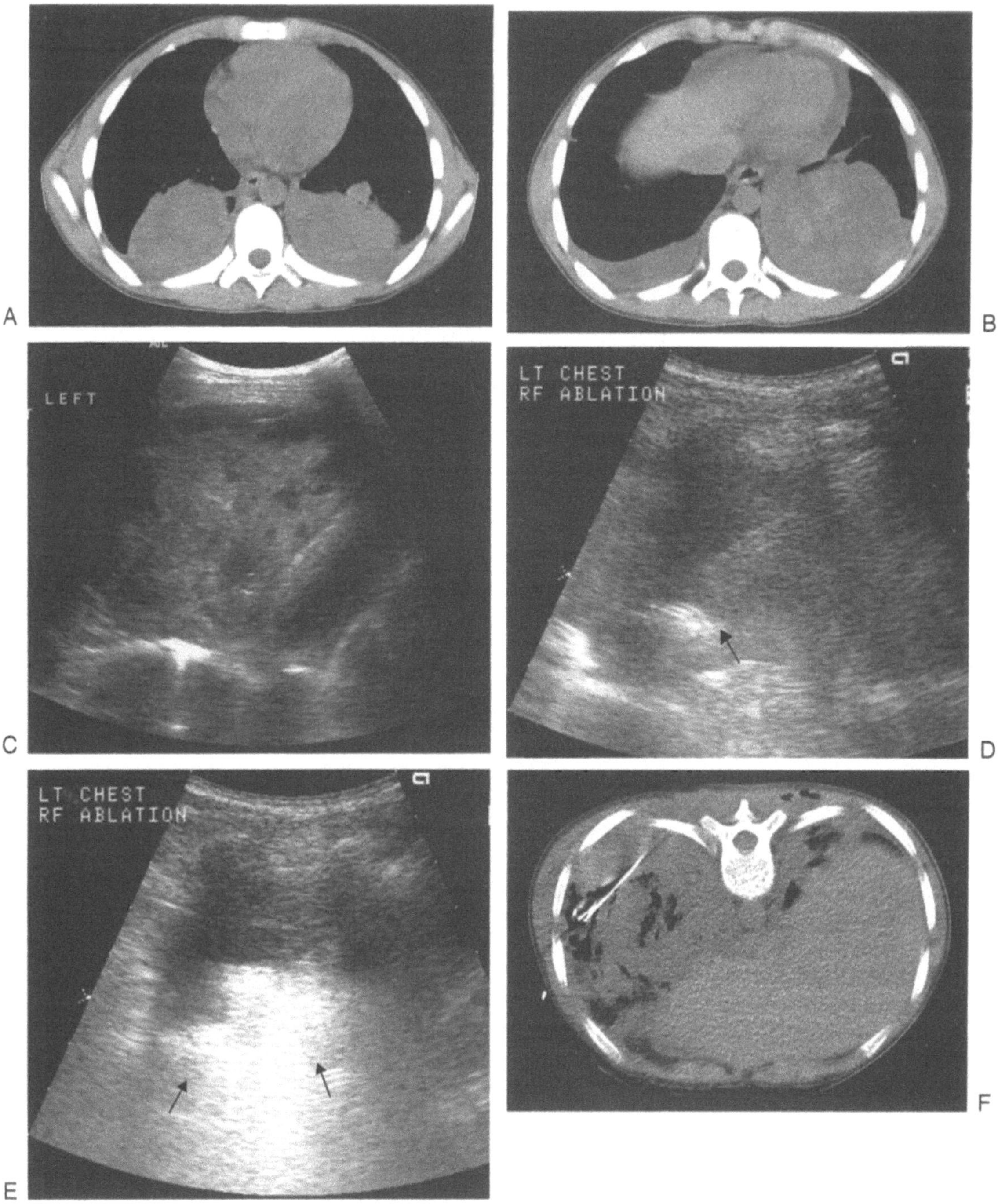

FIGURE 41.5. A 12-year-old boy undergoing palliative RFA for bilateral pulmonary metastatic osteosarcoma. (A,B) CT image of the chest demonstrating bilateral pulmonary metastatic lesions, measuring 5 cm (right) and 8 cm (left). (C) Sonogram of the osteosarcoma prior to RFA. (D) Sonogram during ultrasound (US)-guided RFA of the left metastatic lesion, demonstrating early echogenicity during RFA (arrow). (E) Sonogram in a later stage of RFA demonstrating large area of echogenicity and tumor coagulation (arrows). (F) Prone CT image during second palliative RFA session demonstrating significant bilateral cavitation during RFA.

experience, palliative RFA is currently, and will likely remain, the most frequent indication for lung tumor RFA in children. In the lung, our experience is limited to the treatment of metastatic osteogenic sarcoma in patients who are not operative candidates.

Internally cooled RF electrodes are used with a 200-W RF generator (Radionics; Burlington, MA). Large lesions are treated with a three-electrode cluster to achieve burns reaching a minimum target temperature of 60°C over 12 minutes. We have used both ultrasound and computed tomography (CT) guidance for lung RFA cases, with CT most useful when lung precludes an effective sonographic window. We have provided palliative RFA treatment for metastatic lesions as large as 8 cm (Fig. 41.3). The insulating effect of lung limits the extension of necrosis into adjacent tissue. In large bilateral tumor ablations, core body temperature elevations are maintained at 38° to 39°C with the use of a hypothermic blanket system (Medi-Therm II; Gaymar, Orchard Park, NY), with blanket cooling temperatures as low as 20°C. Our initial experience shows that RFA of pediatric lung lesions is well tolerated. Postprocedural pleuritic pain and nonproductive cough at 12 to 24 hours may occur, and usually last 2 to 3 days and are well managed with narcotic analgesia. Postprocedure fever may develop after 24 hours and lasts 2 to 3 days; blood cultures typically are negative. In palliative treatment of metastatic lung lesions, the tissue most resistant to ablation is adjacent to the heart and rib cage, likely due to the heat-sink effect in these two areas. Follow-up CT scans may demonstrate cavitation of the lesion without pneumothoraces.

Early experience with percutaneous RFA of solid renal masses is promising, with renal cell carcinoma associated with von Hippel–Lindau disease being the most frequent indication in children and young adults (19–21). In this experience, percutaneous RFA is well tolerated and provides an effective nephron-sparing alternative to surgery. This is particularly important with conditions such as von Hippel–Lindau disease, in which patients are predisposed to multifocal renal cell carcinoma. The recent literature has shown that RFA of renal lesions during renal artery balloon occlusion results in larger effective zones of ablation, but with a higher rate of infarction of normal renal tissue peripheral to the treated focus (30). Other pediatric populations that may benefit from RFA of renal masses include those patients with bilateral Wilm's tumor or nephroblastomatosis, or masses arising in solitary kidneys.

Conclusion

Radiofrequency tumor ablation in children is evolving rapidly and offers effective therapeutic options for a variety of pediatric disorders (31,32). Radiofrequency ablation is well tolerated in children and has few complications. As the pediatric experience grows, new opportunities for interdisciplinary treatment regimens that include RFA will develop, defining clear roles for this versatile minimally invasive therapy.

References

1. Goldberg SN, Dupuy DE. Image-guided radiofrequency tumor ablation: challenges and opportunities—part I. J Vasc Intervent Radiol 2001;12:1021–1032.
2. Dupuy DE, Goldberg SN. Image-guided radiofrequency tumor ablation: challenges and opportunities—part II. J Vasc Intervent Radiol 2001;12:1135–1148.
3. Rosenthal DI, Hornicek FJ, Wolfe MW, Jennings LC, Gephart MC, Mankin HJ. Changes in the management of osteoid osteoma. J Bone Joint Surg 1998;80:815–821.
4. Woertler K, Vestring T, Boettner F, Winkelmann W, Heindel W, Lindner N. Osteoid osteoma: CT-guided percutaneous radiofrequency ablation and follow-up in 47 patients. J Vasc Intervent Radiol 2001;12:717–722.
5. Ahmed M, Goldberg SN. Thermal ablation therapy for hepatocellular carcinoma. J Vasc Intervent Radiol 2002;13:S231–S243.
6. Livraghi T, Solbiati L, Meloni MF, Gazelle GS, Halpern EF, Goldberg SN. Treatment of focal liver tumors with percutaneous radiofrequency ablation: complications encountered in a multicenter study. Radiology 2003;226:441–451.

7. Campbell RM, Strieper MJ, Frias PA, Danford DA, Kugler JD. Current status of radiofrequency ablation for common pediatric supraventricular tachycardias. J Pediatr 2002;140:150–155.
8. Hsieh IC, Yeh SJ, Wen MS, Wang CC, Lin FC, Wu D. Radiofrequency ablation for supraventricular and ventricular tachycardia in young patients. Int J Cardiol 1996;54:33–40.
9. Manolis AS, Vassilikos V, Maounis TN, Chiladakis J, Cokkinos DV. Radiofrequency ablation in pediatric and adult patients: comparative results. J Intervent Cardiol Electrophysiol 2001;5:443–453.
10. Van Hare GF, Dubin AM, Collins KK. Invasive electrophysiology in children: state of the art. J Electrocardiol 2002;35 (suppl):165–174.
11. Cable BB, Mair EA. Radiofrequency ablation of lymphangiomatous macroglossia. Laryngoscope 2001;111:1859–1861.
12. Plant RL. Radiofrequency treatment of tonsillar hypertrophy. Laryngoscope 2002;112:20–22.
13. Tsao K, Feldstein VA, Albanese CT, et al. Selective reduction of a cardiac twin by radiofrequency ablation. Am J Obstet Gynecol 2002; 187:635–640.
14. Sydorak RM, Feldstein V, Machin G, et al. Fetoscopic treatment for discordant twins. J Pediatr Surg 2002;37:1736–1739.
15. Lam YH, Tang MH, Shek TW. Thermocoagulation of fetal sacrococcygeal teratoma. Prenat Diagn 2002;22:99–101.
16. Paek BW, Jennings RW, Harrison MR, et al. Radiofrequency ablation of human fetal sacrococcygeal teratoma. Am J Obstet Gynecol 2001; 184:503–507.
17. Iannitti DA, Dupuy DE, Mayo-Smith WW, Murphy B. Hepatic radiofrequency ablation. Arch Surg 2002;137:422–426; discussion 427.
18. Rosenthal DI, Marota JJ, Hornicek FJ. Osteoid osteoma: elevation of cardiac and respiratory rates at biopsy needle entry into tumor in 10 patients. Radiology 2003;226:125–128.
19. Gervais DA, McGovern FJ, Arellano RS, McDougal WS, Mueller PR. Renal cell carcinoma: cliniical experience and technical success with radiofrequency ablation of 42 tumors. Radiology 2003;226:417–424.
20. Gervais DA, McGovern FJ, Wood BJ, et al. Radiofrequency ablation of renal cell carcinoma: early clinical experience. Radiology 2000;217: 665–672.
21. Roy-Choudhury SH, Cast JE, Cooksey G, Puri S, Breen DJ. Early experience with radiofrequency ablation of small solid renal masses. AJR 2003; 180:1055–1061.
22. Goldberg SN, Solbiati L, Halpern EF, Gazelle GS. Variables affecting proper system grounding for radiofrequency ablation in an animal model. J Vasc Intervent Radiol 2000;11:1069–1075.
23. Ramnath RR, Rosenthal DI, Cates J, Gebhardt M, Quinn RH. Intracortical chondroma simulating osteoid osteoma treated by radiofrequency. Skeletal Radiol 2002;31(10):597–602.
24. Chopra S, Dodd GD, Chanin MP, Chintapalli KN. Radiofrequency ablation of hepatic tumors adjacent to the gallbladder: feasibility and safety. AJR 2003;180:697–701.
25. Livraghi T, Lazzaroni S, Meloni MF. Radiofrequency thermal ablation of hepatocellular carcinoma. Eur J Ultrasound 2001;13:159–166.
26. Ahmed M, Lobo SM, Weinstein J, et al. Improved coagulation with saline solution pretreatment during radiofrequency tumor ablation in a canine model. J Vasc Intervent Radiol 2002; 13:717–724.
27. Bloomston M, Binitie O, Fraiji E, et al. Transcatheter arterial chemoembolization with or without radiofrequency ablation in the management of patients with advanced hepatic malignancy. Am Surg 2002;68:827–831.
28. Shankar S, vanSonnenberg E, Morrison PR, Tuncali KT, Silverman SG. Combined radiofrequency and direct alcohol infusion for percutaneous tumor ablation. AJR 2004;183:1425–1429.
29. Dupuy DE, Zagoria RJ, Akerley W, Mayo-Smith WM, Kavanagh PV, Safran H. Percutaneous radiofrequency ablation of malignancies in the lung. AJR 2000;174:57–59.
30. Kariya Z, Yamakado K, Nakatuka A, Onaoda M, Kobayasi S, Takeda K. Radiofrequency ablation with and without balloon occlusion of the renal artery: an experimental study in porcine kidneys. J Vasc Intervent Radiol 2003;14:241–245.
31. Hoffer FA. Pediatric applications of radiofrequency ablation. Sem Interv Radiol 2003;20: 323–331.
32. Hoffer FA. Biopsy, needle localization, and radiofrequency ablation for pediatric patients. Tech Vasc Interv Radiol 2004;6:192–196.

42
Comments from Patients and Their Families

Eric vanSonnenberg

Introduction

To round out the comprehensive ablation story, we thought who better to tell it than the patients and families themselves. Finding the initial few patients whom we broached the idea to contribute to be receptive, if not enthusiastic, we decided to include a whole chapter devoted to this perspective on ablation. Thus included are the views on ablation from six patients (with family input). We asked the patients to be candid, and edited and redacted only names to ensure privacy.

Patient: RR

Dr. vanSonnenberg asked me if I, as his patient, would contribute my thoughts in this text. I was very pleased that he asked. I feel that the ablation procedure, a minimally invasive treatment, has certainly extended my life. Of course, I cannot be considered in remission for five more years. But, according to what I have learned, I have a reasonable possibility of living a complete life span.

I am a male patient at Dana-Farber Cancer Institute, 73 years of age, generally in good health, slightly overweight, and I exercise almost every day. Incidentally, my father, at this writing, is still alive at 101 years of age. I'm trying to catch up with him.

It started when I received a phone call from my primary care physician. He said: "Bob, there was blood in two of the fecal samples that you mailed in. I have scheduled you for a colonoscopy." How can that be? I had a sigmoidoscopy only three years earlier. I had watched the monitor and heard the doctor say, "It's clean and pink. Looks good." I had every right to think that the sigmoidoscopy gave me a clean bill of health, didn't I?

I went in for the colonoscopy that was scheduled. I was nervous. Was blood in the stool serious? Again, I chose to watch the monitor. I saw the probe stop and I could see that there was "something" that didn't seem to belong there. I asked the doctor if he found something. The answer was, "Yes, but you are not in a condition right now for me to discuss it with you. We will wait a little while until the sedative wears off. Then we will review our findings."

Later my wife and I and the doctors sat down to discuss the findings. The doctor said to me, "You have colon cancer." I felt as though I was hit in the face with a sledgehammer! "We suggest that you consider surgery very soon." Another sledgehammer! Now I was scared! The surgeon explained what needed to be done. Evidently, she had watched the monitor during the procedure. She said that the tumor had penetrated the colon wall, and that several of the lymph nodes were involved. Another sledgehammer! The news got worse with every passing moment. Why me? I eat the proper foods. I work out at the gym almost every day. Why me?

We scheduled the surgery right then. I was scheduled for the next day. Instead of going home I went to Pre-Op for preparation. She operated the next morning.

More bad news the next day, after the colectomy. She told me that there were indications that the cancer had spread to my liver. However, before the liver surgery was scheduled, a chest x-ray showed a series of spots on my right lung. More testing was not conclusive. So, thoracic surgery was scheduled for August.

I was scheduled for the liver surgery one month later. Please note that I glossed over a rather difficult recovery due to an infection in, or around, the colon. I could not have food so I was fed intravenously. Needle biopsies and numerous other tests were done to determine the cause of the infection. After a while, I was given some light food. That turned out to be a mistake and they had to pump out my stomach. Not too pleasant.

I was scheduled for surgery on the liver at the appropriate time. A positron emission tomography (PET) scan indicated that there were three tumors in the liver. My wife told me afterward that she thought that everything had gone well, because the surgical procedure lasted over three hours. Unfortunately, that was not the case.

The liver surgeon spoke to my wife when he came out of the operating amphitheater. He told her that he could not do anything for me. He discovered that two of the tumors were too close to major blood vessels and that another one of the tumors was too small to locate. He told us that if he accidentally cut one of the blood vessels it would be very serious and potentially fatal. My wife then asked why the operation had taken so long. The surgeon told us that, during the procedure, he had called in two other surgeons to ascertain if they had any suggestions for removing the tumors. They didn't.

My oncologist told me that the chemotherapy was controlling the cancer cells and that they had shrunk almost in half. But to me the future looked bleak. Very bleak. Then he told me that there was a new technique. Sign me up! It sounded like a potential alternative to an almost certain slow and possibly painful end.

My closest friend was diagnosed with colon cancer a few weeks before I was. His brother and his daughter were both physicians. They researched various techniques used to destroy tumors. One of the methods was called ablation. My friend, Stu, and I spoke two or three times a week and compared notes. He provided me with a paper from *Imaging and Therapeutic Technology* (RSNA, RG volume 20, number 1, January–February 2000). The information was from numerous national and international universities. It gave me a little insight as to what Dr. Eric vanSonnenberg does. Not being a physician, there were many technical words and phrases that I did not understand in the paper. But I did get a little understanding about the procedure and it was apparently low risk.

However, I did know that the most effective way to eliminate cancer tumors was to surgically remove them. That was confirmed in the paper. But, only a percentage of cancers could be removed surgically. This, also, was confirmed in the text. The paper said that in only one in three cases would ablation be feasible. I was the one in three. I was very scared, but I felt that having the ablation done could not be any worse than doing nothing other than chemotherapy.

Finally the day came. I went into the hospital still not really knowing what to expect. I had recent memories of the difficulty after the liver surgery. I had trouble sitting up because the muscles had been surgically cut. It took a while before they were restored. What would be the results of this new ablation procedure? Will it cure my cancer? What are the aftereffects? What are the risks?

My first ablation procedure was done on October 31, 2000. When I woke, in the recovery room, surprisingly, I felt great! No pain! I was told that I would spend the night in the hospital. However, the next day, after a test and a computed tomography (CT) scan, I could go home. It sounded too good to be true. It was true. I went home the next day and I went back to work in a few days. I felt fine. No pain. Minor bandage. To me it was incredible. At one time my oncologist said that they were constantly working on new technology—something like Star Wars.

It would be some months before we would know the results of that ablation. The burns would have to heal before the PET scan and other tests could be done.

In May 2001, a PET scan and CT scan detected a tumor in my right lung. The new technology, the PET scan, discovered the very small tumor in my lung. Dr. vanSonnenberg contemplated using the ablation technique on the lung. However, he considered the risks and decided that surgery would be a safer procedure. I assumed that there was not enough information or experience to proceed with an ablation on the lung.

On June 15, 2001, the second thoracic surgery was performed. That, also, had limited success. Again, a surgeon was not able to get the entire cuff around the cell. So, I experienced a month of radiation on the lung. This was to complete the attack on the cuff.

In September of 2001, I was surveyed, again, by a PET scan and a CT scan. I was told that there was a possibility that the tumors had re-appeared. But, Dr. Fuchs, my oncologist reassured me, that one cell was the one that they originally could not see and the other was a recurrence at the site of one that had been ablated. Dr. vanSonnenberg, at that time, could not take a complete circumferential cuff because of the proximity of a major blood vessel. An extensive needle biopsy was performed, I assume, to confirm the existence of the cells and to verify the type.

So, a second ablation procedure was scheduled for August 22, 2002. From this patient's point of view my trepidation was significantly lower. I definitely felt more confident. My experiences with surgery versus the ablation procedure left me with a great deal of confidence in the ablation technique. My confidence was justified. The recovery was the same as before. . . . a "piece of cake."

When I spoke with Dr. vanSonnenberg afterward, he said that he was not positive that he was able to ablate a sufficient cuff around the small tumor. He said that it was extremely close to my diaphragm. There could be serious results if it was damaged. I asked the doctor what would happen if a tumor reappeared at that site. He said, simply: "We'll go in again." That did not frighten me at all.

Patient and Wife: DM and BM

The Patient's Wife

I am the patient's wife. We have been married since 1975, and our son, Jonathan was born in 1983. I was 37 when our son was born, and my husband was 40. I am now 56. I am an architect for the U.S. Courts, reviewing large projects and designing smaller ones. It is an ideal job for me, and I hope to continue working at it for at least another 10 years. Our son has just started college, at Cornell University, and we will be faced with large expenses for some time.

I have always considered my husband the healthy spouse: not overweight, athletic, with much physical energy. Therefore, it was a terrific shock when he was initially diagnosed with colon cancer in 1995. We were in the process of interviewing prep schools for our son, and it was very difficult to maintain a calm and cheerful demeanor. However, his surgery was considered successful, and I made the incorrect assumption that any future cancers would occur in his colon and could easily be removed, much as the first had been. I knew about the statistics of metastases, but the percentages given to us for recurrence were comfortably low, especially for a cancer that had been identified in its early stages, as his had. I know now that the statistics are skewed, because metastases occur much more frequently in men than in women. I think that oncologists should tell their patients this.

When we went to Europe in 1997, we already had indications that something was amiss: his carcinoembryonic antigen (CEA) levels had been rising. Our oncologist was very watchful, and when the recurrence was confirmed in 1998, she started him immediately on standard chemotherapy. Oddly enough, the physician we consulted with for a second opinion at the Dana-Farber Cancer Institute said that she believed in starting treatments only when the cancer became symptomatic. It is difficult for laypersons to know which approach to choose. There does seem to be an enormous burden on the patient and family to do their own research and plot their own treatment; this has so far worked for us, as we are well-educated people, living in the Boston area (which has major medical institutions), and we have Internet access. But even we do not know if we have access to all available information.

I found out about the results of the conclusive CT scan when I was at a meeting in Providence, R.I. I have no idea how I got home that afternoon. I screamed for some time, and my husband comforted me, then somehow we got into the car to pick up our son at summer camp. I cried on and off for several weeks, but the human spirit is very resilient. Soon, life developed a new routine—treatments and recovering from treatments. But the grief did affect me at work; one day, after a shouting match with a colleague, I called my doctor and headed over to her office. She prescribed Zoloft, clonazepam, and trazodone. I think these drugs have saved my life.

The first approach to controlling the metastases was radiation therapy; it produced good effects, and most of all it was successful, in my mind, because it introduced us to Dr. Anthony Howes, who spoke honestly but optimistically of all the research and treatments that were coming online. The first round of chemotherapy, 5-fluorouracil (5-FU) with leucovorin, produced few bad side effects, and life continued as usual. The second drug, irinotecan, was more invasive, causing hair loss, diarrhea, and the inability to taste food. Each time, we were given no idea how long the positive effects of the treatment would be. Whether this was done so as not to scare us, or because different patients react differently, we did not learn. My husband kept working as an architect throughout this ordeal, arranging his treatments for Friday afternoons so that he could go home immediately afterward. I went with him to the first few, but soon it became routine, and we both felt better about letting him go alone. When the second round of chemo stopped being effective, his oncologist remained optimistic (at least outwardly), and sent him to Dana-Farber to speak with Dr. vanSonnenberg and Dr. Enzinger. Dr. Enzinger recommended that he have the ablation and then return to him for discussion of other treatments.

It was in the time span during which the first ablation was delayed, due to an insurance nightmare, that we began reading about the drug C-225 in newspapers and the popular magazine *Science News*. We telephoned our primary oncologist, and asked if she thought he would qualify for the upcoming trials to be held in Boston and several other cities in the U.S. She verified that he would qualify with Dr. Enzinger. Dr. Enzinger cheered us along as my husband went through a trial of C-225, and apparently had above-average positive results. It is important here to note that it was my husband and I who approached the doctor with questions about the availability of such a trial; no one suggested it to us. As I have said, we had an insurance nightmare during which a lengthy battle ensued, which is described below, but the upshot was that the local BCBS (Federal Employees Service) had not even approached the government agency, OPM, that rules on allowed procedures, but had assumed it was experimental. My husband wrote a brilliant letter, with the help of his physicians, proving that it was not at all experimental. It is a terrible health insurance system that is in place in this country, and it is heartbreaking that it punishes the people with the least amount of spare energy to fight for their treatment.

Now we are considering phase I trials, but my hopes are with continued radiofrequency ablations (RFAs). He is healthy and looks as good as he ever has; everyone comments on it. I like to think that our love and my ability to make him laugh will keep him alive. I have never loved him more.

I have not spoken about our son and his dealings with his father's potentially fatal illness. I know it has affected him deeply, and he has been able to work some of that out in his writing and his art. He argues with his father, which is normal, and I resist the strong impulse to tell him that he may regret his harsh words sooner than he thinks.

The Patient

I asked myself, "Why, when Dr. vanSonnenberg asked me to discuss the goals I had for the ablation, did I sit dumbfounded?" It was early August 2002, one day after my 59th birthday, and two weeks after I had left the Brigham and Women's Hospital, mostly recovered from my second radiofrequency ablation, this time for two large tumors in my liver. Was it not obvious to everyone that I wanted to continue living? Was this not the goal? Or did I not answer because I felt it too presumptuous to have goals? Maybe I could have adopted the posture of the boardroom executive and announced, "Yes! By 2003 we want to be tumor free!"

A more truthful explanation might be that I simply did not think of a specific goal for my ablation. I have metastases from colon cancer, which first became evident two years after the surgery that removed the original tumor and a section of my colon. This was, now, almost seven years ago. After four years of chemotherapy, perhaps I had become too suspicious of goals. Maybe my family and I had been through the success/failure or happiness/sadness cycle of chemotherapy so many times that the confidence to set goals eluded me, because so often one can only wait for the next CT scan to see if treatment has had any effect on the tumors. One is grateful if one can make it from CT scan to CT scan without suffering greatly from some of the side effects of the drugs. In this way, one gradually loses one's sense of reality, or the awareness and alertness that comes with knowing that one is actually in a continual battle with a terrorist. So, I simply muttered something about how I didn't know how successful the procedure had been, as if I could have established a goal after the fact, and in my shyness, like the student who has not done his homework, blurted out something that might have been consistent with the results.

Initially I had learned of RFA casually, while attending a seasonal cocktail party at the home of Dr. Peter Mueller and his wife Dr. Susan Mueller with whom my wife and I had become friends, since our sons were classmates and baseball teammates in high school. At this time, I didn't know I would be a future candidate for the procedure, and I listened as Peter, who was unaware that I had cancer, described some of his work to another guest. Later, my oncologist informed me that the conventional chemotherapy drugs I had been receiving were no longer working. In the brief time that elapsed between this disappointing news and her telling me about RFA, I had begun to feel the grip of despair. She mentioned another patient who was helped by RFA. Helped how much? I didn't ask. I knew it wouldn't necessarily be the same for me, and, should it have been the case, I didn't want to hear any stories about how the operation had been successful but the patient had died. I telephoned Peter to inform him that I would be having an appointment with Dr. vanSonnenberg, who he then informed me was an old friend. Even though Dr. Mueller, by this time, had elucidated some of the uses for RFA, the idea of using high-frequency radio waves still seemed fantastic to me and I went to my first meeting with Dr. vanSonnenberg and his assistant, Dr. Shankar, in awe, thinking that if I were a candidate for this procedure, it would be my last hope. They explained in detail the process and equipment used, the risks, the preparation required, an estimate of the amount of total tumor they thought could be killed, and the recovery. Immediately I thought there would be tumor remaining that could continue to grow, but felt reassured to hear that the process could be repeated. The thought of the risks was sobering, partly because of the location of the tumors in my specific case. However, their track record was excellent, and I felt I needed to have confidence in their experience. I wanted this to work and did not think twice about doing it due to the risks.

The night before my first ablation was to take place Dr. vanSonnenberg's assistant, Dr. Shankar, telephoned me to say that our insurance company had denied coverage of the operation. He was hopeful that the situation would reverse itself and indicated that this would most likely happen once the insurance company had received further clarification from the hospital. Surely, it would be resolved by the end of the week. I became depressed, and during subsequent calls from the doctor later in the week, I remained motionless in the lounge chair while he and my wife discussed the situation further. The thought of the insurance company's waiting until the "midnight hour" to pass along this news was upsetting and foreboding. The next day, the insurance company telephoned and sent a letter to inform me of the denial of coverage and to inform me of my right to appeal their decision. I composed a lengthy appeal letter with the support of all of my cancer doctors, who had given advice on the use of RFA, and Mr. William McMullen of the Dana-Farber Cancer Institute. Along with a letter on my behalf from Dr. vanSonnenberg, we then sent this in to the appeals office of the insurance company. The appeal was denied. My wife and I evaluated our options. Since our family health insurance is purchased through her employer, we naively thought that my switching to a different insurance company, one that *would* provide coverage, would solve the problem. After making a few inquiries we came to understand three things:

1. Switching, in Massachusetts, could be accomplished only during a specific time period each year, and we were not in that "window" of time.
2. Other insurance company spokesmen either did not know if their company covered RFA or were not at liberty to say.
3. It was illegal to change insurance companies in Massachusetts, if you were insured through your spouse's insurance plan at work.

I was beginning to understand what people mean when they say there is something wrong with the system. So what happened to create the situation that allows me to discuss my ablations? My wife gives some details in her section. We were informed after losing the appeal at the local level that we still had the option of appealing to a higher level in Washington, D.C. I am happy to say the higher level appeal was successful.

If you want to have an ablation you must first have a magnetic resonance imaging (MRI) scan. One is required before the ablation, and one afterward. This is the main task required of the patient, and one that I must approach with a dauntless and focused attitude. For me, the MRI experience is simply an extension of the feeling of incarceration that gradually comes over one as one enters the hospital. Why incarceration? Because as you enter the environment of the hospital you must gradually surrender so much, beginning with the beautiful day, and descend into the mysterious underground environment of the building. One might arrive first at a subterranean waiting room with a television as the only link to the outside world, then be transferred to a smaller waiting room with magazines as the only link. At this point one is asked to change into patients' clothing, and after a brief wait is led down an interior corridor to a room resembling a kitchenette where a large padded chair awaits among various pieces of emergency equipment and apparatus. You sit in the chair, have an intravenous device inserted in your arm, and then are escorted to the room that houses the MRI machine. The machine looks like an enormous square, shiny, white metal doughnut standing maybe seven or eight feet high, five feet wide, and perhaps six feet deep. The doughnut hole diameter is about the dimension of my body measured across from elbow to elbow (I am an average-size American male, about 5 ft. 10 in.), and is located in the middle of the machine about three feet above the floor. A padded stretcher resembling a cupped surf board is positioned on a track and centered on the hole. The stretcher movement is controlled by electricity, and when activated, can move into and out of the hole in the doughnut with you on it in a supine position. I have always gone in feet first on my back. This is when you arrive at one of those moments in your life for which you have had no preparation. This is when you lie, flat and straight, in the tube (which is the physical presence represented by the hole on the exterior) with tubes attached to your intravenous device trailing down the tube and out the hole, with ear plugs fitted snugly in each ear, with both arms held tightly against your body, strapped in tightly so as to prevent movement, and find out, if you didn't previously know, if you are claustrophobic.

My first time in the MRI machine was with my eyes open. The inside of the tunnel has tiny lamps fitted to the top of the tube in positions that seemed to me to be similar to those in an airliner. So, if you can imagine yourself as being very tiny, it is almost like what you might see upon waking aboard a night flight to Europe. It wasn't until I began having subsequent MRIs that I began to feel panic about being confined even though the total time in the tube for me was only about fifteen minutes. After talking about this feeling with Dr. vanSonnenberg, he suggested that I close my eyes for the duration in the tube, which I have been doing lately and this technique combined with counting the number of times the magnet is turned on (which I have memorized from having done this about five times) in the process of making the image, allows me to make it through the experience with no panic. The technician, who operates the machine, and with whom one must communicate by way of built-in microphone and speaker, can make a great difference in one's disposition while inside. A few with cheerful dispositions are very good at this, by reassuring the patient and constantly keeping him or her informed about what is happening or how much is left to do.

Preparing for the ablation is exactly the same, except one is escorted not to the MRI machine but to a CT scan machine. This machine is similar in appearance to the MRI machine, yet not nearly as large, and the doughnut hole is larger, with no appreciable tube. Consequently, when one begins to enter the hole, which is done head first in this machine, one quickly exits the other side. The CT scan machine is used extensively in planning the trajectory of the RFA probe that punctures the skin and enters the organ and tumor, and in revealing its precise location. The patient is anesthetized for the duration of the procedure, which can vary in time with the amount of work to be done. In my case, this was about three hours for the first ablation and five-and-a-half hours for the second.

Recovery from the procedure is the same as it would be for any surgical operation. After my first ablation, I was wheeled to the recovery area, then to the MRI machine, and then to a room for an overnight stay. My roommate was a man perhaps ten to fifteen years older than I and talkative. After expressing some initial curiosity, he gave up on me once I told him it was painful for me to talk, but not before each of us had agreed to come to the rescue of the other in the event of an emergency by using the call button to signal the nurse. He was a veteran. After the second ablation, I was sent to a cardiac floor after the initial time in the recovery area, then sent to the MRI sometime within the next two days after the doctors were satisfied that I was not having any cardiac issues. My roommate this time was an unpleasant, belligerent person, about the same age as the first roommate. This one was not, I'm convinced, aware of my presence. He kept his TV on all night long, woke up shouting during the middle of the night, had some sort of psychotic fit, and had to be restrained in his bed with straps. He was hospitalized for a broken leg, which I thought explained his presence (but this was the cardiac floor) and the entourage of loud obsequious female orderlies. Ostensibly present to help him change position and use the bed pan, they responded in equal lewdness to all of his rancorous remarks and generally enjoyed themselves as if they were at a garden party. I pressed frantically on the call button, which was out of order. The hospital, on this occasion, was hell.

After each of my ablations, and a period of recovery, I have returned to Dana-Farber for a follow-up appointment with Dr. vanSonnenberg in the radiology area. Each time he has led me deep into the area behind the front desk and into the room where the radiologists sit before their computer screens and analyze the images transferred electronically from CT scan machines. Since the machine is used extensively in locating the probes that must be inserted in the tumor, it is possible with computer software, which links all of the slice-like images taken by the CT scan machine, to scroll through an image of the entire body (only the abdomen in my case) as if you were looking at a series of cross sections. Imagine ordering some sliced roast beef at the deli, which is then reassembled as a whole as you view each piece. Sitting side by side with Dr. vanSonnenberg, we reviewed the images of before and after. As he began typing in commands on the keyboard I secretly wondered if I would become queasy when looking at my own body this way, but when the images finally came up on the screen my fear gave way to fascination. I would ask, "What is that?" He would reply, "That's bone," or "This is dead tumor here, that's what we want," or "These white spots here are your gallstones," or "This dark area here is air, and this is bowel; here's your stomach." I had been informed by his assistant, Dr. Shankar, that lung tumors could also be ablated and so I asked, "What about the two tumors in my lungs?" to which he replied, "We didn't look at those," which I took as an indication that the operation had lasted long enough without going to another area. He said ablation worked well for me and that if I lived another fifty years they could continue doing these over that time span. If the tumors grow back, I was told, we would do this again, and chemotherapy can be used for anything new. I left Dr. vanSonnenberg's office with a smile on my face, feeling like a stalwart member of the radiofrequency ablation fraternity, happy to be alive!

Nowadays I think of ablation goals at the oddest times. Recently, I helped my son move into his college dorm to begin his freshman year of college. Along with his mother, the three of us had breakfast at one of those off-campus student-frequented restaurants that serves two dozen variations of bagels with eggs. I remembered how one of my doctors described the process of ablating a tumor as a cooking process, and then it occurred to me that here was a place where one could set definite goals and make real choices. Here, at school, one could order the "Big Sur," a toasted bagel with a "nuked" (nuked is a word we use at home for referring to something that has been cooked in the microwave oven) egg sandwiched between salsa and pepper jack cheese, or the "Melissa," a saucy creation with cooked apples and a nuked egg, or a choice of many others. So maybe, I thought, I could think of the goals for my ablation as "The Big Dave": two liver tumors, nuked beyond recognition, hold the bleeding, easy on the pain, served with tender loving care.

Patient: BP

I am a 77 year young man. In 1984 colon cancer was discovered and the sigmoid section of my colon was removed. In June 1989 the cancer had spread to my right lung, and the middle lobe was resected. In 1993 it spread to my left adrenal gland, and that was removed without affecting the kidney. In 1996 the tumor went to my left lung and was successfully resected. Since 1996 the colon cancer has not recurred, and CEA tests have been normal. I have never had chemotherapy, and, until 2003, had not received radiation.

In 2000 I was told that I have aortic stenosis. The valve is nearly closed, but I elected not to have surgery. In February 2002 I contracted endocarditis and was hospitalized for two weeks of antibiotics therapy, and slowly recovered at home.

On November 15, 2002, I had a thorough semiannual checkup that included a CT scan, which revealed a 3-cm tumor on my liver. I then consulted with a hepatologist, who did nothing, and asked me to return in three months. This made no sense to me. I indicated that I did not want to wait so long without definitively knowing what this was. He agreed to see me in two months. At that time, a biopsy indicated that this was a primary liver cancer, not a metastasis from the colon cancer. This doctor recommended chemoembolization, which I declined.

I sought a second opinion from Dr. Eric vanSonnenberg, by which time the tumor had doubled in size. He recommended radiofrequency ablation, which successfully destroyed the tumor without delay. This procedure was simple, not stressful, and pain free. The doctor's professional manner, impressive credentials, and concern for me as an individual gave me great confidence and relieved me from a growing fear that this situation was getting out of hand. I do not like to think about what may have happened had I not seen Dr. vanSonnenberg.

Acknowledgments

I would like to thank Mr. and Mrs. Lank for referring me to Dr. vanSonnenberg.

Patient: JC

Subject

65 years old, married 43 years, four sons and six grandchildren. Owner of computer and sensor development/manufacturing company.

Education

BS Electrical Engineering (1959) MBA (1963).

Cancer History

12/93: Cancer found on routine physical; left hemicolectomy

1/94–1/95: Outpatient chemotherapy

1/00–12/02: CEA rising from 6 to 63

12/01: Spiral CT showed tumor in left lower lobe. Mediastinal biopsy confirmed metastatic colon cancer. Also lymph nodes on right and left chest. All pathology from 12/01 and 12/93 compared by Massachusetts General Hospital Department of Pathology and Brigham and Women's Hospital Department of Pathology.

1/02: Chemotherapy at Dana-Farber Cancer Institute (Drs. Charles Fuchs and Jeffrey Meyerhardt). Also volunteered for Iressa trial. After 3 to 5 weeks I had pain in my right upper quadrant, which resulted in a radiologic intervention to drain the abscess from my appendix (Brigham and Women's Department of Radiology). Chemotherapy was interrupted for 3 weeks and Iressa discontinued.

4/02–8/02: Continued with chemotherapy (95-FU, Lavamisol and irinotecan).

8/23/02: While on vacation, repeat of right upper quadrant symptoms, and repeat radiologic intervention done at Albany Medical Center.

9/13/02: Appendectomy by Dr. Richard Swanson at Brigham and Women's Hospital. Pathology report noted cancer cells in the appendix specimen. Chemotherapy stopped 4 weeks.

10/02: Chemotherapy not as effective on lung tumor, so changed to 5-FU, oxaliplatin.

3/03: Effectiveness of oxaliplatin diminishing

4/03: Dr. Meyerhardt consulted Dr. vanSonnenberg about RFA for the left lower lobe lesion in my lung.

5/29/03: Radiofrequency ablation performed by Drs. Sri Shanker and Eric vanSonnenberg at Brigham and Women's Hospital with thoracic surgeon Dr. Michael Jaklitch in attendance.

Patient's Comments

I wanted to be aggressive against the cancer and RFA was an immediate process that, if successful, could really help me. It was also significantly less invasive than surgery, therefore offering a better recovery potential.

I was concerned that the tumor was close to my aorta and perhaps on the aorta. Could they get it all? Would I die in the process?

As an electrical engineer, the RFA process fascinated me. I had never heard of it. I researched it and could find articles on RFA on the liver, but none on the lung. One article by Gazelle and Goldberg was very helpful as it described the tools, salinity effects, process, etc. It made sense to me, but it appeared very precise and tricky to achieve a conversion of RF energy to such a precise heat energy targeted to such a small area.

When the procedure was over and I saw the probes, I was intrigued about their design, the materials used, etc.

Prior to the procedure, I was confused. When talking to Dr. Jaklitch, the thoracic surgeon, after he saw my CT scans, he said he could "go in and get the whole thing." I didn't know that this alternative existed. Without more information I could not change horses in midstream. I was confident in Dr. vanSonnenberg and in my own research on the RFA process.

As a patient, I think the following improvements could be made:

1. If regular surgery is an option, it should be explained at the earliest opportunity and in detail. If surgery is better than RFA, the patient needs to know why and how. Also, what are the comparative risks and benefits of each option?
2. The radiologist doing the procedure should provide the patient with a written description of the procedure, including the anesthesia process, the risks, and the tumor location.
3. The radiologist should give the patient a good description of the recovery process. What should the patient expect? Discharge from the hospital one day after the procedure does not allow for an adequate postoperative preparation.

Patient: WBS

Survival is only one of many competing interests that influence thought and action.

William James

"Ten percent of liver metastases patients have resectable disease, and surgical resection has yielded a 20% to 40% five-year survival rate." This statement appeared on one of the pages yielded by the National Cancer Institute's Web site in March 1999 when I typed the following search words: resection of hepatic metastatic colon cancer.

In June 1998, 12 inches of my ascending colon were removed surgically because a moderately differentiated colonic adenocarcinoma had invaded the pericolonic fat in my colon. One year later, I learned that the disease had spread to my liver, and surgical resection was the most common therapy for the disease; however, it was a procedure from which recovery would be difficult for a person of my age—I was 80 years old.

My vocations were in the fields of engineering and architecture, and I was, and still am, accustomed to gathering information and making decisions for myself. However, there is one exception to this rule: when it comes to medical decisions, I usually follow the recommendations of my doctors. This time I did not; with a 20% to 40% 5-year survival rate, the odds were too great. So I went back to the Web.

Survival was uppermost in my mind, and soon I had a three-ring binder overflowing with Web-based reports on the results of chemo and percutaneous ablation studies, articles from newspapers and magazines, and notes on suggestions from friends. After reading all of the material, I concluded that things did not look good for me; cancer cells were in my bloodstream and taking root in new places. It was time I gave thought to avenues other than those that would just lead to my survival.

Clinical studies offered such an avenue. Here I would be able to contribute to science, and, if the treatment worked, so much the better. I went back to the computer and there I found a study that caught my eye. It was at Brigham and Women's Hospital (BWH) in Boston; its purpose was to evaluate the effectiveness of using a needle-like probe to apply cold cell killing temperatures to a tumor. It was called "MR-guided cryoablation of liver tumors." The bottom line—I would be a guinea pig for tools that make iceballs of body parts.

I Go for It

I contacted the principal investigator for the study and, soon thereafter, my wife and I drove the 170 miles to the hospital, where I underwent physical exams and imaging studies and completed reams of paperwork. Parking and lodging were close by and their costs were reasonable. The personnel were friendly and informative.

The findings of the exams and imaging studies were that I had a medical history of kidney stones, polyneuropathy, monoclonal gammopathy of unknown significance, and myelodysplasia, and that I presently had one hepatic metastatic colon cancer tumor that measured 4×4.5 cm. All of these diseases notwithstanding, I was eligible for the study.

My first surprise was learning that radiologists would perform the procedure. I thought radiologists just operated imaging machines and read the pictures they produced. I soon learned that it was this expertise that made it possible to perform the type of cryoablation procedure that I was to receive.

I was given a form that thoroughly described the purpose of the research, the study procedures, and possible risks and discomforts. There was a place for me to indicate my willingness to participate in the study and place my signature. I signed it knowing I had made the right decision.

Not for the Claustrophobic

My participation in the study began with some misgivings. The first was the location of the treatment facility. One reaches the areas in BWH where the CT and MR machines are installed by taking a down elevator to below-grade floors and walking a long hall with a low ceiling, the occasional fire door, and walls hung with abstract prints. While it is well-lighted, the light is not the kind of light I like; I am a natural-light person.

The reception and imaging areas exhibited the same characteristics as the hall, but they received additional light from the cheerful and accommodating people that worked there. The machines themselves are another story—they can be intimidating. Spelunkers and cave dwellers will be right at home in an MR machine. I told myself that I had to compare this with an operating room, and, thankfully, the machines won hands down.

Actually, I had experienced CT and MR machines on more than one occasion before I went to BWH, but this time someone was going to poke at me while I was lying in them. As to their being in the basement, this seems to be where imaging machines are installed in hospitals. Being a pragmatist, I began to warm up to the environment.

My Tumor Is Frosted

Three days after my 81st birthday, with a light heart, I took the elevator down, walked the hall, donned the gown, boarded a gurney, and greeted the anesthesiologist. After he explained the procedure he would follow, the radiologists came in. They described what they were going to do, and asked if I had any questions. I said I was ready and a sedative was administered. I kissed my wife, was taken to the MR machine, and soon thereafter was in la-la land.

The next thing I knew, I was lying on a gurney and wondering who had inserted the catheter for draining my urine. My wife was at my side, and for the next few hours I dozed, ate some yogurt, and sensed the coming on of slight discomfort in my belly. I was moved to a hospital room where I spent the night trying to get comfortable—I wish someone would invent a different way to collect patients' urine when they are asleep. At 4 a.m., I was taken to the basement and put in the MR machine. Both the technician and I were grumpy, and the whole thing was a traumatic experience.

But I lived, and later in the morning, the radiologists came to my room and told me that they were happy with the results of the cryo procedure. For several reasons, they had stopped after treating 80% to 90% of the tumor: I had been "under" for 5 hours; the untreated portion of the tumor was so close to the diaphragm that freezing it was risky; and, finally, they wanted to have some MR scans done to see whether the procedure was working. I no longer felt like a guinea pig; these men really wanted to kill my tumor.

Probably because I have myelodysplasia, my red blood cell count dropped to the high 20s after the procedure. The next day it was in the low 30s (where it had been when I was admitted). I was discharged with the same discomfort in my belly, a lack of energy, and Band-Aids where the probes had entered my abdomen.

We drove home, and this time I occupied the passenger seat of our car. I slept soundly that night, and the next day I rested while listening to a books-on-tape version of a Civil War story titled *The Killer Angels*. I could not help reflecting on the quality of medical treatment during the 1860s; I went so far as to compare it with the surgical removal of a metastatic tumor versus killing the cells with a probe.

Following Up

The next week, I felt great and went back to Boston for a checkup. The MR machine showed that healing was progressing, and within the portion that had been treated was an area that may not have been frozen; it measured 1 × 2 cm.

Two months later, I went back for another cryo treatment. The procedure and its risks, benefits, and alternatives were discussed with me; the fact that it was experimental therapy was noted, and I gave my written consent to going ahead. The procedure followed the same lines as the first. Again, I recovered with no significant aftereffects. An MR scan 4 months later showed a 4.1 × 3.4 cm crescent-shaped area that might be residual or recurrent neoplasm. A biopsy performed a month later read positive for malignancy.

Seven months after the first treatment, the team concluded that my liver function was normal; the active portion of the tumor was smaller; an increasing CEA might indicate increasing tumor activity in other areas; the tumor was still resectable; and more cryotherapy in the vicinity of the diaphragm would be dangerous. It was suggested that, if I wanted further percutaneous treatments, they would like to give RFA a try. There were two drawbacks: I would not be in a clinical study, and because the tumor was close to the diaphragm the RFA treatment might just be a way to keep the tumor at bay.

There were other persons in the cryo study and more to come, so the investigators could not tell me whether they had achieved their goal. However, I left the study believing that all of the tumor would have been killed if it had not been so close to the diaphragm. As to whether I had achieved my purpose in becoming a participant in the study, I believed I had contributed to science and had received a bonus in the form of a reduction in the size of my tumor. The latter benefit gave me some time to pursue a clinical study of a different nature.

My Experiences with Radiofrequency Ablation

My choices for a new clinical study appeared to me to be limited to ones that were chemo oriented. Believing that chemo would be time-consuming and debilitating, especially so with my myelodysplasia problem, I began looking for a study that was close to home where I could, more comfortably, put up with the effects of chemo. I found none, and took up BWH's offer of RF therapy.

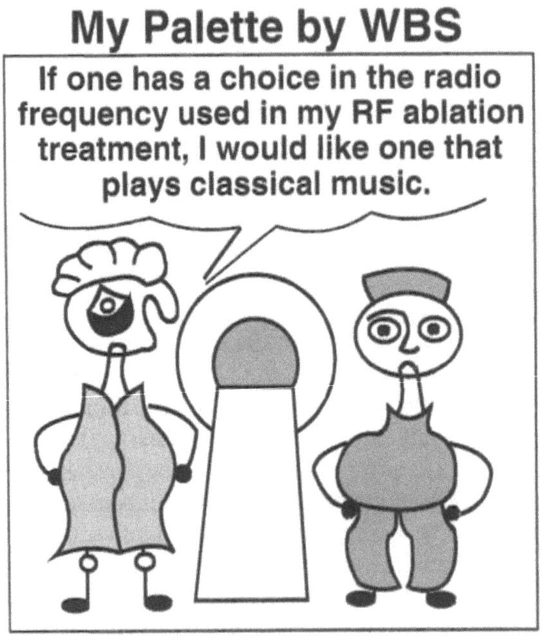
My Palette by WBS
If one has a choice in the radio frequency used in my RF ablation treatment, I would like one that plays classical music.

FIGURE 42.1. An engineer patient's KF preference.

I gathered enough information on RFA to know how it worked and what would be done once I climbed on the table of the CT machine. I learned that RF therapy sometimes is done on an outpatient basis with local anesthesia. This was not for me; I wanted general anesthesia and a short hospital stay. The most optimistic report I found on RFA said it yields 65% to 75% efficacy in the control of tumor growth in metastases. Those were odds I could live with.

Ten months after I had entered the cryo study, I returned to Boston where the anesthesiologist and radiologist explained what they were going to do, the risks, and so forth. I asked some questions (Fig. 42.1). I found the CT machine to be less intimidating than the MR, and was relaxed knowing the radiologist was not exploring a new field of science. I signed the usual release forms, and the treatment was administered.

The CT machine saw a 3.5 × 4.2 cm lesion on the right lobe of the liver near the dome of the diaphragm. The radiologists performed two 12-minute RF applications. I recovered from the anesthesia with no complications, spent that night and the next day trying to satisfy the hospital's fluid discharge requirements, and, having done so, went home the third day.

Two weeks later, a CT scan showed a 6 × 4 cm abnormal area with a 1.3 × 1.3 cm area that the radiologist believed was residual tumor. The radiologist noted that, at best, these dimensions were "guesstimates" because so much had happened to that area of my liver, it was difficult to distinguish between what might still be alive and what was dead.

Three months after the RF treatment, a CT scan showed the live portion of the tumor was bilobed; one lobe (near the vena cava) measured 2.7 × 2.4 cm, and the second lobe (near the diaphragm) measured 2.9 × 2.6 cm. The tumor was being held at bay.

The radiologist said that with another treatment, they might kill all of the cells in the two lobes except those in a small portion near the diaphragm; so 5 months after the first RF treatment, and 13 months after I received my first percutaneous treatment, I went back for what would prove to be my last experience with percutaneous ablation.

It was a nice warm day in June 2000 and all went well with the RF procedure. However, this time my recovery was slower; my hemotocrit count had dropped to the middle 20s right after I came home, and would not rise again. This condition may not have been caused by the RF procedure—low hemotocrit counts are also a product of myelodysplasia.

Since Then

In July my oncologist started me on weekly shots of Procrit in an effort to bring my blood count back to the middle to low thirties. Occasionally, the count would exceed 36 and I would stop for a while, but only for a short while—myelodysplasia had begun to take its toll. On top of that, a PET scan in September showed an "intense tracer uptake in a large area of the right hepatic lobe and in the anterior aspect of the right lower chest wall plus a small area of uptake in the posterior aspect of the right hilum of the lung." The lower right chest wall is adjacent to the points of entry on my abdomen for the cryo needles. The consent form I had signed for admittance to the cryo study noted that spreading tumor cells along the path of the needle is exceedingly rare. My mother believed I was one-in-a-million, so it is befitting that my tumor cells would hitch a ride on the cryo needle.

While time seemed to be getting short, I had not lost sight of my desire to participate in another clinical study. I found one that I believed I could weather and, just before Thanksgiving, I went to Memorial Sloan-Kettering Cancer Center to talk about hepatic arterial infusion of chemo substances using an implanted pump. My hopes were dashed when the administrator said the cryo and RF treatments made me ineligible.

It is now October 2002. During the past two years, survival became the dominant interest that influenced my thoughts and actions. I tried chemo by injection (it all but knocked my socks off); treated bouts of erratic heart beat and shingles; battled two squamous cell eruptions on my head; lost much of the use of my left hand and arm from reflex sympathetic dystrophy; strapped on a truss to hold two hernias in check; underwent surgery and radiation in an effort to remove the lesion on my chest wall; punched another hole in my belt to help with the problems that come with a 25-pound weight loss; and grimaced many times over while Procrit was being administered and blood was being drawn for CBCs.

All the while, rogue cells in my body keep doing their thing and reminding me that maybe now is the time to let nature take her course. On the other hand, maybe it isn't.

Patient: MH

Fiancé: PW

My fiancé passed away on March 20, 2002, of a chondrosarcoma that had finally found its way to his lungs. My story is not your traditional success story in that he did not survive, but our travels in the realm of cancer taught us both some invaluable lessons about medicine, accessibility of treatment options, the health care industry, the brutal reality of insurance arguments, and most importantly, ourselves. We traveled through a world of healing together, and although he did not survive the illness, he healed unlike any other. Our journey through this world of cancer has taught me more than I possibly could have imagined.

We learned that in order to heal, we must love every part of the sickness, or gift, as we later referred to it, including the very real and very loud aspect of pain. We traveled down many roads to try and understand the idea of pain and why its presence is so difficult. It is a way that the body communicates, and cannot just be masked or ignored. It needs to be heard and addressed for any healing to occur. Although this was an extraordinarily difficult lesson, it forced us both to look very closely at our priorities and make progressive choices for improving our quality of life. It is not enough to simply fight for more days. The true fight is in how to enrich those days.

He had been in remission from a non-Hodgkin's lymphoma in the stomach for fifteen years when he was diagnosed with a chondrosarcoma in the left shoulder approximately one year before we met the team at Dana-Farber Cancer Institute. The first year after he was diagnosed was a year of surgeries, appointments, sickness, chemotherapy, nutrition counseling, more sickness, more chemotherapy, hospital stays, new doctors, rehabilitation, stem cell transplants, more chemotherapy, more sickness, and more chemotherapy. We were told from the beginning that sarcomas rarely react to chemotherapy, and yet it was the treatment of choice time and time again. The side effects of these treatments consumed him, and he grew to fear his own mind during the time he was subject to these sessions. After a year and a half of this treatment, he was left with the original tumor in his shoulder, a new tumor in his pelvis, several tumors in his lungs, intense pain in his pelvic area, and absolutely no immune system.

Still, he was only 24 years old and had a huge will to live. I was committed to doing everything that I could to support him. Throughout our many hospital visits I was always surprised at the physicians' need to remind us of "the reality of the situation," or to be more frank, that he should be prepared to die. This was the priority, rather than the discussion of treatment plans. It felt as though our hope was perceived as denial.

In truth, our reality was far different from that of the physicians. Although we were completely aware of the possibility of death, he was still alive and should be treated as such. We could not understand the change in attitude after he was bestowed the title of terminal—a label that haunted us every day. In our world, that label meant we fight harder and use our time to the fullest. In the world we suddenly found ourselves, it meant not only slowing down but giving up. It was as if the entire Western medicine industry shut down. Their efforts were exhausted, and they wanted no part of any new, alternative, or unconventional ideas, regardless of their apparent success. The insurance companies ignored our pleas for help in our desire to try anything other than the two mainstream and obviously ineffective choices of treatment—chemotherapy and radiation. This did not sit well with us at all. I watched him wake up every morning to the immense emotional pain, caused in part by the fear of dying, accompanied by the infamous physical pain. We were never told about radiofrequency ablation as a pain management source, let alone a possible treatment method. This we were fortunate enough to discover on our own. We began our own search, with a true physical yelp leading the way. I made it my sole mission, as any teammate would do in my situation, to get him out of pain.

We had already spent a year and a half chasing it with a wide variety of narcotics and never receiving relief. He was constantly fighting the drowsiness, depression, constipation, and delirium that the drugs were offering. Every day we were increasing the dosages of methadone, fentanyl, oxycodone, Neurontin, and Dilaudid. Our physicians were simply handing over stronger and stronger prescriptions. Despite our faith, we felt as though we were spinning out of control, the illness was starting to give the impression that it was taking over. The only other options we were given were more chemotherapy or the wildly attractive radiation therapy.

From earlier discussions about the resistance a sarcoma has for radiation, we knew it was being suggested as a last resort. We were told that it would not save his life but perhaps prolong it. It would prolong his life, but, we suddenly realized, what *life*? Is it life when you cannot even get out of bed or go to the bathroom without doubling over in agony? Is it life when every position is uncomfortable and nothing smells or tastes appealing? Is it life when you barely have energy to walk to the next room, let alone spend time with your friends? Is it life when you are filled with crazy dreams from the drugs that you are forced to take every four hours, when the only vacation you have to look forward to is your next trip to the radiation room? He deserved a night of sleep, and I deserved a day free of his winces, pill popping, and screams of frustration.

I stepped up my extensive research regarding pain management and must have explored every search engine available. Finally, I came across an article that was written about a physician, Dr. Sridhar Shankar, at Dana-Farber Cancer Institute, regarding the fairly new world of cryotherapy and radiofrequency ablation. We had enough of simply prolonging the illness, so I composed a letter that would soon lead us into the world of radiofrequency ablation and introduce us to the amazing team at Dana-Farber Cancer Institute. The letter read as follows:

Dear Dr. Shankar,

First let me thank you for the phone conversation we had last Friday afternoon and for your patient voice regarding my seemingly desperate situation. I am sure that you and your facility get many similar calls from stressed patients and you must know that your attention and knowledge is greatly appreciated. I have included a general patient history of my boyfriend's case, along with relevant images that I feel will be helpful to you. I will need these returned to us either by mail or in person, depending on the course of action that is decided on.

Forgive me if I seem long winded, but at this time I feel the need to just fill you in on the basic events of the past year to give you perspective as to why we are looking to you for help.

Last fall my boyfriend was feeling pain in his left shoulder region and went to his primary care physician who diagnosed a pulled muscle, and sent him home with a cortisone shot. The pain persisted and brought him to the hospital. He was given an x-ray and it was determined that there was a mass in his shoulder that was suspected of disease. He had prior non-Hodgkin's lymphoma as an eight-year-old, and was in remission for 15 years. His primary physician then referred him to Memorial Sloan-Kettering Cancer Center, where he began consultations and had a biopsy of his chest on December 27, 2000. The diagnosis was, shockingly, chondrosarcoma of the chest, and the plan was surgery in the beginning of the new year. This never happened.

He experienced shortness of breath, which took him to Memorial Sloan-Kettering ER on December 31, 2000. He stayed at the hospital for approximately one month as an inpatient. They put him on heparin to treat what was thought to be a blood clot in his heart, and an immediate open-heart surgery was performed in early January 2001. This surgery surprisingly showed tumor in the heart (NOT a blood clot) that was successfully removed.

Approximately one week after open-heart surgery, a PET scan and MRI revealed tumor around the spine, with a paralysis scare that took him into surgery. Tumor was removed from around his T2. This was also successful, and he began the recovery process from both surgeries.

About a week into the recovery process, chemotherapy was started to treat the tumor still in his chest region with the original long-term goal of surgery still present. He underwent chemotherapy (Adriamycin and ifosfamide) on and off for about 4 weeks. A follow-up CT scan did reveal some tumor response. The same course of action was continued. After another 4 to 6 weeks, they did another CT and PET scan, and the chest tumor had not only ceased response to the chemotherapy, but a new tumor was discovered (approx. 6 cm) in the pelvis region. This was never mentioned before, even though there was complaint of pain in the lower back. The choice of treatment was the same chemotherapy that had ceased to work on the chest.

At this time we decided to leave Sloan-Kettering and seek out a sarcoma specialist. My fiancé began treatments under the care of Dr. Gerald Rosen of St. Vincent's Cancer Center. Immediately he began more chemotherapy treatments (methotrexate) with some success. He was given four rounds (1-day injection and 1-week recovery) of methotrexate, and then a high dose of carboplatin (4-day injection with a 2-week recovery), including stem cell transplant. This ended about one month ago, and a follow-up PET scan showed no response.

The next plan scheduled for the new year is radiation therapy, with surgery still hanging in there as the goal, but now in the pelvis and the chest. This does not sit well with us, and we fear that time is crucial.

So, with two major surgeries behind us, multiple rounds of intense chemotherapy still haunting us, fear of paralysis or limb salvage, the pressure for radiation, and a 24-year-old still waking up in pain every day, we are looking to cryotherapy/thermotherapy to provide any sort of push in the right direction. As you can tell, time is valuable to us and please be aware of how incredibly grateful we are that you have even taken the time to read this letter and offer any advice you can.

Over the phone you asked me to give my expectations as to what I thought you could do. I would not be true to myself or my heart if I did not tell you I expect tumor shrinkage, cease in pain, and a future of remission. However, that being said, I honestly believe that everything happens for a reason, and that finding your facility and your research is simply just another step in our path as we continue to experience the world of cancer.

I thank you again for you attention to our case, and please call us as soon as possible with any questions, concerns, advice, and/or recommendations. I will give you a follow-up call to make sure the films were received. I wish you success in your endeavors.

Respectfully yours,
PW

This letter was well-received and for the first time we felt like we were not fighting this alone. We immediately booked two train tickets to Boston and along with his pillows to sit on, as many of our imaging studies and medical reports that we could carry, and our incredible optimism, we were off to the Dana-Farber

Cancer Institute to learn more about radiofrequency ablation.

We arrived and were instantly impressed with the professional greeting we received, an attitude that truly never ceased throughout our entire time there. We met with Dr. Eric vanSonnenberg and began our first step to pain control. Dr. vanSonnenberg and Dr. Shankar took the time to sit with us, so that we could discuss our options. As we gained knowledge about the basic events surrounding the procedure, we also gained hope for a future: a crucial and often overlooked tool in pain management. We were amazed at the possibilities that ablation offered. As we discussed, it would actually heat the tumor from the inside and essentially dehydrate the cancer cells. The cells would die, and the body would rid them in the natural fashion. This in turn would cause the tumor to shrink and, it was hoped, help with the pain. This was a treatment that entailed no vomiting, lack of appetite, prolonged side effects, or amputation (as surgery would have called for). It would involve a few days in the hospital, as the cancer was very involved, and a Band-Aid on his hip. We found ourselves suddenly filled with enthusiasm as we plotted a game plan we could believe in.

The tumor that we focused on, as it was causing the most pain, was located in his pelvis. It involved his pelvic bone and was creating a great deal of pressure on his testicles. He found it impossible to sit for any period of time and carried a pillow everywhere. The tumor was also pushing on the sciatic nerve, which sent shooting pains down his entire leg. He had a very high tolerance for pain and lived with a constant level-4 pain (on a scale of 1 to 10) throughout his experience with sarcoma. At this time, however, he was fighting with a pain that was rising to levels above 7 and 8, despite the constant increase in medications. He was trying to cope with the everyday struggles, while he became weaker and weaker in mind and body. Physical pain and the emotional stress that joins with the fears of having a terminal illness create a devastating perception of the self and the world around you. With each passing day and with each cry for help, he was trying to trust each moment. This was getting harder and harder, as the illness was getting larger and more severe. The need for pain management was crucial for the quality of his moments, and we began counting the days until the ablation.

The morning of the ablation was full of anticipation, excitement, and fear. He and I, along with his family, were briefed again on the sequence of events, and then the prep for anesthesia. I helped him as he climbed onto the gurney and was pushed into the CT scanner. The procedure lasted approximately four hours, involved two tiny incisions about an inch wide, and six different ablations, each of them the size of a large apple. Immediately after the procedure I met him in the recovery room and although still very stiff, he was fine. He was very pleasant and able to speak to me about his experience. We were taken to a hospital room where we stayed for two nights of healing and monitoring vitals. The recovery process from the ablation was nothing compared to our prior experience, and he was walking around the next morning and had a huge appetite. He was given a follow-up MRI that showed a great deal of dead tumor that would take some time to pass through. He was still in a great deal of pain, but the pain itself was significantly different.

By the time we found our friends at Dana-Farber, were fit into the mainstream schedule of the hospital, and fought with the insurance companies to help us receive treatment, he had multiple tumors and his disease was incredibly advanced. The ablation was successful in a variety of ways. He no longer had pain down his leg and he was able to sit up and walk around with less difficulty. The tumor also significantly decreased in size for the first time since the diagnosis. Unfortunately, it was growing at such a rapid pace that the remaining part inside his bone was still causing pressure. The ablation, however, allowed him to maintain his state of mind, which was the most important aspect to him, and he was given a sense of hope that would carry him through his days. He experienced apparent relief, and he was able to laugh again. He had energy to continue his alternative medicines, visit with friends and family, and make conscious choices regarding his next course of action. We had about two weeks after that first ablation and were actually planning another on the remaining part of the tumor when the lungs had other plans. The tumors in his lungs were causing him to experience shortness of breath and we found ourselves traveling down another path. I wish that I could say that this procedure saved his life, but instead, I can only wish that this information leads to other stories of that sort. It was not that the ablation did not work. Unfortunately, we just found our miracle a little too late.

We live in a world where we are taught to give our complete trust to those who know "more"; to give away our own power simply because the efforts of the "experts" have been exhausted. We discovered, the hard way, that everyone who enters a hospital needs an advocate. We discovered that you also need a great deal of money to receive treatments deemed "unconventional" that could advance your prognosis and help keep you out of pain. Inspired by his courage and faith, by his sheer determination to lead an uplifting and fulfilling life, I agreed to share our story. I want everyone to know what is available to them—all of the options, treatments, and possibilities, not just those currently being advocated by mainstream physicians and insurance companies. My wish is that anyone in a similar situation (and I am aware that this includes millions of people every day) could access any and all information that will help them to honor, in sickness and in health, every moment of their lives.

Index

S

MIX
Papier aus verantwortungsvollen Quellen
Paper from responsible sources
FSC® C105338

If you have any concerns about our products,
you can contact us on
ProductSafety@springernature.com

In case Publisher is established outside the EU,
the EU authorized representative is:
Springer Nature Customer Service Center GmbH
Europaplatz 3, 69115 Heidelberg, Germany

Printed by Libri Plureos GmbH
in Hamburg, Germany